New Frontiers in Ophthalmology

New Frontiers in Ophthalmology

Edited by **Ray George**

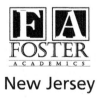

New Jersey

Published by Foster Academics,
61 Van Reypen Street,
Jersey City, NJ 07306, USA
www.fosteracademics.com

New Frontiers in Ophthalmology
Edited by Ray George

© 2016 Foster Academics

International Standard Book Number: 978-1-63242-448-8 (Hardback)

This book contains information obtained from authentic and highly regarded sources. Copyright for all individual chapters remain with the respective authors as indicated. All chapters are published with permission under the Creative Commons Attribution License or equivalent. A wide variety of references are listed. Permission and sources are indicated; for detailed attributions, please refer to the permissions page and list of contributors. Reasonable efforts have been made to publish reliable data and information, but the authors, editors and publisher cannot assume any responsibility for the validity of all materials or the consequences of their use.

The publisher's policy is to use permanent paper from mills that operate a sustainable forestry policy. Furthermore, the publisher ensures that the text paper and cover boards used have met acceptable environmental accreditation standards.

Trademark Notice: Registered trademark of products or corporate names are used only for explanation and identification without intent to infringe.

Printed in the United States of America.

Contents

	Preface	IX
Chapter 1	**Dry Eye Disease Following Refractive Surgery: A 12-Month Follow-Up of SMILE versus FS-LASIK in High Myopia** Bingjie Wang, Rajeev K. Naidu, Renyuan Chu, Jinhui Dai, Xiaomei Qu and Hao Zhou	1
Chapter 2	**Effect of Glyceraldehyde Cross-Linking on a Rabbit Bullous Keratopathy Model** Mengmeng Wang	9
Chapter 3	**Vision Health-Related Quality of Life in Chinese Glaucoma Patients** Lei Zuo, Haidong Zou, Jianhong Zhang, Xinfeng Fei and Xun Xu	14
Chapter 4	**The Ocular Biometry of Adult Cataract Patients on Lifeline Express Hospital Eye-Train in Rural China** Xiaoguang Cao, Xianru Hou and Yongzhen Bao	23
Chapter 5	**The Polymorphisms with Cataract Susceptibility Impair the EPHA2 Receptor Stability and Its Cytoprotective Function** Jin Yang, Dan Li, Qi Fan, Lei Cai, Xiaodi Qiu, Peng Zhou and Yi Lu	30
Chapter 6	**Human Serum Eye Drops in Eye Alterations: An Insight and a Critical Analysis** Maria Rosaria De Pascale, Michele Lanza, Linda Sommese and Claudio Napoli	39
Chapter 7	**Preservation of the Photoreceptor Inner/Outer Segment Junction in Dry Age-Related Macular Degeneration Treated by Rheohemapheresis** Eva Rencová, Milan Bláha, Jan Studnička, Vladimír Bláha, Miriam Lánská, Ondřej Renc, Alexander Stepanov, Věra Kratochvílová and Hana Langrová	53
Chapter 8	**One-Year Results of Simultaneous Topography-Guided Photorefractive Keratectomy and Corneal Collagen Cross-Linking in Keratoconus Utilizing a Modern Ablation Software** A. M. Sherif, M. A. Ammar, Y. S. Mostafa, S. A. Gamal Eldin and A. A. Osman	60
Chapter 9	**The Measurement of Intraocular Biomarkers in Various Stages of Proliferative Diabetic Retinopathy Using Multiplex xMAP Technology** Stepan Rusnak, Jindra Vrzalova, Marketa Sobotova, Lenka Hecova, Renata Ricarova and Ondrej Topolcan	67
Chapter 10	**Local Relationship between Global-Flash Multifocal Electroretinogram Optic Nerve Head Components and Visual Field Defects in Patients with Glaucoma** Chan Hee Moon, Jungwoo Han, Young-Hoon Ohn and Tae Kwann Park	73

Chapter 11	**Effect of Storage Temperature on Key Functions of Cultured Retinal Pigment Epithelial Cells** Lara Pasovic, Jon Roger Eidet, Berit S. Brusletto, Torstein Lyberg and Tor P. Utheim	81
Chapter 12	**Choroidal Thickness in Patients with Mild Cognitive Impairment and Alzheimer's Type Dementia** Mehmet Bulut, Aylin Yaman, Muhammet Kazim Erol, Fatma Kurtuluş, Devrim Toslak, Berna Doğan, Deniz Turgut Çoban and Ebru Kaya Başar	91
Chapter 13	**Comparison of Two Botulinum Neurotoxin A Injection Patterns with or without the Medial Lower Eyelid in the Treatment of Blepharospasm** Hui Yang, Jing Lu, Xiujuan Zhao, Xiaohu Ding, Zhonghao Wang, Xiaoyu Cai, Yan Luo and Lin Lu	98
Chapter 14	**Outcomes of 23-Gauge Vitrectomy Combined with Phacoemulsification, Panretinal Photocoagulation, and Trabeculectomy without Use of Anti-VEGF Agents for Neovascular Glaucoma with Vitreous Hemorrhage** Hua Yan	104
Chapter 15	**Evaluation of Dry Eye and Meibomian Gland Dysfunction in Teenagers with Myopia through Noninvasive Keratograph** Xiu Wang, Xiaoxiao Lu, Jun Yang, Ruihua Wei, Liyuan Yang, Shaozhen Zhao and XilianWang	111
Chapter 16	**Analysis of the Retinal Nerve Fiber Layer in Retinitis Pigmentosa Using Optic Coherence Tomography** Medine Aslı Yıldırım, Burak Erden, Mehmet Tetikoğlu, Özlem Kuru and Mustafa Elçioğlu	116
Chapter 17	**Size of the Optic Nerve Head and Its Relationship with the Thickness of the Macular Ganglion Cell Complex and Peripapillary Retinal Nerve Fiber Layer in Patients with Primary Open Angle Glaucoma** Nobuko Enomoto, Ayako Anraku, Kyoko Ishida, Asuka Takeyama, Fumihiko Yagi and Goji Tomita	121
Chapter 18	**Endothelial Cell Loss after Phacoemulsification according to Different Anterior Chamber Depths** Hyung Bin Hwang, Byul Lyu, Hye Bin Yim and Na Young Lee	127
Chapter 19	**Responses of Multipotent Retinal Stem Cells to IL-1β, IL-18, or IL-17** Shida Chen, Defen Shen, Nicholas A. Popp, Alexander J. Ogilvy, Jingsheng Tuo, Mones Abu-Asab, Ting Xie and Chi-Chao Chan	134
Chapter 20	**Risk Factors for Refractory Diabetic Macular Oedema after Sub-Tenon's Capsule Triamcinolone Acetonide Injection** Toshiyuki Oshitari, Yuta Kitamura, Sakiko Nonomura, Miyuki Arai, Yoko Takatsuna, Eiju Sato, Takayuki Baba and Shuichi Yamamoto	143
Chapter 21	**Intraoperative Corneal Thickness Changes during Pulsed Accelerated Corneal Cross-Linking Using Isotonic Riboflavin with HPMC** Ahmed M. Sherif, Nihal A. El-Gheriany, Yehia M. Salah El-Din, Lamiaa S. Aly, Amr A. Osman, Michael A. Grentzelos and George D. Kymionis	147

Chapter 22	**Acute-Onset Vitreous Hemorrhage of Unknown Origin before Vitrectomy: Causes and Prognosis** Dong Yoon Kim, Soo Geun Joe, Seunghee Baek, June-Gone Kim, Young Hee Yoon and Joo Yong Lee	151
Chapter 23	**Effects of Zeaxanthin on Growth and Invasion of Human Uveal Melanoma in Nude Mouse Model** Xiaoliang L. Xu, Dan-Ning Hu, Codrin Iacob, Adrienne Jordan, Sandipkumar Gandhi, Dennis L. Gierhart and Richard Rosen	159
Chapter 24	**Childbearing May Increase the Risk of Nondiabetic Cataract in Chinese Women's Old Age** Manqiong Yuan, Yaofeng Han, Ya Fang and Cheng-I Chu	167
Chapter 25	**High Levels of 17β-Estradiol Are Associated with Increased Matrix Metalloproteinase-2 and Metalloproteinase-9 Activity in Tears of Postmenopausal Women with Dry Eye** Guanglin Shen and Xiaoping Ma	175
Chapter 26	**Safety and Efficacy of Adding Fixed-Combination Brinzolamide/Timolol Maleate to Prostaglandin Therapy for Treatment of Ocular Hypertension or Glaucoma** Anton Hommer, Douglas A. Hubatsch and Juan Cano-Parra	183
Chapter 27	**Risk Factors in Normal-Tension Glaucoma and High-Tension Glaucoma in Relation to Polymorphisms of Endothelin-1 Gene and Endothelin-1 Receptor Type A Gene** Dominika Wróbel-Dudzińska, Ewa Kosior-Jarecka, Urszula Łukasik, Janusz Kocki, Agnieszka Witczak, Jerzy Mosiewicz and Tomasz Żarnowski	190
Chapter 28	**Scheimpflug Imaging Parameters Associated with Tear Mediators and Bronchial Asthma in Keratoconus** Dorottya Pásztor, Bence Lajos Kolozsvári, Adrienne Csutak, András Berta, Ziad Hassan, Beáta Andrea Kettesy, Péter Gogolák, and Mariann Fodor	202
Chapter 29	**Usefulness of Surgical Media Center as a Cataract Surgery Educational Tool** Tomoichiro Ogawa, Takuya Shiba and Hiroshi Tsuneoka	209
Chapter 30	**Visual and Refractive Outcomes of a Toric Presbyopia-Correcting Intraocular Lens** Alice T. Epitropoulos	217
Chapter 31	**A Head-Mounted Spectacle Frame for the Study of Mouse Lens-Induced Myopia** Yangshun Gu, Baisheng Xu, Chunfei Feng, Yang Ni, QinWu, Chixin Du, Nan Hong, Peng Li, Zhihua Ding and Bo Jiang	223
Chapter 32	**Apelin Protects Primary Rat Retinal Pericytes from Chemical Hypoxia-Induced Apoptosis** Li Chen, Yong Tao, Jing Feng and Yan Rong Jiang	230

Chapter 33 **Novice Reviewers Retain High Sensitivity and Specificity of Posterior Segment Disease Identification with iWellnessExam™** 244
Samantha Slotnick, Catherine Awad, Sanjeev Nath and Jerome Sherman

Permissions

List of Contributors

Preface

This book aims to highlight the current researches and provides a platform to further the scope of innovations in this area. This book is a product of the combined efforts of many researchers and scientists from different parts of the world. The objective of this book is to provide the readers with the latest information in the field.

This book contains some path-breaking studies in the field of Ophthalmology. Some of the diverse topics covered in it address the varied branches that fall under this category. Ophthalmology is the subfield of medicine that deals with physiology, diseases and treatment of the human eyes. Cataracts, cornea, glaucoma, etc are some popular diseases studied and treated under the discipline of ophthalmology. The extensive content of this book provides the readers with a thorough understanding of the subject. It is a compilation of chapters that discuss the most vital concepts and emerging trends in the field of ophthalmology. Scientists, doctors and students actively engaged in this field will find this book full of crucial and unexplored concepts.

I would like to express my sincere thanks to the authors for their dedicated efforts in the completion of this book. I acknowledge the efforts of the publisher for providing constant support. Lastly, I would like to thank my family for their support in all academic endeavors.

Editor

Dry Eye Disease following Refractive Surgery: A 12-Month Follow-Up of SMILE versus FS-LASIK in High Myopia

Bingjie Wang,[1] Rajeev K. Naidu,[2] Renyuan Chu,[1] Jinhui Dai,[1] Xiaomei Qu,[1] and Hao Zhou[1]

[1]Key Myopia Laboratory of Chinese Health Ministry, Department of Ophthalmology, Eye & ENT Hospital, Fudan University, No. 83, Fenyang Road, Shanghai 200031, China
[2]The University of Sydney, Camperdown, NSW 2006, Australia

Correspondence should be addressed to Hao Zhou; zhouhaoeent@163.com

Academic Editor: George Kymionis

Purpose. To compare dry eye disease following SMILE versus FS-LASIK. *Design.* Prospective, nonrandomised, observational study. *Patients.* 90 patients undergoing refractive surgery for myopia were included. 47 eyes underwent SMILE and 43 eyes underwent FS-LASIK. *Methods.* Evaluation of dry eye disease was conducted preoperatively and at 1, 3, 6, and 12 months postoperatively, using the Salisbury Eye Evaluation Questionnaire (SEEQ) and TBUT. *Results.* TBUT reduced following SMILE at 1 and 3 months ($p < 0.001$) and at 1, 3, and 6 months following FS-LASIK ($p < 0.001$). TBUT was greater following SMILE than FS-LASIK at 3, 6, and 12 months ($p < 0.001$, $p < 0.001$, and $p = 0.009$, resp.). SEEQ scores increased (greater symptoms) following SMILE at 1 month ($p < 0.001$) and 3 months ($p = 0.003$) and at 1, 3, and 6 months following FS-LASIK ($p < 0.001$). SMILE produced lower SEEQ scores (fewer symptoms) than FS-LASIK at 1, 3, and 6 months ($p < 0.001$). *Conclusion.* SMILE produces less dry eye disease than FS-LASIK at 6 months postoperatively but demonstrates similar degrees of dry eye disease at 12 months.

1. Introduction

Dry eye disease is a common ocular surface disease and plays a significant role in the ocular comfort and visual performance of patients, with the potential to have a great impact on their quality of life [1–6]. Dry eye is known to be a frequently reported and observed finding following refractive surgery, particularly in the period immediately following surgery [7–12]. With refractive surgery cases increasing in number, dry eye is becoming an increasing challenge for refractive surgeons to overcome, with a large proportion of patients experiencing dry eye symptoms to varying degrees [3, 10, 13–18]. Dry eye has also been associated with a delayed wound healing response and may predispose patients to refractive regression in moderate to severe cases [7, 15].

While the pathophysiology of this complication is still evolving, a number of theories have been proposed to explain why dry eye occurs following refractive surgery, including exacerbation of preexisting dry eye disease [12], medicamentosa from postoperative medications [19, 20], and damage to conjunctival goblet cells increasing tear hyperosmolarity and inflammation [19, 21–23]. The interaction between the ocular surface and eyelids is an important factor in maintaining tear production and flow, which is also altered following surgery [10, 24]. Perhaps the biggest factor, however, is the impact surgery has on corneal nerves and sensation [19, 21, 25, 26]. Intact corneal sensation is required for adequate blink frequency and tear production, and corneal denervation resulting from disruption and damage to corneal nerves has been shown to play a significant role in the development of dry eye disease following refractive surgery [27–29].

Laser-assisted in situ keratomileusis (LASIK) continues to be a popular refractive surgical option [18, 30]; however, almost half of all LASIK patients continue to report dry eye symptoms following surgery [8]. The introduction of the femtosecond laser (FS) has seen FS-LASIK become a more accurate and safe surgical option, with a reduced rate of dry eye disease, which is likely due to reduced neurotrophic effects on the corneal nerves during formation of the corneal flap [22]. A recent advancement in refractive surgery has been small-incision lenticule extraction (SMILE), which was established as a "flapless" procedure in which an intrastromal lenticule is cut by a femtosecond laser and manually extracted through a peripheral corneal tunnel incision. The refractive predictability, safety, and patient satisfaction of SMILE are comparable to FS-LASIK. SMILE has the benefit of being minimally invasive, with a lesser degree of damage to the cornea and corneal nerves, and may therefore result in fewer complications and reduced symptoms of dry eye [9]. The key difference between FS-LASIK and SMILE and their impact on corneal innervation may lie in the fact that FS-LASIK affects the epithelium and anterior stroma, thus resulting in greater resection of the sensory nerves of the cornea [19–21], while SMILE affects the posterior stromal bed with relatively greater preservation of the corneal subbasal nerve plexus [9].

Few studies exist in the literature investigating the long-term effects of refractive surgery, specifically comparing both SMILE and FS-LASIK, on the development of dry eye syndromes. In this prospective observational study, we present the findings of the objectively measured clinical signs and subjective reporting of dry eye symptoms following SMILE versus FS-LASIK for the correction of myopia in a large group of demographically similar patients over a period of 12 months postoperatively.

2. Methods

2.1. Setting and Design. This institutional, prospective, observational study was approved prospectively by the institutional review board of The Eye and ENT Hospital of Fudan University. Written informed consent was obtained from all patients prior to participating in the study. The study adhered to the guidelines and principles of the Declaration of Helsinki.

2.2. Patients. Patients who attended The Eye and ENT Hospital of Fudan University, Shanghai, China, between the period of January 2012 and January 2014, for refractive treatment of their myopia were recruited.

Inclusion criteria included patient aged over 18 years, Spherical Equivalent (SE) refractive error ≥ -6.00 D, a stable refractive error in the last 2 years, no contraindications to laser refractive surgery, and no previous history of dry eye disease. Additionally, prior to surgery, patients completed a dry eye questionnaire (The Salisbury Eye Evaluation) and only those who yielded a total score of 0 were included. Patients were excluded if they had undergone any ocular surgery in the past 6 months or were using medication that could interfere with the ocular surface. A complete dilated ophthalmic examination was performed to assess the patient's suitability for either SMILE or FS-LASIK. Central corneal thickness (CCT) was determined with a Pentacam system (Typ70700; Oculus; Wetzlar, Germany). After the nature of the two procedures was explained, the patients chose the type of surgery they wished to undergo.

In total, 90 patients who completed 12 months of follow-up were included in this study. 47 patients underwent SMILE procedures (SMILE group) while 43 patients underwent FS-LASIK procedures (FS-LASIK group). The mean age of patients undergoing SMILE was 25.21 ± 6.51 years old, which was not significantly different than the mean age of patients undergoing FS-LASIK, which was 24.72 ± 6.53 years old ($p = 0.722$). The mean preoperative SE was -7.46 ± 1.11 D in the SMILE group and -7.44 ± 1.13 D in the FS-LASIK group, with no significant difference between the two groups. The mean preoperative TBUT was 9.87 ± 1.57 seconds in the SMILE group and 9.56 ± 1.35 seconds in the FS-LASIK group, again with no significant difference between the two groups ($p = 0.948$). Written informed consent was obtained from each patient after the details of the study were fully explained.

2.2.1. Tear-Film Breakup Time (TBUT). TBUT was assessed prior to surgery and was repeated at 1 month, 3 months, 6 months, and 12 months after surgery. TBUT was assessed with fluorescein paper strips that were wetted with unpreserved saline solution. One drop was instilled in each eye in the lower conjunctival sac, and the patient was instructed to blink several times. A cobalt filter was attached to a slit-lamp biomicroscope, and the time it took from a complete blink until the first signs of a break in the tear film was recorded. The test was repeated 3 times and averaged. The same observer performed the test.

2.2.2. The Salisbury Eye Evaluation Questionnaire for Dry Eye Symptoms. The Salisbury Eye Evaluation Questionnaire, translated into Chinese, was given to each subject for self-evaluation of dry eye symptoms before operation and at 1, 3, 6, and 12 months after operation. The questionnaire contains 6 items pertaining to dry eye symptoms. Questions include the following: (1) Do your eyes ever feel dry? (2) Do you ever feel a gritty or sandy sensation in your eye? (3) Are your eyes ever red? (4) Do your eyes ever have a burning sensation? (5) Do you notice much crusting on your lashes? (6) Do your eyes ever get stuck shut in the morning? The subject answers each question on the questionnaire based on how often they experience these symptoms as rarely, sometimes, often, or all the time. Symptoms that were experienced often or all the time were given a score of 1, and the other two responses were given a score of 0. The scores were added up to give a total score for each subject.

2.3. Surgical Technique. All surgeries were performed under local anesthesia by one surgeon (Hao Zhou) with patients undergoing either SMILE or FS-LASIK.

SMILE was performed using the VisuMax femtosecond laser system (Carl Zeiss Meditec) with a repetition rate of 500 kHz, pulse energy of 185–190 nJ, intended cap thickness of 100–120 μm, cap diameter of 7.5 mm, lenticule diameter of 6.1 to 6.6 mm (depending on the refractive error), and a 90°-angle side cut with a circumferential length of 2.1 mm at the superior position.

FS-LASIK was performed with the VisuMax system for flap creation followed by Mel 80 excimer laser (Carl Zeiss Meditec) for stromal ablation, with an intended flap thickness of 95 μm and pulse energy of 185 nJ. The hinge was located at the superior position.

A standard postoperative topical steroid (Fluorometholone 0.1%) was tapered over 30 days; topical antibiotic

Table 1: Demographic data of the subjects included in this study.

	Mean ± standard deviation		p value
	SMILE ($n = 47$)	FS-LASIK ($n = 43$)	
Age (y)	25.21 ± 6.51	24.72 ± 6.53	0.722
Gender (F/M)	30/17	27/16	0.157
Preop SE (D)	−7.46 ± 1.11	−7.44 ± 1.13	0.948
Preop CCT (μm)	546.49 ± 25.52	544.88 ± 24.28	0.761
Preop TBUT (sec)	9.87 ± 1.57	9.56 ± 1.35	0.313

Table 2: Lenticule thickness/ablation depth.

	Mean ± standard deviation		p value
	SMILE ($n = 47$)	FS-LASIK ($n = 43$)	
Lenticule thickness/Ablation depth (μm)	138.63 ± 8.56	137.77 ± 13.31	0.711

Table 3: TBUT between SMILE and FS-LASIK.

Postop TBUT (sec)	Mean ± standard deviation		p value
	SMILE ($n = 47$)	FS-LASIK ($n = 43$)	
1 month	6.28 ± 1.35	6.53 ± 1.24	0.348
3 months	8.21 ± 0.95	7.42 ± 0.96	<0.001
6 months	9.57 ± 0.93	8.19 ± 1.45	<0.001
12 months	9.83 ± 0.99	9.30 ± 0.89	0.009

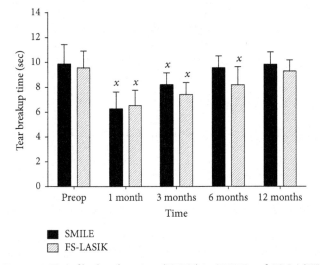

Figure 1: Tear-film breakup time (TBUT) in SMILE and FS-LASIK groups before operation, 1, 3, 6, and 12 months after operation. "x": statistically significantly less than preoperative values, $p < 0.05$.

(Tobramycin 0.003%) QID for 7 days, and unpreserved ocular lubricant 4 times a day was prescribed for a month.

2.4. Statistical Analysis.
In all cases, only data from the first eye (right eye) on which the procedure was performed was used in the statistical analysis. The sample size of this study was determined based on the standard deviation reported from a previous study [9], with the significance level set at $\alpha = 0.05$ (two tailed) and a power of 90%, and a sample size of at least 38 was required in each group. Allowing for a 10% dropout rate, at least 84 subjects were required. All statistical analyses were performed with a statistics program (SPSS 19.0 IBM Corporation, Armonk, NY, USA). Independent-samples t-test was used to compare the differences between groups. One-way repeated measures ANOVA test was used to compare TBUT change and SEEQ score change within groups over time. Tukey's honestly significant difference (HSD) post hoc test was performed to evaluate the differences in parameters between groups. Spearman's correlation test was used to assess relationship between TBUT and SEEQ scores. $p < 0.05$ was considered significant.

3. Results

In total, 90 patients were recruited for the study, with a total of 90 eyes (the first eye to have surgery performed for each patient) included in the analysis. There were a total of 47 eyes in the SMILE group and 43 eyes in the FS-LASIK group. There were no significant differences between the two groups preoperatively in terms of age, SE refractive error, central corneal thickness (CCT), or preoperative TBUT. Demographic data for all subjects included in this study is outlined in Table 1.

Objective surgical changes in corneal parameters were similar between the two groups, with no significant difference in lenticule thickness/ablation depth between the two groups (Table 2).

3.1. Tear-Film Breakup Time (TBUT).
Preoperatively, there was no significant difference in TBUT between the SMILE and FS-LASIK groups (9.87 ± 1.57 seconds and 9.56 ± 1.35 seconds, resp., $p = 0.313$). One-way ANOVA showed that there was a statistically significant difference in TBUT between preoperative values and the different follow-up time periods, for both SMILE ($F(4, 230) = 79.673$, $p < 0.001$) and FS-LASIK ($F(4, 210) = 55.531$, $p < 0.001$).

Post hoc tests showed that, at 1 and 3 months after operation, there was a statistically significant decrease in TBUT from preoperative values in the SMILE group (6.28 ± 1.35, $p < 0.001$, and 8.21 ± 0.95, $p < 0.001$, resp.), before returning to preoperative values by 6 and 12 months (9.57 ± 0.93, $p = 0.740$, and 9.83 ± 0.99, $p = 1.00$, resp.). In the FS-LASIK group, TBUT was statistically significantly reduced from preoperative values at 1 month, 3 months, and 6 months postoperatively (6.53 ± 1.24, $p < 0.001$, 7.41 ± 0.96, $p < 0.001$, and 8.18 ± 1.45, $p < 0.001$, resp.), before returning to preoperative values at 12 months (9.30 ± 0.89, $p = 0.826$) (Figure 1).

Between the two procedures, TBUT was not statistically significantly different at 1 month postoperatively ($p = 0.348$); however, at 3, 6, and 12 months postoperatively, TBUT was statistically significantly greater in the SMILE group than the FS-LASIK group ($p < 0.001$, $p < 0.001$, and $p = 0.009$, resp.) (Table 3).

3.2. Salisbury Eye Evaluation Questionnaire.
The Salisbury Eye Evaluation Questionnaire (SEEQ) was used to assess a patient's subjective reporting of dry eye symptoms, with a

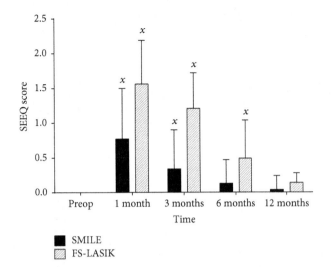

FIGURE 2: Salisbury Eye Evaluation Questionnaire results in SMILE and FS-LASIK groups at 1, 3, 6, and 12 months after operation. "x": statistically significantly greater than preoperative values, $p < 0.05$.

TABLE 4: SEEQ scores between SMILE and FS-LASIK.

Postop SEEQ	Mean ± standard deviation		p value
	SMILE ($n = 47$)	FS-LASIK ($n = 43$)	
1 month	0.77 ± 0.73	1.56 ± 0.63	<0.001
3 months	0.34 ± 0.56	1.21 ± 0.51	<0.001
6 months	0.13 ± 0.34	0.49 ± 0.55	<0.001
12 months	0.04 ± 0.20	0.14 ± 0.14	0.109

higher score indicating a greater degree of experienced dry eye symptoms. Preoperative scores were 0, per the inclusion criteria. One-way ANOVA testing found a statistically significant difference in SEEQ scores within groups over the time period of review for both SMILE ($F(4, 230) = 23.127$, $p < 0.001$) and FS-LASIK ($F(4, 210) = 91.161$, $p < 0.001$).

Post hoc tests showed that, in the SMILE group, SEEQ scores were statistically significantly higher at 1 month ($p < 0.001$) and 3 months ($p = 0.003$) after operation than preoperative values. By 6 and 12 months, this difference was no longer statistically significant ($p = 0.640$ and $p = 0.991$, resp.). For FS-LASIK, post hoc test evaluation found that SEEQ scores at 1 month, 3 months, and 6 months after operation were statistically significantly higher than preoperative values ($p < 0.001$ for all 3 follow-up time periods). By 12 months, this difference was no longer found ($p = 0.636$) (Figure 2).

Postoperatively at the 1-, 3-, and 6-month follow-up intervals, the SEEQ score was higher in the FS-LASIK group than the SMILE group ($p < 0.001$ for all 3 follow-up time intervals). 12 months after operation, this difference was no longer statistically significant ($p = 0.109$) (Table 4).

Spearman's correlation test revealed a moderate negative correlation between SEEQ scores and TBUT at 1 month after operation for the SMILE group ($r_s = -0.599$, $p < 0.001$) as well as in the FS-LASIK group ($r_s = -0.518$, $p < 0.001$).

4. Discussion

Dry eye disease continues to be a common complication of refractive surgery, affecting not only the ocular comfort of patients, but also their visual quality [8, 31]. This can have a direct impact on their overall satisfaction and quality of life following surgery. Although a frequently noted condition, dry eye disease remains a complex syndrome with a wide-ranging spectrum of clinical signs and subjective symptoms that do not always show a great degree of correlation [4, 32].

While there exist several clinical measures to diagnose and monitor the severity of dry eye disease, it is difficult to fully understand the impact it has on a patient, as many patients that show early clinical signs of dry eye disease may be asymptomatic, while others may report symptoms greater than their clinical signs may suggest, or without any tissue damage at all [32]. Assessment of dry eye disease should, therefore, consist of both clinical examination and subjective self-reporting of symptoms by patients, ideally through the use of a dry eye questionnaire. The purpose of this study was to investigate and compare the long-term dry eye outcomes up to 12 months following SMILE and FS-LASIK for the correction of high myopia, using both clinical (TBUT) and subjective (SEEQ) measures of dry eye disease.

Dry eye symptoms are often considered a transient occurrence, occurring in the vast majority of patients in the short-term following refractive surgery [9, 15, 17]. Many studies have shown an increase in dry eye symptoms in the period immediately following refractive surgery, which often improves within three to nine months postoperatively [7, 9–11, 13–17, 19, 21, 22, 30, 31, 33–36]. In the present study, we investigated the objectively measured clinical signs and subjective reporting of dry eye symptoms following SMILE and FS-LASIK for the correction of high myopia in a large group of demographically similar patients over a longer period of 12 months postoperatively. The main outcome measures of interest were the TBUT as a clinical marker for dry eye disease and the Salisbury Eye Evaluation Questionnaire as a subjective indicator of a patient's experience of dry eye symptoms, with a comparison of both measures between two highly affective refractive procedures, SMILE and FS-LASIK. The use of both of these measures provides a good representation of dry eye disease. TBUT has been shown to be both sensitive and accurate as a noninvasive method of dry eye diagnosis [37], and dry eye questionnaires have been shown to represent the true degree of morbidity of the disease as experienced by patients [2, 4, 32, 37].

The present study demonstrated that both the SMILE and FS-LASIK procedures resulted in changes in both the clinical and subjective markers of dry eye, with a transient increase in dry eye disease in both groups. A reduction in TBUT was observed for both the SMILE and FS-LASIK groups following surgery at 1 and 3 months postoperatively. However, this change was only transient, as the TBUT had recovered to preoperative levels for patients that underwent SMILE by 6 months postoperatively, whereas for patients that underwent FS-LASIK, this recovery did not occur until 12 months postoperatively.

These results suggest that SMILE may be superior to FS-LASIK, inducing a shorter duration of tear-film disturbance and leading to a quicker recovery of tear-film function postoperatively. Our results also indicate that this advantage of the SMILE procedure was noted subjectively with the patient's experience of dry eye symptoms, as demonstrated by the results of the SEEQ. Patients in the SMILE group reported lower SEEQ scores (fewer dry eye symptoms) compared to patients in the FS-LASIK group at 1, 3, and 6 months postoperatively, before equalizing at 12 months postoperatively. Therefore, patients who underwent SMILE were less prone to dry eye symptoms, as assessed with both clinical and subjective measures, than those who underwent FS-LASIK in the first 6 months following surgery, but they demonstrated similar degrees of dry eye disease after 12 months of follow-up.

Several hypotheses have been proposed to explain the pathophysiology underlying the development of dry eye disease following refractive surgery. Changes in corneal innervation and sensitivity induced by refractive surgery are key in understanding the pathogenesis of dry eye disease and revolve around the idea that corneal sensitivity is reduced due to transection of the corneal nerves, thus resulting in dysfunction of the cornea-lacrimal gland functional unit [19, 21]. Transection of the sensory nerves of the cornea, as it occurs during FS-LASIK, is thought to lead to a decrease in the innervation to the autonomic nerve fibres supplying the lacrimal gland that would otherwise stimulate tear production via the neural reflex arc [19, 21]. This change may result in tear-film dysfunction via a number of mechanisms, including changes in the composition of the tears, ocular surface changes, and decreased blink frequency [21, 23].

There has been increasing evidence supporting the theory that damage to the corneal nerve density occurs following refractive surgery, particularly affecting the subbasal nerve plexus [19, 21, 24, 27, 38–40]. The main consequence of this change in nerve density is a reduction in corneal sensitivity. This results in a hypoesthetic cornea and is likely the key factor in the development of postrefractive dry eye disease [13, 23, 25, 26, 35, 41, 42]. With the aid of in vivo confocal microscopy, Denoyer et al. demonstrated that SMILE preserved the corneal subbasal nerve plexus better than LASIK [9]. They found a greater nerve density, number of long nerve fibres and nerve fibre branchings in patients that underwent SMILE compared to those that underwent LASIK. They also found that corneal sensitivity was greater in the SMILE group in the short-term but found no significant difference between SMILE and LASIK after 6 months after surgery [9]. This loss in nerve fibre density does start to regenerate months after surgery, with almost complete recovery by 2 to 5 years postoperatively [21, 43–45].

The degree of injury to corneal nerves is understandably expected to be different between the two surgical procedures, owing to the differing nature of each procedure. The two procedures differ in the method of ablation and the layers of the cornea affected, with FS-LASIK affecting the epithelium and anterior stroma, with the creation of a flap, while SMILE mainly affects the posterior stromal bed, only requiring a small tunnel incision [26]. Our results demonstrated a clear difference in the degree of injury and in the time to recovery of tear function between SMILE and FS-LASIK, as assessed by the TBUT. SMILE not only showed a more rapid recovery of tear function, with a return in TBUT to preoperative levels at 6 months compared to 12 months for FS-LASIK, but also showed a significantly lower degree of loss in TBUT compared to FS-LASIK at 3, 6, and 12 months postoperatively. Recent studies have demonstrated that SMILE preserves corneal sensitivity better than LASIK but demonstrated that both procedures eventually result in the recovery of corneal sensitivity to levels seen in healthy controls [9, 21, 25, 30, 43]. This may help to explain the transient nature and the long-term return of TBUT and SEEQ scores to preoperative levels in both groups after 12 months.

Li et al., who examined corneal sensitivity and dry eye following SMILE and FS-LASIK surgery, found that corneal sensitivity was less reduced and thus better in patients that underwent SMILE at all postoperative time intervals compared to those patients that underwent FS-LASIK [41]. The present study found that patients who underwent SMILE not only recovered tear-film function quicker than those who underwent FS-LASIK, but also were less symptomatic in the first 6 months. We also found a moderate correlation between the TBUT and SEEQ scores at 1 month postoperatively in both the SMILE and FS-LASIK groups; however, this correlation did not persist, suggesting that the clinical signs do not always correlate with reported symptoms. This discrepancy between clinical signs and patient symptoms has been previously noted, as Demirok et al. demonstrated that although both SMILE and FS-LASIK resulted in a decrease in corneal sensation up to 3 months postoperatively, there was no change in dry eye symptoms at any point in their patients [25].

Ocular surface changes, including those to the conjunctiva, induced by the two procedures would also differ. Coupled with the effects of hypoesthesia of the cornea, these changes may help to further explain the difference in the development of dry eye disease between SMILE and FS-LASIK patients. Contour changes may impact the distribution of tears over the corneal surface and are likely to pose a greater problem following FS-LASIK than SMILE due to disruption of the epithelium during the formation of the epithelial flap [11, 22]. Damage to and loss of mucin-producing conjunctival goblet cells have been shown to occur following LASIK, resulting in tear-film instability through a reduction of the mucin layer of the tear film [19, 21, 23]. This change may, however, return to baseline after 6 months and may contribute to the transient nature of the postrefractive dry eye disease. An increase in the osmolarity of tears following refractive surgery has also been demonstrated to occur after LASIK [19, 33, 34]. Hyperosmolarity of the tears occurs due to decreased blinking and increased evaporative loss of tears, reduced secretion of tears from the lacrimal gland, and the loss of goblet cells producing the mucin layer of the tear film [19]. This hyperosmolar environment results in the triggering of an inflammatory cascade with an upregulation of inflammatory cytokines, leading to continuing ocular surface irritation, a reduction in TBUT, and the development of dry eye symptoms [33].

FS-LASIK has been proven to be a safe and successful procedure for the surgical correction of refractive error over a number of years [8, 46]. SMILE, although in its clinical infancy, is now proving to also be a safe and successful alternative for the correction of refractive error and may provide a more superior and safer refractive outcome than FS-LASIK [36]. Extensive literature exists demonstrating the safety, efficacy, and complications of FS-LASIK, including a substantial amount of literature investigating the development of ocular surface and dry eye disease following FS-LASIK [8, 10, 11, 17, 19, 22, 23, 47]. Recently, there have been limited studies investigating the development of dry eye following SMILE, as well as studies comparing the two procedures [9, 25, 36, 41]. The majority of the literature, however, has focused on the short-term dry eye outcomes following SMILE and FS-LASIK, looking at the development of dry eye disease up to 3 to 9 months postoperatively. The present study advances on the current literature by investigating and comparing the clinical and subjective dry eye outcomes of patients undergoing SMILE and FS-LASIK over a longer period of follow-up, with measures up to 12 months postoperatively. One other advantage of the present study is that all patients investigated had a moderate to high degree of myopia prior to surgery. This is significant as the large majority of patients undergoing refractive surgery each year are myopic, and the greater the degree of myopia, the greater the amount of stromal ablation or lenticular extraction required [8, 12, 16]. This is a potential area of future research, investigating the development of dry eye disease in relation to the degree of refractive error.

Future advancements can be made on this study to further investigate both the clinical and subjective dry eye outcomes following SMILE and FS-LASIK. The present study was limited in the scope of assessments it conducted, looking at only 2 clinical indicators of dry eye: one objective measure using the TBUT and one subjective evaluation of patient symptoms using the SEEQ. A more comprehensive combination of assessments, as suggested by the Dry Eye Workshop and other studies, would provide a more accurate diagnosis of dry eye disease [5, 24, 37–39]. This would include a measure of tear osmolarity, corneal sensitivity, TBUT, a measure of tear function such as the Schirmer's test, and with advances in technology even the use of confocal microscopy. Also, a more rigorous questionnaire should be utilised, such as the 12-item Ocular Surface Disease Index (OSDI) or the 57-item Impact of Dry Eye on Everyday Life (IDEEL) questionnaires, which have been shown to be more accurate indicators of dry eye disease [2, 47, 48]. The SEEQ had the advantage of being quick and easy to administer, with only 6 items, but has been shown to be outdated and having a low correlation with dry eye signs [47].

The present study demonstrated that SMILE resulted in a lesser degree of dry eye disease and a faster recovery of tear function compared to FS-LASIK in the short-term following surgery in those patients with no preexisting dry eye disease. This was found using both clinical and subjective measures of dry eye and also demonstrated that the long-term outcome was not significantly different between the two procedures after 12 months of follow-up postoperatively. This short-term change, however, can have a great impact on a patients' overall satisfaction with their surgical and visual outcome and may influence their quality of life. Further studies may aim to determine preventative measures that may be taken to help prevent or reduce the development of dry eye disease in patients undergoing refractive surgery and help better monitor and manage those that do.

Conflict of Interests

The authors declare that there is no conflict of interests regarding the publication of this paper.

Acknowledgment

This study was supported by the Science and Technology Commission of Shanghai Municipality, Grant no. 134119a5100.

References

[1] I. K. Gipson, "Research in dry eye: report of the research subcommittee of the International Dry Eye WorkShop (2007)," *The Ocular Surface*, vol. 5, no. 2, pp. 179–193, 2007.

[2] L. Abetz, K. Rajagopalan, P. Mertzanis, C. Begley, R. Barnes, and R. Chalmers, "Development and validation of the impact of dry eye on everyday life (IDEEL) questionnaire, a patient-reported outcomes (PRO) measure for the assessment of the burden of dry eye on patients," *Health and Quality of Life Outcomes*, vol. 9, article 111, 2011.

[3] H. Brewitt and F. Sistani, "Dry eye disease: the scale of the problem," *Survey of Ophthalmology*, vol. 45, supplement 2, pp. S199–S202, 2001.

[4] J. R. Grubbs Jr., S. Tolleson-Rinehart, K. Huynh, and R. M. Davis, "A review of quality of life measures in dry eye questionnaires," *Cornea*, vol. 33, no. 2, pp. 215–218, 2014.

[5] H. D. Perry and E. D. Donnenfeld, "Dry eye diagnosis and management in 2004," *Current Opinion in Ophthalmology*, vol. 15, no. 4, pp. 299–304, 2004.

[6] M. A. Lemp, C. Baudouin, J. Baum et al., "The definition and classification of dry eye disease: report of the definition and classification subcommittee of the international Dry Eye WorkShop (2007)," *Ocular Surface*, vol. 5, no. 2, pp. 75–92, 2007.

[7] M. V. Netto, R. R. Mohan, R. Ambrósio Jr., A. E. K. Hutcheon, J. D. Zieske, and S. E. Wilson, "Wound healing in the cornea: a review of refractive surgery complications and new prospects for therapy," *Cornea*, vol. 24, no. 5, pp. 509–522, 2005.

[8] K. D. Solomon, L. E. Fernández de Castro, H. P. Sandoval et al., "LASIK world literature review: quality of life and patient satisfaction," *Ophthalmology*, vol. 116, no. 4, pp. 691–701, 2009.

[9] A. Denoyer, E. Landman, L. Trinh, J. Faure, F. Auclin, and C. Baudouin, "Dry eye disease after refractive surgery: comparative outcomes of small incision lenticule extraction versus LASIK," *Ophthalmology*, vol. 122, no. 4, pp. 669–676, 2015.

[10] D. Garcia-Zalisnak, D. Nash, and E. Yeu, "Ocular surface diseases and corneal refractive surgery," *Current Opinion in Ophthalmology*, vol. 25, no. 4, pp. 264–269, 2014.

[11] D. Raoof and R. Pineda, "Dry eye after laser in-situ keratomileusis," *Seminars in Ophthalmology*, vol. 29, no. 5-6, pp. 358–362, 2014.

[12] A. A. M. Torricelli, S. J. Bechara, and S. E. Wilson, "Screening of refractive surgery candidates for lasik and PRK," *Cornea*, vol. 33, no. 10, pp. 1051–1055, 2014.

[13] N. S. Jabbur, K. Sakatani, and T. P. O'Brien, "Survey of complications and recommendations for management in dissatisfied patients seeking a consultation after refractive surgery," *Journal of Cataract and Refractive Surgery*, vol. 30, no. 9, pp. 1867–1874, 2004.

[14] B. A. Levinson, C. J. Rapuano, E. J. Cohen, K. M. Hammersmith, B. D. Ayres, and P. R. Laibson, "Referrals to the Wills Eye Institute Cornea Service after laser in situ keratomileusis: reasons for patient dissatisfaction," *Journal of Cataract and Refractive Surgery*, vol. 34, no. 1, pp. 32–39, 2008.

[15] E. Y. W. Yu, A. Leung, S. Rao, and D. S. C. Lam, "Effect of laser in situ keratomileusis on tear stability," *Ophthalmology*, vol. 107, no. 12, pp. 2131–2135, 2000.

[16] S. D. Hammond Jr., A. K. Puri, and B. K. Ambati, "Quality of vision and patient satisfaction after LASIK," *Current Opinion in Ophthalmology*, vol. 15, no. 4, pp. 328–332, 2004.

[17] A. E. Levitt, A. Galor, J. S. Weiss et al., "Chronic dry eye symptoms after LASIK: parallels and lessons to be learned from other persistent post-operative pain disorders," *Molecular Pain*, vol. 11, article 21, 2015.

[18] M. D. Hammond, W. P. Madigan Jr., and K. S. Bower, "Refractive surgery in the United States Army, 2000–2003," *Ophthalmology*, vol. 112, no. 2, pp. 184–190, 2005.

[19] G. R. Nettune and S. C. Pflugfelder, "Post-LASIK tear dysfunction and dysesthesia," *The Ocular Surface*, vol. 8, no. 3, pp. 135–145, 2010.

[20] A. M. Alfawaz, S. Algehedan, S. S. Jastaneiah, S. Al-Mansouri, A. Mousa, and A. Al-Assiri, "Efficacy of punctal occlusion in management of dry eyes after laser in situ keratomileusis for myopia," *Current Eye Research*, vol. 39, no. 3, pp. 257–262, 2014.

[21] C. Chao, B. Golebiowski, and F. Stapleton, "The role of corneal innervation in LASIK-induced neuropathic dry eye," *The Ocular Surface*, vol. 12, no. 1, pp. 32–45, 2014.

[22] M. Q. Salomão, R. Ambrósio Jr., and S. E. Wilson, "Dry eye associated with laser in situ keratomileusis: mechanical microkeratome versus femtosecond laser," *Journal of Cataract & Refractive Surgery*, vol. 35, no. 10, pp. 1756–1760, 2009.

[23] R. Solomon, E. D. Donnenfeld, and H. D. Perry, "The effects of LASIK on the ocular surface," *The Ocular Surface*, vol. 2, no. 1, pp. 34–44, 2004.

[24] M. S.-B. Zeev, D. D. Miller, and R. Latkany, "Diagnosis of dry eye disease and emerging technologies," *Clinical Ophthalmology*, vol. 8, pp. 581–590, 2014.

[25] A. Demirok, E. B. Ozgurhan, A. Agca et al., "Corneal sensation after corneal refractive surgery with small incision lenticule extraction," *Optometry and Vision Science*, vol. 90, no. 10, pp. 1040–1047, 2013.

[26] S. Wei and Y. Wang, "Comparison of corneal sensitivity between FS-LASIK and femtosecond lenticule extraction (ReLEx flex) or small-incision lenticule extraction (ReLEx smile) for myopic eyes," *Graefe's Archive for Clinical and Experimental Ophthalmology*, vol. 251, no. 6, pp. 1645–1654, 2013.

[27] A. Kheirkhah, U. S. Saboo, T. B. Abud et al., "Reduced corneal endothelial cell density in patients with dry eye disease," *American Journal of Ophthalmology*, vol. 159, no. 6, pp. 1022.e2–1026.e2, 2015.

[28] C. F. Marfurt, J. Cox, S. Deek, and L. Dvorscak, "Anatomy of the human corneal innervation," *Experimental Eye Research*, vol. 90, no. 4, pp. 478–492, 2010.

[29] L. J. Müller, C. F. Marfurt, F. Kruse, and T. M. T. Tervo, "Corneal nerves: structure, contents and function," *Experimental Eye Research*, vol. 76, no. 5, pp. 521–542, 2003.

[30] M. O'Doherty, M. O'Keeffe, and C. Kelleher, "Five year follow up of laser in situ keratomileusis for all levels of myopia," *British Journal of Ophthalmology*, vol. 90, no. 1, pp. 20–23, 2006.

[31] W. Sekundo, K. Bönicke, P. Mattausch, and W. Wiegand, "Six-year follow-up of laser in situ keratomileusis for moderate and extreme myopia using a first-generation excimer laser and microkeratome," *Journal of Cataract and Refractive Surgery*, vol. 29, no. 6, pp. 1152–1158, 2003.

[32] K. K. Nichols, J. J. Nichols, and G. L. Mitchell, "The lack of association between signs and symptoms in patients with dry eye disease," *Cornea*, vol. 23, no. 8, pp. 762–770, 2004.

[33] L. Battat, A. Macri, D. Dursun, and S. C. Pflugfelder, "Effects of laser in situ keratomileusis on tear production, clearance, and the ocular surface," *Ophthalmology*, vol. 108, no. 7, pp. 1230–1235, 2001.

[34] A. Denoyer, G. Rabut, and C. Baudouin, "Tear film aberration dynamics and vision-related quality of life in patients with dry eye disease," *Ophthalmology*, vol. 119, no. 9, pp. 1811–1818, 2012.

[35] J. S. Kung, C. S. Sáles, and E. E. Manche, "Corneal sensation and dry eye symptoms after conventional versus inverted side-cut femtosecond LASIK: a prospective randomized study," *Ophthalmology*, vol. 121, no. 12, pp. 2311–2316, 2014.

[36] Y. Xu and Y. Yang, "Dry eye after small incision lenticule extraction and LASIK for myopia," *Journal of Refractive Surgery*, vol. 30, no. 3, pp. 186–190, 2014.

[37] "Methodologies to diagnose and monitor dry eye disease: report of the Diagnostic Methodology Subcommittee of the International Dry Eye WorkShop (2007)," *The Ocular Surface*, vol. 5, no. 2, pp. 108–152, 2007.

[38] Y. Qazi, S. Aggarwal, and P. Hamrah, "Image-guided evaluation and monitoring of treatment response in patients with dry eye disease," *Graefe's Archive for Clinical and Experimental Ophthalmology*, vol. 252, no. 6, pp. 857–872, 2014.

[39] E. Villani, C. Baudouin, N. Efron et al., "In vivo confocal microscopy of the ocular surface: from bench to bedside," *Current Eye Research*, vol. 39, no. 3, pp. 213–231, 2014.

[40] B. J. Thomas, A. Galor, A. A. Nanji et al., "Ultra high-resolution anterior segment optical coherence tomography in the diagnosis and management of ocular surface squamous neoplasia," *The Ocular Surface*, vol. 12, no. 1, pp. 46–58, 2014.

[41] M. Li, J. Zhao, Y. Shen et al., "Comparison of dry eye and corneal sensitivity between small incision lenticule extraction and femtosecond LASIK for myopia," *PloS ONE*, vol. 8, no. 10, Article ID e77797, 2013.

[42] B. S. Shaheen, M. Bakir, and S. Jain, "Corneal nerves in health and disease," *Survey of Ophthalmology*, vol. 59, no. 3, pp. 263–285, 2014.

[43] M. P. Calvillo, J. W. McLaren, D. O. Hodge, and W. M. Bourne, "Corneal reinnervation after LASIK: prospective 3-year longitudinal study," *Investigative Ophthalmology and Visual Science*, vol. 45, no. 11, pp. 3991–3996, 2004.

[44] J. C. Erie, J. W. McLaren, D. O. Hodge, and W. M. Bourne, "Recovery of corneal subbasal nerve density after PRK and LASIK," *American Journal of Ophthalmology*, vol. 140, no. 6, pp. 1059.e1–1064.e1, 2005.

[45] C. Wang, Y. Peng, S. Pan, and L. Li, "Effect of insulin-like growth factor-1 on corneal surface ultrastructure and nerve regeneration of rabbit eyes after laser in situ keratomileusis," *Neuroscience Letters*, vol. 558, pp. 169–174, 2014.

[46] C. McAlinden, "Corneal refractive surgery: past to present," *Clinical and Experimental Optometry*, vol. 95, no. 4, pp. 386–398, 2012.

[47] "The epidemiology of dry eye disease: report of the Epidemiology Subcommittee of the International Dry Eye WorkShop (2007)," *The Ocular Surface*, vol. 5, no. 2, pp. 93–107, 2007.

[48] S. Vitale, L. A. Goodman, G. F. Reed, and J. A. Smith, "Comparison of the NEI-VFQ and OSDI questionnaires in patients with Sjögren's syndrome-related dry eye," *Health and Quality of Life Outcomes*, vol. 2, article 44, 2004.

Effect of Glyceraldehyde Cross-Linking on a Rabbit Bullous Keratopathy Model

Mengmeng Wang

Hebei Provincial Eye Hospital, Hebei Provincial Ophthalmology Key Lab, Hebei Provincial Institute of Ophthalmology, Xingtai, Hebei 054001, China

Correspondence should be addressed to Mengmeng Wang; wangmengmg@163.com

Academic Editor: Vito Romano

Background. To evaluate the effects of corneal glyceraldehyde CXL on the rabbit bullous keratopathy models established by descemetorhexis. *Methods.* Fifteen rabbits were randomly divided into five groups. Group A ($n = 3$) is the control group. The right eyes of animals in Groups B, C, D, and E ($n = 3$, resp.) were suffered with descemetorhexis procedures. From the 8th day to the 14th day postoperatively, the right eyes in Groups C and D were instilled with hyperosmolar drops and glyceraldehyde drops, respectively; the right eyes in Group E were instilled with both hyperosmolar drops and glyceraldehyde drops. Central corneal thickness (CCT), corneal transparency score, and histopathological analysis were applied on the eyes in each group. *Results.* Compared with Group A, statistically significant increase in CCT and corneal transparency score was found in Groups B, C, D, and E at 7 d postoperatively ($P < 0.05$) and in Groups C, D, and E at 14 d postoperatively ($P < 0.05$). *Conclusion.* Chemical CXL technique using glyceraldehyde improved the CCT and corneal transparency of the rabbit bullous keratopathy models. Topical instillation with glyceraldehyde and hyperosmolar solutions seems to be a good choice for the bullous keratopathy treatment.

1. Introduction

Bullous keratopathy is a condition of overhydration (edema) of the cornea, resulting from endothelial failure [1]. It is characterized by both stromal and epithelial edema; the increase of corneal thickness signifies the aggravation of hydration. The most common reasons associated with this disease include detachment of Descemet's membrane [2], Fuchs endothelial dystrophy [3], and postoperative bullous keratopathy [4]. Clinically, many therapeutic methods have been used to treat bullous keratopathy.

Collagen cross-linking (CXL), introduced by Wollensak et al. [5, 6], is an effective approach to increase the biomechanical strength of the corneal and scleral tissue [7]. By means of a highly localized photopolymerization, corneal CXL can create additional chemical bonds inside the corneal stroma, compact the anterior corneal stroma, and decrease the central corneal thickness [8]. Cross-linking might become a useful tool in the temporary treatment of bullous keratopathy [9]. Glyceraldehyde ($C_3H_6O_3$) is a simple aldotriose sugar. As a chemical cross-linking agent, glyceraldehyde not only provided excellent efficacy of increasing scleral rigidity by up to 419% [7] but also showed low toxicity on in vitro corneal epithelial and endothelial cell lines [10].

The purpose of the present study was to evaluate the effects of corneal glyceraldehyde CXL on the rabbit bullous keratopathy models, which were established by descemetorhexis.

2. Methods

2.1. Animals. Fifteen New Zealand adult albino rabbits weighing 2.0–3.0 kg were obtained from the Laboratory Animal Center of Peking University. Before recruiting into the experiment, all rabbits were given a complete ophthalmological and systemic examination to exclude any ocular and body disease. All procedures in the present study were approved by the Ethics Committee of Peking University and were in accordance with the Association for Research in

TABLE 1: Treatment protocols for the eyes in each group.

Groups	Eyes	Descriptions
A	$n = 3$	Sham operated control
B	$n = 3$	Descemetorhexis
C	$n = 3$	Descemetorhexis + hyperosmolar eye drops
D	$n = 3$	Descemetorhexis + glyceraldehyde eye drops
E	$n = 3$	Descemetorhexis + hyperosmolar eye drops + glyceraldehyde eye drops

TABLE 2: Characteristics of 15 rabbits in central corneal thickness (CCT) and corneal transparency score.

Groups	Animals	CCT, μm			Corneal transparency score		
		Pre	7 d	15 d	Pre	7 d	15 d
A	1	373	375	378	0	0	0
	2	354	350	357	0	0	0
	3	391	385	390	0	0	0
B	4	346	1020	975	0	4	4
	5	368	871	804	0	3	2
	6	359	905	783	0	4	3
C	7	375	879	497	0	3	1
	8	337	1010	652	0	4	2
	9	380	935	585	0	4	2
D	10	352	986	614	0	4	2
	11	347	1019	657	0	4	3
	12	359	873	489	0	3	1
E	13	338	1014	496	0	4	1
	14	343	902	449	0	4	1
	15	389	1040	534	0	4	2

Pre, before descemetorhexis surgery; 7 d, 7 days after descemetorhexis surgery; 15 d, 15 days after descemetorhexis surgery.

Vision and Ophthalmology (ARVO) Statement for the Use of Animals in Ophthalmic and Vision Research.

2.2. Grouping and Treatment Protocols. According to the treatment protocols shown in Table 1, these animals were randomly divided into five groups. Group A is the sham operated control group (only corneal incision, without descemetorhexis, $n = 3$). To establish the bullous keratopathy, the right eyes of animals in the other four groups were suffered with detachment of Descemet's membrane using a descemetorhexis technique [11]. In Group B ($n = 3$), no treatment was applied for the bullous keratopathy postoperatively. In Group C ($n = 3$), hyperosmolar drops (5.00% NaCl) were instilled in the eyes 4 times daily from the 8th day to the 14th day postoperatively. In Group D ($n = 3$), glyceraldehyde drops (0.5 M glyceraldehyde (DL-glyceraldehyde, Wako Pure Chemical Industries, Ltd., Osaka, Japan) and 0.02% benzalkonium chloride [BAC, Wako Pure Chemical Industries, Ltd., Osaka, Japan] in 0.90% NaCl) were instilled in the eyes 4 times daily from the 8th day to the 14th day postoperatively. In Group E ($n = 3$), both hyperosmolar drops and glyceraldehyde drops were combined to be instilled in the eyes 4 times daily from the 8th day to the 14th day postoperatively.

2.3. Descemetorhexis Procedure. All operations were performed by the same surgeon (M.W.) under sterile conditions. After the general and topical anesthesia, the right eyes of animals in Groups B, C, D, and E had a self-sealing clear corneal incision (2.0 mm in length and 3.0 mm in width) at the 12 o'clock surgical position of peripheral cornea. A hook was used to strip the surrounding edges of Descemet's membrane (DM) inward toward the center and then they were removed from the anterior chamber. Chloramphenicol eye drops were applied 4 times daily for 3 days preoperatively and 7 days postoperatively.

2.4. Pre- and Postoperative Examinations. Preoperatively and at the 7th and 15th day postoperatively, both central corneal thickness (CCT) and corneal transparency were measured on the right eyes of all animals to check their corneal conditions. Ultrasound pachymetry was performed for the CCT using Nidek UP-1000 ultrasonic pachymeter (NIDEK CO., LTD., Gamagori, Aichi, Japan). Corneal transparency was measured by slit lamp biomicroscopy and graded according to a previously published scale [12] from 0 to 4 (0 = no edema, totally transparent; 1+ = slight corneal edema, slight loss of transparency; 2+ = moderate edema, iris details seen; 3+ = intense edema, some iris details seen; and 4+ = very opaque, no iris details seen). All examinations were performed on the animals after their general and topical anesthesia by an independent masked examiner.

2.5. Histopathological Analysis. All animals were euthanized using an overdose of pentobarbital at the 15th day postoperatively. The right eyes were immediately enucleated for histopathological analysis. The cornea was bisected vertically in the center at the 12 o'clock position. One-half of the cornea was fixed in 4% neutral buffered formalin; 5.0 μm thin paraffin sections were stained with hematoxylin and eosin (H&E). The specimens were evaluated using a light microscope (Leica DM750, Leica Microsystems GmbH, Wetzlar, Germany) at 100- to 400-fold magnification.

2.6. Statistical Analysis. Statistical analysis was performed with JMP 9 statistical package (SAS Institute, Inc., Cary, NC, USA) software. Categorical variables were compared using Pearson's chi-square test. When parametric analysis was possible, one-way ANOVA with Tukey's HSD test was used to compare the results among the different groups/time points; when parametric analysis was not possible, the Kruskal-Wallis test with Steel-Dwass test was used instead. Results with $P < 0.05$ were considered statistically significant.

3. Results

Table 2 shows the characteristics of 15 included rabbits in CCT and corneal transparency score preoperatively and postoperatively. The preoperative transparency scores of all

TABLE 3: Central corneal thickness (CCT) of each group at different time points pre- and postoperatively.

Groups	CCT			P values	P values of post hoc comparison		
	Pre	7 d	15 d	Among three time points	Pre versus 7 d	7 d versus 15 d	Pre versus 15 d
A	372.67 ± 18.50	370.00 ± 18.03	375.00 ± 16.70	0.9428	NS	NS	NS
B	357.67 ± 11.06	932.00 ± 78.08*	854.00 ± 105.31*	0.0002	0.0002	NS	0.0005
C	364.00 ± 23.52	941.33 ± 65.73*	618.50 ± 47.38*,§	<0.0001	<0.0001	0.0008	0.0115
D	352.67 ± 6.03	959.33 ± 76.57*	586.67 ± 87.27*,§	<0.0001	<0.0001	0.0012	0.0125
E	356.67 ± 28.11	985.33 ± 73.33*	493.00 ± 42.58§	<0.0001	<0.0001	<0.0001	0.0407

Pre, before descemetorhexis surgery; 7 d, 7 days after descemetorhexis surgery; 15 d, 15 days after descemetorhexis surgery; NS, no significance. *Statistically significant difference compared with the value in Group A at the same time point; §statistically significant difference compared with the value in Group B at the same time point.

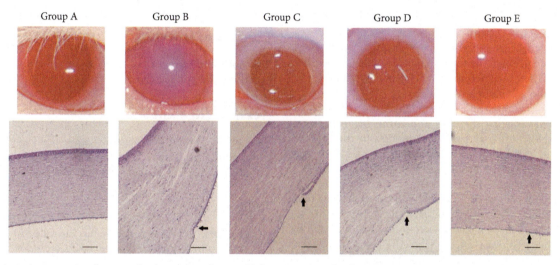

FIGURE 1: Anterior segment photographs (upper) and corneal photomicrographs (lower, H&E stain; original magnification ×200, bar = 100 μm) of rabbits in each group at 15 days postoperatively. Arrows show the edges of the Descemet membrane in eyes after descemetorhexis procedures.

eyes in four groups were 0, which means they were totally transparent. There was no transparency change in Group A at all time points. At the 7th day after descemetorhexis procedures, the transparency scores in Groups B, C, D, and E were increased from 0 to 3+ in 3 eyes and from 0 to 4+ in 9 eyes. At the end of the study, the transparency scores were ranging between 2+ and 4+ in Group B and between 1+ and 2+ in Group E.

Table 3 shows the mean CCT values of each group at different preoperative and postoperative time points. Statistically significant increase in CCT was found in Groups B, C, D, and E at 7 days postoperatively and in Groups B, C, and D at 15 days postoperatively ($P < 0.05$). Compared with the CCT value in Group B, statistically significant improvements were found in Groups C, D, and E at end of this study ($P < 0.05$). Although the mean value in Group E was thicker than Group A, there was no statistically significant difference between the two groups at the end of this study ($P = 0.3435$).

As was shown in Table 2 and Figure 1, corneal opaque and edema were observed in the corneal stroma 7 days after descemetorhexis procedures, which suggested the bullous keratopathy. Corneal transparency scores were reduced in all eyes of Groups B, C, D, and E at 7 days postoperatively. According to the anterior segment photographs and corneal photomicrographs, corneal transparency and edema condition were observed much better in Groups C and E than in Group B at the end of the study.

4. Discussion

Although bullous keratopathy is one of the leading indications, immediate keratoplasty is not a reality in many countries. It has to cost patients a few weeks to years for a suitable corneal tissue from a donor [13]. Thus, several options have been proposed for the bullous keratopathy treatment when patients are waiting for their surgical procedures. Topical hypertonic solutions could yield short-term relief of visual acuity and corneal clarity by reducing the epithelial edema [14]. Recently, a physical CXL technique using ultraviolet (UVA) and riboflavin has been developed to provide temporary improvements in corneal transparency, corneal thickness, and ocular pain [9, 15, 16]. Because of their similar biomechanical efficiency [7], a chemical CXL technique using glyceraldehyde was substituted for the physical CXL technique in the present study as a new attempt for the bullous keratopathy treatment.

In previous studies, transcorneal freezing was performed using a cryoprobe or a brass dowel cooled in liquid nitrogen for establishing the bullous keratopathy models [17, 18]. The cryoprobe or brass dowel should be kept on the corneal surface until the endothelium was affected. After the transcorneal freezing procedures, the severity of endothelial dysfunction could not be accurately reflected by evaluating the postoperative CCT and corneal clarity because of the destruction in overall corneal layers. In the present study, a descemetorhexis technique was performed for establishing the rabbit bullous keratopathy models, which was not intraoperative damage to the epithelium and stroma. It was found that the average values of postoperative CCT were almost 2-3 times thicker than the preoperative levels. The corneal edema and opacity were observed in all rabbit eyes with descemetorhexis procedures at 7 days postoperatively. All these biological and histopathological results proved the efficiency of the descemetorhexis technique in establishing the rabbit bullous keratopathy models.

Both hyperosmolar and glyceraldehyde were proved to be effective in reducing the CCT and corneal transparency scores of rabbit bullous keratopathy models in the present study ($P < 0.05$). Although there was no statistically significant difference among three treatment groups (Groups C, D, and E), the largest improvement in CCT and corneal transparency scores was observed in Group E. It seemed that the hyperosmolar effect of 5.00% NaCl solution and the CXL effect of glyceraldehyde solution were combined in Group E. When the hyperosmolar effect makes the corneal collagen fibers gather together, CXL effect could be much easier to be applied. To verify this combination and improve the topical solution, more bullous keratopathy animals and examination parameters should be included for long-term studies in the future.

The present chemical CXL technique using glyceraldehyde for the bullous keratopathy treatment has the following advantages. First, the toxicity level of glyceraldehyde has preliminarily been proven to be lowest among several chemical CXL agents [10]. Until now, no side effect was reported in previous glyceraldehyde CXL studies involving human [7], porcine [19], guinea pig [20], and rabbit [21, 22] eyes. Second, compared with the invasive physical CXL surgery, no corneal deepithelialization during the glyceraldehyde CXL may yield less postoperative discomfort [23] and complications (such as haze, infective keratitis, and reduction of corneal thickness) [24]. Third, chemical CXL technique is more convenient to be applied. Topical glyceraldehyde solution can be instilled by patients themselves several times daily for a long treatment period.

Nevertheless, the following limitations of the current study should be noted. First, the limited animal sample cannot elaborate information about the long-term efficacy and safety of the current CXL technique. Second, the current rabbit bullous keratopathy model was still different from human cases in clinical settings. Third, because of the lack of corneal glyceraldehyde CXL previously, the only glyceraldehyde concentration (0.5 M) in the present study was chosen according to several scleral CXL studies [19–22]. Finally, although a 24-hour exposure to glyceraldehyde has been proved to be safe for cultured human corneal epithelial cells and bovine corneal endothelial cells [10], long-term safety of this agent was still unknown. Further studies using more animal models and human cases are needed to set up a long-term safe and effective protocol of corneal glyceraldehyde CXL for bullous keratopathy treatment.

In sum, chemical CXL technique using glyceraldehyde improved the CCT and corneal transparency of the rabbit bullous keratopathy models established by descemetorhexis. Topical instillation with glyceraldehyde and hyperosmolar solutions seems to be a good choice for bullous keratopathy patients as a temporary therapeutic measure when they are waiting for the keratoplasty.

Conflict of Interests

The author declares that there is no conflict of interests regarding the publication of this paper.

Acknowledgment

The author thanks Dr. Christine Carole C. Corpuz (Eye Can Philippines, Inc., San Juan, Metro Manila, Philippines) for her English editing and critical review of this paper.

References

[1] A. J. Bron, "UV-riboflavin cross-linking of the cornea in bullous keratopathy: appraising the rationale," *Cornea*, vol. 30, no. 6, pp. 724–726, 2011.

[2] R. E. Braunstein, S. Airiani, M. A. Chang, and M. G. Odrich, "Corneal edema resolution after 'descemetorhexis'," *Journal of Cataract & Refractive Surgery*, vol. 29, no. 7, pp. 1436–1439, 2003.

[3] A. P. Adamis, V. Filatov, B. J. Tripathi, and R. A. M. C. Tripathi, "Fuchs' endothelial dystrophy of the cornea," *Survey of Ophthalmology*, vol. 38, no. 2, pp. 149–168, 1993.

[4] N. Szentmáry, B. Szende, and I. Süveges, "Epithelial cell, keratocyte, and endothelial cell apoptosis in Fuchs' dystrophy and in pseudophakic bullous keratopathy," *European Journal of Ophthalmology*, vol. 15, no. 1, pp. 17–22, 2005.

[5] G. Wollensak, E. Spoerl, and T. Seiler, "Riboflavin/ultraviolet-A-induced collagen crosslinking for the treatment of keratoconus," *American Journal of Ophthalmology*, vol. 135, no. 5, pp. 620–627, 2003.

[6] G. Wollensak, E. Spoerl, and T. Seiler, "Stress-strain measurements of human and porcine corneas after riboflavin-ultraviolet-A-induced cross-linking," *Journal of Cataract and Refractive Surgery*, vol. 29, no. 9, pp. 1780–1785, 2003.

[7] G. Wollensak and E. Spoerl, "Collagen crosslinking of human and porcine sclera," *Journal of Cataract and Refractive Surgery*, vol. 30, no. 3, pp. 689–695, 2004.

[8] R. Arora, A. Manudhane, R. K. Saran, J. Goyal, G. Goyal, and D. Gupta, "Role of corneal collagen cross-linking in pseudophakic bullous keratopathy: a clinicopathological study," *Ophthalmology*, vol. 120, no. 12, pp. 2413–2418, 2013.

[9] G. Wollensak, H. Aurich, C. Wirbelauer, and D.-T. Pham, "Potential use of riboflavin/UVA cross-linking in bullous keratopathy," *Ophthalmic Research*, vol. 41, no. 2, pp. 114–117, 2009.

[10] M. Kim, A. Takaoka, Q. V. Hoang, S. L. Trokel, and D. C. Paik, "Pharmacologic alternatives to riboflavin photochemical

corneal cross-linking: a comparison study of cell toxicity thresholds," *Investigative Ophthalmology & Visual Science*, vol. 55, no. 5, pp. 3247–3257, 2014.

[11] G. R. J. Melles, R. H. J. Wijdh, and C. P. Nieuwendaal, "A technique to excise the descemet membrane from a recipient cornea (descemetorhexis)," *Cornea*, vol. 23, no. 3, pp. 286–288, 2004.

[12] R. C. Ghanem, M. R. Santhiago, T. B. Berti, S. Thomaz, and M. V. Netto, "Collagen crosslinking with riboflavin and ultraviolet-A in eyes with pseudophakic bullous keratopathy," *Journal of Cataract and Refractive Surgery*, vol. 36, no. 2, pp. 273–276, 2010.

[13] P. C. Rocon, L. P. Ribeiro, R. F. Scárdua et al., "Main causes of nonfulfillment of corneal donation in five hospitals of a Brazilian State," *Transplantation Proceedings*, vol. 45, no. 3, pp. 1038–1042, 2013.

[14] M. S. Insler, D. W. Benefield, and E. V. Ross, "Topical hyperosmolar solutions in the reduction of corneal edema," *Contact Lens Association of Ophthalmologists Journal*, vol. 13, no. 3, pp. 149–151, 1987.

[15] G. Wollensak, H. Aurich, D.-T. Pham, and C. Wirbelauer, "Hydration behavior of porcine cornea crosslinked with riboflavin and ultraviolet A," *Journal of Cataract & Refractive Surgery*, vol. 33, no. 3, pp. 516–521, 2007.

[16] R. R. Krueger, J. C. Ramos-Esteban, and A. J. Kanellopoulos, "Staged intrastromal delivery of riboflavin with UVA cross-linking in advanced bullous keratopathy: laboratory investigation and first clinical case," *Journal of Refractive Surgery*, vol. 24, no. 7, pp. S730–S736, 2008.

[17] S. B. Han, H. Ang, D. Balehosur et al., "A mouse model of corneal endothelial decompensation using cryoinjury," *Molecular Vision*, vol. 19, pp. 1222–1230, 2013.

[18] T. Mimura, S. Yamagami, T. Usui, N. Honda, and S. Amano, "Necessary prone position time for human corneal endothelial precursor transplantation in a rabbit endothelial deficiency model," *Current Eye Research*, vol. 32, no. 7-8, pp. 617–623, 2007.

[19] G. Wollensak, "Thermomechanical stability of sclera after glyceraldehyde crosslinking," *Graefe's Archive for Clinical and Experimental Ophthalmology*, vol. 249, no. 3, pp. 399–406, 2011.

[20] Y. Wang, Q. Han, F. Han, Y. Chu, and K. Zhao, "Experimental study of glyceraldehyde cross-linking of posterior scleral on FDM in guinea pigs," *Zhonghua Yan Ke Za Zhi*, vol. 50, no. 1, pp. 51–59, 2014.

[21] G. Wollensak and E. Iomdina, "Long-term biomechanical properties after collagen crosslinking of sclera using glyceraldehyde," *Acta Ophthalmologica*, vol. 86, no. 8, pp. 887–893, 2008.

[22] G. Wollensak and E. Iomdina, "Crosslinking of scleral collagen in the rabbit using glyceraldehyde," *Journal of Cataract and Refractive Surgery*, vol. 34, no. 4, pp. 651–656, 2008.

[23] V. C. Ghanem, R. C. Ghanem, and R. de Oliveira, "Postoperative pain after corneal collagen cross-linking," *Cornea*, vol. 32, no. 1, pp. 20–24, 2013.

[24] S. Dhawan, K. Rao, and S. Natrajan, "Complications of corneal collagen cross-linking," *Journal of Ophthalmology*, vol. 2011, Article ID 869015, 5 pages, 2011.

Vision Health-Related Quality of Life in Chinese Glaucoma Patients

Lei Zuo,[1,2] Haidong Zou,[3] Jianhong Zhang,[2] Xinfeng Fei,[2] and Xun Xu[1]

[1]*Department of Ophthalmology, Shanghai General Hospital, Nanjing Medical University, Shanghai 200080, China*
[2]*Department of Ophthalmology, Branch of Shanghai First People's Hospital, Shanghai 200081, China*
[3]*Department of Ophthalmology, Shanghai General Hospital, Shanghai Jiao Tong University, Shanghai 200080, China*

Correspondence should be addressed to Xun Xu; drxuxun@sjtu.edu.cn

Academic Editor: Gianluca Scuderi

This cross-sectional study evaluated VRQOL in Chinese glaucoma patients and the potential factors influencing VRQOL. The VRQOL was assessed using the Chinese-version low vision quality of life questionnaire. Visual field loss was classified by the Hodapp-Parrish-Anderson method. The correlations of VRQOL to the best corrected visual acuity and the VF loss were investigated. The potential impact factors to VRQOL of glaucoma patients were screened by single factor analysis and were further analyzed by multiple regression analysis. There were significant differences in VRQOL scores between mild VF loss group and moderate VF loss group, moderate VF loss group and severe VF loss group, and mild VF loss group and severe VF loss group according to the better eye. In multiple linear regression, the binocular weighted average BCVA significantly affected the VRQOL scores. Binocular MD was the second influencing factor. In logistic regression, binocular severe VF loss and stroke were significantly associated with abnormal VRQOL. Education was the next influencing factor. This study showed that visual acuity correlated linearly with VRQOL, and VF loss might reach a certain level, correlating with abnormal VRQOL scores. Stroke was significantly associated with abnormal VRQOL.

1. Introduction

Glaucoma, a group of eye diseases that permanently damage visual function [1], can impact patient quality of life [2] adversely [3–5]. Ophthalmologists have been working on the best treatment for glaucoma patients and mitigating the adverse impact. Previous studies have investigated the life quality of glaucoma patients, suggesting a relationship between visual field defects and impaired quality of life in patients with glaucoma [6–8]. Furthermore, the association between rates of binocular visual field loss and vision-related quality of life in glaucoma was observed [9]; special attention was paid to the quality of life of young patients with glaucoma [10]; and Globe et al. noticed that self-reported systemic comorbid diseases were associated with self-reported visual function [11]. Understanding of influencing factor to quality of life of the patients will ultimately benefit glaucoma treatment.

Epidemiologic studies in China showed that the overall prevalence rate of primary glaucoma was 0.56% and that of populations over 50 years of age was 2.07% [12]. The blindness rate of glaucoma was 9.04–10% [13]. Lee et al. [14] investigated the association between clinical parameters and quality of life in Chinese primary open angle glaucoma patients (using the Glaucoma Quality of Life-15 Questionnaire (GQL-15)). Kong et al. [15] found that the level of understanding about glaucoma was associated with psychological disturbance and quality of life (using the 25-Item National Eye Institute Visual Function Questionnaire (NEI-VFQ 25) [16]).

In the present study, we assessed vision health-related quality of life (VRQOL) [17] in Chinese glaucoma patients using Chinese-version low vision quality of life questionnaire (CLVQOL) [18] and made comprehensive analysis on screening the potential influencing factors (such as visual field damage, glaucoma type (primary open angle or angle close), age, and self-reported comorbidities) to VRQOL. The CLVQOL questionnaire was originally acquired from the low vision health-related quality of life questionnaire (LVQOL) [17] and translated into a Chinese version that was modified and culturally adapted for the Chinese patients [18]. We hoped our results could provide reference for clinical better understanding of glaucoma patients and developing suitable therapeutic strategy for them.

2. Methods

2.1. Study Patients. There were 202 glaucoma patients who met eligibility criteria and agreed to participate in the study, and these patients were enrolled at the glaucoma clinic at the Branch of Shanghai First People's Hospital from January 1, 2013, through June 31, 2013. The investigation was approved by the hospital ethics committee. All methods adhered to the Declaration of Helsinki. All participants gave their written informed consent.

The inclusion criteria were adult patients (18 years old and above) with glaucoma diagnosis based on glaucomatous disc cupping and reproducible visual field damage detected by automated static perimetry (the Humphrey Visual Field Analyzer) in one or both eyes [4, 19]. There were 2 kinds of glaucoma: primary open angle glaucoma and primary angle closure glaucoma [19] in our study. The exclusion criteria were as follows: (1) secondary glaucoma; (2) any other coexisting ocular condition that could impair visual function (e.g., clinically significant cataract, macular degeneration, or any other ophthalmic condition); (3) incisional ocular surgery or laser treatment in past except antiglaucoma surgery and laser therapy; and (4) disability in a visual field test due to cognitive impairment.

At each follow-up visit, patients underwent a comprehensive ophthalmic examination, including review of medical history, best-corrected visual acuity, slit lamp biomicroscopy, intraocular pressure measurement using noncontact tonometry, gonioscopy, stereoscopic optic disc photography (Canon, CR-1 Mark II), visual fields test, and optic nerve head assessment in optical coherence tomography (Stratus OCT, Carl Zeiss Meditec, CA). The type of local ophthalmic medication was also noted.

2.2. Binocular Visual Fields. Visual fields (VF) test was performed using the Humphrey Visual Field Analyzer (Humphrey Instruments, Zeiss, CA). Humphrey central 30-2 threshold test plotted the central 30 degrees of visual field in both eyes. Only reliable tests (≤33% fixation losses and false-negative results and ≤15% false-positive results) were included. Visual fields were reviewed and excluded in the presence of artifacts such as eyelid or rim artifacts, fatigue effects, inattention, or inappropriate fixation. Visual fields were also reviewed for the presence of abnormalities that could indicate diseases other than glaucoma, such as homonymous hemianopia.

Mean deviation (MD) scores were used to assess the severity of VF loss. For the purpose of the statistical analysis, the binocular VF loss was classified into 3 groups according to MD: group 1 (mild: −6 dB < MD < −3 dB), group 2 (moderate: −12 dB < MD < −6 dB), or group 3 (severe: MD < −12 dB) (the Hodapp-Parrish-Anderson method [20]), which was used for the better eye and worse eye. According to spearman correlation and linear regression, monocular data of MD values was transformed to binocular data using a formula for binocular summation, as suggested by Nelson-Quigg et al. [21]:

$$\text{Binocular Sensitivity} = \sqrt{(\text{Sensitivity R eye})^2 + (\text{Sensitivity L eye})^2}. \quad (1)$$

2.3. Visual Function Questionnaire. The VRQOL was evaluated using the CLVQOL questionnaire [17, 18]. The scale consists of four scales: general vision and lighting (reading road signs or watching TV), mobility (outdoor activities and crossing a street with traffic), psychological adjustment (expectations on quality of life and perceived visual acuity), and reading and fine work and activities of daily living (reading the clock, reading one's own handwriting, and daily activities), including 25 items. Each item was scored using a numeric scale ranging from 0 (worst) to 5 (best). The total highest score was 125, and the higher the score, the better the quality of life [17, 18]. The questionnaires were completed through face-to-face patient interviews conducted by two well-trained investigators.

2.4. Demographic and Clinical Variables. Demographic and clinical questionnaires were also administered to patients concurrent with the CLVQOL questionnaire. These questionnaires contained a survey of demographics, history of glaucoma, marital status, residence, educational level, and history of topical antiglaucomatous treatment.

Self-reported systemic comorbidities were investigated as follows: hypertension, diabetes mellitus, stroke, and other systemic comorbidities such as asthma, cancers, and heart disease.

Visual acuity was measured using the Snellen visual acuity chart. The best corrected visual acuity (BCVA) (subjective optometry) was converted into the minimum angle of resolution (logMAR) vision. When Snellen visual acuity was less than 0.01, the visual acuity of "counting fingers" perception was defined as logMAR2.2, "hand-motion" as logMAR2.3, and "light perception" as logMAR2.5 [22]. Monocular data of logMAR BCVA was transformed to binocular weighted average BCVA with the weight of the better eye and the worse eye taken as 0.75 and 0.25, respectively (as recommended by Scott et al. [23]).

2.5. Statistical Analysis. Descriptive statistics included the mean and standard deviation (SD) for variables. The Spearman correlation was used to analyze the correlation between the binocular weighted average logMAR BCVA and the VRQOL scores and between the binocular MD and the VRQOL scores. When equal variances were assumed, the 1-way ANOVA or χ^2 test was used to process the impact of demographic and clinical variables on the VRQOL scores change. When equal variances were not assumed, a nonparametric test or Fisher's exact 2-tailed test was used.

After single factor analysis of demographic and clinical variables, the statistically significant or nearly significant results were screened out. Then multiple linear regression was used to analyze the impact of linear variables on the VRQOL

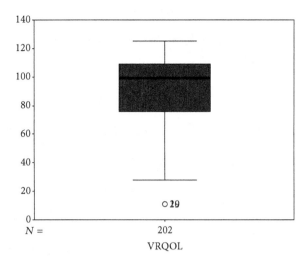

Figure 1: Boxplot showing the range of visual health-related quality of life (VRQOL).

score changes. Logistic regression was used to analyze dichotomous variables; VRQOL scores were considered to be the dependent variable. These variables were categorized into dichotomous variables as follows: marital status (married (yes/no)), residence (urban (yes/no)), education (more than secondary school degree (yes/no)), both eyes MD < −12 dB (yes/no), at least 3 years glaucoma history (yes/no), stroke (yes/no), diabetes mellitus (yes/no), and VRQOL (at least mean value (yes/no)).

The level of statistical significance was set at 0.05. All statistical analyses were performed using SPSS 11.0 (SPSS Inc., Chicago, IL, USA).

3. Results

3.1. Patient Demographic Characteristics and Clinical Variables with VRQOL. There were 92 men and 110 women enrolled in this study, with a mean age (mean (SD)) of 69.49 (12.04) years, ranging from 31 to 89 years. The mean VRQOL score was 92.08 (23.97), ranging from 11 to 125 (Figure 1). VRQOL differences between 50–59 years and 60–69 years and between 50–59 years and 70–79 years were significant ($P = 0.032, 0.018$); differences in VRQOL between other age groups were not significant (all $P > 0.10$). When VRQOL of patients with different education levels (level 1 = illiterate and primary school, level 2 = secondary school, and level 3 = more than secondary school) were compared, there was a significant difference in VRQOL between level 1 and level 3 ($P = 0.027$); VRQOL differences between the other levels were not significant (all $P > 0.10$). When VRQOL of patients with different glaucoma durations (≤3 months, 3–12 months, 1–3 years, and >3 years) were compared, the difference was found to be significant between the VRQOL scores of patients who had been diagnosed with glaucoma within the past 3 months and those of patients with a 3-year course ($P = 0.045$); no remarkable differences were observed in VRQOL scores of other durations of glaucoma (all $P > 0.10$) (Table 1).

3.1.1. Spearman Correlation. The Spearman correlation coefficient between the binocular weighted average logMAR BCVA and VRQOL scores was 0.572 ($P < 0.001$), and correlation coefficient between the binocular MD and VRQOL scores was −0.490 ($P < 0.001$) (Table 2).

Binocular VF Loss and VRQOL. When VRQOL results of patients in the 3 VF loss groups according to the better eye were compared, there were significant differences between group 1 and group 2, group 2 and group 3, and group 1 and group 3 (all $P = 0.014, 0.016, <0.001$). When the VRQOL of the 3 groups according to the worse eye were compared, there was no difference between group 1 and group 2 ($P = 0.509$), but there was a significant difference between group 2 and group 3 and group 1 and group 3 ($P = 0.015, 0.001$) (Table 3).

Glaucoma Type and VRQOL. When VRQOL, binocular weighted logMAR BCVA, and binocular MD of different glaucoma type groups were compared, there were no differences (all $P > 0.10$) (Table 4).

3.2. Analysis of Multiple Impact Factors after Screening

Denied Factors. These included gender, the type of glaucoma, the number of antiglaucoma instillations, and previous antiglaucoma surgery/laser. These factors were not analyzed further.

Possible Impact Factors. These included age, education, marital status, glaucoma duration, and systemic comorbidity (diabetes mellitus, stroke). These factors were analyzed further.

Positive Factors. These included binocular weighted average logMAR BCVA, binocular visual field loss, and residence. These factors were analyzed further.

In multiple linear regression, binocular weighted BCVA impacted VRQOL scores significantly ($P < 0.001$), and binocular MD was the next factor ($P = 0.063$).

In logistic regression, severe binocular VF loss (both eyes MD < −12 dB) and stroke were significantly associated with abnormal VRQOL ($P = 0.004, 0.016$). More than secondary school degree was the secondary factor ($P = 0.052$) (Table 5).

Example of 2 Patients

Patient A. Patient A was a married 72-year-old female, with primary angle closure glaucoma; her residence was urban area; her education level was secondary school; and her medical history was as follows: 10 years after bilateral trabeculectomy, not using any antiglaucoma eye drop; MD: right eye: −5.75 dB, left eye: −6.63 dB; logMAR BCVA: right eye: 0.00, left eye: 0.00; and VRQOL score: 107.

Patient B. Patient B was a married 65-year-old male, with primary open angle glaucoma; his residence was urban area; his education level was more than secondary school; and his medical history was as follows: glaucoma duration for 11 years; using ≥3 kinds of antiglaucoma eye drop; self-reported systemic comorbidity: diabetes mellitus; MD: right

TABLE 1: Patient's demographic characteristics and clinical variables.

Variable	Number of patients	VRQOL score mean (SD)	P values
All	202	92.08 (23.97)	
Binocular weighted average BCVA		0.48 (0.52), 0.00 to 2.35	
BCVA for better eye		0.37 (0.49), 0.00 to 2.30	<0.001
<0.3 (>20/40)	122	102.80 (15.87)	
0.3 to 1.0 (20/200 to 20/40)	62	86.90 (20.42)	
>1.0 (<20/200)	18	44.00 (17.41)	
BCVA for worse eye		0.81 (0.81), 0.00 to 2.50	<0.001
<0.3 (>20/40)	60	105.53 (14.0)	
0.3 to 1.0 (20/200 to 20/40)	88	94.16 (17.94)	
>1.0 (<20/200)	54	73.74 (29.84)	
Binocular MD (dB value)		18.14 (12.09), 3.82 to 45.28	
MD for better eye (dB)		−8.76 (8.23), −31.00 to 1.37	<0.001
>−6	106	101.94 (16.25)	
−6 to −12	46	91.35 (19.19)	
<−12	50	71.84 (29.03)	
MD for worse eye (dB)		−15.28 (9.88), −33.19 to −2.98	0.001
>−6	48	104.17 (13.57)	
−6 to −12	44	100.18 (18.87)	
<−12	110	83.5 (26.10)	
Age (year)		69.49 (12.04), 31 to 89	0.151
≤49	14	98.29 (19.59)	
50–59	26	106.69 (15.13)	
60–69	52	89.23 (24.20)	
70–79	60	87.77 (23.34)	
≥80	50	90.88 (27.48)	
Gender			0.812
Male	92	91.43 (28.08)	
Female	110	92.62 (20.15)	
Education			0.079
Illiterate and primary school	36	81.67 (26.05)	
Secondary school	50	90.52 (23.01)	
Secondary school+	116	95.98 (23.06)	
Residence			0.002
Rural area	12	56.83 (27.72)	
Urban area	190	94.31 (22.05)	
Marital status (married)			0.085
Yes	152	95.07 (21.84)	
No	50	83.00 (28.94)	
Duration of glaucoma			0.222
≤3 months	20	105.00 (19.75)	
3–12 months	36	92.94 (21.50)	
1–3 years	44	94.32 (21.97)	
>3 years	102	88.27 (25.85)	
Previous antiglaucoma surgery/laser			0.867
Yes	42	93.90 (16.82)	
No	160	91.60 (25.58)	
Antiglaucoma eye drop (type)			0.869
0	56	91.57 (21.21)	
1	62	95.03 (20.57)	
2	68	90.29 (28.11)	
≥3	16	90.00 (29.52)	
Self-reported systemic comorbidity			0.072
No	70	93.00 (21.10)	
High blood pressure	56	99.71 (15.84)	
Diabetes mellitus	28	83.50 (24.41)	
Stroke	16	74.63 (25.73)	
Other systemic diseases	32	92.81 (34.68)	

VRQOL: visual health-related quality of life; SD: standard deviation; BCVA: best corrected visual acuity; MD: mean defect.

TABLE 2: Correlation between Chinese-version low vision quality of life (CLVQOL) questionnaire score and visual severity score.

	Spearman correlation	P value
BCVA		
Better eye	−0.614	<0.001
Worse eye	−0.483	<0.001
Binocular weighted average	−0.572	<0.001
MD		
Better eye	0.467	<0.001
Worse eye	0.491	<0.001
Binocular	−0.490	<0.001
PSD		
Better eye	−0.211	0.053
Worse eye	−0.078	0.487
VFI		
Better eye	0.447	<0.001
Worse eye	0.443	<0.001
CDR		
Better eye	−0.280	0.006
Worse eye	−0.313	0.003

VRQOL = vision health-related quality of life; BCVA = best corrected visual acuity; MD = mean defect; PSD = pattern standard deviation; VFI = visual field index; CDR = cup to disk ration.

eye: −27.52 dB, left eye: −29.76 dB; logMAR BCVA: right eye: 0.92, left eye: 0.83; and VRQOL score: 59.

4. Discussion

This cross-sectional study evaluated VRQOL in Chinese glaucoma patients and the potential factors influencing VRQOL. Here, we observed the demographic characteristics and clinical data of 202 Chinese glaucoma patients and analyzed the correlation between these variables and VRQOL.

4.1. Relationship between VRQOL and Visual Health in Glaucoma Patients. Spearman correlation analysis showed that VRQOL and binocular weighted average BCVA were closely related. In multiple linear regression, binocular weighted BCVA had a significant effect on VRQOL. VA and VRQOL of glaucoma patients were shown to have a direct linear correlation [14].

When binocular MD was regarded as a linear variable, the effect on VRQOL showed a trend toward significance. However, when binocular VF loss (binocular MD < −12 dB (yes/no)) was regarded as a dichotomous variable using logistic regression, the association with abnormal VRQOL was significant. This showed that binocular VF loss should reach a certain level, which could greatly affect the VRQOL of glaucoma patients [4–7].

After VF loss was further divided into groups according to VF loss stage [20, 24, 25], a significant relationship between VRQOL and VF loss stage was observed using the four subscales and in the better eye [26]. There was a significant influence on "mobility" subscale and "reading, fine work, and activities of daily living" subscale and total VRQOL scores with mild VF loss in the better eye that changed to moderate VF loss. However, there was a significant influence on the same subscales and total VRQOL scores with moderate VF loss of the worse eye that changed to severe VF loss. These results suggested that the better eye was more sensitive to visual field damage than the worse eye. As these results are shown, it is reasonable to believe that glaucoma patients sometimes neglect early VF damage.

In our study, the high correlation of the CDR with VRQOL was not found (better eye: 0.281, worse eye: 0.313) Our research suggested that the CDR had no significant relationship with patient quality of life [9, 27], and patients paid more attention on visual acuity and visual field results rather than OCT, though the defects of retinal nerve fiber layer were the important signal to be concerned by eye doctors.

4.2. The Effects of Glaucoma Patient Demographic Characteristics on VRQOL. The current research found that the relationship between age and VRQOL in glaucoma patients was more complicated than previous studies [6, 9]. The relationship might be influenced by the patients' psychological and environmental factors. Young people face pressures from life, study, and work, and if there was visual function damage or the threat of damage, the psychological impact would be great (Gupta et al. [28] used the Time-Tradeoff method to observe utility values among glaucoma patients and found that juveniles were willing to give up more years to spend the rest of their living years with perfect vision and free of glaucoma, compared with adult patients). However, elderly people, especially after retirement, showed a partial reduction in the pressures mentioned above. This reduction in pressures would be beneficial for the VRQOL. The coincidence degree of decline in VRQOL of glaucoma patients with age growth might be worse than other age related eye diseases [29, 30].

Labiris et al. [27] indicated that a higher educational background was positively correlated with higher vision-specific QOL scores, but Lisboa et al. [9] found that an educational level of at least high school completion had no significant effect on vision-related QOL. In a single analysis of the present study, the VRQOL score of glaucoma patients with an educational level of more than a secondary school degree was higher than that of the illiterate or primary school educational level of patients. In multiple linear regression, there was no linear relationship between education and VRQOL. However, using logistic regression, when education was regarded as dichotomous variable and was analyzed together with other variables, we found that more than a secondary school degree educational level was a nearly significant impact factor on abnormal VRQOL in glaucoma patients. Therefore, education that reaches a certain level could somewhat improve the VRQOL of glaucoma patients.

There was a significant effect of residence on VRQOL of glaucoma patients, and the effect of marital status showed a trend toward significance in single analysis of our study. It seemed that VRQOL of glaucoma patients living in urban areas was better than that of patients living in rural areas, and

TABLE 3: Relationship between vision health-related quality of life (VRQOL) score calculated for separate factors and visual fields (VF) loss.

	VRQOL score% (SD)	Mild VF loss P value	Moderate VF loss P value	Severe VF loss P value
Better eye				
General vision and lighting (GL)				
Mild VF loss	76.17 (15.57)	—	0.114	0.001*
Moderate VF loss	68.94 (17.14)	0.114	—	0.096
Severe VF loss	56.11 (25.91)	0.001*	0.096	—
Mobility (M)				
Mild VF loss	85.44 (15.16)	—	0.012*	<0.001*
Moderate VF loss	77.04 (15.52)	0.012*	—	0.017*
Severe VF loss	59.84 (24.72)	<0.001*	0.017*	—
Psychological adjustment (PA)				
Mild VF loss	79.35 (12.90)	—	0.066	0.001*
Moderate VF loss	71.50 (17.75)	0.066	—	0.126
Severe VF loss	61.60 (23.20)	0.001*	0.126	—
Reading, fine work, and activities of daily living (RFA)				
Mild VF loss	84.31 (16.22)	—	0.026*	<0.001*
Moderate VF loss	74.78 (19.87)	0.026*	—	0.026*
Severe VF loss	55.38 (30.33)	<0.001*	0.026*	—
Total VRQOL				
Mild VF loss	81.55 (13.00)	—	0.014*	<0.001*
Moderate VF loss	73.08 (15.35)	0.014*	—	0.016*
Severe VF loss	57.47 (23.22)	<0.001*	0.016*	—
Worse eye				
General vision and lighting (GL)				
Mild VF loss	75.60 (13.97)	—	0.664	0.020*
Moderate VF loss	78.17 (19.91)	0.664	—	0.006*
Severe VF loss	63.94 (22.31)	0.020*	0.006*	—
Mobility (M)				
Mild VF loss	89.32 (11.36)	—	0.366	<0.001*
Moderate VF loss	84.72 (15.88)	0.366	—	0.003*
Severe VF loss	69.32 (22.16)	<0.001*	0.003*	—
Psychological adjustment (PA)				
Mild VF loss	81.25 (12.25)	—	0.271	0.005*
Moderate VF loss	78.20 (14.25)	0.271	—	0.050
Severe VF loss	67.65 (20.35)	0.005*	0.050	—
Reading, fine work, and activities of daily living (RFA)				
Mild VF loss	86.96 (14.56)	—	0.241	0.001*
Moderate VF loss	81.00 (17.07)	0.241	—	0.057
Severe VF loss	67.65 (27.31)	0.001*	0.057	—
Total VRQOL				
Mild VF loss	83.33 (10.86)	—	0.509	0.001*
Moderate VF loss	80.14 (15.10)	0.509	—	0.015*
Severe VF loss	66.85 (20.88)	0.001*	0.015*	—

VF loss was classified according to mean deviation (MD) into mild VF loss: −6 dB < MD < −3 dB, moderate VF loss: −12 dB < MD < −6 dB, and severe VF loss: MD < −12 dB; MD was determined using the Humphrey central 30-2 threshold test (*$P < 0.05$).

TABLE 4: Visual function score of different glaucoma type groups.

	Number of patients	Binocular weighted average BCVA mean (SD)	Binocular MD (dB value) mean (SD)	VRQOL score mean (SD)
Primary angle closure glaucoma	118	0.50 (0.53)	16.58 (12.70)	92.02 (23.83)
Primary open angle glaucoma	84	0.47 (0.52)	20.33 (10.96)	92.17 (24.46)

BCVA: best correct visual acuity; SD: standard deviation; MD: mean deviation; VRQOL: vision health-related quality of life.

TABLE 5: Multiple impact factors that influence VRQOL score of glaucoma patients.

	Mean (SD) or number	t or b	P
Age (year)	69.49 (12.04)	−0.793	0.430
Glaucoma duration (year)	5.72 (6.79)	−1.380	0.171
Education (year)	10.61 (4.28)	0.099	0.921
Binocular MD (dB value)	18.14 (12.09)	−1.878	0.063**
Binocular weighted average logMAR BCVA	0.48 (0.52)	−10.699	<0.001*
Married (yes/no)	152/50	−0.603	0.311
Urban (yes/no)	190/12	1.606	0.232
More than secondary school degree (yes/no)	116/86	0.951	0.052**
Both eyes MD < −12 dB (yes/no)	58/144	−1.556	0.004*
At least 3 years of glaucoma history (yes/no)	102/100	−0.304	0.538
Diabetes mellitus (yes/no)	28/174	−0.714	0.301
Stroke (yes/no)	16/186	−2.240	0.016*

VRQOL = vision health-related quality of life; SD = standard deviation; MD = mean deviation; BCVA = best corrected visual acuity (*$P < 0.05$, **$0.05 < P < 0.10$).

VRQOL of married glaucoma patients was probably better than that of patients who were unmarried. Multivariable regression showed that when these 2 factors were analyzed together with items such as education, visual field loss, and systemic comorbidity, there were no significant effects. Thus, residence and marital status might not be as important as other factors when they were considered together [9, 27].

4.3. The Influence of Medical Conditions and Other Factors on VRQOL of Glaucoma Patients. Our cross-sectional study showed that the change in the VRQOL value with the change in glaucoma duration was not statistically significant. Glaucoma patients' VRQOL was closely related to vision activity and visual field damage, and VRQOL and duration of the disease had no direct relationship.

This study indicated that there were no differences between the VRQOL of primary angle close glaucoma and primary open angle glaucoma [8]. Our results showed that the patients are not interested in whether their glaucoma type is the open or closed angle type, but rather their concern is the impact of the disease on their quality of life.

In this study, previous glaucoma surgery/laser had no impact on the VRQOL scores of glaucoma patients. The number of antiglaucoma eye drops also had no impact. This result was similar to that of previous reports, whose aim did not involve evaluating the side effects of glaucoma treatments [14, 27].

This study showed that whether VRQOL scores reached mean value was significantly influenced by stroke. In the Los Angeles Latino Eye Study, systemic comorbidity weighted index of glaucoma patients was analyzed. They indicated that the weighted index of stroke or brain hemorrhage was 2.06, that of diabetes mellitus was 1.80, and that of high blood pressure was 1.06. Stroke or brain hemorrhage had the greatest effect on glaucoma patients' VRQOL compared with other self-reported systemic comorbidities [11]. Our study similarly found that stroke could significantly affect the VRQOL of glaucoma patients. An explanation for this might be that stroke was significantly associated with visual impairment and low physical function [11]. Additionally, glaucoma patients in our study with high blood pressure had relatively high VRQOL, refracting their insufficient attention to hypertension.

5. Limitations

Our study has limitations. First, sample size was relatively small, and all patients were recruited from a single eye institute; this might cause selection bias. Second, our study was cross-sectional study; however, information obtained from longitudinal observation is likely to reduce the interindividual variability and possible effects of compensatory mechanisms and provides more robust evaluation on the association between variables and VRQOL [9, 31, 32]. Third, if more than one questionnaire (e.g., the Short-Form 36 Health Survey (SF-36) [33], which is used to assess the general health status of glaucoma patients [34], and the Glaucoma Symptom Scale (GSS) [35], a measure to assess the symptoms associated with glaucoma and its management [36]) is used simultaneously for the survey, the effects of glaucoma on the patient could be understood on different levels [37], and further studies could be performed to observe the difference [38] between

CLVQOL and NEI VFQ-25 [16] or between CLVQOL and the Visual Activities Questionnaire (VAQ) [39], exploring which questionnaire can more exactly describe VRQOL for Chinese glaucoma patients.

In the analysis of the survey results, we should also note that normal variations in personality characteristics will influence how patients report their VRQOL [40].

Media opacity such as cataract can influence VRQOL; patients with obvious cataract were excluded from the study, but we did not use any classification (e.g., Lens Opacity Classification System III (LOCS III) [41]). It was limitation in the study.

In summary, the clinical eye doctors could treat, guide, and help glaucoma patients, manage therapeutic strategy to preserve or improve visual ability, and prevent visual field impairment. Ophthalmologists should also keep their patients well informed of the necessary knowledge about glaucoma [42], reduce their risk of stroke, and thereby protect their VRQOL.

Conflict of Interests

The authors declare that there is no conflict of interests regarding the publication of this paper.

References

[1] C. J. Bassi and J. C. Galanis, "Binocular visual impairment in glaucoma," *Ophthalmology*, vol. 98, no. 9, pp. 1406–1411, 1991.

[2] WHO, *The Development of the WHO Quality of Life Assessment Instrument*, vol. 1, World Health Organization, Geneva, Switzerland, 1993.

[3] R. Varma, P. P. Lee, I. Goldberg, and S. Kotak, "An assessment of the health and economic burdens of glaucoma," *American Journal of Ophthalmology*, vol. 152, no. 4, pp. 515–522, 2011.

[4] P. Nelson, P. Aspinall, O. Papasouliotis, B. Worton, and C. O'Brien, "Quality of life in glaucoma and its relationship with visual function," *Journal of Glaucoma*, vol. 12, no. 2, pp. 139–150, 2003.

[5] R. McKean-Cowdin, Y. Wang, J. Wu, S. P. Azen, and R. Varma, "Impact of visual field loss on health-related quality of life in glaucoma: the Los Angeles Latino Eye Study," *Ophthalmology*, vol. 115, no. 6, pp. 941–948.e1, 2008.

[6] M. Qiu, S. Y. Wang, K. Singh, and S. C. Lin, "Association between visual field defects and quality of life in the United States," *Ophthalmology*, vol. 121, no. 3, pp. 733–740, 2014.

[7] A. van Gestel, C. A. B. Webers, H. J. M. Beckers et al., "The relationship between visual field loss in glaucoma and health-related quality-of-life," *Eye*, vol. 24, no. 12, pp. 1759–1769, 2010.

[8] S.-M. Saw, G. Gazzard, K.-G. A. Eong, F. Oen, and S. Seah, "Utility values in Singapore Chinese adults with primary open-angle and primary angle-closure glaucoma," *Journal of Glaucoma*, vol. 14, no. 6, pp. 455–462, 2005.

[9] R. Lisboa, Y. S. Chun, L. M. Zangwill et al., "Association between rates of binocular visual field loss and vision-related quality of life in patients with glaucoma," *JAMA Ophthalmology*, vol. 131, no. 4, pp. 486–494, 2013.

[10] V. Gupta, P. Dutta, O. V. Mary, K. S. Kapoor, R. Sihota, and G. Kumar, "Effect of glaucoma on the quality of life of young patients," *Investigative Ophthalmology & Visual Science*, vol. 52, no. 11, pp. 8433–8437, 2011.

[11] D. R. Globe, R. Varma, M. Torres, J. Wu, R. Klein, and S. P. Azen, "Self-reported comorbidities and visual function in a population-based study: the Los Angeles Latino Eye Study," *Archives of Ophthalmology*, vol. 123, no. 6, pp. 815–821, 2005.

[12] J. Zhao, R. Sui, L. Jia, and L. B. Ellwein, "Prevalence of glaucoma and normal intraocular pressure among adults aged 50 years or above in Shunyi county of Beijing," *Zhonghua Yan Ke Za Zhi*, vol. 38, no. 6, pp. 335–339, 2002.

[13] L. Xu, J.-H. Chen, J.-J. Li et al., "The prevalence and its screening methods of primary open angle glaucoma in defined population-based study of rural and urban in Beijing," *Zhonghua Yan Ke Za Zhi*, vol. 40, no. 11, pp. 726–732, 2004.

[14] J. W. Y. Lee, C. W. S. Chan, J. C. H. Chan, Q. Li, and J. S. M. Lai, "The association between clinical parameters and glaucoma-specific quality of life in Chinese primary open-angle glaucoma patients," *Hong Kong Medical Journal*, vol. 20, no. 4, pp. 274–278, 2014.

[15] X. M. Kong, W. Q. Zhu, J. X. Hong, and X. H. Sun, "Is glaucoma comprehension associated with psychological disturbance and vision-related quality of life for patients with glaucoma? A cross-sectional study," *BMJ Open*, vol. 4, no. 5, Article ID e004632, 2014.

[16] C. M. Mangione, S. Berry, and P. P. Lee, "Identifying the content area for the National Eye Institute vision function questionnaire (NEI-VFQ): results from focus groups with visually impaired persons," *Archives of Ophthalmology*, vol. 116, pp. 227–238, 1998.

[17] J. S. Wolffsohn and A. L. Cochrane, "Design of the low vision quality-of-life questionnaire (LVQOL) and measuring the outcome of low-vision rehabilitation," *American Journal of Ophthalmology*, vol. 130, no. 6, pp. 793–802, 2000.

[18] H. Zou, X. Zhang, X. Xu, L. Bai, and J. S. Wolffsohn, "Development and psychometric tests of the Chinese-version Low Vision Quality of Life Questionnaire," *Quality of Life Research*, vol. 14, no. 6, pp. 1633–1639, 2005.

[19] D. Vaughan, T. Asbury, and P. Riordan-Eva, *General Ophthalmology*, Appleton & Lange, 15th edition, 1999.

[20] E. Hodapp, R. K. Parrish, and D. Anderson, *Clinical Decisions in Glaucoma*, Mosby-Year Book, St. Louis, Mo, USA, 1993.

[21] J. M. Nelson-Quigg, K. Cello, and C. A. Johnson, "Predicting binocular visual field sensitivity from monocular visual field results," *Investigative Ophthalmology and Visual Science*, vol. 41, no. 8, pp. 2212–2221, 2000.

[22] J. T. Holladay and T. C. Prager, "Mean visual acuity," *American Journal of Ophthalmology*, vol. 111, no. 3, pp. 372–374, 1991.

[23] I. U. Scott, W. E. Smiddy, W. Feuer, and A. Merikansky, "Vitreoretinal surgery outcomes: results of a patient satisfaction/functional status survey," *Ophthalmology*, vol. 105, no. 5, pp. 795–803, 1998.

[24] K. M. Kulkarni, J. R. Mayer, L. L. Lorenzana, J. S. Myers, and G. L. Spaeth, "Visual field staging systems in glaucoma and the activities of daily living," *American Journal of Ophthalmology*, vol. 154, no. 3, pp. 445.e3–451.e3, 2012.

[25] R. P. Mills, D. L. Budenz, P. P. Lee et al., "Categorizing the stage of glaucoma from pre-diagnosis to end-stage disease," *American Journal of Ophthalmology*, vol. 141, no. 1, pp. 24–30, 2006.

[26] H. Sawada, T. Fukuchi, and H. Abe, "Evaluation of the relationship between quality of vision and the visual function index in Japanese glaucoma patients," *Graefe's Archive for Clinical and Experimental Ophthalmology*, vol. 249, no. 11, pp. 1721–1727, 2011.

[27] G. Labiris, A. Katsanos, M. Fanariotis, F. Zacharaki, D. Chatzoulis, and V. P. Kozobolis, "Vision-specific quality of life in Greek glaucoma patients," *Journal of Glaucoma*, vol. 19, no. 1, pp. 39–43, 2010.

[28] V. Gupta, P. Dutta, O. V. Mary, K. S. Kapoor, R. Sihota, and G. Kumar, "Effect of glaucoma on the quality of life of young patients," *Investigative Ophthalmology and Visual Science*, vol. 52, no. 11, pp. 8433–8437, 2011.

[29] A. M. Bhorade, M. S. Perlmutter, B. Wilson et al., "Differences in vision between clinic and home and the effect of lighting in older adults with and without glaucoma," *JAMA Ophthalmology*, vol. 131, no. 12, pp. 1554–1562, 2013.

[30] R. Klein and B. E. K. Klein, "The prevalence of age-related eye diseases and visual impairment in aging: current estimates," *Investigative Ophthalmology & Visual Science*, vol. 54, no. 14, pp. ORSF5–ORSF13, 2013.

[31] F. A. Medeiros, C. P. B. Gracitelli, E. R. Boer, R. N. Weinreb, L. M. Zangwill, and P. N. Rosen, "Longitudinal changes in quality of life and rates of progressive visual field loss in glaucoma patients," *Ophthalmology*, vol. 122, no. 2, pp. 293–301, 2015.

[32] C. P. Gracitelli, R. Y. Abe, A. J. Tatham et al., "Association between progressive retinal nerve fiber layer loss and longitudinal change in quality of life in glaucoma," *JAMA Ophthalmology*, vol. 133, no. 4, pp. 384–390, 2015.

[33] J. E. Ware Jr. and C. D. Sherbourne, "The MOS 36-item short-form health survey (SF-36). I. Conceptual framework and item selection," *Medical Care*, vol. 30, no. 6, pp. 473–483, 1992.

[34] R. K. Parrish, S. J. Gedde, I. U. Scott et al., "Visual function and quality of life among patients with glaucoma," *Archives of Ophthalmology*, vol. 115, no. 11, pp. 1447–1455, 1997.

[35] B. L. Lee, P. Gutierrez, M. Gordon et al., "The glaucoma symptom scale: a brief index of glaucoma-specific symptoms," *Archives of Ophthalmology*, vol. 116, no. 7, pp. 861–866, 1998.

[36] G. C. M. Rossi, G. M. Pasinetti, L. Scudeller, M. Raimondi, S. Lanteri, and P. E. Bianchi, "Risk factors to develop ocular surface disease in treated glaucoma or ocular hypertension patients," *European Journal of Ophthalmology*, vol. 23, no. 3, pp. 296–302, 2013.

[37] B. L. Lee and M. R. Wilson, "Health-related quality of life in patients with cataract and glaucoma," *Journal of Glaucoma*, vol. 9, no. 1, pp. 87–94, 2000.

[38] B. W. Gillespie, D. C. Musch, L. M. Niziol, and N. K. Janz, "Estimating minimally important differences for two vision-specific quality of life measures," *Investigative Ophthalmology & Visual Science*, vol. 55, no. 7, pp. 4206–4212, 2014.

[39] M. E. Sloane, K. Ball, C. Owsley et al., "The visual activities questionnaire: developing an instrument for assessing problems in everyday visual tasks," in *Technical Digest, Noninvasive Assessment of the Visual System*, vol. 1, pp. 26–29, 1992.

[40] K. J. Warrian, G. L. Spaeth, D. Lankaranian, J. F. Lopes, and W. C. Steinmann, "The effect of personality on measures of quality of life related to vision in glaucoma patients," *British Journal of Ophthalmology*, vol. 93, no. 3, pp. 310–315, 2009.

[41] L. T. Chylack Jr., J. K. Wolfe, D. M. Singer et al., "The lens opacities classification system III. The Longitudinal Study of Cataract Study Group," *Archives of Ophthalmology*, vol. 111, no. 6, pp. 831–836, 1993.

[42] X. Kong, X. Chen, X. Sun, M. Xiao, L. Zuo, and W. Guo, "Glaucoma club: a successful model to educate glaucoma patients," *Clinical & Experimental Ophthalmology*, vol. 37, no. 6, pp. 634–636, 2009.

The Ocular Biometry of Adult Cataract Patients on Lifeline Express Hospital Eye-Train in Rural China

Xiaoguang Cao, Xianru Hou, and Yongzhen Bao

Peking University People's Hospital, Ophthalmology Department, Key Laboratory of Vision Loss and Restoration, Ministry of Education, Beijing Key Laboratory for the Diagnosis and Treatment of Retinal and Choroid Diseases, Beijing 100044, China

Correspondence should be addressed to Yongzhen Bao; drbaoyz@sina.com

Academic Editor: Qin Long

Aims. To describe and explore the distribution of ocular biometric parameters of adult cataract patients in rural China. *Methods.* Three Lifeline Express Hospital Eye-Train missions of Peking University People's Hospital in China were chosen. 3828 adult cataract patients aged 29 to 88 years with axial length (AL) less than 27.0 mm were enrolled. The ocular biometry including visual acuity (VA), intraocular pressure, AL, corneal power ($K1$ and $K2$), and corneal endothelial counting (CEC) were collected and analysis. Corneal radius (CR) was calculated from the corneal power. *Results.* The participants in Zhoukou of these three missions had the worse preoperative VA ($p < 0.001$), the lowest $K1$ ($p < 0.001$), $K2$ ($p < 0.001$), and K ($p < 0.001$) and the highest $|K1 - K2|$ ($p < 0.001$), moreover AL/CR more closely to 3.0. The AL, $|K1 - K2|$, and AL/CR were normally distributed. But the $K1$, $K2$, K, and CEC were not normal distributions. Except $K1$, all parameters were positively skewed and peaked. *Conclusion.* Our study provides normative ocular biometry in a large, representative rural Chinese population. The AL is normally distributed with a positive skew and big kurtosis. The corneal powers are not normal distribution. The corneal astigmatism might have a significant effect on the visual acuity.

1. Introduction

According to China's Ministry of Health, China has approximately 4 million cataract victims, with 500,000 new cases being diagnosed each year [1]. As a developing country, especially in rural China, poverty and limited access to health care, due to the uneven distribution of health care sources, can make it very difficult for these people to obtain proper treatment [2]. Cataract surgical rate (CSR) is still very low in rural China. Moreover, a lot of these cataract surgeries were charge-free. Lifeline Express Hospital Eye-Train (LEHET), the first charge-free cataract surgery project founded in 1997, is a quite important way to restore vision for the low-income rural people in China.

Independent of cost or other factors, the first expectation from surgeons and patients is good postoperative visual outcomes. To meet these expectations, attention to accurate biometry measurements is critical [3]. The biometry is indispensable to the surgeons and patients as it might indicate the prognosis and safety of the coming operation. In the biometric parameters, axial length (AL) and corneal curvature are the most important. However, the distribution and determinants of AL have been assessed in only a few population-based studies of older persons [4–10], of which there is still no study of rural Chinese population, especially in Middle China, having cities with extremely long history.

In 2011 and 2012, our hospital (Peking University People's Hospital, PUPH) had three missions of LEHET in Middle China. In this study, we explored the biometric parameters of adult cataract patients who had cataract surgeries on LEHET in these missions and all were rural people.

2. Methods

2.1. Recruitment of Patients, Preoperative Assessment, and Exclusion Criteria. Our hospital, PUPH, had four missions of LEHET, Zhoukou in Henan province and Songyuan in Jilin province in 2011, Yuncheng in Shanxi province and Sanmenxia in Henan province in 2012. The sites were selected by the office of LEHET, and they were blind to our hospital

Table 1: CSR of China 2010.

Province	Population	Cataract surgeries	Charge-free cataract surgeries for low-income people	CSR	Charge-free CSR	Ratio of charge-free cataract surgeries for low-income people
Beijing	19,612,368	11961	1402	610	71	11.72%
Shanxi	35,712,101	15902	4929	445	138	31.00%
Henan	94,029,939	36935	9915	393	105	26.84%

CSR: cataract surgical rate.

Table 2: Demographic characteristics of the three groups.

	Zhoukou ($n = 991$)	Yuncheng ($n = 1240$)	Sanmenxia ($n = 1497$)	p
Age (years)	69.20 ± 8.10	69.73 ± 7.84	69.49 ± 8.20	0.293
Sex Male/female	355/636	502/838	562/935	0.640
Eye operated on Right/left	538/453	697/643	749/748	0.113

p values were calculated with ANOVA.

before the mission start. Songyuan in Jilin province was excluded from this study as the incompleted data. Yuncheng (N 35.03; E 111.01; altitude: 369.53 m) in Shanxi province and Zhoukou (N 33.62; E 114.66; altitude: 50.50 m) in Henan province have thousands of years of history. Most residents in these two cities are rural people and live there since birth. Sanmenxia (N 34.77; E 111.20; altitude: 376.08 m) in Henan province was built in the 1950s and also is a rural city. Residents in this new city partly immigrated from the whole of China, such as Northeast China and West China. In 2011, the pure annual income of rural people was 5601.40 CNY (about 889.11 USD) in Shanxi province and 6604.03 CNY (1048.26 USD) in Henan province, much lower than Beijing 14735.68 CNY (about 2339.00 USD) cited from China Statistical Yearbook 2012 [2]. Based on the Sixth National Census of China 2010 (http://www.stats.gov.cn/) [11] and the 2010 annual survey data of China Disabled Persons' Federation (http://www.cdpf.org.cn) [12], cataract surgical rate (CSR) was calculated as in Table 1.

Any patients who wanted to have the charge-free cataract operations on LEHET registered at the base hospital (a local hospital selected by the office of LEHET). After the systemic and ocular examinations and signing the informed consent at the base hospital, the patients were sent to LEHET. Preoperatively on LEHET, all patients underwent a complete ophthalmological examination, that is, measurement of presenting visual acuity (VA) by means of Snellen charts (performed by the nurses from the base hospital), intraocular pressure evaluation (IOP) by noncontact tonometer (Canon TX-10/TX-F, Tokyo, Japan) by the trained nurses from PUPH, slit lamp examination (Topcon SL-1E, Tokyo, Japan), and fundus examination (90 Dioptre, Volk Optical, Mentor, OH) with dilated pupil by the ophthalmologists from PUPH. Corneal curvature by Auto-Keratometer (Nikon Speedy-K, Tokyo, Japan), axial length (AL) and B-scan by ultrasonic system (ODM-2100, MEDA, Tianjing, China), and corneal endothelial counting (CEC) by Specular Microscope (Topcon SP-3000P, Tokyo, Japan) were performed by the trained technicians from PUPH on the patients suitable for operation. The flatter ($K1$) and steeper corneal curvature ($K2$) were read directly from the Auto-Keratometer, and K was calculated as the average of $K1$ and $K2$. Corneal radius (CR) was calculated from the formula CR (millimeter, mm) = 1000 × 0.3375/K (Diopter, D). The SRK/T formula for normal or long axial length (AL more than 25.00 mm) and Hoffer Q formula for short axial length (AL less than 22.00 mm) were used to calculate the power of intraocular lens (IOL) and the estimated postoperative refractive errors were less than ±0.25 D except patients with high myopia. LEHET was equipped with Specular Microscope, SP-3000P, in the first half of year 2012; the patients of Zhoukou and part of Yuncheng had no CEC measurement.

Exclusion criteria for this study are as follows: age less than 20 years, AL equal to or more than 27.00 mm, and history of intraocular surgery.

The study was in accordance with the tenets of the Declaration of Helsinki and has been approved by the institutional review board of PUPH. Written informed consent was obtained from all patients.

2.2. Statistical Analysis. The Student t-test was used to compare age and chi-square test was used to compare the female ratio between the groups. A p value less than 0.05 was considered to be statistically significant. Statistical analysis was performed using Statistical Product and Service Solutions software (SPSS version 20.0, Armonk, New York, USA).

3. Results

The demographic characteristics of the three missions are shown in Table 2. Totally, 3828 cataract patients (3828 eyes) were enrolled in this study, including 1419 males and 2409

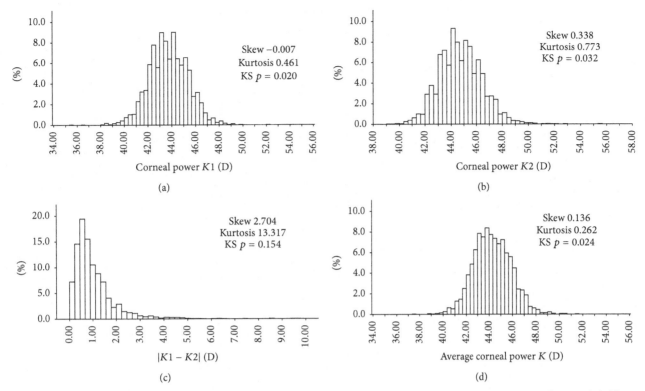

FIGURE 1: The distributions of corneal power in rural China. $K1$ (a), $K2$ (b), $|K1 - K2|$ (c), and average corneal power (K) (d).

females (male : female = 1 : 1.70) and 1984 right eyes and 1844 left eyes. There were no statistically significant differences between missions preoperatively in age, gender, and eye operated on.

As in Table 2, average age of these cataract patients was 69.50 ± 8.05, which was 69.10 ± 8.41 for males and 69.74 ± 7.82 for females ($p = 0.019$), respectively. In detail, the average age was 68.55 ± 8.12 for males and 69.57 ± 8.07 for females in Zhoukou ($p = 0.056$), 69.02 ± 8.33 for males and 70.16 ± 7.50 for females in Yuncheng ($p = 0.010$), and 69.52 ± 8.64 for males and 69.48 ± 7.92 for females in Sanmenxia ($p = 0.933$). Although the average age of females is older than males totally, that of males and females was of no difference for Zhoukou and Sanmenxia, except that of females which was older than that of males in Yuncheng.

As shown in Tables 3, 4, and 5, not only for males or females, but also for total patients, the preoperative VA (LogMAR) of these three groups is as follows: Zhoukou > Yuncheng > Sanmenxia. The patients in Sanmenxia had the best preoperative VA, even in each gender, significantly.

As shown in Tables 3, 4, and 5, there was a statistically significant difference in preoperative IOP between the patients of Yuncheng and Zhoukou, Yuncheng and Sanmenxia. The males, females, and total patients of Yuncheng had lower preoperative IOP compared with those in Zhoukou or Sanmenxia.

As shown in Figure 1 and Tables 3, 4, and 5, the patients of Zhoukou had lower $K1$ and $K2$, significantly. There was no statistically significant difference in $K1$ between those of Yuncheng and Sanmenxia, but $K2$ of Yuncheng was higher than Sanmenxia significantly. Respectively, both the males and females in Zhoukou had lower $K1$ and $K2$. However, for either the males or the females, there was no difference of $K1$ and $K2$ between those in Yuncheng and Sanmenxia.

Average corneal power (K) is an important parameter to calculate the power of IOL. In Figure 1 and Tables 3, 4, and 5, the patients in Zhoukou had lower average corneal power (K) significantly compared with the other two groups, the same for male and female patients in Zhoukou. But there was no significant difference in average corneal power (K) between those in Yuncheng and Sanmenxia, for either the males or the females.

The difference between $K1$ and $K2$ could be used to indicate the corneal astigmatism, which has the effect on the postoperative visual acuity. In Figure 1 and Tables 3, 4, and 5, the difference of $K1$ and $K2$ for the patients was as follows: Zhoukou > Yuncheng > Sanmenxia. That was the same for the females. But for the males except that $|K1-K2|$ of Zhoukou was higher than Sanmenxia significantly, there was no significant difference between Zhoukou and Yuncheng or between Yuncheng and Sanmenxia.

AL is another important parameter to calculate the power of IOL. As seen in Figure 2 and Tables 3, 4, and 5, AL for the patients was as follows: Zhoukou < Sanmenxia < Yuncheng. For the males, AL of Zhoukou was shorter than the other two cities. For the females, AL of Yuncheng was longer than the other two sites. There was no significant difference in AL between Yuncheng and Sanmenxia for males or between Zhoukou and Sanmenxia for females.

The AL/CR ratio is highly correlated with the spherical equivalent as a previous study. As seen in Figure 2 and Tables 3, 4, and 5, the patients in Zhoukou had the smallest AL/CR

TABLE 3: Biological parameters of the three groups.

		Zhoukou	Yuncheng	Sanmenxia	Total	p
Preoperative visual acuity	LogMAR	1.20 ± 0.38	0.95 ± 0.37	0.63 ± 0.43	0.87 ± 0.46	0.000
	Less than 6/60 n (%)	763 (76.99%)	653 (48.73%)	636 (42.48%)	2052 (53.61%)	0.000
	Equal to or better than 6/60 and less than 6/18 n (%)	218 (22.00%)	565 (42.16%)	710 (47.43%)	1493 (39.00%)	0.000
	Equal to or better than 6/18 n (%)	10 (1.01%)	122 (9.10%)	151 (10.09%)	283 (7.39%)	0.000
	Preoperative IOP (mmHg)	14.53 ± 3.44	13.98 ± 2.92	14.78 ± 3.11	14.44 ± 3.15	0.000
Corneal curvature (D)	K1	43.40 ± 1.65	43.89 ± 1.68	43.82 ± 1.56	43.74 ± 1.64	0.000
	K2	44.59 ± 1.79	44.88 ± 1.70	44.75 ± 1.57	44.75 ± 1.68	0.000
	|K1 − K2|	1.20 ± 1.03	0.98 ± 0.81	0.93 ± 0.76	1.02 ± 0.86	0.000
	Average corneal power (K)	44.00 ± 1.64	44.38 ± 1.64	44.29 ± 1.52	44.24 ± 1.60	0.000
	Axial length (AL) (mm)	22.95 ± 1.05	23.17 ± 0.95	23.12 ± 0.92	23.04 ± 1.49	0.000
	AL/CR	2.99 ± 0.14	3.04 ± 0.12	3.03 ± 0.11	3.03 ± 0.12	0.000
	CEC (n/mm^2)	*	2505.63 ± 431.98*	2445.24 ± 419.23	2462.36 ± 423.65*	0.003

p values were calculated with ANOVA or chi-square test.
*LEHET was equipped with Specular Microscope, SP-3000P, in the first half of year 2012; the patients of Zhoukou and part of Yuncheng had no CEC measurement.

Table 4: Biological parameters for males of the three groups.

	Zhoukou	Yuncheng	Sanmenxia	Total	p
Preoperative visual acuity (LogMAR)	1.21 ± 0.38	0.98 ± 0.36	0.66 ± 0.44	0.89 ± 0.46	0.000
Preoperative IOL (mmHg)	14.28 ± 3.46	13.69 ± 2.87	14.50 ± 3.18	14.16 ± 3.17	0.000
Corneal curvature (D)					
$K1$	42.80 ± 1.52	43.37 ± 1.64	43.31 ± 1.44	43.20 ± 1.55	0.000
$K2$	43.86 ± 1.50	44.27 ± 1.64	44.19 ± 1.45	44.13 ± 1.54	0.000
$|K1 - K2|$	1.07 ± 0.85	0.91 ± 0.80	0.87 ± 0.66	0.94 ± 0.77	0.001
Average corneal power (K)	43.33 ± 1.45	43.82 ± 1.59	43.75 ± 1.41	43.67 ± 1.49	0.000
Axial length (AL) (mm)	23.12 ± 0.90	23.44 ± 0.89	23.46 ± 0.88	23.37 ± 0.90	0.000
AL/CR	2.97 ± 0.12	3.04 ± 0.11	3.04 ± 0.11	3.02 ± 0.11	0.000
CEC (n/mm^2)	*	2537.49 ± 450.38*	2437.86 ± 439.39	2467.32 ± 444.71*	0.004

p values were calculated with ANOVA.
*LEHET was equipped with Specular Microscope, SP-3000P, in the first half of year 2012; the patients of Zhoukou and part of Yuncheng had no CEC measurement.

Table 5: Biological parameters for females of the three groups.

	Zhoukou	Yuncheng	Sanmenxia	Total	p
Preoperative visual acuity (LogMAR)	1.19 ± 0.38	0.93 ± 0.37	0.61 ± 0.42	0.85 ± 0.46	0.000
Preoperative IOL (mmHg)	14.67 ± 3.43	14.17 ± 2.93	14.95 ± 3.06	14.60 ± 3.13	0.000
Corneal curvature (D)					
$K1$	43.74 ± 1.63	44.20 ± 1.63	44.13 ± 1.54	44.05 ± 1.61	0.000
$K2$	45.00 ± 1.81	45.24 ± 1.63	45.09 ± 1.54	45.12 ± 1.65	0.016
$|K1 - K2|$	1.27 ± 1.11	1.02 ± 0.82	0.96 ± 0.81	1.06 ± 0.91	0.000
Average corneal power (K)	44.37 ± 1.63	44.72 ± 1.58	44.61 ± 1.49	44.58 ± 1.56	0.000
Axial length (AL) (mm)	22.86 ± 1.11	23.01 ± 0.96	22.91 ± 0.88	22.93 ± 0.97	0.008
AL/CR	3.00 ± 0.15	3.05 ± 0.12	3.03 ± 0.11	3.03 ± 1.29	0.000
CEC (n/mm^2)	*	2484.59 ± 418.72*	2449.66 ± 406.84	2459.30 ± 410.29*	0.174

p values were calculated with ANOVA.
*LEHET was equipped with Specular Microscope, SP-3000P, in the first half of year 2012; the patients of Zhoukou and part of Yuncheng had no CEC measurement.

ratio closer to 3.0, and Yuncheng and Sanmenxia had similar ratio. That is the same for the males and females.

CEC is a very important factor to decide the operation scheme and to predict prognosis. As there was no machine in Zhoukou at that time, we only could compare CEC between those in Yuncheng and Sanmenxia. As shown in Figure 2 and Tables 3, 4, and 5, CEC of Yuncheng was higher than Sanmenxia, which was same result for the males. But for the females, there was no significant difference in CEC between Yuncheng and Sanmenxia.

4. Discussion

This study explored the data of cataract patient, who had the free surgeries on LEHET, on ocular biometry of Chinese population in rural China. And our study provided the normative data on $K1$, $K2$, $|K1 - K2|$, average corneal power (K), AL, AL/CR, and CEC of this population; those were 43.74 ± 1.64 D, 44.75 ± 1.68 D, 1.02 ± 0.86 D, 44.24 ± 1.60 D, 23.04 ± 1.49 mm, 3.03 ± 0.12, and 2462.36 ± 423.65/mm^2, respectively.

Our study showed AL in rural Chinese population was normally distributed with a positive skew and a big kurtosis (1.417). Skew and kurtosis have been reported in the distribution of AL in the Reykjavik Eye study [13], the Singapore Malay Eye study [7], the Singapore Indian Eye study [10], and Fotedar et al.'s study [14]. Hence, this is the first report of the appearance of big kurtosis in the distribution of AL in rural Chinese population.

It is worthwhile comparing our findings with those of the Tanjong Pagar study on adult Chinese population in Singapore, which also used A-scan. The mean AL in that study (23.23 ± 1.17 mm) was a little longer than in our study (23.04 ± 1.49 mm). Moreover, AL in our study is shorter than Latinos (23.38 mm) in Los Angeles with A-scan [8], Malay people (23.55 mm) [7] in Singapore, Indian people (23.45 mm) [10] in Singapore, and Caucasian people (23.44) [14] in the Blue Mountains area in Australia with IOLMaster, longer than another Asian population (22.76 mm) in Myanmar with Ocuscan [9]. The similarity of AL in those studies with A-scan and ours is likely to be explained by the same method of AL measurement. The difference in AL of these studies might be explained by a greater degree of urbanization in Singapore and subsequently a higher rate of axial myopia [10]. Those three studies with IOLMaster indicated that the race might have significant effect on AL compared with region as the similarity of Indian and Caucasian people.

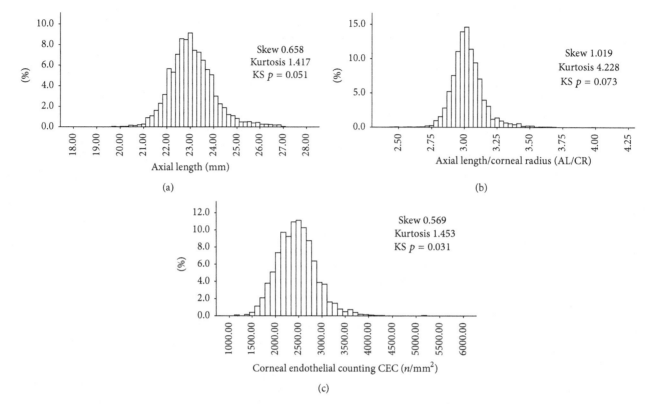

FIGURE 2: The distributions of axial length (AL), axial length/corneal curvature (AL/CR), and corneal endothelial counting (CEC) in rural China. Axial length (AL) (a), axial length/corneal curvature (AL/CR) (b), and corneal endothelial counting (CEC) (c).

The corneal power $K1$, corneal power $K2$, and K (average corneal power) in our study were not normally distributed with different skews and kurtosis. That is similar to the Singapore Malay Eye study [7] and Fotedar et al.'s study [14]. On the contrary, $|K1 - K2|$ in our study was normally distributed with a positive skew (2.704) and a significant kurtosis (13.317). Moreover, the preoperative visual acuities in the three missions of our study had the same trend as $|K1 - K2|$, both of that of males and females are the same. It indicated that the corneal astigmatism might have obvious effect on the visual acuity.

There is evidence that the AL/CR ratio of an emmetropic eye is usually very close to 3.0, and a higher AL/CR ratio was reported to be a risk factor in myopia [15, 16]. However, few studies have reported the AL/CR ratio [10]. Compared with Zhoukou, the patients in Yuncheng and Sanmenxia had similar AL/CR ratio, also in males and in females. The Singapore Indian Eye study [10] showed that the AL/CR ratio correlated more highly with the spherical equivalent than AL alone. This correlation indicated that longer eyes are not necessarily myopic and worse presenting visual acuity, including those that are long because of overall body stature. The patients in Zhoukou, who had shorter AL and AL/CR closer to 3.0, had the worst preoperative visual acuities. This indicated that in rural Chinese population at least in the cataract patients the AL/CR ratio, in other words, the spherical equivalent, had less effect on the visual acuity than $|K1 - K2|$, the corneal astigmatism.

In conclusion, this study provides normative ocular biometry in a large, representative rural Chinese population. The AL is normally distributed with a positive skew and a big kurtosis. The corneal power $K1$, corneal power $K2$, and K (average corneal power) are not with normal distribution. The corneal astigmatism might have a significant effect on the visual acuity.

Conflict of Interests

The authors declare that there is no conflict of interests and that they have no proprietary or commercial interest in any materials discussed in this paper.

Authors' Contribution

Xiaoguang Cao and Xianru Hou contributed to the work equally and should be regarded as co-first authors.

References

[1] Lifeline Express Hospital Eye-Train, Lifeline Express: A Mission of Sight, 2013, http://lxenglish.com/article.php?id=171fb2589f73f2e5b4a6ca52db5737f7_136.

[2] National Bureau of Statistics of China, *China Statistical Yearbook 2012*, 2012, http://www.stats.gov.cn/tjsj/ndsj/2012/indexch.htm.

[3] A. B. Bhatt, A. C. Schefler, W. J. Feuer, S. H. Yoo, and T. G. Murray, "Comparison of predictions made by the intraocular lens master and ultrasound biometry," *Archives of Ophthalmology*, vol. 126, no. 7, pp. 929–933, 2008.

[4] T. Y. Wong, P. J. Foster, T. P. Ng et al., "Variations in ocular biometry in an adult Chinese population in Singapore: the Tanjong Pagar survey," *Investigative Ophthalmology and Visual Science*, vol. 42, no. 1, pp. 73–80, 2001.

[5] J. Francois and F. Goes, "Ultrasonographic study of 100 emmetropic eyes," *Ophthalmologica*, vol. 175, no. 6, pp. 321–327, 1977.

[6] M. G. Villarreal, J. Ohlsson, M. Abrahamsson, A. Sjöström, and J. Sjöstrand, "Myopisation: the refractive tendency in teenagers. Prevalence of myopia among young teenagers in Sweden," *Acta Ophthalmologica Scandinavica*, vol. 78, no. 2, pp. 177–181, 2000.

[7] L. S. Lim, S.-M. Saw, V. S. E. Jeganathan et al., "Distribution and determinants of ocular biometric parameters in an asian population: the Singapore malay eye study," *Investigative Ophthalmology and Visual Science*, vol. 51, no. 1, pp. 103–109, 2010.

[8] C. Shufelt, S. Fraser-Bell, M. Ying-Lai, M. Torres, and R. Varma, "Refractive error, ocular biometry, and lens opalescence in an adult population: the Los Angeles Latino Eye Study," *Investigative Ophthalmology and Visual Science*, vol. 46, no. 12, pp. 4450–4460, 2005.

[9] S. Warrier, H. M. Wu, H. S. Newland et al., "Ocular biometry and determinants of refractive error in rural Myanmar: the Meiktila eye study," *The British Journal of Ophthalmology*, vol. 92, no. 12, pp. 1591–1594, 2008.

[10] C.-W. Pan, T.-Y. Wong, L. Chang et al., "Ocular biometry in an Urban Indian population: the Singapore Indian Eye study (SINDI)," *Investigative Ophthalmology and Visual Science*, vol. 52, no. 9, pp. 6636–6642, 2011.

[11] National Bureau of Statistics of China, *Sixth National Census of China*, National Bureau of Statistics of China, Beijing, China, 2010, http://www.stats.gov.cn/tjsj/pcsj/rkpc/6rp/indexch.htm.

[12] China Disabled Persons' Federation, *Comprehensive Statistical Data—Rehabilitation*, 2010, http://www.cdpf.org.cn/tjsj/ndsj/2010/indexch.htm.

[13] T. Olsen, A. Arnarsson, H. Sasaki, K. Sasaki, and F. Jonasson, "On the ocular refractive components: the Reykjavik Eye Study," *Acta Ophthalmologica Scandinavica*, vol. 85, no. 4, pp. 361–366, 2007.

[14] R. Fotedar, J. J. Wang, G. Burlutsky et al., "Distribution of axial length and ocular biometry measured using partial coherence laser interferometry (IOL Master) in an older white population," *Ophthalmology*, vol. 117, no. 3, pp. 417–423, 2010.

[15] D. A. Goss and P. Erickson, "Meridional corneal components of myopia progression in young adults and children," *American Journal of Optometry and Physiological Optics*, vol. 64, no. 7, pp. 475–481, 1987.

[16] T. Grosvenor and R. Scott, "Comparison of refractive components in youth-onset and early adult-onset myopia," *Optometry and Vision Science*, vol. 68, no. 3, pp. 204–209, 1991.

The Polymorphisms with Cataract Susceptibility Impair the EPHA2 Receptor Stability and Its Cytoprotective Function

Jin Yang,[1,2] Dan Li,[2,3] Qi Fan,[1,2] Lei Cai,[1,2] Xiaodi Qiu,[1,2] Peng Zhou,[4] and Yi Lu[1,2]

[1]Department of Ophthalmology, Eye and ENT Hospital, Fudan University, 83 Fenyang Road, Shanghai 200031, China
[2]Myopia Key Laboratory of Health PR China, Shanghai 200031, China
[3]Research Center, Eye and ENT Hospital, Fudan University, 83 Fenyang Road, Shanghai 200031, China
[4]Department of Ophthalmology, Parkway Health Hong Qiao Medical Center, Shanghai 200336, China

Correspondence should be addressed to Yi Lu; luyieent@126.com

Academic Editor: Jun Zhang

Despite accumulating evidence revealing susceptibility genes for age-related cataract, its pathophysiology leading to visual impairment at the cellular and molecular level remains poorly understood. Recent bioinformatic studies uncovered the association of two single nucleotide polymorphisms in human EPHA2, rs2291806 and rs1058371, with age-related cataract. Here we investigated the role of EPHA2 in counteracting oxidative stress-induced apoptosis of lens epithelial cells. The cataract-associated missense mutations resulted in the destabilization of EPHA2 receptor without altering the mRNA transcription. The cytoprotective and antiapoptotic function of EPHA2 in lens epithelial cells was abolished by the functional polymorphisms. Furthermore, our results suggest that the downstream signaling of activated EPHA2 promotes the antioxidative capacity of lens epithelial cells to eradicate the overproduction of reactive oxygen species. In contrast, the overexpression of EPHA2 with nonsynonymous mutations in the lens epithelial cells offered limited antioxidative protection against oxidative stress. Thus, our study not only sheds the light on the potential cytoprotective function of EPHA2 signaling in lens but also provides the cellular mechanisms underlying the pathogenesis of age-related cataract.

1. Introduction

Cataract, the opacity of crystalline lens, is the leading cause of blindness and visual impairment worldwide. While congenital cataract is largely inherited in a Mendelian manner with high penetrance, both genetic risk and environmental factors contribute to age-related cataract [1, 2]. Cumulative damage of environmental insults exerts oxidative stress on lens epithelial cells with genetic susceptibility and induces cellular apoptosis, a common cellular mechanism underpinning noncongenital cataract [3–5]. Recent genetic and epidemiological studies suggest the association of Eph-receptor tyrosine kinase-type A2 (EPHA2) with human age-related cataract in distinct populations [6–9]. Despite the bioinformatic screening of nonsynonymous single nucleotide polymorphism (SNP) in EPHA2 gene as potential risk variants for cataract [10], the cellular and molecular mechanisms underlying its pathogenesis remain elusive.

As a member of the Eph superfamily of receptor tyrosine kinases, the forward signaling cascade of EPHA2 is primarily mediated by its corresponding ephrin-A ligands [11, 12]. Genetic and pharmacological inhibition of EPHA2 induces apoptosis and abrogates tumorigenic growth of tumor cells [13–16]. EPHA2 protein is expressed in human and mouse lens [6], implying its potential role in maintaining lens clarity during aging by promoting cell viability. The combined application of bioinformatic tools including Soft Intolerant from Tolerant (SIFT), Polymorphism Phenotype (PolyPhen), and I-Mutant identified nonsynonymous rs2291806 and rs1058371 as potential functional polymorphisms [10].

The accrual of oxidative damage to lens epithelial cells at least partially causes age-related cataract [17–19]. Under physiological conditions, reactive oxygen species (ROS) are scavenged and eliminated by superoxide dismutase (SOD) in the mitochondria [20]. Either the overproduction of ROS or the dysfunction of endogenous antioxidants disrupts the redox homeostasis and thus triggers the apoptotic process and pathogenesis of the disease [21, 22]. It was shown that the induction of ROS activated EPHA2 receptor to promote virus entry during Kaposi's sarcoma-associated herpesvirus (KSHV) infection [23], which raises questions about the antioxidant role of EHPA2 signaling. Here we show the cytoprotective function by EPHA2 against oxidative stress-mediated damages as well as the antioxidative capacity of EPHA2 polymorphisms rs2291806 and rs1058371 which predispose the individuals to age-related cataract.

2. Materials and Methods

2.1. Cell Culture. The human lens epithelial cell (HLEC) line SRA 01/04 (transformed by Simian virus 40 large T antigen) was purchased from the American Type Culture Collection [24]. For maintenance, HLECs were cultured in Dulbecco's modified eagle's medium (DMEM; Invitrogen, Carlsbad, CA, USA) with 10% of heat inactivated fetal bovine serum (Invitrogen), 100 U/mL of penicillin (Sigma, St. Louis, MO, USA), and 100 μg/mL of streptomycin (Sigma) in humidified 5% CO_2 at 37°C.

2.2. Plasmid Construction and Cell Transfection. The wild-type human *EPHA2* gene (NM_004431.3) was generated by PCR using the following primers:

forward primer: 5′-CTAGCTAGCATGGAGCTC-CAGGCAGCCCGC-3′,

reverse primer: 5′-ACGCGTCGACTCAGATGG-GGATCCCCACAGT-3′.

The PCR product was then subcloned into Ubi-MCS-3FLAG-SV40-EGFP-IRES-puromycin lentiviral vector. The plasmids encoding EPHA2 polymorphism: rs1058371 (286A>T; forward primer: 5′-GAGGCTGAGCGTATCTTCTTTGAG-CTCAAGTTTACTG-3′, and reversed primer: 5′-CAG-TAAACTTGAGCTCAAAGAAGATACGCTCAGCCTC-3′), rs2291806 (2473G>A; forward primer: 5′-TGGGAG-TTGTCCAACCACAAGGTGATGAAAGCCATCA-3′, and reversed primer: 5′-TGATGGCTTTCATCACCTTGTGGT-TGGACAACTCCCA-3′), and rs3754334 (2874C>T; forward primer: 5′-CGGCCACCAGAAGCGCATTGCCTA-CAGCCTGCTGGGA-3′, and reversed primer: 5′-TCC-CAGCAGGCTGTAGGCAATGCGCTTCTGGTGGCCG-3′), were constructed using Multipoints Mutagenesis Kit (Takara, Dalian, Liaoning, China). The lentiviral plasmid encoding WT or mutated EPHA2 was cotransfected with pMDL, pRev, and pVSVG into 293gp cells to generate high-titers of lentivirus, followed by ultracentrifugation of viral supernatants [25]. HLECs were infected with diluted lentivirus and the green fluorescence signal was examined under a fluorescence light microscope (Olympus Inc., Tokyo, Japan) with digital images captured.

2.3. Real-Time PCR. Total RNA was extracted with Trizol reagent (Invitrogen) from the HLECs 72 h after infection. First strand cDNAs were synthesized from 1.0 μg total RNA by reverse transcription using the RevertAid H Minus First Strand cDNA Synthesis Kit (Hanover, MD, USA). Real-time PCR was performed using the following primers: forward primer 5′-TGGCTCACACACCCGTATG-3′ and reversed primer 5′-GTCGCCAGACATCACGTTG-3′. As an internal control, β-*actin* was amplified using 5′-CATTAAGGAGAA-GCTGTGCT-3′ and 5′-GTTGAAGGTAGTTTCGTGGA-3′ as forward and reverse primers, respectively.

2.4. Western Blotting Analysis. Cell lysates were collected from the HLECs 72 h after infection with lentivirus expressing wild-type EPHA2 or mutants. The protein concentration was determined by BCA assay. The proteins were separated by electrophoresis and transferred to a nitrocellulose membrane. The blocked membrane was incubated overnight with primary antibodies against EPHA2, GFP, or GAPDH (Santa Cruz, CA, USA) at 4°C. Following washing three times in TBST, the membrane was incubated with goat anti-mouse HRP-conjugated secondary antibodies for 30 min at room temperature. After washes with TBST, immunoreactive signals were detected using enhanced chemiluminescence reagent (Pierce). Images were captured with the ChemiDocT-MMP imaging system (Bio-Rad, Hercules, CA, USA). The densitometric intensity of the imaged bands was analyzed by Image-Pro Plus 5.0 (Media Cybernetics, Silver Spring, EUA). Triplicate experiments were performed.

2.5. Cell Viability Assay. Cell viability and proliferation were determined using a Cell Counting Kit-8 (CCK-8) assay (Dojindo Laboratories, Kumamoto, Japan), which is a sensitive measurement of the survival status of cells. HLECs in the logarithmic growth phase were collected and seeded in 96-well plates (1×10^4 cells/well). After culture in the absence of antibiotics for 24 h, cells were infected with lentivirus encoding wild-type EPHA2 or SNP mutants for 72 h. To each well, 100 μL CCK8 solution dissolved in DMEM was added. After incubation for 3 h, the optical density of formazan crystals was measured in an X Mark microplate spectrophotometer (Bio-Rad) at 450 nm. Eight duplicate wells were used for measurement. Triplicate experiments were performed.

2.6. Measurement of Lipid Peroxidation Products. Lipid peroxidation was assessed with malondialdehyde (MDA) assay using Lipid Peroxidation MDA Assay Kit from Beyotime. Briefly, HLECs with lentiviral infection were lysed in 0.1 M Tris/HCl buffer (pH 7.4 containing 0.5% Triton X-100, 5 mM β-mercaptoethanol, and 0.1 mg/mL PMSF) 72 h after transfection. The lysate supernatant (0.1 mL) was mixed with trichloroacetic acid (15%, w/vol), thiobarbituric acid (0.375%, w/vol), and hydrochloric acid (0.25 M) at a 1:1:1:1 ratio. The mixture was heated at 100°C for 30 min, immediately cooled, and then centrifuged (3,500 ×g for 5 min). The absorbance of the supernatant was measured at 532 nm. The amount of thiobarbituric-acid-reacting substance (TBARS) was calculated MDA equivalents as previously described [26]. Triplicate experiments were performed.

2.7. Superoxide Dismutase (SOD) Activity Assay. In this assay, a water-soluble formazan dye is produced from WST-1 upon its reduction by superoxide anion. The rate of the superoxide anion-mediated reduction is linearly related to the xanthine oxidase activity and is inhibited by SOD, and the inhibitory activity of SOD can be determined by a colorimetric method. To perform this assay, HLECs were seeded on 6-well plates, infected with lentivirus, and lysed in ice-cold 0.1 M Tris/HCl buffer 72 h later. The lysates were centrifuged at 14000 ×g at 4°C for 5 min and the supernatant was collected. The SOD activity in the supernatants was determined by measuring the absorbance at 450 nm in a spectrophotometer. Triplicate experiments were performed.

2.8. Total Antioxidant Capacity (TAC) Assay. Total Antioxidant Capacity (TAC) Colorimetric Assay Kit from BioVision was used to measure the endogenous antioxidants. Briefly, HLECs cells were infected with lentivirus in 6-well plates and collected with ice-cold 0.1 M PBS. Cell lysates were centrifuged at 14000 ×g at 4°C for 4 min and the supernatant was harvested. The absorbance of the supernatant was measured at 570 nm in an X Mark microplate spectrophotometer (Bio-Rad). Triplicate experiments were performed.

2.9. Flow Cytometric Detection of Apoptosis Assay. Apoptosis was evaluated by APC-annexin V/7-AAD (BD Pharmingen, California, USA) staining followed by flow cytometric analysis. Cells were plated in 6-well plates at a density of 1×10^5/well and cultured for 48 h with reagents. Then, the cells were gently trypsinized and washed twice with ice-cold PBS. At least 10,000 cells were resuspended in 100 μL 1x binding buffer, stained with 5 μL 7-AAD (25 μg/mL) and 5 μL APC-annexin V at 4°C for 30 min, and immediately analyzed with a FACScanto flow cytometer (BD Bioscience, USA). Each measurement was carried out in triplicate.

2.10. Statistical Analysis. Data were expressed as mean ± standard error and analyzed by one-way ANOVA and *post hoc* Bonferroni's test. The statistical software, Prism 5 (GraphPad software Inc., San Diego, CA, USA), was used. The criterion for statistical significance was $p < 0.05$.

3. Results

3.1. Impaired Protein Stability Caused by Missense Mutation in EPHA2. There are a total of 134 nonsynonymous SNPs identified within the coding region of *EPHA2* gene. A previous bioinformatic analysis suggests that rs2291806 (E825K) and rs1058371 (I96F) are potential functional polymorphisms involved in susceptibility to cataract formation [10]. Multiple sequence alignment of human, macaque, rat, and mouse EPHA2 showed that both amino acids with missense mutations are evolutionarily conserved (Figure 1(a)). To investigate the cytoprotective role of EPHA2 in lens epithelial cells and the molecular mechanism underlying the association of EPHA2 mutation with age-related cataract, we generated the lentiviral plasmids encoding wild-type EPHA2, EPHA2^{E825K}, and EPHA2^{I96F} and prepared the high-titers of corresponding lentivirus for infection. The human lens epithelial cells (HLECs) were subsequently infected with lentivirus expressing either wild-type or mutant EPHA2. The quantification by counting the green fluorescent protein- (GFP-) positive cells showed that ~85% of cells on average were overexpressed by EPHA2 and its missense mutants 72 h after infection (Figures 1(b) and 1(c)).

The abundance of *EPHA2* mRNA in each group after lentiviral infection was evaluated with real-time PCR. There was a 2.5-fold increase in the level of *EPHA2* mRNA following lentivirus-mediated overexpression, as compared with noninfected cells and vector control (Figures 2(a) and 2(b)). Our previous study showed that a synonymous polymorphism within *EPHA2* gene, named rs3754334, is associated with the risk of age-related cataract [27]. Using the synonymous substitution as negative control, we compared the level of mRNA transcripts encoding the wild-type and mutant EPHA2 and found no difference in the transcription (Figure 2(b)).

The missense mutations with apparent effects on function are dominated by compromised protein stability [28]. Thus, we further examined the protein level of EPHA2 without or with amino acid substitution in HLECs by western blot. The results showed that EPHA2^{I96F} and EPHA2^{E825K} mutation significantly impaired the receptor stability while synonymous SNP rs3754334 did not affect the protein expression of EPHA2 (Figure 2(c)). Taken together, these results suggest that the missense mutations in EPHA2 are potentially associated with age-related cataract via compromising the macromolecular stability and its functional network.

3.2. Loss of Cytoprotective Function by Cataract-Associated Mutation in EPHA2. Eph receptors have been shown to play critical roles in tissue boundary formation, neural crest cell migration, axon guidance, bone remodeling, and vascular organization [12]. However, whether the EPHA2 signaling pathway provides cytoprotective effects against oxidative challenge remains largely unclear. To decipher the cellular functions of EPHA2, we overexpressed wild-type EPHA2 in HLECs and examined the cell viability before and after the treatment with 200 μM H_2O_2 to induce oxidative stress (Figure 3(a)). The relative index of cell death was evaluated by

$$\text{Absorbance index} = \frac{\text{The number of starter cells}}{\text{Absorbance value} \times 10000},$$

$$\text{Relative index} = \frac{\text{Absorbance index of experimental group}}{\text{Avergae absorbance index of vector group}}. \quad (1)$$

The absorbance value at 450 nm was determined using CCK8 assay. The relative results of cell viability assay without H_2O_2 stimulation imply that EPHA2 overexpression may enhance the proliferation of lens epithelial cells (Figure 3(b)). The quantitative analysis also showed that overexpression of EPHA2 in HLECs reduced the relative index of cell death and especially ameliorated H_2O_2-induced apoptosis (Figures 3(b) and 3(c)), suggesting the cytoprotective function of EPHA2 in the cultured lens epithelial cells. In addition, we found that

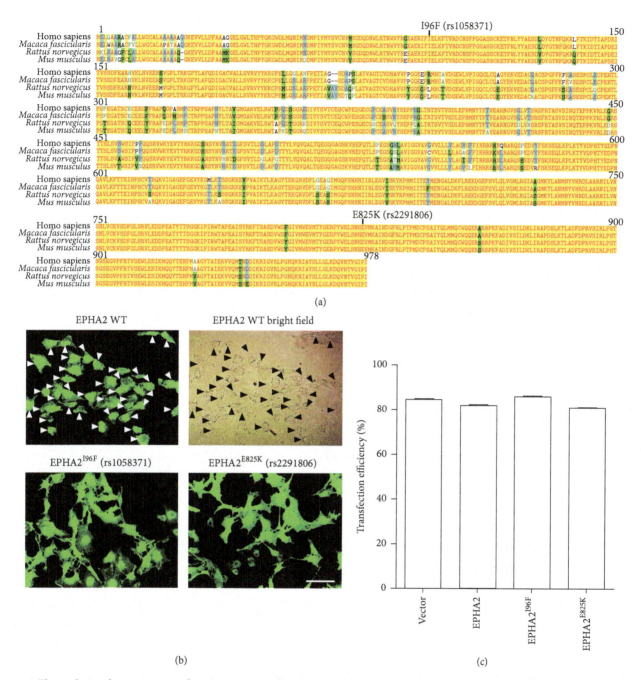

FIGURE 1: The evolutional conservation of cataract-associated SNP and the overexpression of EPHA2 in lens epithelial cells. (a) The protein sequences of human, macaque, rat, and mouse EPHA2 were aligned for multiple comparison. The functional polymorphisms rs1085371 and rs2291806 are highlighted here to show the missense mutation in EPHA2. The sequence alignment shows the evolutional conservation of both amino acids with substitution. (b) The human lens epithelial cells (HLECs) were infected with lentivirus encoding wild-type EPHA2, EPHA2^{I96F}, or EPHA2^{E825K}. The images captured with fluorescent microscopy 72 h after infection are shown here. Scale bar: 50 μm. (c) The infection efficiency was quantified by counting GFP-positive cells and total number of cells. Data are shown as the mean ± SEM.

the cytoprotective effect on oxidative stress was abolished by either EPHA2^{I96F} or EPHA2^{E825K} mutation (Figure 3(c)).

To specifically determine the antiapoptotic effect of EPHA2 in HLECs in vitro, we further performed the staining with APC-annexin V or vital dye 7-AAD on the dissociated cells, followed by fluorescent flow cytometry to analyze the proportion of H_2O_2-induced early and apoptotic cells.

The data indicated that HLECs with wild-type EPHA2 overexpression displayed a striking reduction in both early and late apoptosis, as compared with control cells undergoing cell death together with the diminishing GFP signal (Figure 4). As expected, ectopic expression of either EPHA2^{I96F} or EPHA2^{E825K} in HLECs showed reduced cytoprotective effects against H_2O_2-induced cell death (Figure 4). These data

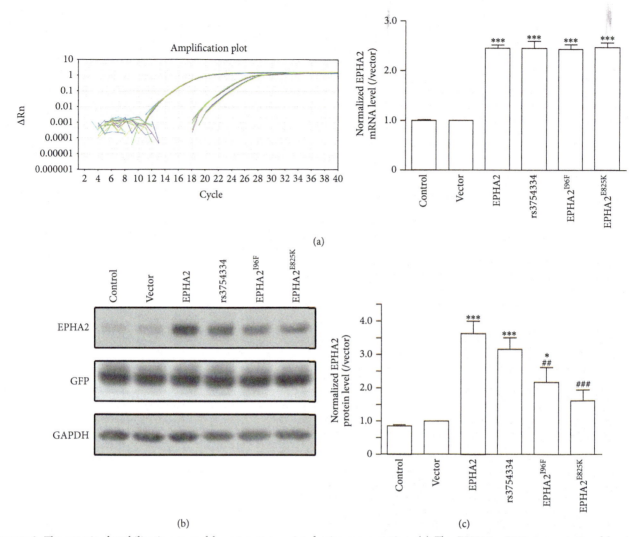

FIGURE 2: The protein destabilization caused by cataract-associated missense mutation. (a) The *EPHA2* mRNA transcriptional level was measured with real-time PCR after HLECs were overexpressed with wild-type or mutant EPHA2 for 48 h. The *EPHA2* mRNA level was normalized with the internal control β-actin and the data are presented as ratio of vector control. (b) The EPHA2 protein expression was tested with western blotting after the lentivirus-mediated overexpression in HLECs. (c) Quantitative analysis shows the impaired protein stability of EPHA2 with missense mutation. The EPHA2 protein level was normalized with the internal control *GAPDH*. Data are shown as the mean ± SEM. $^{*}p < 0.05$, $^{***}p < 0.001$ versus vector control; $^{\#\#}p < 0.01$, $^{\#\#\#}p < 0.001$ versus wild-type EPHA2.

combined demonstrated the protective function of EPHA2 in lens epithelial cells through preventing apoptosis and the neutralization of antiapoptotic effect by two functional polymorphisms.

3.3. Abrogated Antioxidative Effect by Nonsynonymous Polymorphisms with Risk of Cataract. The ROS generated endogenously or induced by environmental stress have long been implicated in cell death and tissue injury in the context of age-related cataract [3–5, 17, 18, 22]. The most efficient enzymatic antioxidants in the lens include SOD, catalase, glutathione peroxidase, and cytosolic glutathion-S-transferase [22, 29]. To investigate the mechanisms underlying the antiapoptotic effect of EPHA2 in the lens, we assessed the levels of lipid peroxidation in the HLECs by MDA assay. Despite the undetectable effect by EPHA2 overexpression under basal conditions, we found that the activation of EPHA2 signaling significantly declined the H_2O_2-induced oxidation of lipids in the lens epithelial cells (Figures 5(a) and 5(b)). Moreover, the SOD activity and the total antioxidative potency were upregulated by overexpression of EPHA2 to counterbalance the production of ROS in HLECs (Figures 5(c) and 5(d)). Interestingly, the antioxidative effect of EPHA2 was consistently abrogated by the identified functional polymorphisms rs2291806 and rs1058371 (Figure 5). Our results showed the antioxidative role of EPHA2 in the lens epithelial cells under the exposure of extrinsic oxidative stress.

4. Discussion

Although genetic studies have hitherto provided a deep insight into the understanding of genetic framework involved

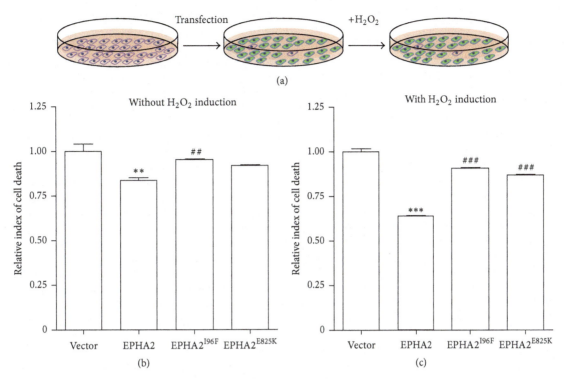

FIGURE 3: The functional polymorphisms abolish EPHA2-mediated cytoprotective effect. (a) The experimental paradigm. The HLECs were seeded and infected with lentivirus expressing wild-type EPHA2, EPHA2^{I96F}, or EPHA2^{E825K}. The infected cells were treated with 200 μM H_2O_2 to mimic the light-induced oxidative stress in lens. (b-c) The cell viability was assayed before and after H_2O_2 treatment following lentivirus-based gene overexpression. The quantification reveals the cytoprotective effect of wild-type EPHA2 and the loss of function in cataract-associated mutants. Data are shown as the mean ± SEM. $**p < 0.01$, $***p < 0.001$ versus vector control; $^{##}p < 0.01$, $^{###}p < 0.001$ versus wild-type EPHA2.

in the age-related cataract, its pathophysiology remains to be elucidated. The putative role of EPHA2 in the etiopathogenesis of age-related cataract has attracted much attention regarding the molecular mechanisms involved in maintaining the clarity of lens by EPHA2. Here we report that EPHA2 signaling protects the lens epithelial cells from oxidative stress-induced cell death. Furthermore, the loss of protein stability in two of the nonsynonymous polymorphisms compromises the antioxidative and antiapoptotic effect of EPHA2.

The previously identified cataract-associated mutations in EPHA2 basically reside in kinase and sterile alpha motif (SAM) domains [2, 12]. It is hypothesized that the loss of EPHA2 function may directly or indirectly impair cellular structural stability, cell-to-cell crosstalk, protein folding, and transcriptional activation, which cause congenital or age-related cataract [6, 12]. Impaired development of lens fiber cells or equatorial cells caused by loss of function in EPHA2 may lead to hereditary cataract, whereas accumulating oxidative stress resulting from both environmental insults and age-dependent reduction of EPHA2 expression in lens could contribute to age-related cataract [6, 12, 17, 30, 31]. Our data suggests that EPHA2 plays a cytoprotective role in lens epithelial cells by promoting cell viability under oxidative stress. In spite of the established regulatory role of Eph/ephrin role in the epithelial morphogenesis and homeostasis [32], we did not find conspicuous differences in the morphology of lens epithelial cells between control and overexpressing cells. Consistent with bioinformatic analysis showing that both rs2291806 and rs1058371 are the least stable among varieties of SNPs [10], our biochemical data confirms that both functional polymorphisms in EPHA2 lead to the destabilization of the receptor and thus neutralize its antiapoptotic role. The decay of mutant EPHA2 is possibly caused by reduced protein solubility and ubiquitin-mediated proteasomal degradation [33]. These results further support that the genetic mutation-mediated protein degradation contributes to apoptosis in age-related degenerative diseases [34, 35].

We further identified the antioxidative effect of EPHA2 by gain-of-function analysis, which underlies its cytoprotective function against environmental insult. Activation of Nrf2 increases the elimination of both exogenous and endogenous toxic chemicals including ROS and Nrf2-dependant signaling regulates the gene expression of EPHA2 [36, 37]. Indeed, our data revealed the upregulation of antioxidative SOD activity and the neutralization of lipid oxidation by EPHA2 activation in the lens epithelial cells. However, the complex transcriptional activation mediated by overexpression of EPHA2 to increase antioxidative capacity still remains to be determined. Importantly, the missense mutations in EPHA2 associated with age-related cataract abolished the EPHA2-mediated enhancement of antioxidative capacity, suggesting the loss of function in both polymorphisms.

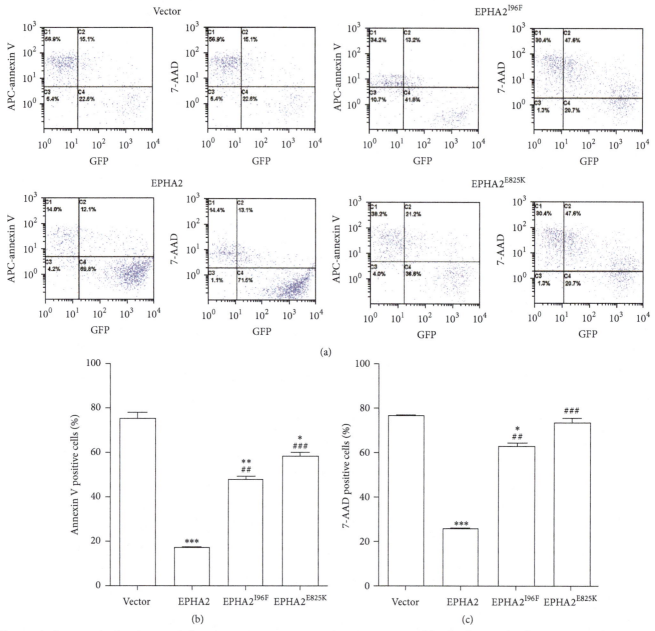

FIGURE 4: Compromised antiapoptotic function in cataract-associated genetic mutants. (a) After lentiviral infection to introduce control vector, EPHA2, EPHA2^{I96F}, or EPHA2^{E825K} into the cells and the administration with 200 μM H_2O_2, the HLECs were digested, dissociated, and stained with either APC-annexin V or 7-AAD, followed by the fluorescence activated cell sorting to analyze the early and late apoptosis. The GFP signal intensity was compromised if the HLECs undergo oxidative stress-induced apoptosis. (b-c) The statistical analysis shows that overexpression of wild-type EPHA2 reduces the proportion of both early and late apoptotic cells. The missense mutations abolish the antiapoptotic effect against oxidative damage. $^*p < 0.05$, $^{**}p < 0.01$, and $^{***}p < 0.001$ versus vector control; $^{\#\#}p < 0.01$, $^{\#\#\#}p < 0.001$ versus wild-type EPHA2.

5. Conclusion

In summary, our study revealed the cytoprotective and antioxidative function of EPHA2 in lens epithelial cells, which coordinate and maintain the lens epithelial structural integrity. The nonsynonymous polymorphisms rs2291806 and rs1058371 disrupt the protein stability and diminish the antiapoptotic effect of EPHA2 in human lens during aging, contributing to age-related cataract. The bioinformatic prediction helps us to identify the functional SNP in disease. The future gain- and loss-of-function studies in the animal model will further elucidate the cytoprotective and antioxidative role of EPHA2 in vivo.

Disclaimer

The authors are responsible for the content and writing of the paper.

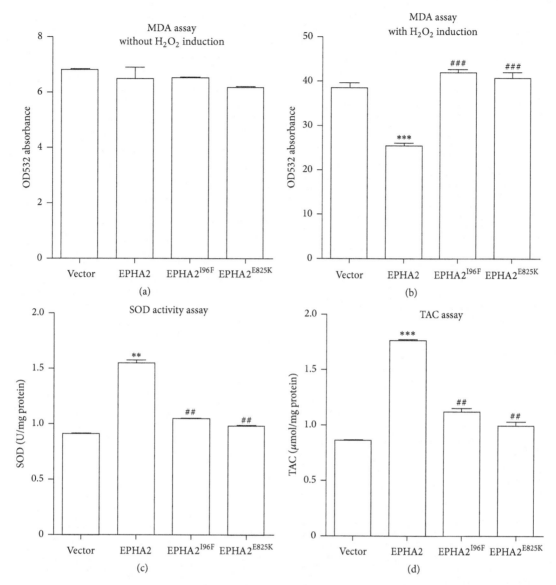

FIGURE 5: The nonsynonymous polymorphisms nullify the antioxidative capacity of EPHA2. (a-b) The lipid oxidation was evaluated with MDA assays in the HLECs before and after H_2O_2 treatment. The overexpression of EPHA2 reduces the absorbance value of cell lysate with H_2O_2 treatment, while the introduction of EPHA2^{I96F} or EPHA2^{E825K} mutant does not decline the lipid oxidation. (c-d) The SOD activity and the total antioxidative capacity were tested with SOD and TAC assay kit, respectively. The data are presented as U/mg or μmol/mg proteins. The upregulation of SOD level and total antioxidant content by EPHA2 is abrogated by the cataract-associated SNPs. $^*p < 0.05$, $^{**}p < 0.01$, and $^{***}p < 0.001$ versus vector control; $^{\#\#}p < 0.01$, $^{\#\#\#}p < 0.001$ compared with wild-type EPHA2.

Conflict of Interests

The authors declare no conflict of interests.

Authors' Contribution

Jin Yang and Dan Li contributed equally to this work.

Acknowledgments

This work was supported by the National Natural Science Foundation of China (NSFC) Grants (81270989 and 81200668) and the Research Fund for the Doctoral Program of Higher Education of China (no. 20120071120089).

References

[1] A. T. Moore, "Understanding the molecular genetics of congenital cataract may have wider implications for age related cataract," *British Journal of Ophthalmology*, vol. 88, no. 1, pp. 2–3, 2004.

[2] J. F. Hejtmancik and M. Kantorow, "Molecular genetics of age-related cataract," *Experimental Eye Research*, vol. 79, no. 1, pp. 3–9, 2004.

[3] A. Charakidas, A. Kalogeraki, M. Tsilimbaris, P. Koukoulomatis, D. Brouzas, and G. Delides, "Lens epithelial apoptosis and cell proliferation in human age-related cortical cataract," *European Journal of Ophthalmology*, vol. 15, no. 2, pp. 213–220, 2005.

[4] G. J. Harocopos, K. M. Alvares, A. E. Kolker, and D. C. Beebe, "Human age-related cataract and lens epithelial cell death," *Investigative Ophthalmology & Visual Science*, vol. 39, no. 13, pp. 2696–2706, 1998.

[5] W.-C. Li, J. R. Kuszak, K. Dunn et al., "Lens epithelial cell apoptosis appears to be a common cellular basis for non-congenital cataract development in humans and animals," *The Journal of Cell Biology*, vol. 130, no. 1, pp. 169–181, 1995.

[6] G. Jun, H. Guo, B. E. K. Klein et al., "EPHA2 is associated with age-related cortical cataract in mice and humans," *PLoS Genetics*, vol. 5, no. 7, Article ID e1000584, 2009.

[7] D. Celojevic, A. Abramsson, M. S. Palmér et al., "EPHA2 polymorphisms in Estonian patients with age-related cataract," *Ophthalmic Genetics*, 2014.

[8] P. Sundaresan, R. D. Ravindran, P. Vashist et al., "EPHA2 polymorphisms and age-related cataract in India," *PLoS ONE*, vol. 7, no. 3, Article ID e33001, 2012.

[9] W. Tan, S. Hou, Z. Jiang, Z. Hu, P. Yang, and J. Ye, "Association of EPHA2 polymorphisms and age-related cortical cataract in a Han Chinese population," *Molecular Vision*, vol. 17, pp. 1553–1558, 2011.

[10] T. A. Masoodi, S. A. Shammari, M. N. Al-Muammar, T. M. Almubrad, and A. A. Alhamdan, "Screening and structural evaluation of deleterious non-synonymous SNPs of ePHA2 gene involved in susceptibility to cataract formation," *Bioinformation*, vol. 8, no. 12, pp. 562–567, 2012.

[11] E. B. Pasquale, "Eph receptors and ephrins in cancer: bidirectional signalling and beyond," *Nature Reviews Cancer*, vol. 10, no. 3, pp. 165–180, 2010.

[12] J. E. Park, A. I. Son, and R. Zhou, "Roles of EphA2 in development and disease," *Genes*, vol. 4, no. 3, pp. 334–357, 2013.

[13] K. R. Amato, S. Wang, A. K. Hastings et al., "Genetic and pharmacologic inhibition of EPHA2 promotes apoptosis in NSCLC," *The Journal of Clinical Investigation*, vol. 124, no. 5, pp. 2037–2049, 2014.

[14] J.-W. Lee, R. L. Stone, S. J. Lee et al., "EphA2 targeted chemotherapy using an antibody drug conjugate in endometrial carcinoma," *Clinical Cancer Research*, vol. 16, no. 9, pp. 2562–2570, 2010.

[15] K. A. Mohammed, X. Wang, E. P. Goldberg, V. B. Antony, and N. Nasreen, "Silencing receptor EphA2 induces apoptosis and attenuates tumor growth in malignant mesothelioma," *American Journal of Cancer Research*, vol. 1, no. 3, pp. 419–431, 2011.

[16] B. Miao, Z. Ji, L. Tan et al., "EPHA2 is a mediator of vemurafenib resistance and a novel therapeutic target in melanoma," *Cancer Discovery*, vol. 5, no. 3, pp. 274–287, 2015.

[17] S. Ottonello, C. Foroni, A. Carta, S. Petrucco, and G. Maraini, "Oxidative stress and age-related cataract," *Ophthalmologica*, vol. 214, no. 1, pp. 78–85, 2000.

[18] O. Ates, H. H. Alp, I. Kocer, O. Baykal, and I. A. Salman, "Oxidative DNA damage in patients with cataract," *Acta Ophthalmologica*, vol. 88, no. 8, pp. 891–895, 2010.

[19] R. J. W. Truscott, "Age-related nuclear cataract—oxidation is the key," *Experimental Eye Research*, vol. 80, no. 5, pp. 709–725, 2005.

[20] K. Kannan and S. K. Jain, "Oxidative stress and apoptosis," *Pathophysiology*, vol. 7, no. 3, pp. 153–163, 2000.

[21] J. P. Kehrer, "Cause-effect of oxidative stress and apoptosis," *Teratology*, vol. 62, no. 4, pp. 235–236, 2000.

[22] R. Thiagarajan and R. Manikandan, "Antioxidants and cataract," *Free Radical Research*, vol. 47, no. 5, pp. 337–345, 2013.

[23] V. Bottero, S. Chakraborty, and B. Chandran, "Reactive oxygen species are induced by Kaposi's sarcoma-associated herpesvirus early during primary infection of endothelial cells to promote virus entry," *Journal of Virology*, vol. 87, no. 3, pp. 1733–1749, 2013.

[24] J. Yang, T.-J. Liu, Y.-X. Jiang, and Y. Lu, "ATRA enhances the bystander effect of suicide gene therapy driven by the specific promoter LEP 503 in human lens epithelial cells," *Molecular Vision*, vol. 18, pp. 2053–2066, 2012.

[25] G. Tiscornia, O. Singer, and I. M. Verma, "Production and purification of lentiviral vectors," *Nature Protocols*, vol. 1, no. 1, pp. 241–245, 2006.

[26] D. Chang, X. Zhang, S. Rong et al., "Serum antioxidative enzymes levels and oxidative stress products in age-related cataract patients," *Oxidative Medicine and Cellular Longevity*, vol. 2013, Article ID 587826, 7 pages, 2013.

[27] J. Yang, J. Luo, P. Zhou, Q. Fan, Y. Luo, and Y. Lu, "Association of the ephreceptor tyrosinekinase-type A2 (EPHA2) gene polymorphism rs3754334 with age-related cataract risk: a meta-analysis," *PLoS ONE*, vol. 8, no. 8, Article ID e71003, 2013.

[28] Z. Wang and J. Moult, "SNPs, protein structure, and disease," *Human Mutation*, vol. 17, no. 4, pp. 263–270, 2001.

[29] K. Rahman, "Studies on free radicals, antioxidants, and cofactors," *Clinical Interventions in Aging*, vol. 2, no. 2, pp. 219–236, 2007.

[30] C. Cheng, M. M. Ansari, J. A. Cooper, and X. Gong, "EphA2 and Src regulate equatorial cell morphogenesis during lens development," *Development*, vol. 140, no. 20, pp. 4237–4245, 2013.

[31] M. A. Coopera, A. I. Sona, D. Komlosb, Y. Suna, N. J. Kleimanc, and R. Zhoua, "Loss of ephrin-A5 function disrupts lens fiber cell packing and leads to cataract," *Proceedings of the National Academy of Sciences of the United States of America*, vol. 105, no. 43, pp. 16620–16625, 2008.

[32] H. Miao and B. Wang, "Eph/ephrin signaling in epithelial development and homeostasis," *International Journal of Biochemistry and Cell Biology*, vol. 41, no. 4, pp. 762–770, 2009.

[33] J. E. Park, A. I. Son, R. Hua, L. Wang, X. Zhang, and R. Zhou, "Human cataract mutations in EPHA2 SAM domain alter receptor stability and function," *PLoS ONE*, vol. 7, no. 5, Article ID e36564, 2012.

[34] E. H. Rannikko, L. B. Vesterager, J. H. A. Shaik et al., "Loss of DJ-1 protein stability and cytoprotective function by Parkinson's disease-associated proline-158 deletion," *Journal of Neurochemistry*, vol. 125, no. 2, pp. 314–327, 2013.

[35] J. A. Sommers, A. N. Suhasini, and R. M. Brosh, "Protein degradation pathways regulate the functions of helicases in the DNA damage response and maintenance of genomic stability," *Biomolecules*, vol. 5, no. 2, pp. 590–616, 2015.

[36] N. M. Reddy, S. R. Kleeberger, M. Yamamoto et al., "Genetic dissection of the Nrf2-dependent redox signaling-regulated transcriptional programs of cell proliferation and cytoprotection," *Physiological Genomics*, vol. 32, no. 1, pp. 74–81, 2007.

[37] Q. Ma, "Advances in mechanisms of anti-oxidation," *Discovery Medicine*, vol. 17, no. 93, pp. 121–130, 2014.

Human Serum Eye Drops in Eye Alterations: An Insight and a Critical Analysis

Maria Rosaria De Pascale,[1] Michele Lanza,[2] Linda Sommese,[1] and Claudio Napoli[1]

[1] U.O.C. Immunohematology, Transfusion Medicine and Transplant Immunology, Regional Reference Laboratory of Transplant Immunology, Azienda Ospedaliera Universitaria (AOU), Second University of Naples, 80100 Naples, Italy
[2] Multidisciplinary Department of Medical, Surgical and Dental Sciences, Second University of Naples, 80100 Naples, Italy

Correspondence should be addressed to Michele Lanza; mic.lanza@gmail.com

Academic Editor: Flavio Mantelli

Human serum contains a physiological plethora of bioactive elements naturally released by activated platelets which might have a significant effect on the regeneration of corneal layers by stimulating the cell growth. This mechanism supported the use of human serum eye drops in some ocular diseases associated with dystrophic changes and alterations of the tear film, such as persistent corneal epithelial defects and dry eye syndrome. We focused our effort on potential benefits and limitations of the use of human serum eye drops when conventional therapies failed. We reviewed the recent literature by reporting published studies from 2010 to 2014. Despite the limited evaluated study populations, most of the clinical studies have confirmed that serum eye drop therapy is effective in corneal healing by reducing ocular symptom, particularly during the short-term follow-up. In addition, three recent published studies have shown the efficacy of the serum eye drop therapy in comparison to traditional ones in intractable patients. Besides, reported ongoing clinical studies confirmed the open debate regarding the use of biologic tools for cornea regeneration. Results from these studies might open novel challenges and perspectives in the therapy of such refractory patients.

1. Introduction

Cornea is mostly composed of collagen and water and is enveloped by epithelium and endothelium [1]. These layers cooperate to ensure tissue homeostasis by providing adequate corneal transparency and reliability [1]. After injury, corneal epithelial cells regenerate and restore the physiologic tissue architecture. In addition, a concomitant nerve regrowth and a controlled neovascularization of the damaged surface may occur [2, 3]. Cellular loss needs replacement by cell growth and migration [3]. The mechanism driving the epithelialization involves a multiplicity of cells stimulated by serum growth factors (GFs) (Table 1) [4–6], mostly contained in platelet-α granules and issued by the same GFs into the blood during stress and tissue repair [4–10]. The great quantity and accessibility of GFs and other signaling proteins in platelets with a consequent inhibition of cell apoptosis and improvement of cell proliferation, differentiation, and migration suggested the extensive use of platelet derivatives for clinical and surgical aims in regenerative medicine (Table 1 and Figure 1) [7, 11]. Indeed, GFs, binding to tyrosine kinase or G protein-coupled receptor families, drive both the inflammatory process and the stroma remodeling through autocrine, juxtacrine, or, most commonly, paracrine means. Thus, the transcription of critical proteins for cell cycle returning to prewounding levels after the tissue healing occurs (Table 1) [12, 13].

Particularly, serum GFs such as epidermal growth factor (EGF), hepatocyte growth factor (HGF), and keratinocyte growth factor (KGF) stimulate corneal wound closure accelerating the healing time. Moreover, transforming growth factor-$\beta1/\beta2$ (TGF $\beta1/\beta2$) induces myofibroblast from fibroblast differentiation coupled to corneal opacification (corneal haze) (Table 1) [14–16]. Moreover, cytokines derived from the trigeminal nerve like substance P, neuropeptide y, catecholamines, and acetylcholine are positively involved in corneal healing [17]. Besides, an aged decreased response to mitogens mediated by alterations in the expression and

TABLE 1: Main growth factors involved in corneal epithelial healing.

Growth factors	Utilized pathway	Cellular target	Cellular effects	Corneal effects	Tear level	Serum level	References
EGF	EGFR/erbB1/HER1, erbB2/HER2/neu, erbB3/HER3, erbB4/HER4	Corneal epithelial cells (limbal region)	It increases epithelial migration and proliferation, inhibits corneal epithelial terminal differentiation, and upregulates activations of B4 integrins.	It stimulates epithelial wound closure accelerating the healing time.	2053 ± 312.4 pg/mL	199.74/±64.74 pg/mL	[16]
TGF-α	EGFR/erbB1/HER1, erbB2/HER2/neu, erbB3/HER3, erbB4/HER4	Corneal epithelial cells	It increases epithelial migration and proliferation and inhibits the expression of keratin K3.	It leads edge extension in epithelial sheet migration during eyelid closure.	84 ± 19 pg/mL	120 to 207 pg/mL	[16, 20, 21]
KGF	Ras-MAPK, PI3K/p70S6	Corneal epithelial cells	It increases epithelial cell proliferation protecting them from hypoxia.	It stimulates epithelial wound closure accelerating the healing time in the limbus zone.	Not provided	10.63 ± 4.98 pg/mL	[56]
HGF	c-Met, Ras-MAPK, PI3K/AKT, p70S6K, EGFR	Corneal epithelial cells, fibroblasts	It increases epithelial cell migration and motility and proliferation and inhibits apoptosis.	It stimulates epithelial wound closure.	200 pgmL^{-1}	573.9 ± 142.8 pgmL^{-1}	[18, 57]
IGF-1	PI3K/AKT	Corneal epithelial cells, fibroblasts	It increases epithelial cell proliferation, inhibits apoptosis, increases chemotaxis, and increases the expression of connexin 43 in corneal fibroblasts.	It stimulates epithelial wound closure improving gap-junctions.	Not provided	173.5 ng/mL	[6]
TGF β1/β2	TGF β-RI, TGF β-RII	Corneal epithelial cells, fibroblasts (limbal and central region)	It inhibits epithelial cells proliferation, increases keratocyte proliferation, and promotes myofibroblast differentiation.	It promotes scar formations, delays reepithelialization, and inhibits angiogenesis.	10 ng/mL	50 ng/mL	[24]
PDGF	PDGF-R	Endothelial cell, fibroblasts, epithelial cells	It increases endothelial cell proliferation, enhances fibroblast migration, and increases chemotaxis of epithelial cells.	It stimulates epithelial wound closure.	95–1330 ng/L	1.70 ng/mL	[22]
FGF-2	FGF-R, heparan sulfate proteoglycans, RTKs	Corneal epithelial cells, fibroblasts (Bowman's and Descemet's membrane)	It increases epithelial, endothelial, and stromal cell proliferation.	It stimulates epithelial wound closure and improves gap-junctions.	Not provided	8.3 ± 1.75 pg/mL	[13]
NGF	TRKA-R	Corneal epithelial cells, endothelial cells, fibroblasts	It increases epithelial cell proliferation and differentiation.	It stimulates epithelial wound closure, improves nerve regrowth, and induces inflammation and vascularization.	8.3 +/− 4.7 ng/ml	18.5 +/− 6.1 ng/mL	[19, 62, 63]

EGF: epidermal growth factor; TGF-α: transforming growth factor α; KGF: keratinocyte growth factor; HGF: hepatocyte growth factor; IGF-1: insulin growth factor 1; TGFβ1/β2: transforming growth factor β1/β2; PDGF: platelet derived growth factor; FGF-2: fibroblastic growth factor 2; NGF: nerve growth factor.

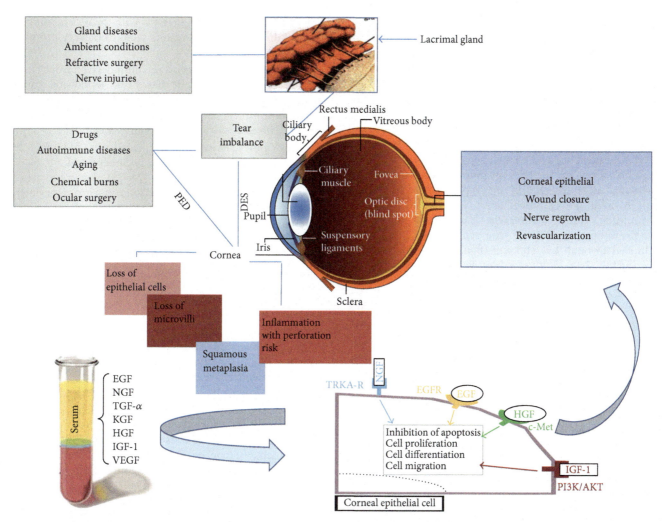

Figure 1: Mechanisms involved in damaged cornea and serum growth factor regeneration pathways. Several corneal injuries can promote pathological conditions such as PED or DES. Action of drugs, autoimmune diseases, aging, chemical insults, and postsurgical lesions can wound the cornea directly or indirectly through the imbalance of the lachrymal gland. Microscopically, these pathogenic conditions result in a loss of epithelial cells and microvilli, epithelial squamous metaplasia, and inflammation of the corneal surface. The corneal healing process can benefit from the promoting action of serum GFs. Once they are released, through tyrosine kinase receptors, they propagate their signal from the plasma membrane to the nucleus. Through explicit pathways and signaling cascades, GFs activate the expression of target genes involved in apoptosis, proliferation, cell differentiation, and migration. This synergistic action establishes regenerative effects with closure of epithelial lesions, revascularization, and neurorepair.

activity of cyclin-dependent kinase inhibitors (p27KIP1, p16INK4A, and p21CIP1) appears to be involved in a lacking or a damaging of cellular repair processes [3].

Toward this context, the lachrymal film plays a critical role such as resource of GFs [18–24] since the lack of tear epitheliotropic support promotes corneal opacity onset with consequent visual impairment [25]. On the other hand, tear upregulation drives corneal epithelial hyperplasia, excessive deposition of extracellular matrix, and hypervascularization with cornea conjunctivalization [8]. Here, we report the different concentrations of each GF in the human serum with respect to tears. The levels of transforming growth factor α (TGF-α), hepatocyte growth factor (HGF), TGFβ1/2, and nerve growth factor (NGF) resulted to be even more elevated in serum than in tears.

Failure of the corneal repair mechanisms leads to a chronic pathologic condition as persistent epithelial defects (PED) or dry eye syndrome (DES) [15]. PED result from several factors such as aging, chemical burns, systemic disorders, and drugs [26] (Figure 1). Nevertheless, DES, associated to tear deficit or tear inefficiency, is able to promote the corneal epithelial instability and inflammation [27, 28] supporting PED syndrome. DES is caused by lacrimal gland imbalance often connected to systemic inflammatory diseases [29–32], such as Sjogren's syndrome [33], rheumatoid arthritis [31], diabetes [34], systemic lupus erythematosus, acne rosacea, and Graves' disease [35]. In addition, hormonal modifications, drugs (e.g., systemic antihistamines, diuretics, and topical beta blockers for glaucoma therapies), and surgeries (e.g., photorefractive keratectomy and laser *in situ* keratomileusis) [36] as well as the repeated use of contact lenses could be involved in DES development [27]. On the basis of mechanistic criteria, International Dry Eye WorkShop has characterized two main subtypes of the disorder (aqueous deficiency and evaporative dry eye) both interested by tear film instability and symptoms of discomfort [28, 37]. Ocular dryness or irritation might increase light sensitivity, foreign body sensation, red eyes, poor vision, and daily life limitations which are the most referred symptoms which have great impact on patient quality of life [37, 38]. The best clinical marker for DES diagnosis and for the severity assessment is represented by the improved tear osmolarity [39]. In addition, tear production is currently evaluated by Schirmer's testing, fluorescein clearance, and fluorescein tear break-up time (TBUT). The ocular surface damage is estimated through dye staining (fluorescein and lissamine green) while the severity of subjective symptoms is assessed by subjective scored questionnaires (like OXFORD score and Ocular Surface Disease Index) [37, 38].

Up to now, there is no gold standard therapy for DES or PED [40–42]. Current therapeutic strategies require the accurate identification of etiologic mechanisms that cause the corneal injury by providing epitheliotropic factors and enhancing tear replacement [26, 43, 44]. When standard therapeutic options fail, the main treatment purpose is the increased patient comfort and corneal moisture through the instillation of artificial tears, corticosteroids, antibiotics, and use of bandage contact lenses [30, 45–47]. However, natural tears have a particular composition of water, salts, hydrocarbons, proteins, and lipids that cannot be restored by pharmacological alternatives [25]. Furthermore, artificial tear substitutes contain chemical preservatives associated with toxic and allergic reactions, especially for those patients with sensitive eyes [6]. Moreover, the repeated instillation of topical corticosteroids could be associated with long-term side effects including cataracts and increased intraocular pressure [48]. For these motivations, alternative therapies like silicone punctal plug insertion, botulinum neurotoxin type A, nutritional supplements (essential fatty acids, including omega-3, linoleic acid, and gamma-linoleic acid), and topical 0.05% solution of cyclosporine A have been proposed [49–55]. However, changes in life style as an increased water intake and reduction of alcohol consumption, indoor humidifiers, and air filters or cleaners have been recommended [56].

A debated aspect of the treatment of corneal diseases is focused on the use of novel regenerative instruments for corneal regeneration [57–60]. The evidence regarding the key role of several GFs for the integrity of the ocular surface (Table 1) fits the use of single recombinant GFs in several human corneal degenerative disorders [57–61]. Nerve growth factor (NGF) alteration in corneal diseases has been largely evaluated; NGF pathway alteration has been tested in an animal model by demonstrating NGF to be involved in corneal healing and in sensory denervation [62]. Moreover, in studies evaluating human being, low tears level of NGF has been proved to be reduced in eyes affected by dry eye [63] and has been proved to be effective in several corneal diseases such as neurotrophic keratitis, immune corneal ulcer, and HSV keratitis and after cataract surgery [64]. Clinical trials are ongoing to evaluate therapy with NGF eye drops in corneal diseases and first results seem to be very promising [65].

In addition, a conditioned medium derived from human uterine cervical stem cells has been tested for corneal epithelial healing [66], and a therapeutically ocular surface medium, routinely used to culture epithelial cells, was suggested as novel eye drops for DES and PED [67].

Among these emerging therapies, the use of biologic eye drops derived from both human peripheral [44, 50, 68–75] and umbilical cord blood serum [76–78] plays a crucial role in several corneal diseases. Previous *in vitro* experiments showed that corneal epithelial cell morphology and cell functions are better maintained by human serum eye drops (SE) than pharmaceutical tear substitutes [79].

The first applications of human SE to support corneal regeneration were performed in 1975 in corneal alkali injury cases [80]; later, in 1984, Fox et al. [81] reported the use of SE in a DES. Later, SE have gained a therapeutic dignity in ophthalmology as a new concept to manage wounded cornea [82, 83]. To date, despite the fact that SE therapy could avoid drug side effects, its use is restricted and is not universally recognized as therapeutic option although several aspects of the whole regenerative medicine are still debated [11].

Here, we critically analyzed the current applications of SE in corneal diseases like DES and PED by focusing on crucial topics for its production and the current legislative restrictions in support of its use. To analyze the SE therapeutic achievement, we reported the most recent published randomized clinical trials (RTCs) and ongoing studies where this kind of treatment has been applied and compared to standard and other emergent treatments in severe ocular conditions.

2. Legislative, Ethical, and Technical Implications on the Use of Serum Eye Drops

The use of SE obtained from patient peripheral whole blood (autologous) or from healthy donor (nonautologous or allogenic) represents a biological therapeutic strategy influencing and promoting the corneal restitution [11, 68, 83]. The rationale for its use arises from its strong similarity to tears, in regard to pH (7.4) and osmolarity (298 mml for tears and 296 mml for serum) [84] as well as its biochemical constitution. In addition, SE offer the same platelet derived antibacterial and anti-inflammatory effect *in vivo* [85].

Despite the fact that multiple studies supported the safety and efficacy of SE over standard treatments, SE have not yet been considered for approval by Food and Drug Administration, in the United States [8].

For this reason, SE are not a recognized treatment and are not covered by most of medical insurances [82]. In addition, despite the improved reliability of current serologic tests for HBs-Ag, anti-HCV, anti-HIV-1/2, and syphilis detection, the use of allogenic SE is associated with the immunologic and infectious implications of donor exposure [86]. However, even though autologous SE should be considered the best choice, patients with absolute contraindications to provide blood as a result of specific diseases or conditions (e.g., bacteremia) or who are unable to tolerate frequent venipunctures are eligible for the treatment with healthy donor SE. The allogenic SE, subjected to severe laboratory checks, can be used as an effective alternative treatment showing comparable clinical results to the autologous one [73, 86].

The established criteria for donor enrollment and for blood collection include hemoglobin level higher than 11 g/dL (hematocrit > 33%) and exclude subjects presenting risk of bacteremia and cardiovascular diseases deferring pregnant women and children. Despite the absence of absolute prohibitions, the use of SE in children is restricted to avoid repeated required venipunctures and limiting instillation of potentially infectious donor sera in such patients [86, 87]. In these cases, if traditional therapy with artificial tears, antibiotics, or steroids is not effective, the topical cyclosporine or the conjunctival flap can be applied to improve the corneal conditions [87].

According to the current protocols, blood samples should be collected with previous informant consent and transferred into a sterile kit or blood bag without anticoagulant and treated under sterile conditions (laminar flow hood) (Table 2). A sufficient time has to be dedicated to the patient to illustrate properly the treatment and the need for repeated blood sampling. As shown in Table 2, the routine production of SE is frequently affected by the lack of recognized procedures [11, 85]. However, the proper management, handling, and storage of final product are essential for the successful treatment avoiding side effects.

To date, many laboratory protocols have been published for SE production with variable dilutions of serum (from 20% to 100%) and with differences in clotting phase, centrifugation time, and speed [88, 89] (Table 2). According to previous studies, clotting time is critical to obtain ideal concentrations of EGF, TGF-β-1, and fibronectin in the collected serum [85]. In addition, a proper serum dilution is recommended to reduce the antiproliferative effect of TGF-β which results five times higher in human serum than in tears [85]. Usually, 0.9% sodium saline or balanced salt solutions are utilized as diluents and preservatives solutions are not usually added to decrease the risk of induced toxicity. For the lack of preservatives, microbial cultures as well as the antibiotic therapy are recommended [85]. Finally, to preserve the biologic activity, the SE should be frozen in blood banks at −70°C until its use or at −20°C for a month and protected from light to prevent the degradation of vitamin A (Table 2).

Depending on clinical conditions, the frequency of instillations of SE may go from every 15 minutes to two times per day; also the duration of the reported treatment widely ranged from 3 days to a maximum of 36 months. In most cases, the improvement appears after a brief period of therapy (from 1 to 4 weeks) [90]. Studies reported one case of corneal immunoglobulin deposition, scleral vasculitis, epithelial erosion, conjunctivitis, decreased corneal sensitivity, inflammatory response, infections, and an isolated case of mycosis [90]. Recently, to avoid immunity complications, Anitua et al. have characterized a plasma rich in GF without IgE and complement suggesting its use in autoimmune diseases [82]. Until now, the few published data on clinical complications associated with SE have demonstrated the safety of this therapy. However, limitations in published studies as discussed below are observed.

3. Clinical Applications and Study Results

As shown in Table 2, several studies investigated the role of SE treatment mostly in corneas affected by DES and PED.

Despite the fact that most of the authors found objective and subjective wellbeing after the treatment with SE, the comparison of clinical results is complex because data have been obtained from nonhomogeneous populations affected by several unrelated corneal diseases. In addition, the technical preparation of SE shows different dilutions obtained with different solutions, clotting phases, centrifugation forces, and time intervals, as well as different storage temperatures and times that can modify the final clinical outcomes and healing times as shown in Table 2.

Recent results have confirmed the efficacy of SE with respect to conventional therapy [91] in patients with severe DES or PED [79, 92] both by improving tear film stability and providing subjective comfort. Moreover, two recent prospective interventional studies [93, 94], on large cohorts of patients with PED treated with SE after ocular surgery, showed a significant or moderate improvement of delayed heal. In particular, Chen et al. [93] showed that 165 patients treated with 20% SE after penetrating keratoplasty drastically reduced postoperative PED when compared to patients that received artificial tears. In addition, Lekhanont et al. [94] evaluated SE for PED in 181 patients showing a high proportion (93.92%) of complete corneal epithelialization in only 4 days with low rate of adverse reactions.

Case reports have been described about the use of SE in other corneal diseases like ocular graft versus host disease [95, 96], bullous keratopathy [97], fulminant bilateral *Haemophilus influenzae* keratitis [98], neurotrophic corneal ulcer [99], anterior tissue necrosis after porous orbital implant [41], and Mooren's ulcer [100]. In all these cases, SE allowed a complete corneal healing with an effective improvement of the clinical conditions.

Despite many promising results, some recent studies have questioned the validity of this treatment. A prospective cross-sectional study on 34 patients did not find that SE could be effective in secondary Sjogren's syndrome due to elevated serum proinflammatory cytokine levels [101]. Moreover, a single prospective study on 17 patients with DES demonstrated the short-term benefit of SE, which persisted up only to three months after the end of therapy [102]. In 2013, Pan et al. [36] performed a meta-analysis identifying four randomized clinical trials, which compared SE with artificial tear treatment or saline solutions in patients with Sjogren's syndrome-related DES, non-Sjogren's syndrome DES, and postoperative DES. In conclusion, they advocated the need of recognized measures to define subjective symptoms and to assess the real effect of SE therapy for DES [36]. The use of SE was compared in randomized trials to unconventional biologic therapies, which have gained a growing interest, such as umbilical cord blood serum (CBS) [103, 104] and amniotic membrane transplant [105]. CBS is collected from umbilical vein after fetal delivery, manipulated, and collected

TABLE 2: Published studies on serum eye drops from 2010 to 2014.

Type of component	Study design	Year	Patient number	Corneal disease	Clotting phase	Centrifugation/time	Dilution	Storage	Results	References
100% AS	Single-center prospective interventional study	2013	181	Corneal epithelial defects after ocular surgery	2 h at RT	3000 g/15 min	None	−20°C three months	It improves corneal healing.	[94]
50% AS	Single-center prospective study	2014	28	Acute and chronic eye pathologies	24–48 h at 4°C	4000 g/10 min	Sterile saline solution	−30°C six months −20°C three months	It stabilizes and improves signs and symptoms in eyes previously treated with conventional therapy.	[91]
20% AS, CBS	Double-blind prospective randomized controlled clinical study	2011	33	Ocular chemical burns of grades III, IV, and V	Not provided	1800 g/10 min	Sterile balanced salt solution	−20.0°C until use	Umbilical cord serum therapy is more effective than AS eye drops or artificial tears in ocular surface restoration after acute chemical injuries.	[112]
20% AS versus AMT	Retrospective study	2014	42	Neurotrophic keratitis Corneal ulcers	2 h	3000 g/15 min	Sterile saline solution	Not provided	Amniotic membrane transplantation is more effective than AS in deep corneal ulcers with postherpes neurotrophic keratitis.	[105]
100% AS	Not provided	2013	10	PED	2 h at RT	3000 g/15 min	None	4°C	Improvement in corneal healing.	[115]
100% AS	Descriptive prospective observational study	2011	15	Various ocular surface disorders	None	10000 rpm/10 min	None	−20°C three months	Redness, burning, sharp pain, and tired eyes improved in 100% of the patients, whereas dryness and sandy/gritty sensation improved in 92% of the patients.	[69]
20% AS, 20% no AS	Prospective interventional study	2010	165	PED after PK	30 min	1500 rpm/5 min	Sterile saline solution	−4°C	AS improves healing in patients with potentially delayed epithelial heal.	[93]
20% AS	Prospective, double-blind randomized crossover study	2014	40	Severe DES	2 h at RT	2600 g/10 min	Sterile saline solution	−20°C	AS eye drops are more effective than conventional eye drops for improving tear film stability and subjective comfort in patients with severe DES.	[92]
100% AS versus normal saline/artificial tears/antibiotics AS	Randomized study	2013	85	DES/SS, DES/no SS, PED	5 min at RT	3000 g/5 min	None versus 50% saline or artificial tears or antibiotic	Not provided	AS was the most effective in decreasing symptoms, corneal epitheliopathy, and promoting fast closure of wound.	[88]

TABLE 2: Continued.

Type of component	Study design	Year	Patient number	Corneal disease	Clotting phase	Centrifugation/time	Dilution	Storage	Results	References
50% AS	Prospective cross-sectional study	2014	34	SS	2 h at RT	3000 g/15 min	Sodium hyaluronate	−70°C until use	AS might not be effective for the treatment of secondary SS because of elevated serum proinflammatory cytokine levels.	[101]
20% AS	Three-month prospective study	2014	17	Severe DES	Not provided	3000 g/15 min	Isotonic buffered saline solution	−20°C four months 4–8°C one week	The positive effect of AS decreased with time but still persisted up to three months after the end of therapy.	[102]
20% AS	Double-blind prospective randomized controlled clinical study	2011	32	Acute chemical burns	Not provided	180 g/10 min	Sterile balanced solution	−20°C until use	Umbilical cord serum was more effective than AS and artificial tears in ocular surface restitution.	[112]
20% AS versus PRP	Retrospective review	2012	28	DES	Not provided	3000 g/15 min 200 g/11 min	Sterile saline solution	−20°C until use	The concentrations of GFs in the PRP and AS were not statistically different. PRP could be an effective, novel treatment option for chronic ocular surface disease.	[70]
20% AS versus conventional artificial tears treatment	Double masked randomized crossover clinical trial	2012	12	Severe DES	2 h at RT	3500 rpm/5 min at 4°C	Sterile saline solution	−20°C	AS achieves better symptom improvement compared to artificial tears in a short-term treatment.	[79]

AS: autologous serum; RT: room temperature; CBS: cord blood serum; AMT: amniotic membrane transplantation; PED: persistent epithelial defects; PK: penetrating keratoplasty; DES: dry eye syndrome; SS: Sjogren's syndrome; PRP: platelet rich plasma; GFs: growth factors.

similarly to peripheral serum [104]. CBS is considered a reliable source of undifferentiated mesenchymal stem cells [106, 107], which are self-renewal elements that are able to replace directly corneal keratocytes [104] and conjunctival, limbal [76], and retinal nerve cells [104]. In addition, CBS contains consistent levels of cytokines, GFs, fibronectin, prealbumin, and fatty oils that provide useful instruments for corneal differentiation [74, 108]. Moreover, CBS includes antibacterial agents as IgG, lysozyme, and complement but lower levels of vitamin A compared to peripheral serum [109]. Despite the reduced immunogenicity of CBS with respect to peripheral serum due to the lower levels of IgM anti-A, anti-B, and IgG2 [78, 107], the use of the first is naturally associated to donor exposure and increased infectious risk and subjected to obstetric factors which could modify GF levels [110].

Some authors tested CBS for PED [77, 103], DES [111], corneal diseases due to chemical burns [112], and surgeries associated [113, 114]. Due to prominent GFs, anti-inflammatory cytokines, and mesenchymal stem cell levels in CBS, some authors demonstrated the main effectiveness of CBS with respect to both conventional treatment and traditional SE in severe corneal diseases [77, 104, 109, 112]. For this reason, clinical ongoing trials are mostly focused on the comparative evaluation of the use of SE and CBS, especially in DES, PED, and ocular GVHD as summarized in Table 3. In six ongoing studies reported on CBS eye drops, four are comparing CBS *versus* traditional SE and only one study analyzes amniotic membrane transplant *versus* SE in 180 patients with PED. Probably, promising results will arise from a large cohort randomized intervention single blind study which has enrolled 165 patients with diabetic retinopathy and penetrating keratoplasty comparing SE with standard treatments like corticosteroids and antibiotics. To date, there are no follow-up studies on SE or CBS eye drops treatment.

4. Future Directions

Several fields of medicine are focusing on a regenerative approach to treat pathologic conditions affected by insensitivity and toxic reactions to standard therapies. In this context, tissue engineering and regenerative medicine are the present and the future aim of clinical therapy, especially where traditional treatments fail or promote severe adverse events.

A number of corneal conditions are often not fully managed by standard treatments and are characterized by intolerances and systemic effects. New treatments have to be considered. Subjective and objective results suggest that biologic therapies for corneal surface alterations like SE treatment could be an effective option. Indeed, the use of biologic eye drops provides the beneficial effects of vitamins, GFs, and cytokines by correcting delayed corneal healing pathways and by restoring balanced mechanisms [76, 78, 79].

However, the technical preparation of human serum for ocular instillation should require a well-equipped laboratory with specialized trained personnel as well as the respect of aseptic and quality procedures. In addition, methods for SE production (clotting time, centrifugation, and concentration) including the proper additive and GF doses should be optimized according to well-established guidelines and standardized quality controlled protocols [9, 36, 111]. Specifically, a proper serum dilution should be performed to reduce the TGF $\beta1/\beta2$ levels (present in more than 5 times in serum compared to tears), which would promote corneal scar formations and a delayed reepithelialization (Table 1) [113]. Additionally, informed consent should be obtained from each patient in case of allogenic somministration to avoid ethical and juridical implications owing to blood transfusion practices and legislative restrictions should be carefully respected to minimize the immunological and infectious risks [11, 84].

5. Conclusions

To date, clinical benefits of SE therapy have been demonstrated by some published studies. Most of the recent analyzed trials have tested the clinical results coming from SE treatment through the comparison with traditional therapeutic approaches such as artificial tears, antibiotics, or corticosteroids [79, 91, 92]. Several randomized studies suggest that SE treatment leads to an improved tear film stability and subjective comfort [29, 69, 83, 88, 91, 93, 94] by determining a faster epithelial healing time and a better corneal transparency without increase of vascularization or fibrosis. Moreover, several data have confirmed the safety and the almost absolute absence of toxic and side effects, especially in severe case of DES or in PED (except those related to an improper handling). A critical point of these published studies concerns the number of patients enrolled which are recurrently less than 100 [4, 13, 16, 35, 38, 39, 43, 84, 85, 95, 96] and the almost absence of long follow-up studies [69]. On the other hand, the evaluation of the ongoing studies on this therapy showed that the newer fields of clinical research are focusing on alternatives to SE like CBS. In this regard, many studies are testing CBS and its therapeutic properties and safety. However, further studies with large populations comparing biological therapies with the traditional ones in corneal diseases are needed to provide the best treatment tailored to the singular patient.

Forthcoming conclusions will guide future efforts useful to clinical advances. They will clarify the therapeutic limits and resources of these emergent biologic therapies for corneal surface alterations, especially for refractory patients.

6. Method of Literature Search

We performed a computerized literature search on studies and trials by using the following search terms in various combinations: serum eye drops, cord blood serum, dry eye, and persistent epithelial defects. This search was achieved without any time and language restrictions in the following databases: PubMed, http://www.controlled-trials.com/, https://www.clinicaltrialsregister.eu/, https://eudract.ema.europa.eu/, and https://www.clinicaltrials.gov/. The complete reference list of the most relevant studies was compared for the methodology of serum eye drops collection, preparation, and

TABLE 3: Ongoing controlled clinical studies on serum eye drops from ClinicalTrials.gov.

Trial registration number	Study type	Patient number	Blood derivatives	Conditions	End-point	Phase
NCT01089985	Interventional	10	AS	Xerophthalmia	Efficacy and safety of AS.	Phase 1
NCT01972438	Randomized Intervention Double-blind	44	Autologous serum versus saline solution	HSCT patients with severe ocular GVHD	Treatment of severe chronic ocular GVHD in HSCT patients unresponsive to standard medical treatment.	Phase 1 Phase 2
NCT01075347	Randomized Intervention Assignment Single-blind	165	Human autoserum versus traditional medications (0.1% betamethasone, 0.3% gentamicin, and 0.4% tropicamide eye drops)	Corneal epithelial defect, diabetic retinopathy, penetrating keratoplasty	Corneal epithelial healing time by slit-lamp examination with fluorescein staining.	Phase 1
NCT00681642	Observational	7	Human autoserum versus cord blood serum	Corneal epithelial defect, dry eye syndrome	Wound healing, cell proliferation and migration by means of wound healing assay evaluation, MTS assay, and Boyden chamber migration assay.	Completed
NCT00442273	Interventional Nonrandomized Double-blind	48	20% autologous serum and umbilical cord serum eye drops	Severe dry eye syndrome	Therapeutic effect between autologous serum and umbilical cord serum eye drops in the treatment of severe dry eye syndrome.	Not provided
NCT00598299	Observational Prospective	100	Human autoserum versus cord blood serum	Corneal epithelial defect, dry eye syndrome	Corneal wound healing assay evaluation, MTS assay, and Boyden chamber migration assay	Completed
NCT01168375	Intervention	80	Umbilical cord serum	Corneal epithelial defect following diabetic vitrectomy	Measurement of corneal epithelial defect in days 3, 5, 7, and 12 by slit lamp.	Phase 1
NCT01016158	Interventional Randomized Single-blind	NP	20% umbilical cord serum eye drops	Recurrent corneal erosion	Efficacy 20% umbilical cord serum eye drops.	Completed
NCT01234623	Randomized	30	Cord blood serum	GVHD, Sjogren's Disease	Healing of corneal epithelial defects, ameliorating the painful subjective symptoms.	Phase 1
NCT02291731	Interventional Single-blind	Not provided	20% autologous serum eye drops and silicone-hydrogel contact lens (CLs)	Corneal diseases	Clinical effect of combination of topical 20% autologous serum eye drops and CLs in the treatment of recalcitrant PEDs and the recurrence rate of epithelial breakdown with or without continued use of autologous serum eye drops for 2 weeks after total reepithelialization.	Currently recruiting
NCT01122303	Observational	20	20% autologous serum eye drops	SJS, nonautoimmune dry eye	Comparisons of the concentrations of EGF, TGF-β1, TGF-β2, and fibronectin in 20% AS between SJS patients with dry eye and nonautoimmune dry eye patients.	Unknown
NCT00238862	Randomized single group Open label	180	Autologous serum 20% versus amniotic membrane transplantation	PED	Corneal reepithelialization, persistent corneal reepithelialization.	Completed

TABLE 3: Continued.

Trial registration number	Study type	Patient number	Blood derivatives	Conditions	End-point	Phase
NCT02153515	Single group Open label	60	Autologous serum finger prick of blood	Dry eyes, PED, ulcers	Ulcers time healing (within 4 weeks) Improving of corneal and conjunctival staining, Schirmer's test, tear break-up time, or symptoms ocular comfort index questionnaire (dry eyes).	Phase 3
NCT00779987	Interventional study Double-blind	12	20% autologous serum solution	Dry eye	Score reduction in the OSDI between patients treated with autologous serum and conventional artificial tears.	Phase 2

HCST: hematopoietic stem cell transplant; GVHD: chronic graft versus host disease; CLs: silicone-hydrogel contact lens; PED: persistent epithelial defects; SJS: Steven Johnson Syndrome; OSDI: Ocular Surface Disease Index; EGF: epidermal growth factor; TGF-β1: transforming growth factor β1; TGF-β2: transforming growth factor β2; MTS: 3-(4,5-dimethylthiazol-2-yl)-5-(3-carboxymethoxyphenyl)-2-(4-sulfophenyl)-2Htetrazolium.

storage. Clinical trials reported in Table 2 were selected from studies published in the last 5 years (2010–2014).

Conflict of Interests

The authors have no financial interests with any concept material or devices listed in this paper.

Authors' Contribution

Maria Rosaria De Pascale and Michele Lanza equally contributed to this work.

Acknowledgment

The authors would like to acknowledge Dr. Maria Vasco for illustrations (Figure 1).

References

[1] T. Lai and S. Tang, "Cornea characterization using a combined multiphoton microscopy and optical coherence tomography system," *Biomedical Optics Express*, vol. 5, no. 5, pp. 1494–1511, 2014.

[2] J.-H. Chang, N. K. Garg, E. Lunde, K.-Y. Han, S. Jain, and D. T. Azar, "Corneal neovascularization: an Anti-VEGF therapy review," *Survey of Ophthalmology*, vol. 57, no. 5, pp. 415–429, 2012.

[3] N. C. Joyce, "Cell cycle status in human corneal endothelium," *Experimental Eye Research*, vol. 81, no. 6, pp. 629–638, 2005.

[4] B. Czarkowska-Paczek, I. Bartlomiejczyk, and J. Przybylski, "The serum levels of growth factors: PDGF, TGF-beta and VEGF are increased after strenuous physical exercise," *Journal of Physiology and Pharmacology*, vol. 57, no. 2, pp. 189–197, 2006.

[5] I. Flisiak, M. Szterling-Jaworowska, A. Baran, and M. Rogalska-Taranta, "Effect of psoriasis activity on epidermal growth factor (EGF) and the concentration of soluble EGF receptor in serum and plaque scales," *Clinical and Experimental Dermatology*, vol. 39, no. 4, pp. 461–467, 2014.

[6] R. Kucera, I. Treskova, J. Vrzalova et al., "Evaluation of IGF1 serum levels in malignant melanoma and healthy subjects," *Anticancer Research*, vol. 34, no. 9, pp. 5217–5220, 2014.

[7] P. Blair and R. Flaumenhaft, "Platelet alpha-granules: basic biology and clinical correlates," *Blood Reviews*, vol. 23, no. 4, pp. 177–189, 2009.

[8] J. Imanishi, K. Kamiyama, I. Iguchi, M. Kita, C. Sotozono, and S. Kinoshita, "Growth factors: importance in wound healing and maintenance of transparency of the cornea," *Progress in Retinal and Eye Research*, vol. 19, no. 1, pp. 113–129, 2000.

[9] J. K. Lee and T. H. Kim, "Changes in cytokines in tears after endoscopic endonasal dacryocystorhinostomy for primary acquired nasolacrimal duct obstruction," *Eye*, vol. 28, no. 5, pp. 600–607, 2014.

[10] T. L. Moskal, S. Huang, L. M. Ellis, H. A. Fritsche Jr., and S. Chakrabarty, "Serum levels of transforming growth factor alpha in gastrointestinal cancer patients," *Cancer Epidemiology Biomarkers and Prevention*, vol. 4, no. 2, pp. 127–131, 1995.

[11] M. R. De Pascale, L. Sommese, A. Casamassimi, and C. Napoli, "Platelet derivatives in regenerative medicine: an update," *Transfusion Medicine Reviews*, vol. 29, no. 1, pp. 52–61, 2015.

[12] J.-P. Montmayeur, M. Valius, J. Vandenheede, and A. Kazlauskas, "The platelet-derived growth factor beta receptor triggers multiple cytoplasmic signaling cascades that arrive at the nucleus as distinguishable inputs," *The Journal of Biological Chemistry*, vol. 272, no. 51, pp. 32670–32678, 1997.

[13] J. Schechter, M. Wallace, J. Carey, N. Chang, M. Trousdale, and R. Wood, "Corneal insult affects the production and distribution of FGF-2 within the lacrimal gland," *Experimental Eye Research*, vol. 70, no. 6, pp. 777–784, 2000.

[14] E. Anitua, M. Sanchez, J. Merayo-Lloves, M. de La Fuente, F. Muruzabal, and G. Orive, "Plasma rich in growth factors (PRGF-Endoret) stimulates proliferation and migration of primary keratocytes and conjunctival fibroblasts and inhibits and reverts TGF-β1-induced myodifferentiation," *Investigative Ophthalmology & Visual Science*, vol. 52, no. 9, pp. 6066–6073, 2011.

[15] M. E. Fini and B. M. Stramer, "How the cornea heals: cornea-specific repair mechanisms affecting surgical outcomes," *Cornea*, vol. 24, supplement 8, pp. S2–S11, 2005.

[16] J. L. Peterson, E. D. Phelps, M. A. Doll, S. Schaal, and B. P. Ceresa, "The role of endogenous epidermal growth factor receptor ligands in mediating corneal epithelial homeostasis," *Investigative Ophthalmology and Visual Science*, vol. 55, no. 5, pp. 2870–2880, 2014.

[17] F. Castro-Muñozledo, "Review: corneal epithelial stem cells, their niche and wound healing," *Molecular Vision*, vol. 24, no. 19, pp. 1600–1613, 2013.

[18] Q. Li, J. Weng, R. R. Mohan et al., "Hepatocyte growth factor and hepatocyte growth factor receptor in the lacrimal gland, tears, and cornea," *Investigative Ophthalmology & Visual Science*, vol. 37, no. 5, pp. 727–739, 1996.

[19] K. S. Park, S. S. Kim, J. C. Kim et al., "Serum and tear levels of nerve growth factor in diabetic retinopathy patients," *American Journal of Ophthalmology*, vol. 145, no. 3, pp. 432–437, 2008.

[20] G. B. van Setten, S. Macauley, M. Humphreys-Beher et al., "Detection of transforming growth factor-alpha mRNA and protein in rat lacrimal glands and characterization of transforming growth factor-alpha in human tears," *Journal of Physiology and Pharmacology*, vol. 57, no. 2, pp. 189–197, 2006.

[21] G. B. van Setten, "Basic fibroblast growth factor in human tear fluid: detection of another growth factor," *Graefe's Archive for Clinical and Experimental Ophthalmology*, vol. 234, no. 4, pp. 275–277, 1996.

[22] M. Vesaluoma, A. M. Teppo, C. Grönhagen-Riska et al., "Platelet-derived growth factor-BB (PDGF-BB) in tear fluid: a potential modulator of corneal wound healing following photorefractive keratectomy," *Investigative Ophthalmology & Visual Science*, vol. 37, no. 1, pp. 166–173, 1996.

[23] S. E. Wilson and H. D. Perry, "Long-term resolution of chronic dry eye symptoms and signs after topical cyclosporine treatment," *Ophthalmology*, vol. 114, no. 1, pp. 76–79, 2007.

[24] K. Yoshino, R. Garg, D. Monroy, Z. Ji, and S. C. Pflugfelder, "Production and secretion of transforming growth factor beta (TGF-β) by the human lacrimal gland," *Current Eye Research*, vol. 15, no. 6, pp. 615–624, 1996.

[25] B. Klenkler, H. Sheardown, and L. Jones, "Growth factors in the tear film: role in tissue maintenance, wound healing, and ocular pathology," *Ocular Surface*, vol. 5, no. 3, pp. 228–239, 2007.

[26] L. R. Katzman and B. H. Jeng, "Management strategies for persistent epithelial defects of the cornea," *Saudi Journal of Ophthalmology*, vol. 28, no. 3, pp. 168–172, 2014.

[27] C. Cursiefen, "Dry eye," *Der Ophthalmologe*, vol. 110, no. 6, pp. 498–499, 2013.

[28] M. Hessen and E. K. Akpek, "Dry eye: an inflammatory ocular disease," *Journal of Ophthalmic & Vision Research*, vol. 9, no. 2, pp. 240–250, 2014.

[29] M. M. Choudhary, R. A. Hajj-Ali, and C. Y. Lowder, "Gender and ocular manifestations of connective tissue diseases and systemic vasculitides," *Journal of Ophthalmology*, vol. 2014, Article ID 403042, 8 pages, 2014.

[30] C. F. Henrich, P. Y. Ramulu, and E. K. Akpek, "Association of dry eye and inflammatory systemic diseases in a tertiary care-based sample," *Cornea*, vol. 33, no. 8, pp. 819–825, 2014.

[31] M. C. Moura, P. T. S. Zakszewski, M. B. G. Silva, and T. L. Skare, "Epidemiological profile of patients with extra-articular manifestations of rheumatoid arthritis from the city of Curitiba, south of Brazil," *Revista Brasileira de Reumatologia*, vol. 52, no. 5, pp. 679–694, 2012.

[32] S. J. Patel and D. C. Lundy, "Ocular manifestations of autoimmune disease," *American Family Physician Journal*, vol. 66, no. 6, pp. 991–998, 2002.

[33] K. A. Beckman, "Detection of early markers for Sjögren syndrome in dry eye patients," *Cornea*, vol. 33, no. 12, pp. 1262–1264, 2014.

[34] V. Achtsidis, I. Eleftheriadou, E. Kozanidou et al., "Dry eye syndrome in subjects with diabetes and association with neuropathy," *Diabetes Care*, vol. 37, no. 10, pp. e210–e211, 2014.

[35] B. Yañez-Soto, M. J. Mannis, I. R. Schwab et al., "Interfacial phenomena and the ocular surface," *Ocular Surface*, vol. 12, no. 3, pp. 178–201, 2014.

[36] Q. Pan, A. Angelina, A. Zambrano et al., "Autologous serum eye drops for dry eye," *The Cochrane Database of Systematic Reviews*, vol. 8, Article ID CD009327, 2013.

[37] C. G. Begley, R. L. Chalmers, L. Abetz et al., "The relationship between habitual patient-reported symptoms and clinical signs among patients with dry eye of varying severity," *Investigative Ophthalmology & Visual Science*, vol. 44, no. 11, pp. 4753–4761, 2003.

[38] M. S.-B. Zeev, D. D. Miller, and R. Latkany, "Diagnosis of dry eye disease and emerging technologies," *Clinical Ophthalmology*, vol. 8, pp. 581–590, 2014.

[39] B. D. Sullivan, L. A. Crews, E. M. Messmer et al., "Correlations between commonly used objective signs and symptoms for the diagnosis of dry eye disease: clinical implications," *Acta Ophthalmologica*, vol. 92, no. 2, pp. 161–166, 2014.

[40] M. Dogru and K. Tsubota, "Pharmacotherapy of dry eye," *Expert Opinion on Pharmacotherapy*, vol. 12, no. 3, pp. 325–334, 2011.

[41] J. Hefner and H. Reinshagen, "Conservative treatment of dry eye," *Klinische Monatsblätter für Augenheilkunde*, vol. 231, no. 11, pp. 1093–1096, 2014.

[42] V. Valim, V. F. M. Trevisani, J. M. de Sousa, V. S. Vilela, and R. Belfort Jr., "Current approach to dry eye disease," *Clinical Reviews in Allergy & Immunology*, 2014.

[43] R. R. Pfister, "Clinical measures to promote corneal epithelial healing," *Acta Ophthalmologica Supplement*, vol. 202, pp. 73–83, 1992.

[44] K. Tsubota, "Ocular surface treatment before last in situ keratomileusis in patients with severe dry eye," *Journal of Refractive Surgery*, vol. 20, no. 3, pp. 270–275, 2004.

[45] T. G. Coursey and C. S. de Paiva, "Managing Sjögren's syndrome and non-Sjögren syndrome dry eye with anti-inflammatory therapy," *Clinical Ophthalmology*, vol. 8, pp. 1447–1458, 2014.

[46] B. Colligris, A. Crooke, F. Huete-Toral, and J. Pintor, "An update on dry eye disease molecular treatment: advances in drug pipelines," *Expert Opinion on Pharmacotherapy*, vol. 15, no. 10, pp. 1371–1390, 2014.

[47] S. Schrader, T. Wedel, R. Moll, and G. Geerling, "Combination of serum eye drops with hydrogel bandage contact lenses in the treatment of persistent epithelial defects," *Graefe's Archive for Clinical and Experimental Ophthalmology*, vol. 244, no. 10, pp. 1345–1349, 2006.

[48] K.-Y. Wu, H.-Z. Wang, and S.-J. Hong, "Effects of antibiotics and corticosteroid eyedrops on cellular proliferation in cultured human corneal keratocytes," *The Kaohsiung Journal of Medical Sciences*, vol. 22, no. 8, pp. 385–389, 2006.

[49] S. Shi, W. Chen, X. Zhang, H.-X. Ma, and L. Sun, "Effects of silicone punctal plugs for tear deficiency dry eye patients," *Chinese Journal of Ophthalmology*, vol. 49, no. 2, pp. 151–154, 2013.

[50] A.-M. Ervin, R. Wojciechowski, and O. Schein, "Punctal occlusion for dry eye syndrome," *Cochrane Database of Systematic Reviews*, no. 9, Article ID CD006775, 2010.

[51] A. A. Bukhari, "Botulinum neurotoxin type A versus punctal plug insertion in the management of dry eye disease," *Oman Journal of Ophthalmology*, vol. 7, no. 2, pp. 61–65, 2014.

[52] A. Liu and J. Ji, "Omega-3 essential fatty acids therapy for dry eye syndrome: a meta-analysis of randomized controlled studies," *Medical Science Monitor*, vol. 20, pp. 1583–1589, 2014.

[53] A. Oleñik, "Effectiveness and tolerability of dietary supplementation with a combination of omega-3 polyunsaturated fatty acids and antioxidants in the treatment of dry eye symptoms: results of a prospective study," *Clinical Ophthalmology*, vol. 8, pp. 169–176, 2014.

[54] E. Toker and E. Asfuroğlu, "Corneal and conjunctival sensitivity in patients with dry eye: the effect of topical cyclosporine therapy," *Cornea*, vol. 29, no. 2, pp. 133–140, 2010.

[55] A. A. M. Torricelli, M. R. Santhiago, and S. E. Wilson, "Topical cyclosporine A treatment in corneal refractive surgery and patients with dry eye," *Journal of Refractive Surgery*, vol. 30, no. 8, pp. 558–564, 2014.

[56] N. P. Walsh, M. B. Fortes, P. Raymond-Barker et al., "Is whole-body hydration an important consideration in dry eye?" *Investigative Ophthalmology & Visual Science*, vol. 53, no. 10, pp. 6622–6627, 2012.

[57] S. E. Wilson, Q. Liang, and W. J. Kim, "Lacrimal gland HGF, KGF, and EGF mRNA levels increase after corneal epithelial wounding," *Investigative Ophthalmology & Visual Science*, vol. 37, no. 5, pp. 727–739, 1996.

[58] F. N. Syed-Picard, Y. Du, K. L. Lathrop, M. M. Mann, M. L. Funderburgh, and J. L. Funderburgh, "Dental pulp stem cells: a new cellular resource for corneal stromal regeneration," *Stem Cells Translational Medicine*, vol. 4, no. 3, pp. 276–285, 2015.

[59] M. H. Frank and N. Y. Frank, "Restoring the cornea from Limbal stem cells," *Regenerative Medicine*, vol. 10, no. 1, pp. 1–4, 2015.

[60] S. Rauz and V. P. Saw, "Serum eye drops, amniotic membrane and limbal epithelial stem cells—tools in the treatment of ocular surface disease," *Cell and Tissue Banking*, vol. 11, no. 1, pp. 13–27, 2010.

[61] J. M. Lou-Bonafonte, E. Bonafonte-Marquez, S. Bonafonte-Royo, and P. A. Martínez-Carpio, "Posology, efficacy, and safety of epidermal growth factor eye drops in 305 patients: logistic regression and group-wise odds of published data," *Journal of Ocular Pharmacology and Therapeutics*, vol. 28, no. 5, pp. 467–472, 2012.

[62] A. Lambiase, L. Aloe, F. Mantelli et al., "Capsaicin-induced corneal sensory denervation and healing impairment are reversed by NGF treatment," *Investigative Ophthalmology & Visual Science*, vol. 53, no. 13, pp. 8280–8287, 2012.

[63] A. Lambiase, A. Micera, M. Sacchetti, M. Cortes, F. Mantelli, and S. Bonini, "Alterations of tear neuromediators in dry eye disease," *Archives of Ophthalmology*, vol. 129, no. 8, pp. 981–986, 2011.

[64] A. Lambiase, M. Sacchetti, and S. Bonini, "Nerve growth factor therapy for corneal disease," *Current Opinion in Ophthalmology*, vol. 23, no. 4, pp. 296–302, 2012.

[65] M. P. Ferrari, F. Mantelli, M. Sacchetti et al., "Safety and pharmacokinetics of escalating doses of human recombinant nerve growth factor eye drops in a double-masked, randomized clinical trial," *BioDrugs*, vol. 28, no. 3, pp. 275–283, 2014.

[66] M. A. Bermudez, J. Sendon-Lago, N. Eiro et al., "Corneal epithelial wound healing and bactericidal effect of conditioned medium from human uterine cervical stem cells," *Investigative Ophthalmology & Visual Science*, vol. 56, no. 2, pp. 983–992, 2015.

[67] S. L. Watson, G. Geerling, and J. K. G. Dart, "Clinical study of therapeutic ocular surface medium for persistent epithelial defect," *Ophthalmic Research*, vol. 51, no. 2, pp. 82–87, 2014.

[68] A. A. Azari and C. J. Rapuano, "Autologous serum eye drops for the treatment of ocular surface disease," *Eye & Contact Lens*, vol. 41, no. 3, pp. 133–140, 2015.

[69] A. J. Botella, J. F. M. Peiró, K. Márques, N. M. Cambero, and J. S. Otaolaurruchi, "Effectiveness of 100% autologous serum drops in ocular surface disorders," *Farmacia Hospitalaria*, vol. 35, no. 1, pp. 8–13, 2011.

[70] K. M. Kim, Y.-T. Shin, and H. K. Kim, "Effect of autologous platelet-rich plasma on persistent corneal epithelial defect after infectious keratitis," *Japanese Journal of Ophthalmology*, vol. 56, no. 6, pp. 544–550, 2012.

[71] T. Kojima, R. Ishida, M. Dogru et al., "The effect of autologous serum eyedrops in the treatment of severe dry eye disease: a prospective randomized case-control study," *American Journal of Ophthalmology*, vol. 139, no. 2, pp. 242–246, 2005.

[72] Y. Matsumoto, M. Dogru, E. Goto et al., "Autologous serum application in the treatment of neurotrophic keratopathy," *Ophthalmology*, vol. 111, no. 6, pp. 1115–1120, 2004.

[73] K.-S. Na and M. S. Kim, "Allogeneic serum eye drops for the treatment of dry eye patients with chronic graft-versus-host disease," *Journal of Ocular Pharmacology and Therapeutics*, vol. 28, no. 5, pp. 479–483, 2012.

[74] S. Kamal, S. Kumar, and R. Goel, "Autologous serum for anterior tissue necrosis after porous orbital implant," *Middle East African Journal of Ophthalmology*, vol. 21, no. 2, pp. 193–195, 2014.

[75] S. D. Schulze, W. Sekundo, and P. Kroll, "Autologous serum for the treatment of corneal epithelial abrasions in diabetic patients undergoing vitrectomy," *American Journal of Ophthalmology*, vol. 142, no. 2, pp. 207–211, 2006.

[76] L. P.-K. Ang, T. P. Do, Z. M. Thein et al., "Ex vivo expansion of conjunctival and limbal epithelial cells using cord blood serum-supplemented culture medium," *Investigative Ophthalmology & Visual Science*, vol. 52, no. 9, pp. 6138–6147, 2011.

[77] E. Erdem, M. Yagmur, I. Harbiyeli, H. Taylan-Sekeroglu, and R. Ersoz, "Umbilical cord blood serum therapy for the management of persistent corneal epithelial defects," *International Journal of Ophthalmology*, vol. 18, no. 5, pp. 807–810, 2014.

[78] H. M. Reza, B.-Y. Ng, F. L. Gimeno, T. T. Phan, and L. P.-K. Ang, "Umbilical cord lining stem cells as a novel and promising source for ocular surface regeneration," *Stem Cell Reviews and Reports*, vol. 7, no. 4, pp. 935–947, 2011.

[79] C. A. Urzua, D. H. Vasquez, A. Huidobro, H. Hernandez, and J. Alfaro, "Randomized double-blind clinical trial of autologous serum versus artificial tears in dry eye syndrome," *Current Eye Research*, vol. 37, no. 8, pp. 684–688, 2012.

[80] R. A. Ralph, M. G. Doane, and C. H. Dohlman, "Clinical experience with a mobile ocular perfusion pump," *Archives of Ophthalmology*, vol. 93, no. 10, pp. 1039–1043, 1975.

[81] R. I. Fox, R. Chan, J. B. Michelson, J. B. Belmont, and P. E. Michelson, "Beneficial effect of artificial tears made with autologous serum in patients with keratoconjunctivitis sicca," *Arthritis & Rheumatism*, vol. 27, no. 4, pp. 459–461, 1984.

[82] E. Anitua, F. Muruzabal, M. De la Fuente, J. Merayo-Lloves, and G. Orive, "Effects of heat-treatment on plasma rich in growth factors-derived autologous eye drop," *Experimental Eye Research*, vol. 119, pp. 27–34, 2014.

[83] B. H. Jeng and W. J. Dupps Jr., "Autologous serum 50% eye drops in the treatment of persistent corneal epithelial defects," *Cornea*, vol. 28, no. 10, pp. 1104–1108, 2009.

[84] A. Partal and E. Scott, "Low-cost protocol for the production of autologous serum eye drops by blood collection and processing centres for the treatment of ocular surface diseases," *Transfusion Medicine*, vol. 21, no. 4, pp. 271–277, 2011.

[85] H. R. Lee, Y. J. Hong, S. Chung et al., "Proposal of standardized guidelines for the production and quality control of autologous serum eye drops in Korea: based on a nationwide survey," *Transfusion*, vol. 54, no. 7, pp. 1864–1870, 2014.

[86] C.-C. Chiang, J.-M. Lin, W.-L. Chen, and Y.-Y. Tsai, "Allogeneic serum eye drops for the treatment of severe dry eye in patients with chronic graft-versus-host disease," *Cornea*, vol. 26, no. 7, pp. 861–863, 2007.

[87] F. M. C. Medina, R. S. de Castro, S. C. Leite, E. M. Rocha, and G. D. M. Rocha, "Management of dry eye related to systemic diseases in childhood and longterm follow-up," *Acta Ophthalmologica Scandinavica Journal*, vol. 85, no. 7, pp. 739–744, 2007.

[88] Y. K. Cho, W. Huang, G. Y. Kim, and B. S. Lim, "Comparison of autologous serum eye drops with different diluents," *Current Eye Research*, vol. 38, no. 1, pp. 9–17, 2013.

[89] J. S. López-García, I. García-Lozano, L. Rivas, N. Ramírez, R. Raposo, and M. T. Méndez, "Autologous serum eye drops diluted with sodium hyaluronate: clinical and experimental comparative study," *Acta Ophthalmologica*, vol. 92, no. 1, pp. e22–e29, 2014.

[90] C. Yamada, K. E. King, and P. M. Ness, "Autologous serum eyedrops: literature review and implications for transfusion medicine specialists," *Transfusion*, vol. 48, no. 6, pp. 1245–1255, 2008.

[91] F. Semeraro, E. Forbice, O. Braga, A. Bova, A. Di Salvatore, and C. Azzolini, "Evaluation of the efficacy of 50% autologous serum eye drops in different ocular surface pathologies," *BioMed Research International*, vol. 2014, Article ID 826970, 11 pages, 2014.

[92] A. R. C. Celebi, C. Ulusoy, and G. E. Mirza, "The efficacy of autologous serum eye drops for severe dry eye syndrome: a randomized double-blind crossover study," *Graefe's Archive for Clinical and Experimental Ophthalmology*, vol. 252, no. 4, pp. 619–626, 2014.

[93] Y.-M. Chen, F.-R. Hu, J.-Y. Huang, E. P. Shen, T.-Y. Tsai, and W.-L. Chen, "The effect of topical autologous serum on graft

re-epithelialization after penetrating keratoplasty," *American Journal of Ophthalmology*, vol. 150, no. 3, pp. 352.e2–359.e2, 2010.

[94] K. Lekhanont, P. Jongkhajornpong, L. Choubtum, and V. Chuckpaiwong, "Topical 100% serum eye drops for treating corneal epithelial defect after ocular surgery," *BioMed Research International*, vol. 2013, Article ID 521315, 7 pages, 2013.

[95] A. I. Fernando, B. J. L. Burton, G. T. Smith, and M. C. Corbett, "Autologous serum drop-dependent re-epithelialisation following penetrating keratoplasty in chronic graft vs host disease," *Eye*, vol. 19, no. 7, pp. 823–825, 2005.

[96] B. Mixon, J. Mixon, E. K. Isbey et al., "Autologous serum eye drops for severe dry eye syndrome in a patient with chronic graft-versus-host disease: a case report," *International Journal of Pharmaceutical Compounding*, vol. 18, no. 5, pp. 370–377, 2014.

[97] A. Mataftsi, A. Bourtoulamaiou, K. Anastasilakis, N. G. Ziakas, and S. A. Dimitrakos, "Management of bullous keratopathy-related ulcer with autologous serum," *Eye & Contact Lens*, vol. 39, no. 4, pp. e19–e20, 2013.

[98] E. Sanz-Marco, M. J. Lopez-Prats, S. Garcia-Delpech, P. Udaondo, and M. Diaz-Llopis, "Fulminant bilateral *Haemophilus influenzae* keratitis in a patient with hypovitaminosis A treated with contaminated autologous serum," *Clinical Ophthalmology*, vol. 11, no. 5, pp. 71–73, 2011.

[99] S.-W. Moon, D.-J. Yeom, and S.-H. Chung, "Neurotrophic corneal ulcer development following cataract surgery with a limbal relaxing incision," *Korean Journal of Ophthalmology*, vol. 25, no. 3, pp. 210–213, 2011.

[100] P. Lavaju, M. Sharma, A. Sharma, and S. Chettri, "Use of amniotic membrane and autologous serum eye drops in Mooren's ulcer," *Nepalese Journal of Ophthalmology*, vol. 5, no. 1, pp. 120–123, 2013.

[101] J. Hwang, S.-H. Chung, S. Jeon, S.-K. Kwok, S.-H. Park, and M.-S. Kim, "Comparison of clinical efficacies of autologous serum eye drops in patients with primary and secondary Sjögren syndrome," *Cornea*, vol. 33, no. 7, pp. 663–667, 2014.

[102] K. Jirsova, K. Brejchova, I. Krabcova et al., "The application of autologous serum eye drops in severe dry eye patients; subjective and objective parameters before and after treatment," *Current Eye Research*, vol. 39, no. 1, pp. 21–30, 2014.

[103] R. B. Vajpayee, N. Mukerji, R. Tandon et al., "Evaluation of umbilical cord serum therapy for persistent corneal epithelial defects," *British Journal of Ophthalmology*, vol. 87, no. 11, pp. 1312–1316, 2003.

[104] K. C. Yoon, "Use of umbilical cord serum in ophthalmology," *Chonnam Medical Journal*, vol. 50, no. 3, pp. 82–85, 2014.

[105] E. Turkoglu, E. Celik, and G. Alagoz, "A comparison of the efficacy of autologous serum eye drops with amniotic membrane transplantation in neurotrophic keratitis," *Seminars in Ophthalmology*, vol. 29, no. 3, pp. 119–126, 2014.

[106] A. Erices, P. Conget, and J. J. Minguell, "Mesenchymal progenitor cells in human umbilical cord blood," *British Journal of Haematology*, vol. 109, no. 1, pp. 235–242, 2000.

[107] P.-F. Choong, P.-L. Mok, S.-K. Cheong, and K.-Y. Then, "Mesenchymal stromal cell-like characteristics of corneal keratocytes," *Cytotherapy*, vol. 9, no. 3, pp. 252–258, 2007.

[108] M. W. Varner, N. E. Marshall, D. J. Rouse et al., "The association of cord serum cytokines with neurodevelopmental outcomes," *American Journal of Perinatology*, vol. 30, no. 2, pp. 115–122, 2015.

[109] K.-C. Yoon, H. Heo, S.-K. Im, I.-C. You, Y.-H. Kim, and Y.-G. Park, "Comparison of autologous serum and umbilical cord serum eye drops for dry eye syndrome," *American Journal of Ophthalmology*, vol. 144, no. 1, pp. 86.e2–92.e2, 2007.

[110] P. Versura, M. Buzzi, G. Giannaccare et al., "Cord blood serum-based eye drops: the impact of donor haematological and obstetric factors on the variability of epidermal growth factor levels," *Blood Transfusion*, vol. 12, supplement 1, pp. s44–s50, 2014.

[111] P. Versura, V. Profazio, M. Buzzi et al., "Efficacy of standardized and quality-controlled cord blood serum eye drop therapy in the healing of severe corneal epithelial damage in dry eye," *Cornea*, vol. 32, no. 4, pp. 412–418, 2013.

[112] N. Sharma, M. Goel, T. Velpandian, J. S. Titiyal, R. Tandon, and R. B. Vajpayee, "Evaluation of umbilical cord serum therapy in acute ocular chemical burns," *Investigative Ophthalmology & Visual Science*, vol. 52, no. 2, pp. 1087–1092, 2011.

[113] S. Sriram, D. J. Gibson, P. Robinson et al., "Assessment of anti-scarring therapies in ex vivo organ cultured rabbit corneas," *Experimental Eye Research*, vol. 125, pp. 173–182, 2014.

[114] K.-C. Yoon, H.-J. Oh, J.-W. Park, and J. Choi, "Application of umbilical cord serum eyedrops after laser epithelial keratomileusis," *Acta Ophthalmologica*, vol. 91, no. 1, pp. e22–e28, 2013.

[115] M. A. Arain, A. J. Dar, and L. Adeeb, "Autologous serum eye drops for the treatment of persistent corneal epithelial defects," *Journal of the College of Physicians and Surgeons Pakistan*, vol. 23, no. 10, pp. 737–739, 2013.

Preservation of the Photoreceptor Inner/Outer Segment Junction in Dry Age-Related Macular Degeneration Treated by Rheohemapheresis

Eva Rencová,[1] Milan Bláha,[2] Jan Studnička,[1] Vladimír Bláha,[3] Miriam Lánská,[2] Ondřej Renc,[4] Alexander Stepanov,[1] Věra Kratochvílová,[1] and Hana Langrová[1]

[1]*Department of Ophthalmology, Lékařská Fakulta, Fakultní Nemocnice, Sokolská 581, 500 09 Hradec Králové, Czech Republic*
[2]*Fourth Department of Internal Medicine–Hematology, Lékařská Fakulta, Fakultní Nemocnice, Sokolská 581, 500 09 Hradec Králové, Czech Republic*
[3]*Department of Gerontology and Metabolic Care, Lékařská Fakulta, Fakultní Nemocnice, Sokolská 581, 500 09 Hradec Králové, Czech Republic*
[4]*Department of Radiology, Lékařská Fakulta, Fakultní Nemocnice, Sokolská 581, 500 09 Hradec Králové, Czech Republic*

Correspondence should be addressed to Milan Bláha; blaham@email.cz

Academic Editor: Bartosz Sikorski

Aim. To evaluate the long-term effect of rheohemapheresis (RHF) treatment of age-related macular degeneration (AMD) on photoreceptor IS/OS junction status. *Methods.* In our study, we followed 24 patients with dry AMD and drusenoid retinal pigment epithelium detachment (DPED) for a period of more than 2.5 years. Twelve patients (22 eyes) were treated by RHF and 12 controls (18 eyes) were randomized. The treated group underwent 8 RHF standardized procedures. We evaluated best-corrected visual acuity, IS/OS junction status (SD OCT), and macular function (multifocal electroretinography) at baseline and at 2.5-year follow-up. *Results.* RHF caused a decrease of whole-blood viscosity/plasma viscosity at about 15/12%. BCVA of treated patients increased insignificantly ($P = 0.187$) from median 74.0 letters (56.2 to 81.3 letters) to median 79.0 letters (57.3 to 83.4 letters), but it decreased significantly from 74.0 letters (25.2 to 82.6 letters) to 72.5 letters (23.4 to 83.1 letters) in the control group ($P = 0.041$). The mfERG responses in the region of eccentricity between 1.8° and 7° were significantly higher in treated patients ($P = 0.04$). *Conclusions.* RHF contributed to sparing of photoreceptor IS/OS junction integrity in the fovea, which is assumed to be a predictive factor for preservation of visual acuity.

1. Introduction

Retinal changes associated with the development of age-related macular degeneration (AMD) have become even more important than once described [1]. Even prompt therapy of the wet form of AMD with antivascular, endothelial, growth factor drugs has been shown to ameliorate vision loss [2]. If diagnosis is established earlier—during the dry form of AMD, there is a better chance that visual acuity can be maintained. However, treatment options are still limited at this stage.

Rheohemapheresis (formally known as rheopheresis) has been investigated over the past decade as a possible method of positively affecting AMD in its dry-form stage. Rheohemapheresis is a method of double plasma filtration performed in order to eliminate high-molecular-weight substances—especially proteins such as fibrinogen, α_2-macroglobulin, immunoglobulin M (IgM), thrombomodulin, and low-density (LDL) cholesterol [3–6]. This method leads to the improvement of rheological parameters (reduction of plasma and whole blood viscosity), as well as the improvement of erythrocyte aggregation and their flexibility [6, 7]. It can also lead to a significant improvement of blood flow in the choroid, which is reduced in patients with AMD. Therefore, visual functions can improve [3, 7–9].

When treating our patients suffering from the dry form of AMD accompanied by reticular drusen or even drusenoid detachment of the retinal pigment epithelium, we noticed positive morphological changes of the retina after rheohemapheresis treatment, including the preservation of the photoreceptor inner/outer segment (IS/OS) junction, as well as stabilisation or even improvement of retinal function: best-corrected visual acuity (BCVA) and electroretinography results. A description of the above changes and their correlation is the subject of this work.

2. Methods and Subjects of the Study

At our department, we have seven years of experience in treating AMD using rheohemapheresis. So far, 61 patients with the dry form of AMD, soft drusen, confluent soft drusen, and drusenoid pigment epithelium detachment (DPED) have been treated. We perform long-term monitoring of morphological and functional changes in the retina [12, 13].

The interrelationship of morphological changes in the photoreceptor inner and outer segment (IS/OS) junction retinal layer as well as changes in visual acuity and retinal function (electroretinography) was evaluated in the group of 24 patients (40 eyes) who were long-term followed (for 2.5 years or longer). All patients had the dry form of AMD with the presence of drusenoid pigment epithelium detachment. Twelve of these patients (22 eyes) with an average age of 64.3 years (range: 64–83 years) were treated with RHF. Twelve controls (18 eyes) with an average age of 65.6 years (range: 64–83 years) were randomized. Ophthalmologic inclusion criteria were high-risk, preangiogenic form of AMD with soft drusen, reticular drusen, confluent soft drusen, and DPED— in accordance with the EUREYE Study [14]—and ability to complete the series of 8 rheohemapheresis procedures within 10 weeks. Exclusion criteria were any retinal or choroidal disorders other than AMD, optic nerve disorders, glaucoma, conditions limiting the examination of the fundus, and acute bleeding in the studied eye. General exclusion criteria for rheohemapheresis treatment were the usual exclusion criteria of extracorporeal circulation or therapeutic hemapheresis and the absence of peripheral veins suitable for establishing an extracorporeal circuit.

Rheohemapheresis was performed in the treatment group, as described in detail in our previous work [3, 13]. After plasma separation (blood-cell separator, COBE Spectra or Optia, Terumo, Lakewood, CO, USA), the separated plasma was pumped through the rheofilter (Evaflux, Kawasumi, Tokyo, Japan) to remove high-molecular-weight factors. Using this filter, we repeatedly (8 times over the period of 10 weeks) removed a precisely defined spectrum of high-molecular-weight substances, such as fibrinogen, LDL cholesterol, and α_2-macroglobulin, from the blood of the patient, thus reducing blood viscosity in an attempt to improve the perfusion of the retina and the choroid.

Fundus photography and fluorescein angiography were performed using a digital fundus camera (Zeiss FF 450, Jena, Germany). The DPED area was measured in mm^2 by fundus photography using VISUPAC software (Zeiss Meditec AG, Jena, Germany), which is acceptable for measuring the area of retinal affections [15]. Spectral domain- (SD-) OCT (Cirrus HD-OCT, Zeiss Meditec, Jena, Germany) with an axial resolution of 6 μm was used to evaluate central retinal thickness. Thickness in the central point of the 1 mm fixation zone was evaluated using 6 radial scans. SD-OCT enabled us to distinguish between DPED and the vascular type of retinal pigment epithelium detachment. A detailed image of the photoreceptor IS/OS junction was obtained using a 5-line raster scan, which precisely shows the shape, coherence, and defects of the photoreceptor IS/OS junction as well as the detachment of this layer from the retinal pigment epithelium (RPE). See Figure 1.

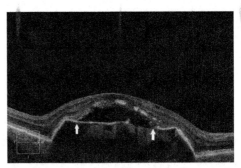

FIGURE 1: SD-OCT of a patient from the control group—preangiogenic dry from of AMD. SD-OCT of the right eye of a patient from the control group with the dry form of AMD 2.5 years after the start of follow-up, showing persistent DPED. DPED symmetrically transitions into the detachment of the IS/OS photoreceptor junction, localized between the two arrows, where the beginning and end of junction detachment are indicated. In addition, the detached IS/OS photoreceptor junction shows uneven reflectivity and thickness of the retinal layer, a sign of incipient degenerative changes of the IS/OS junction, which are considered to be the result of the lack of junction nutrition due to its increased distance from the RPE [10, 11].

Multifocal ERG (mfERG; RETI-port plus mfERG System, Roland Consult GmbH, Brandenburg, Germany) was performed according to the standards of the International Society for Clinical Electroretinography and Vision (ISCEV) [16, 17]. mfERG traces were recorded from the central 60° of the retina using a resolution of 61-scaled hexagons. We evaluated the amplitudes of the positive peak component from the first-order kernel analysis of the central element, representing the foveal response (0°–1.8°) of the four rings centered on the fovea: 1st ring (1.8°–7.0°), 2nd ring (5°–13°), 3rd ring (11°–22°), and 4th ring (17°–30°). All examinations were performed at baseline and at 2.5-year follow-up.

For statistical analysis, we used nonparametric tests (the Kruskal-Wallis test, Mann-Whitney U test, and chi-square approximation). The study protocol was approved by the Institutional Ethics Committee and the reported investigations were in accordance with the principles of the current version of the Helsinki Declaration.

3. Results

3.1. BCVA. BCVA was evaluated as the number of correctly read ETDRS letters. Median best-corrected visual acuity (BCVA) before rheohemapheresis in the treatment group was

74.0 letters (56.2 to 81.3 letters; 95% CI) and increased to 79.0 letters (57.3 to 83.4 letters; 95% CI), ($P = 0.187$) after 2.5 years. In the control group, mean BCVA decreased from 74.0 letters (25.2 to 82.6 letters; 95% CI) at baseline to 72.5 letters (23.4 to 83.1 letters) after 2.5 years ($P = 0.041$). While the difference in BCVA between the treatment groups was insignificant at baseline ($P = 0.457$), BCVA was significantly higher in the treatment group after 2.5 years ($P = 0.021$).

3.2. DPED.

At baseline, mean DPED was 3.68 ± 4.45 mm^2 in treated patients and 4.12 ± 6.64 mm^2 in controls, reaching the central fovea in all cases. After 2.5 years, the mean DPED area decreased significantly to 0.71 ± 1.27 mm^2 in the rheohemapheresis group ($P < 0.001$), whereas it increased significantly to 9.19 ± 9.51 mm^2 in the controls ($P < 0.01$). The differences in size of the DPED area were only insignificant at baseline ($P = 0.605$) and significant after 2.5 years ($P < 0.001$). Reduction of the size of the DPED area after rheohemapheresis was found in 19/22 rheohemapheresis-treated eyes (86.4%), as opposed to only 3/18 eyes (16.7%) in the control group. Enlargement of the DPED area occurred as part of the natural progress of AMD over the same period of 2.5 years in 15/18 (83.3%) eyes in the control group, compared to only 3/22 eyes (13.6%) of treated patients.

3.3. IS/OS Receptor Junction

3.3.1. At the Beginning of Follow-Up.
The study and control groups were comparable.

(i) In the group of treated patients, the photoreceptor IS/OS junction was attached to the DPED in 6/22 (27.3%) eyes. (DPED was accompanied by a detachment of the photoreceptor IS/OS junction in the remaining 16/22 eyes, i.e., 72.7%, without defect in 15/22 eyes and with defect in 1 eye).

(ii) In the control group, the photoreceptor IS/OS junction was attached to the DPED in 6/18 (33.3%) (DPED was accompanied by a detachment of the photoreceptor IS/OS junction in the remaining 12/18 eyes (66.6%), without defect in 4 eyes and with defect in 8 eyes).

3.3.2. At the End of Follow-Up

(1) The Group of Patients. In the group of treated patients, where the photoreceptor IS/OS junction was intact in 6/22 (27.3%) eyes, it remained without defect even after 2.5 years.

Attachment of the originally detached IS/OS junction occurred in 16 eyes. However, in 7 cases of the attached IS/OS junction, there was a certain residual defect. In one additional eye with the IS/OS junction at baseline, the defect of this layer significantly improved after attachment.

Summary. Overall, IS/OS junction defects were demonstrated in 8/22 eyes (31.8%). Defects reached the central foveola in 4

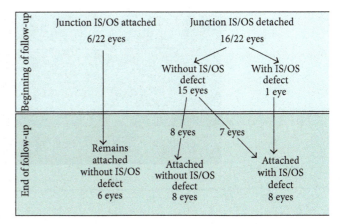

SCHEME 1: Follow-up results of patients treated with RHF.

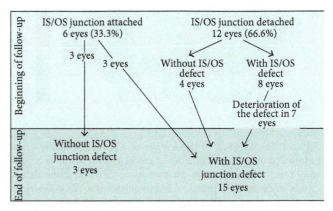

SCHEME 2: Follow-up results in the control group.

eyes (8.8%), thus negatively affecting photoreceptor function and vision. See Scheme 1.

(2) In the Control Group. Integrity of the IS/OS junction layer was preserved in only 3/18 eyes (16.7%) after 2.5 years and IS/OS junction defects were diagnosed in 15/18 eyes (83.3%), 12 of which reached the foveolar region and adversely affected vision. See Scheme 2.

(3) Transition into the Wet Form of AMD. It is important to note that none of the treated patients progressed into the wet form during the 2.5-year follow-up. In the control group, 6 eyes with detachment of the IS/OS junction at baseline developed choroidal neovascularization (CNV) (confirmed by fluorescein angiography).

3.4. Multifocal ERG.

The amplitudes of foveal responses and responses in the most peripheral areas of the retina, as shown on the multifocal ERG, changed only slightly during the entire follow-up period in both groups of patients. In the parafoveal and paramacular regions of eccentricity between 1.8° and 13°, we only found an insignificant increase of activity in treated patients. Activity in the same region decreased slightly in the control group. The differences were statistically nonsignificant between groups of patients in both periods

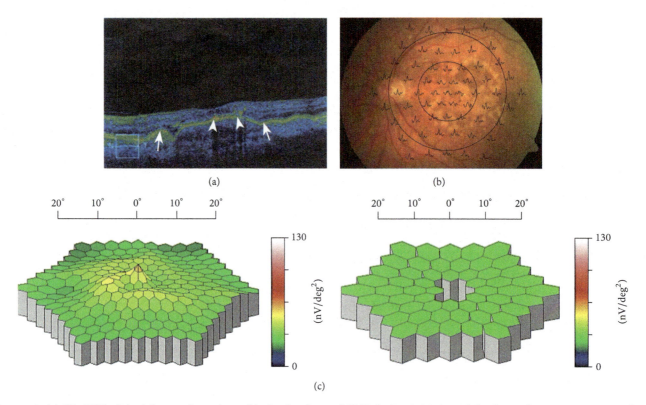

FIGURE 2: (a) SD-OCT of the left eye of a patient with the dry form of AMD before initiation of rheohemapheresis treatment. A large photoreceptor IS/OS junction defect marked by arrows at its beginning and end. Only the top of the surface DPED under the central foveola shows remnants of previous photoreceptor IS/OS junction detachment (indicated by arrowheads) in the form of degraded degenerated material of the original junction. The photoreceptor IS/OS junction is normally attached to the RPE only peripherally from the arrows. Visual acuity at this stage was 20/80 (0.25). (b) Multifocal electroretinography. Superposition of mfERG responses to the fundus of the left eye of the patient from (a). (c) A three-dimensional image of the electrical activity of the retina. Left: A three-dimensional image of the electrical activity of the retina of the left eye of the patient from (a) and (b) compared to the normal-for-age image on the right (decrease of foveal and parafoveal responses below the normal range, i.e., grey-colored central depressions bordered by green, i.e., within normal range responses).

of examination, except for the activity in the region of eccentricity between 1.8° and 7°, which was significantly higher in treated patients ($P = 0.04$) at 2.5-year follow-up. The implicit times of the majority of responses increased after 2.5 years in all patients. At baseline, they were significantly longer in the controls (P values ranging from < 0.05 to < 0.01), with the exception of the foveal response. At 2.5 years, the foveal response was significantly longer in the control group ($P = 0.035$).

In general, retinal activity remained stable or even improved in treated patients with early decrease or complete disappearance of DPED and detachment of the photoreceptor IS/OS junction, along with preservation of its integrity or development of only small defects in the parafoveal region (Figures 2(a), 2(b), 2(c), 3(b), and 3(c)). In contrast, in patients with long-lasting or persistent DPED with detachment of the IS/OS junction and development of its defects or even development of CNV, retinal activity was even reduced.

4. Discussion

The photoreceptor IS/OS junction layer is currently receiving attention from many researchers [10, 18–22]. According to Baba et al. [19], the state of this thin hyper-reflective layer, which lies above the RPE layer, directly correlates with BCVA after successful macular hole repair. BCVA deterioration has proved to be an early indicator of transformation to the wet form of AMD [1]. We have verified the direct correlation of the state of the IS/OS photoreceptor junction and BCVA on patients with Stargardt disease [18]. Disruption of the IS/OS junction is associated with poor vision in uveitic macular edema and retinitis pigmentosa [22, 23].

As a result of our findings, we can add the IS/OS junction as another indicator of the risk of transformation to the wet form of AMD. The detachment of the photoreceptor IS/OS junction (Figure 1) is usually located at the top of the area affected by drusenoid retinal pigment epithelium detachment (DPED). Sikorski et al. found that rupture of IS/OS photoreceptor junction detachment is directly associated with the emergence of submacular neovascularization [10]. Schuman et al. reported thinning of the IS/OS photoreceptor layer and the progress of its changes over drusen and DPED [20].

In the present study, we found reattachment of the photoreceptor IS/OS junction layer in the study group. After the 2.5-year follow-up, 8 eyes were reattached without IS/OS junction defect after RHF; the IS/OS junction defect was

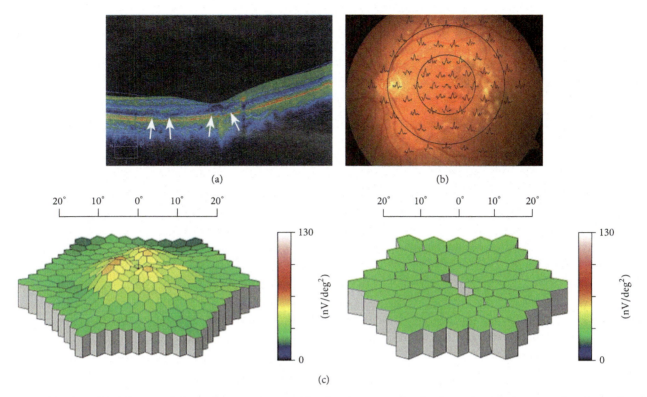

Figure 3: (a) SD-OCT of the same left eye shown in Figure 2(a), taken 2.5 years after rheohemapheresis treatment. Dry form of AMD. In addition to the perfect attachment of the original DPED, there is evident attachment and restoration of the previously detached and degeneratively damaged photoreceptor IS/OS junction, with the exception of two small defects in the central fovea and to the left of it (these defects are located between both the left and right pair of arrows). To the right of the central defect, there is also a small portion of the IS/OS junction which is not visible because it becomes a part of the vertically oriented optical shadow under a dense particle. The remainder of the original junction degeneration is offset towards the inner part of the retina into its plexiform layer. The abovementioned vertical optical shadow does not preclude the presence of the junction section already attached to its intact neighboring sections. Clear morphologic rectification of the position and structure of the photoreceptor IS/OS junction corresponds to the restoration of visual acuity of this eye (BCVA 20/25 (0.8) and improvement of mfERG). (b) Multifocal electroretinogram—responses after RHF. Superposition of mfERG responses to the fundus of the left eye of the patient from (a). (c) A three-dimensional image of the electrical activity of the retina after RHF. Left: A three-dimensional image of the electrical activity of the retina of the left eye of the patient from (a) with increased parafoveal activity, compared to the normal-for-age image on the right (increase of parafoveal activity moves back into the normal range, illustrated by the change from grey depressions to green columns in the parafoveal region).

partially reattached in another 8 of the treated eyes. However, in only 4 of these eyes (18.1% of the entire sample), the defect reached the central fovea. The fact that, after rheohemapheresis, patients only rarely developed the photoreceptor IS/OS junction defect affecting the central foveola and that mean visual acuity actually slightly improved in the majority of these patients is considered an obvious interdependence.

In control patients, we did not observe full restoration (reattachment) of a photoreceptor IS/OS junction layer when detached at the baseline. Drusenoid retinal pigment epithelium detachment usually progresses (which was observed in 7 eyes); otherwise, rupture occurs—caused by submacular neovascularization development, as has also been observed by other authors [24, 25]. The photoreceptor IS/OS junction layer rupture is usually apparent in patients with neovascularization. The remaining fluid as well as the fluid under the detached drusenoid retinal pigment epithelium then spreads into the inner retinal layers and can cause macular edema.

In the control group, we observed 6 cases (33.3%) of submacular choroidal neovascularization. The following is one possible mechanism of its development: the existing DPED was later accompanied by a detached layer adjoined to it from above (i.e., by detachment of the photoreceptor IS/OS junction). DPED and IS/OS layer detachment gradually grew in size and eventually ruptured due to the development of submacular choroidal neovascularization. As evidence of progression to the wet form of AMD, fluid inside and underneath the inner retinal layer appeared on SD-OCT. These findings are supported by the findings of occult submacular choroidal neovascularization using fluorescein angiography.

Patients with preservation of photoreceptor IS/OS junction integrity or development of only small, paracentral defects by early decrease or complete disappearance of the DPED area also exhibited slightly increased retinal activity, which led to significantly higher parafoveal activity in treated patients using mfERG (see Section 3.4). We found a significantly higher amplitude of parafoveal responses in eccentricity between 1.8° and 7° in treated patients 2.5 years after initiation of the treatment ($P = 0.04$). In contrast, in patients with development of IS/OS junction defects or even progression of the disease to its wet form, central retinal activity and visual acuity were even reduced. Development of photoreceptor IS/OS junction defects in the control group probably contributed to the slight decrease of electrical retinal activity in the parafoveal and paramacular regions of eccentricity between 1.8° and 13° using mfERG. This may be due to the long-term accumulation of fluid between the RPE and IS/OS junctions, which causes "stretching" of photoreceptor outer segments, thus leading to their malfunction even without the development of associated RPE atrophy [10]. Insignificant changes of foveal activity could result from the greater vulnerability of foveal cones.

Our study has some limitations. The question of treating the dry form of AMD by rheohemapheresis has not yet been fully answered. Case series, two controlled trials and five completed randomized controlled trials, have reported the efficacy of rheohemapheresis in treating dry AMD [6]. These studies (inclusive of our two [3, 26]) have shown an improvement in the number of lines that can be read on ETDRS charts, improvement in the Pepper Visual Skills for reading tests, a decrease in viscosity parameters, shortening of arteriovenous passage times, and improvement in electroretinograms. The studies have shown improvements shortly after completion of treatment, lasting up to four years [6, 18]. Considerable confusion has been aroused by the preliminary results from the Mira 1 study—an extensive, sham-controlled, randomized, multicenter trial conducted in the USA. Its encouraging first results were later challenged and a clear positive effect was not proved [27, 28]. However, analysis revealed that 37% of treated patients and 29% of control patients were protocol violators who did not fulfill the trial's inclusion criteria of AMD leading to bias in the study's final outcome. Excluding those subjects who had vision loss due to other causes, this trial demonstrated significant improvement with treatment but the trial was underpowered by US FDA licensure. The largest controlled trial to date was conducted by the RheoNet registry. Two hundred and seventy-nine patients with dry AMD were treated and compared to 55 untreated controls. In the treated group, visual acuity gain greater than or equal to one ETDRS line was seen in 42% compared to an improvement in 26% of controls. Vision loss greater than or equal to one ETDRS line was seen in 17% of the treated patients versus 40% of controls. These were statistically significant differences. The ASFA (American Society for Apheresis) issues directives (guidelines) for individual procedures in various diseases; according to the latest criteria from 2013, rheohemapheresis is newly classified as a category IB treatment (first line therapy) [6].

The second limitation of this study is obviously the small number of patients, despite the relatively long follow-up. The clinical impression of the importance of the IS/OS layer was established at the beginning of our research 7 years ago, but only patients with follow-up times longer than 2.5 years, that is, in the case of 40 eyes (22 eyes in the study group and 18 control eyes), were randomized for assessment of morphological and functional changes to the IS/OS layer. Our results will need to be confirmed on a larger number of patients in the future.

5. Conclusion

With the use of rheohemapheresis, preservation of photoreceptor IS/OS junction layer coherence in the fovea of patients with high-risk dry AMD can be achieved, even when drusenoid retinal pigment epithelium detachment is already present. After rheohemapheresis, there was a significant morphological improvement of the damaged IS/OS layer, as evidenced by reduction of the scope of the defect or reattachment of the detached IS/OS layer either with or even without the defect of this layer. After 2.5 years of follow-up, better visual acuity, reduced DPED size, and improvement of some functional parameters (electroretinography findings) were observed in the study group.

Conflict of Interests

The authors declare that there is no conflict of interests regarding the publication of this paper.

Acknowledgment

This research was supported by the grant of the Ministry of Health, Czech Republic, no. NT14037-3/2013.

References

[1] T. R. Friberg, R. A. Bilonick, and P. M. Brennen, "Risk factors for conversion to neovascular age-related macular degeneration based on longitudinal morphologic and visual acuity data," *Ophthalmology*, vol. 119, no. 7, pp. 1432–1437, 2012.

[2] U. Chakravarthy, A. P. Adamis, E. T. Cunningham Jr. et al., "Year 2 efficacy results of 2 randomized controlled clinical trials of pegaptanib for neovascular age-related macular degeneration," *Ophthalmology*, vol. 113, no. 9, pp. 1508.e1–1508.e25, 2006.

[3] E. Rencová, M. Bláha, J. Studnička et al., "Haemorheopheresis could block the progression of the dry form of age-related macular degeneration with soft drusen to the neovascular form," *Acta Ophthalmologica*, vol. 89, no. 5, pp. 463–471, 2011.

[4] H. Borberg, "26 years of LDL—apheresis: a review of experience," *Transfusion and Apheresis Science*, vol. 41, no. 1, pp. 49–59, 2009.

[5] R. Klingel, C. Fassbender, T. Faßbender, and B. Göhlen, "Clinical studies to implement Rheopheresis for age-related macular degeneration guided by evidence-based-medicine," *Transfusion and Apheresis Science*, vol. 29, no. 1, pp. 71–84, 2003.

[6] J. Schwartz, J. L. Winters, A. Padmanabhan et al., "Guidelines on the use of therapeutic apheresis in clinical practice-evidence-based approach from the Writing Committee of the American Society for Apheresis: the sixth special issue," *Journal of Clinical Apheresis*, vol. 28, no. 3, pp. 145–284, 2013.

[7] M. Bláha, E. Rencová, and H. Langrová, "The importance of rheological parameters in the therapy of the dry form of age-related macular degeneration with rheohaemapheresis," *Clinical Hemorheology and Microcirculation*, vol. 50, no. 4, pp. 245–255, 2012.

[8] R. Klingel, C. Fassbender, A. Heibges et al., "RheoNet registry analysis of rheopheresis for microcirculatory disorders with a focus on age-related macular degeneration," *Therapeutic Apheresis and Dialysis*, vol. 14, no. 3, pp. 276–286, 2010.

[9] M. J. Koss, P. Kurz, T. Tsobanelis et al., "Prospective, randomized, controlled clinical study evaluating the efficacy of Rheopheresis for dry age-related macular degeneration. Dry AMD treatment with Rheopheresis Trial-ART," *Graefe's Archive for Clinical and Experimental Ophthalmology*, vol. 247, no. 10, pp. 1297–1306, 2009.

[10] B. L. Sikorski, D. Bukowska, J. J. Kaluzny, M. Szkulmowski, A. Kowalczyk, and M. Wojtkowski, "Drusen with accompanying fluid underneath the sensory retina," *Ophthalmology*, vol. 118, no. 1, pp. 82–92, 2011.

[11] B. Kousal, J. Záhlava, S. Vejvalková et al., "Molecular-genetic cause and clinical feature in two patients with Stargardt disease," *Česká a Slovenská Oftalmologie*, vol. 70, no. 6, pp. 228–233, 2014.

[12] J. Studnička, E. Rencová, M. Bláha et al., "Long-term outcomes of rheohaemapheresis in the treatment of dry form of age-related macular degeneration," *Journal of Ophthalmology*, vol. 2013, Article ID 135798, 8 pages, 2013.

[13] M. Blaha, E. Rencova, H. Langrova et al., "Rheohaemapheresis in the treatment of nonvascular age-related macular degeneration," *Atherosclerosis Supplements*, vol. 14, no. 1, pp. 179–184, 2013.

[14] C. A. Augood, J. R. Vingerling, P. T. de Jong et al., "Prevalence of age-related maculopathy in older Europeans: the European Eye Study (EUREYE)," *Archives of Ophthalmology*, vol. 124, no. 4, pp. 529–535, 2006.

[15] J. E. Grunwald, E. Daniel, G. Ying et al., "Photographic assessment of baseline fundus morphologic features in the Comparison of Age-Related Macular Degeneration Treatments Trials," *Ophthalmology*, vol. 119, no. 8, pp. 1634–1641, 2012.

[16] M. F. Marmor, D. C. Hood, D. Keating et al., "Guidelines for basic multifocal electroretinography (mfERG)," *Documenta Ophthalmologica*, vol. 106, no. 2, pp. 105–115, 2003.

[17] D. C. Hood, M. Bach, M. Brigell et al., "ISCEV guidelines for clinical multifocal electroretinography (2007 edition)," *Documenta Ophthalmologica*, vol. 116, no. 1, pp. 1–11, 2008.

[18] E. Rencová, J. Studnicka, J. Marák, H. Dvoráková, and H. Langrová, "The coincidence of the junction layer of inner and outer photoreceptors segments (IS/OS) defects localization on SD OCT and functional defects in case of Stargardt disease—a case report," *Česká a slovenská oftalmologie*, vol. 68, no. 2, pp. 84–86, 2012.

[19] T. Baba, S. Yamamoto, M. Arai et al., "Correlation of visual recovery and presence of photoreceptor inner/outer segment junction in optical coherence images after successful macular hole repair," *Retina*, vol. 28, no. 3, pp. 453–458, 2008.

[20] J. S. Schuman, C. A. Puliafito, and J. G. Fujimoto, *Optical Coherence Tomography in Ocular Diseases*, Slack Inc, Thorofare, NJ, USA, 2nd edition, 2004.

[21] Y. Mitamura, K. Hirano, T. Baba, and S. Yamamoto, "Correlation of visual recovery with presence of photoreceptor inner/outer segment junction in optical coherence images after epiretinal membrane surgery," *British Journal of Ophthalmology*, vol. 93, no. 2, pp. 171–175, 2009.

[22] L. Iannetti, G. Spinucci, A. Abbouda, D. De Geronimo, P. Tortorella, and M. Accorinti, "Spectral-domain optical coherence tomography in uveitic macular edema: morphological features and prognostic factors," *Ophthalmologica*, vol. 228, no. 1, pp. 13–18, 2012.

[23] S. Aizawa, Y. Mitamura, A. Hagiwara, T. Sugawara, and S. Yamamoto, "Changes of fundus autofluorescence, photoreceptor inner and outer segment junction line, and visual function in patients with retinitis pigmentosa," *Clinical & Experimental Ophthalmology*, vol. 38, no. 6, pp. 597–604, 2010.

[24] W. Roquet, F. Roudot-Thoraval, G. Coscas, and G. Soubrane, "Clinical features of drusenoid pigment epithelial detachment in age related macular degeneration," *British Journal of Ophthalmology*, vol. 88, no. 5, pp. 638–642, 2004.

[25] F. Alten, C. R. Clemens, C. Milojcic, and N. Eter, "Subretinal drusenoid deposits associated with pigment epithelium detachment in age-related macular degeneration," *Retina*, vol. 32, no. 9, pp. 1727–1732, 2012.

[26] M. Bláha, E. Rencová, J. Studnicka et al., "Cascade filtration in the therapy of the dry form of age-related macular degeneration," *Therapeutic Apheresis and Dialysis*, vol. 13, no. 5, pp. 453–454, 2009.

[27] J. S. Pulido, J. L. Winters, and D. Boyer, "Preliminary analysis of the final multicenter investigation of rheopheresis for age related macular degeneration (AMD) trial (MIRA-1) results," *Transactions of the American Ophthalmological Society*, vol. 104, pp. 221–231, 2006.

[28] J. Pulido, D. Sanders, J. L. Winters, and R. Klingel, "Clinical outcomes and mechanism of action for rheopheresis treatment of age-related macular degeneration (AMD)," *Journal of Clinical Apheresis*, vol. 20, no. 3, pp. 185–194, 2005.

One-Year Results of Simultaneous Topography-Guided Photorefractive Keratectomy and Corneal Collagen Cross-Linking in Keratoconus Utilizing a Modern Ablation Software

A. M. Sherif, M. A. Ammar, Y. S. Mostafa, S. A. Gamal Eldin, and A. A. Osman

Department of Ophthalmology, Faculty of Medicine, Cairo University, Cairo 12411, Egypt

Correspondence should be addressed to A. M. Sherif; asherif1975@yahoo.com

Academic Editor: David P. Piñero

Purpose. To evaluate effectiveness of simultaneous topography-guided photorefractive keratectomy and corneal collagen cross-linking in mild and moderate keratoconus. *Methods.* Prospective nonrandomized interventional study including 20 eyes of 14 patients with grade 1-2 keratoconus that underwent topography-guided PRK using a Custom Ablation Transition Zone (CATz) profile with 0.02% MMC application immediately followed by standard 3 mw/cm^2 UVA collagen cross-linking. Maximum ablation depth did not exceed 58 μm. Follow-up period: 12 months. *Results.* Progressive statistically significant improvement of UCVA from 0.83 ± 0.37 logMAR preoperative, reaching 0.25 ± 0.26 logMAR at 12 months ($P < 0.001$). Preoperative BCVA (0.27 ± 0.31 logMAR) showed a progressive improvement reaching 0.08 ± 0.12 logMAR at 12 months ($P = 0.02$). Mean Kmax reduced from 48.9 ± 2.8 to 45.4 ± 3.1 D at 12 months ($P < 0.001$), mean Kmin reduced from 45.9 ± 2.8 D to 44.1 ± 3.2 D at 12 months ($P < 0.003$), mean keratometric asymmetry reduced from 3.01 ± 2.03 D to 1.25 ± 1.2 D at 12 months ($P < 0.001$). The safety index was 1.39 at 12 months and efficacy index 0.97 at 12 months. *Conclusion.* Combined topography-guided PRK and corneal collagen cross-linking are a safe and effective option in the management of mild and moderate keratoconus. *Precis.* To our knowledge, this is the first published study on the use of the CATz ablation system on the Nidek Quest excimer laser platform combined with conventional cross-linking in the management of mild keratoconus.

1. Introduction

Keratoconus is a chronic bilateral noninflammatory corneal degeneration, characterized by localized corneal thinning and corneal steepening, leading to irregular astigmatism and impaired visual acuity [1].

Corneal collagen cross-linking has found a broad international application for keratoconus in recent years [2, 3]. The combination of ultraviolet A (UVA) light with riboflavin as a photosensitizing agent produces interfibrillar cross-linking between corneal stromal collagen fibers, thus increasing corneal rigidity and halting the ectatic process. The spherocylindrical change that it causes is limited [4].

Several adjuvant therapies in combination with CXL have been proposed in an effort to develop a technique that can offer patients keratectasia corneal stability together with improved functional vision, including intracorneal rings [5] and phakic intraocular lenses [6].

Topography-guided PRK to correct ametropia and irregular astigmatism in form fruste and frank keratoconus was introduced over a decade ago [7–9] with good results. However, concerns were raised about the long-term complications, being a tissue subtraction technique.

The mechanism of topography-guided ablation is the fitting of an ideal corneal shape (usually a sphere) under the present topography map with the ablation of tissue in between.

Topography-guided PRK flattens not only some of the cone peaks but also an arcuate broader area of the cornea away from the cone, usually in the superior nasal periphery; this ablation pattern will resemble part of a hyperopic treatment and thus will cause some amount of steepening, or elevation adjacent to the cone, effectively normalizing the cornea [10].

Kanellopoulos and Binder were the first to combine CXL with topography-guided PRK in the management of keratoconus. They introduced a two-step procedure with CXL performed first and topography-guided PRK after a 1-year interval [2].

However, the fact that cross-linked corneas may have a different ablation rate from normal corneas—which could lead to unpredictable PRK results—and the hypothesis that the removal of the cross-linked corneal tissue by the PRK procedure could decrease the stiffening effects of the CXL treatment in addition to the increased possibility of haze formation after PRK were serious limitations [3].

Since then, several studies have evaluated the simultaneous use of topography-guided PRK followed immediately by CXL in progressive keratoconus [9, 11–13].

The aim of this study is to evaluate the effectiveness of combined corneal collagen cross-linking and topography-guided PRK in cases of mild and moderate keratoconus using an advanced ablation software with the Quest laser platform (Nidek, Gamagori, Japan).

2. Materials and Methods

This nonrandomized prospective clinical study was conducted on 20 eyes of 14 Caucasian patients in between February 2012 and December 2013. The study was conducted within the tenets of the Declaration of Helsinki after the approval of the institutional review board. A written informed consent was obtained from all patients.

All cases were performed at Eye Care Center for refractive surgery, Cairo, Egypt.

Inclusion criteria included grade 1 or 2 stable keratoconus (Amsler-Krumeich classification) [10] documented by topography with a corneal thickness not less than 450 μm and above 18 years of age. Exclusion criteria included patients below 18 years of age, advanced (stage 3 or 4 Amsler-Krumeich classification), BSCVA worse than 1 logMAR, central corneal scars, cases that underwent previous refractive surgery, and patients with history of herpetic eye disease or who were pregnant or lactating.

Preoperative examination included complete ocular examination included the following: assessment of uncorrected visual acuity (UCVA) and best spectacle corrected visual acuity (BSCVA), slit-lamp examination, intraocular pressure (IOP) measurement using Goldman's applanation tonometry, assessment of manifest and cycloplegic refraction, and fundus examination using indirect ophthalmoscopy.

Corneal topography was performed using Optical Path Difference (OPD scan II) scanning System (Nidek, Gamagori, Japan). The device collects corneal topography, ocular wavefront, autorefraction, and pupillometric data. The topography is Placido-based, collecting data from more than 6800 points. Axial map data were collected. Measurements were repeated at least 3 times, and the best image was chosen for the final analysis (the best one was being defined as the image with the best quality peaks for individual points). Soft contact lenses were stopped one week before topography while rigid gas permeable and hard contact lenses were stopped 2 weeks before topography.

Corneal pachymetry was done using PacScan 300P ultrasound pachymeter (Sonomed Escalon, NY, USA) with map mode to measure 5 points at the cornea (centre, superior, inferior, temporal, and nasal area). Measurement accuracy and repeatability are assured by each scan actually consisting of 256 individual measurements and an automatic measurement algorithm to ensure that only scans with proper probe alignment are accepted.

Surgeries were performed by 2 surgeons (Y. S. Mostafa and A. M. Sherif).

2.1. Operative Steps

Step 1 (topography-guided PRK). After topical anaesthesia, the epithelium was mechanically removed within an 8.5 mm diameter using hockey knife. Topography-guided PRK was performed with the aim to normalize the cornea, by reducing irregular astigmatism and also treating part of the refractive error. Custom Ablation Transition Zone (CATz) ablation profile (Quest, Nidek, Japan) was used. The CATz algorithm delivers aspheric treatment zones combined with the treatment of corneal elevation irregularities or corneal wavefront at the surgeon's choice. The treatment was planned using the Final Fit software version 1.11T3,4 (Nidek, Co., Ltd.) based on the curvature and elevation maps from the Placido disc system of the linked topography device OPD scan II.

To ensure minimal tissue removal, the effective optical zone diameter was decreased to 5.5 mm. The transition zone was 1.5 mm. Correction of up to 70% of cylinder in addition to up to 40% of the spherical component—without exceeding a maximal ablation depth limit of 50 μm—was attempted. Corneal target asphericity was set to −0.5 and no tilt correction was attempted. An example of the ablation pattern is shown in Figure 6.

After completion of ablation, 0.02% mitomycin C was applied for 30 seconds, followed by copious irrigation with balanced salt solution.

Step 2 (corneal collagen cross-linking). For the next 20 minutes, 0.1% riboflavin 5-phosphate plus 20% Dextran T 500 ophthalmic solution (Ribolink Isotonic, Optos, Australia) was applied topically every 2 minutes. The solution appeared to "soak" into the corneal stroma rapidly, as it was centrally devoid of Bowman's layer. Following the initial riboflavin administration, collagen cross-linking was performed by projecting Ultraviolet (UV) light at 370 nm wavelength (365 to 375 nm) and 3 mW/cm^2 radiance at 4.5 cm onto the surface of the cornea for 30-minute X link cross-linking system (Opto Global, Australia). The device has an accurate internal power meter and feedback loop control deliver consistent UV irradiation during the entire procedure and eliminates the need for periodic calibration.

A bandage contact lens was placed on the cornea at the completion of the procedure and was removed at 3–5 days following complete reepithelialization.

Postoperative treatment included the topical antibiotic moxifloxacin (Vigamox, Alcon) four times a day for the first week and topical nonsteroidal anti-inflammatory drops Nepafenac 0.1% (Nevanac, Alcon Research Ltd., Fort Worth, TX) for 3 to 5 days until complete epithelial healing. This was followed by an antibiotic/steroid combination (Tobradex, Alcon) to be tapered over 60 days. 1000 mg Vitamin C was given orally for 30 days.

Postoperative examinations were performed by 2 independent observes (M. A. Ammar and A. A. Osman).

Patients were assessed 1 month, 3 months, 6 months, and 12 months after surgery. On each visit, the patients were examined for uncorrected visual acuity (UCVA), best corrected visual acuity (BCVA), epithelial healing, and haze formation according to Fantes haze grading system using slit lamp [14] and corneal topography was performed using OPD scan II. Total eye aberrometry was not recorded in all cases and thus was not included in the results. Examples of pre- and postoperative topography maps are shown in Figure 5.

2.2. Statistical Methods. Data management and analysis were performed using Statistical Package for Social Sciences (SPSS) version 17.

Data were summarized using means and standard deviations. To examine the changes between the different time periods for normally distributed variables, a one-way repeated measures analysis of variance was conducted. For nonnormally distributed variables, the analyses were performed by the Friedman test, a nonparametric repeated measures one-way analysis of variance. Pairwise comparisons were done using the Wilcoxon Signed test after adjusting the P values using the Bonferroni corrections. P values ≤ 0.05 were considered significant.

The main outcome measures of the study were UCVA and BCVA.

Secondary outcome measures were Kmax, Kmin, and keratometric asymmetry. The data were obtained from the axial maps of the OPD scan.

In addition, the safety and efficacy indices were calculated [15].

The predictability index was not included because we were not sure about the fine accuracy of the subjective spherical equivalent and because the aim was more of surface regularization rather than spherocylindrical correction.

3. Results

The study included 20 eyes of 14 patients: 11 eyes belonged to males (55%) and 9 eyes belonged to females (45%). The age of patients ranged from 18 to 29 years with a mean of 23.6 ± 3.2.

The results are summarized in Table 1.

The mean ablation depth was $48.09 \pm 9.6\,\mu m$ (range 23.3–57.3 μm).

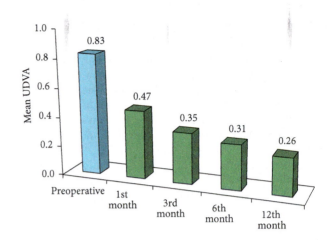

Figure 1: Preoperative and postoperative uncorrected distance visual acuity.

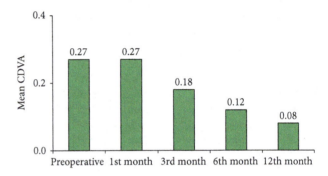

Figure 2: Preoperative and postoperative best corrected distance visual acuity.

The mean target cylindrical correction was 1.25 ± 0.85 D (range 0–3.25 D).

The preoperative and 1-, 3-, 6-, and 12-month postoperative sphere, cylindrical, and spherical equivalent data are shown in Table 2.

There was a statistically significant difference between the mean preoperative logMAR UCVA (0.83 ± 0.37) (0.21 ± 0.19 decimals) and 1-month postoperative logMAR UCVA (0.47 ± 0.23) (0.41 ± 0.27 decimals) ($P < 0.001$). UCVA continued to improve progressively until the end of the 12-month follow-up period (0.25 ± 0.26 logMAR) (0.63 ± 0.25 decimals) ($P < 0.001$) shown in Figure 1.

The preoperative mean logMAR BCVA (0.27 ± 0.31) (0.62 ± 0.29 decimals) showed an insignificant change ($P = 0.99$) one month postoperatively (0.27 ± 0.29 logMAR) (0.61 ± 0.28 decimal) and continued to improve over the follow-up period, reaching 0.18 ± 0.21 logMAR at 3 months ($P = 0.108$), 0.12 ± 0.19 logMAR (0.82 ± 0.29 decimal) at 6 months ($P = 0.04$), and 0.08 ± 18 logMAR (0.89 ± 0.27 decimal) at 12 months ($P = 0.02$) (as shown in Figure 2).

Two eyes (20%) showed no improvement in BCVA in lines, 10 eyes (50%) gained one line, 10% gained two lines, 10% gained 3 lines, and one eye (5%) gained 4 lines in BCVA. One eye (5%) lost one line in BCVA at the 12th month follow-up

TABLE 1: Summary of results.

Parameter	Preoperatively	1 month postoperatively	3 months postoperatively	6 months postoperatively	12 months postoperatively
LogMAR UDVA Mean ± SD	0.830 ±.37	0.47 ±0.32	0.35 ±0.25	0.31 ±0.26	0.26 ±0.25
P value		**0.003**	**<0.001**	**<0.001**	**<0.001**
LogMAR CDVA Mean ± SD	.27 ±0.31	0.27 ±0.29	0.18 ±0.21	0.12 ±0.19	0.08 ±0.18
P value		0.99	0.108	**0.04**	0.02
Kmax in D Mean ± SD	48.9 ±2.8	45.6 ±3.2	45.6 ±3.2	45.5 ±3.1	45.4 ±3.1
P value		**<0.001**	**<0.001**	**<0.001**	**<0.001**
Kmin in D Mean ± SD	45.9 ±2.8	44.4 ±2.9	44.3 ±3.0	44.3 ±3.1	44.1 ±3.2
P value		0.004	**0.003**	0.003	0.003
Median cylindrical error in D	2.13	1.25	**1.0**	1.00	**1.13**
P value		**<0.001**	**<0.001**	**<0.001**	**<0.001**

LogMAR = logarithm of the minimal angle of resolution, UDVA = uncorrected distance visual acuity, CDVA = corrected distance visual acuity, Kmax = maximum keratometry, Kmin = minimum keratometry, and D = diopter.

TABLE 2: Pre- and postoperative sphere, cylindrical and spherical equivalent values.

	Sph. preoperative	Sph. 1 m	Sph. 3 m	Sph. 6 m	Sph. 12 m	Cyl. preoperative	Cyl. 1 m	Cyl. 3 m	Cyl. 6 m	Cyl. 12 m	SE preoperative	SE 1 m	SE 3 m	SE 6 m	SE 12 m
Case 1	1.5	0.75	0.5	0.5	0.5	1.5	0.75	0.75	0.5	0.5	2.25	1.13	0.88	0.75	0.75
Case 2	2.5	1	1	0.75	0.75	1.5	1	0.5	0.5	0.5	3.25	1.5	1.25	1	1
Case 3	3	1.5	1.5	1.5	1.5	2.25	1.5	1.25	1	1.25	4.13	2.25	2.13	2.13	2.13
Case 4	1	0.25	0	0	0	1.5	0.75	0.75	1	0.5	1.75	0.63	0.37	0.5	0.25
Case 5	2.5	1.75	1.5	1.25	1	8.5	6.75	6	5.5	5.5	6.75	5.13	4.5	4	3.75
Case 6	1.5	0.25	0.5	0.25	0.25	2.75	1.5	2	2.25	2	2.88	1	1.5	1.38	1.25
Case 7	1.5	0.75	0.75	0.5	0.5	1.75	0.75	1	0.75	0.5	2.38	1.13	1.25	0.88	0.75
Case 8	1.75	0.75	0.5	0.5	0.5	0.75	1.25	0.5	0.5	0.5	2.13	1.38	0.75	0.75	0.75
Case 9	2	0.75	0.75	1	1	1.5	1	0.75	1.25	1.25	2.75	1.25	1.13	1.63	1.63
Case 10	0.75	0.75	0.75	0.5	0.75	6.5	3.25	5	4.5	4	4	2.38	3.25	3	2.75
Case 11	1	0.75	0.75	0.75	0.75	4	4	4	3.75	3.5	3	2.75	2.75	2.63	2.25
Case 12	0.5	0.5	0.5	0.5	0.5	2	1	0.75	0.5	0.5	1.5	1	0.87	0.75	0.75
Case 13	1.75	0.75	0.75	0.5	0.5	0.75	1	0.5	0.5	0.25	2.13	1.25	1	0.75	0.63
Case 14	1.5	1	1	1	1	2.75	1.5	1	1	0.5	2.88	1.75	1.5	1.5	1.25
Case 15	1.25	0.75	1	0.75	0.75	1.5	1	1.25	1	0.75	2	1.25	1.63	1.25	1.12
Case 16	1	0.75	0.5	0.5	0.5	2.5	2	2.25	1.75	2	2.25	1.75	1.63	1.5	1.68
Case 17	2	1.5	1.25	1.25	1	3	2.5	2.5	2.25	2	3.5	2.75	2.5	2.38	2
Case 18	0.5	0.25	0	0	0.25	4.75	1.25	1.25	1	1.25	2.63	0.88	0.68	0.5	0.68
Case 19	0.75	0.25	0.25	0.5	0.25	0.75	0.75	0.5	0.5	0.5	1.13	0.63	0.5	0.75	0.5
Case 20	1.25	1	1	0.75	0.75	4.5	1.25	1	1.25	1	3.5	1.63	1.5	1.38	1.25

Sph.: sphere, cyl.: cylinder, and SE: spherical equivalent; all are in minus dioptric form.

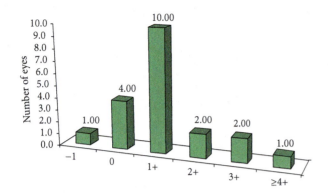

Figure 3: Gain/loss of lines of CDVA.

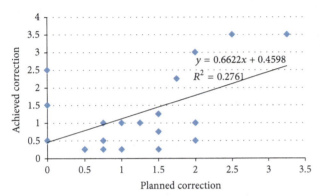

Figure 4: Linear regression analysis graph of planned and achieved cylindrical correction.

in comparison to preoperative BCVA due to grade 3 haze (as shown in Figure 3).

The efficacy index (postoperative mean decimal UDVA divided by preoperative mean decimal BCDVA) was 0.66 one month after surgery, improved to 0.88 at 6 months, and continued to improve at 12 months, reaching 0.97.

The safety index (postoperative mean decimal BCDVA divided by preoperative mean decimal BCDVA) showed a progressive improvement from 0.96 at one month, reaching 1.31 at 6 months and settling at 1.39 at 12 months.

The mean of planned cylindrical correction was 1.25 ± 0.85 D and the mean achieved cylindrical correction was 1.29 ± 1.08 D at 12 months (as shown in Figure 4).

The median of the preoperative cylinder was reduced from 2.13 D to 1.25 D at one month ($P < 0.001$). It remained stable over the follow-up period (1 D at 3, 6 months ($P < 0.001$) and 1.13 D at 12 months ($P < 0.001$)).

The mean keratometric asymmetry was reduced from 3.01 ± 2.03 D preoperatively to 1.25 ± 1.2 D at 12 months ($P < 0.001$).

The improvement in mean Kmax and mean Kmin was stable over the 12-month follow-up period as shown in Table 1.

No serious complications were recorded during the follow-up period. 30% of cases had mild haze 1 month after surgery that was gradually reduced with topical steroids, reaching 20% at 3 months, 10% at 6 months, and 5% at 12 months.

4. Discussion

This study evaluated simultaneous topography-guided PRK and corneal CXL for treatment of early cases of keratoconus.

It has been possible to use topography-guided excimer laser treatments in highly irregular corneas that are beyond the limits of wavefront measuring devices, making this approach more efficient in treating highly irregular astigmatism, such as in keratoconus, as its measurements are based solely on the cornea surface reflection [10].

Sequential CXL-Topo-guided PRK one year apart was first introduced to address the refractive element of keratoconus using PRK and the biomechanical aspect using CXL [2]. However several later studies reported better results with simultaneous Topo PRK and CXL regarding UCVA, BCVA, keratometry reduction, and haze [3, 16].

In our study, the preoperative mean UCVA was 0.83 ± 0.37 which improved at the 1st month postoperatively to 0.47 ± 0.32 with a P value of <0.001 which was statistically significant. It continued to improve over the following months, reaching 0.26 ± 0.25 at the last follow-up (12th month).

These results are better than the results of Lin et al. [10] in 2012 and comparable to the results reported by Alessio et al. in 2013 [11], Mukherjee et al. in 2013 [12], and Kanellopoulos in 2009 [3] and slightly worse than the results of Kymionis et al. in 2009 [17].

The preoperative mean BCVA was 0.27 ± 0.31 which showed a gradual improvement over the follow-up period reaching 0.12 ± 0.19 ($P = 0.04$) at 6 months. At the last follow-up (12th month) the mean BCVA was 0.08 ± 0.18 ($P = 0.02$).

20% of eyes in our study showed no improvement in BCVA in Snellen chart lines, 50% of eyes gained one line, 10% gained two lines, 10% gained 3 lines, and one eye (5%) gained 4 lines in BCVA.

These results are comparable to the results reported by Kymionis et al. [17], Kanellopoulos [3], and Stojanovic et al. in 2010 [13].

While one eye (5%) lost one line in BCVA at the 12th month postoperative follow-up in comparison to preoperative BCVA, Lin et al. reported that 12.5% of eyes lost 1 line and 4% lost >2 lines of BCVA [10]. However, Alessio et al. [11] and Mukherjee et al. [12] reported no loss of lines of BCVA.

The reduction in mean Kmax in our study was around 3.3 D, similar to the results of Kymionis et al. [17], Chan et al. [5], Alessio et al. [11], and Mukherjee et al. [12].

Regarding corneal haze, only one eye (5%) had visually significant haze (grade 3). Eight eyes (40%) had trace haze (grade 1) and 55% of eyes had no haze at all at the end of the 12-month follow-up. This concurs with other studies on simultaneous collagen cross-linking and topography-guided PRK [16, 18].

Previous studies [3, 11–13, 16–18] evaluated the technique of simultaneous topography-guided PRK with CXL in keratoconus with encouraging results and few postoperative complications.

To our knowledge, there are no previously published studies describing the use of the CATz software of the Quest Nidek excimer laser system for topography-guided PRK in combination with collagen cross-linking in keratoconus. Our

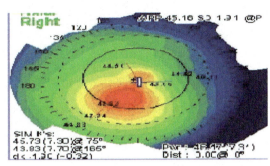
(a) Preoperative topography with OPD scan II (Case 1)

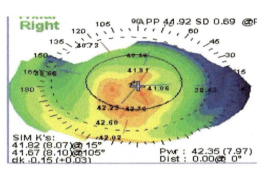
(b) 1-year postoperative topography with OPD scan II (Case 1)

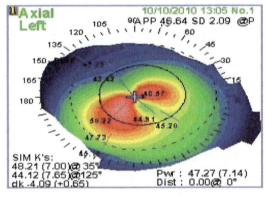
(c) Preoperative topography with OPD scan II (Case 2)

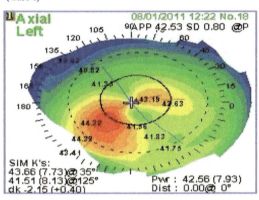
(d) 1-year postoperative topography with OPD scan II (Case 2)

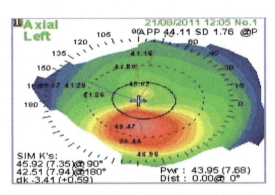
(e) Preoperative topography with OPD scan II (Case 3)

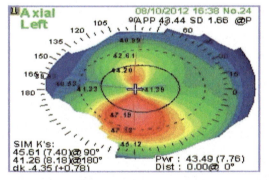
(f) 1-year postoperative topography with OPD scan II (Case 3)

FIGURE 5: Comparative topography maps before and after surgery.

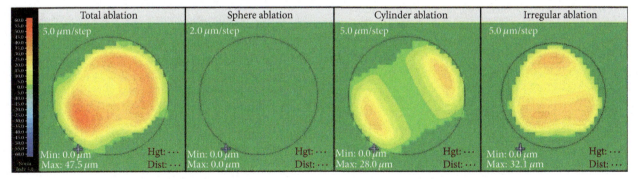
FIGURE 6: The ablation profile in CATz (Quest, Nidek excimer laser machine).

results showed significant progressive improvement of UCVA and BCVA and low risk of haze throughout the 12-month follow-up period.

One of the limitations of the study was that the maximum ablation depth of 50 μm was exceeded in two cases (53.5 μm and 57.3 μm). In addition, rigid gas permeable and hard contact lenses were stopped 2 weeks only before surgery which may be too short for some corneas. In addition, the follow-up period in our study was 12 months and due to the reports of progressive excessive corneal flattening [19, 20] which may lead to hyperopic shift up to several years after CXL [21], further studies with longer follow-up periods are needed to further evaluate the long-term outcomes of this technique.

Disclosure

This study was carried out at Eye Care Center, Cairo, Egypt.

Conflict of Interests

The authors declare that there is no conflict of interests regarding the publication of this paper.

Acknowledgment

The authors acknowledge Professor Jorge L. Alio, Alicante, Spain, for his help with the revision of the scientific content of the paper.

References

[1] M. Romero-Jiménez, J. Santodomingo-Rubido, and J. S. Wolffsohn, "Keratoconus: a review," *Contact Lens and Anterior Eye*, vol. 33, no. 4, pp. 157–166, 2010.

[2] A. J. Kanellopoulos and P. S. Binder, "Collagen cross-linking (CCL) with sequential topography-guided PRK: a temporizing alternative for keratoconus to penetrating keratoplasty," *Cornea*, vol. 26, no. 7, pp. 891–895, 2007.

[3] A. J. Kanellopoulos, "Comparison of sequential vs same-day simultaneous collagen cross-linking and topography-guided PRK for treatment of keratoconus," *Journal of Refractive Surgery*, vol. 25, no. 9, pp. S812–S818, 2009.

[4] G. Wollensak, E. Spoerl, and T. Seiler, "Riboflavin/ultraviolet-A-induced collagen crosslinking for the treatment of keratoconus," *American Journal of Ophthalmology*, vol. 135, no. 5, pp. 620–627, 2003.

[5] C. C. K. Chan, M. Sharma, and B. S. B. Wachler, "Effect of inferior-segment Intacs with and without C3-R on keratoconus," *Journal of Cataract and Refractive Surgery*, vol. 33, no. 1, pp. 75–80, 2007.

[6] L. Izquierdo Jr., M. A. Henriquez, and M. McCarthy, "Artiflex phakic intraocular lens implantation after corneal collagen cross-linking in keratoconic eyes," *Journal of Refractive Surgery*, vol. 27, no. 7, pp. 482–487, 2011.

[7] J. L. Alió, J. I. Belda, A. A. Osman, and A. M. M. Shalaby, "Topography-guided laser in situ keratomileusis (TOPOLINK) to correct irregular astigmatism after previous refractive surgery," *Journal of Refractive Surgery*, vol. 19, no. 5, pp. 516–527, 2003.

[8] F. Carones, L. Vigo, and E. Scandola, "Wavefront-guided treatment of abnormal eyes using the LADARVision platform," *Journal of Refractive Surgery*, vol. 19, no. 6, pp. S703–S708, 2003.

[9] R. Shetty, S. D'Souza, S. Srivastava, and R. Ashwini, "Topography-guided custom ablation treatment for treatment of keratoconus," *Indian Journal of Ophthalmology*, vol. 61, no. 8, pp. 445–450, 2013.

[10] D. T. C. Lin, S. Holland, J. C. H. Tan, and G. Moloney, "Clinical results of topography-based customized ablations in highly aberrated eyes and keratoconus/ectasia with cross-linking," *Journal of Refractive Surgery*, vol. 28, no. 11, pp. 841–848, 2012.

[11] G. Alessio, M. L'Abbate, C. Sborgia, and M. G. La Tegola, "Photorefractive keratectomy followed by cross-linking versus cross-linking alone for management of progressive keratoconus: Two-year follow-up," *American Journal of Ophthalmology*, vol. 155, no. 1, pp. 54–65, 2013.

[12] A. N. Mukherjee, V. Selimis, and I. Aslanides, "Transepithelial photorefractive keratectomy with crosslinking for keratoconus," *Open Ophthalmology Journal*, vol. 7, pp. 63–68, 2013.

[13] A. Stojanovic, J. Zhang, X. Chen, T. A. Nitter, S. Chen, and Q. Wang, "Topography-guided transepithelial surface ablation followed by corneal collagen cross-linking performed in a single combined procedure for the treatment of keratoconus and pellucid marginal degeneration," *Journal of Refractive Surgery*, vol. 26, no. 2, pp. 145–152, 2010.

[14] F. E. Fantes, K. D. Hanna, G. O. Waring III, Y. Pouliquen, K. P. Thompson, and M. Savoldelli, "Wound healing after excimer laser keratomileusis (photorefractive keratectomy) in monkeys," *Archives of Ophthalmology*, vol. 108, no. 5, pp. 665–675, 1990.

[15] D. D. Koch, T. Kohnen, S. A. Obstbaum, and E. S. Rosen, "Format for reporting refractive surgical data," *Journal of Cataract and Refractive Surgery*, vol. 24, no. 3, pp. 285–287, 1998.

[16] G. D. Kymionis, G. A. Kontadakis, G. A. Kounis et al., "Simultaneous topography-guided PRK followed by corneal collagen cross-linking for keratoconus," *Journal of Refractive Surgery*, vol. 25, no. 9, pp. S807–S811, 2009.

[17] G. D. Kymionis, D. M. Portaliou, G. A. Kounis, A. N. Limnopoulou, G. A. Kontadakis, and M. A. Grentzelos, "Simultaneous topography-guided photorefractive keratectomy followed by corneal collagen cross-linking for keratoconus," *American Journal of Ophthalmology*, vol. 152, no. 5, pp. 748–755, 2011.

[18] H. Sakla, W. Altroudi, G. Muñoz, and C. Albarrán-Diego, "Simultaneous topography-guided partial photorefractive keratectomy and corneal collagen crosslinking for keratoconus," *Journal of Cataract and Refractive Surgery*, vol. 40, no. 9, pp. 1430–1438, 2014.

[19] M. R. Santhiago, N. T. Giacomin, C. S. Medeiros, D. Smadja, and S. J. Bechara, "Intense early flattening after corneal collagen cross-linking," *Journal of Refractive Surgery*, vol. 31, no. 6, pp. 419–422, 2015.

[20] S. A. Greenstein, K. L. Fry, and P. S. Hersh, "Effect of topographic cone location on outcomes of corneal collagen cross-linking for keratoconus and corneal ectasia," *Journal of Refractive Surgery*, vol. 28, no. 6, pp. 397–405, 2012.

[21] G. D. Kymionis, K. I. Tsoulnaras, D. A. Liakopoulos, T. A. Paraskevopoulos, A. I. Kouroupaki, and M. K. Tsilimbaris, "Excessive corneal flattening and thinning after corneal cross-linking: single-case report with 5-year follow-up," *Cornea*, vol. 34, no. 6, pp. 704–706, 2015.

The Measurement of Intraocular Biomarkers in Various Stages of Proliferative Diabetic Retinopathy Using Multiplex xMAP Technology

Stepan Rusnak,[1] Jindra Vrzalova,[2,3] Marketa Sobotova,[1] Lenka Hecova,[1] Renata Ricarova,[1] and Ondrej Topolcan[2,3]

[1]Department of Ophthalmology, University Hospital Pilsen, Alej Svobody 80, 304 60 Plzen, Czech Republic
[2]Department of Nuclear Medicine, Laboratory of Immunoanalysis, University Hospital Pilsen, Dr. E. Benese 13, 305 99 Plzen, Czech Republic
[3]Central Radioisotopic Laboratory, Faculty of Medicine in Pilsen, Charles University in Prague, Dr. E. Benese 13, 305 99 Plzen, Czech Republic

Correspondence should be addressed to Marketa Sobotova; sobotovam@fnplzen.cz

Academic Editor: Ricardo Giordano

Purpose. To determine the intraocular levels of growth factors and cytokines in patients with various degrees of severity of proliferative diabetic retinopathy (PDR) using multiplex xMAP technology. *Methods.* A prospective cohort study of 61 eyes from 56 patients who were divided into 3 groups based on the severity of PDR. Patients in group number 1 are those who presented PDR with no need of repeated surgical intervention; patients in group number 2 had repeated vitreous bleeding; and patients in group number 3 had refractory neovascular glaucoma. The concentrations of proangiogenic, antiangiogenic, inflammatory, and neurotrophic factors were measured in intraocular fluid. The results were also compared with levels of factors measured in 50 eyes from 50 patients prior to senile cataract surgery (control group). *Results.* Patients with refractory neovascular glaucoma (the highest clinical severity group) had higher levels of interleukin 6 (IL-6) (median1 37.19; median3 384.74; $P = .00096$), transforming growth factor beta 1 (TGFβ-1) (median1 49.00; median3 414.40; $P = .0017$), and vascular endothelial growth factor (VEGF) (median1 211.62; median3 352.82; $P = .0454$) compared with other PDR patients. *Conclusions.* Results of our study imply that levels of IL-6, TGFβ-1, and VEGF correlate with the severity of PDR.

1. Introduction

Diabetes mellitus is one of the most common endocrine disorders in the world; it affected roughly 6% of the global population ca. in the year 2000, and it is estimated that it will affect 300 million people in 2025 [1]. Diabetic retinopathy affects 35% of the patients in the diabetic population [2] and is the main cause of permanent vision loss in the working population [3]. Proliferative diabetic retinopathy (PDR) is characterized by the pathological formation of retinal blood vessels. Despite progress in diagnostics and therapies, PDR leads to a terminal stage of therapeutically unmanageable neovascularization that is characterized by the development of secondary neovascular glaucoma in a number of cases.

Retinal hypoxia is a major driving force for retinal neovascularization that increases hypoxia inducible factor (HIF) levels and launches a cascade of the production of cytokines and growth factors. Since the discovery of the proangiogenic role of vascular endothelial growth factor (VEGF) in PDR, changes in the levels of a number of other proangiogenic factors, such as those in the insulin-like growth factor family (IGF), hepatocyte growth factor (HGF), basic fibroblast growth factor (b-FGF), platelet-derived growth factor (PDGF), proinflammatory cytokines, and angiopoietin, have been demonstrated. However, the intraocular synthesis of angiogenic factors is counterbalanced by the synthesis of antiangiogenic factors, including γ-interferon inducible protein 10 (IP-10), the pigment epithelium-derived factor

(PEDF), transforming growth factor beta (TGFβ), thrombospondin (TSP), endostatin, angiostatin, and somatostatin [4, 5]. Fluorescein angiography, or more recently ultra widefield fluorescein angiography, is used to determine the scope of neovascularization or ischemia [6]. This method is an image-processing technique for angiographic mapping of the retina. It enables the most recent stage of retinal angiogenesis to be described, but it is not an objective risk assessment technique. The measurement of intraocular biomarkers is emerging as a novel possibility for patient stratification. Because neovascularization results from an imbalance in proangiogenic and antiangiogenic factors, a multiplex analytical tool for monitoring the levels of several factors in a small sample volume is necessary to describe this process. A combination of immunoanalysis and flow cytometry [7], called xMAP technology, is one of the most promising multiplex technologies in clinical research to date.

In our study, the concentration levels of epidermal growth factor (EGF), interleukin 6 (IL-6), VEGF, tumor necrosis factor alfa (TNF-α), interleukin 8 (IL-8), IP-10, monocyte chemoattractant protein 1 (MCP-1), PDGF, TGFβ-1, fractalkine, interleukin 10 (IL-10), interferon gamma (IFN-γ), fibroblast growth factor 2 (FGF-2), brain-derived neurotrophic factor (BDNF), ciliary neurotrophic factor (CNTF), and RANTES in samples of the aqueous humour from a group of PDR patients were measured using xMAP technology. The PDR cohort was further divided into three subgroups on the basis of clinical severity and these subgroups were compared with a control group. Our aim was to demonstrate that a biomarker panel measurement using multiplex immunoanalysis is applicable as a diagnostic and prognostic method in ophthalmology.

2. Materials and Methods

2.1. Patient Cohort. Patients undergoing treatment for PDR at the University Hospital in Pilsen during 2008–2010 were enrolled in this institutional prospective cohort study.

The patients with PDR were divided into groups according to the severity of their pathologies. Group 1 included 41 eyes from 37 patients with PDR who had no need for repeated surgical intervention (for better understanding, this group consists of 26 patients with PDR and vitreous bleeding, 5 patients with PDR and tractional retinal detachment, 5 patients with PDR, vitreous bleeding, and tractional retinal detachment, 4 patients with PDR and exudative maculopathy, and 1 patient with PDR with fibroproliferation), group 2 was composed of 11 eyes of nine patients who had repeated vitreous bleeding, and group 3 included 10 eyes from 10 patients with refractory neovascular glaucoma, which represents the most severe stage of the disease. The control group (group 0) was composed of 50 eyes from 50 preoperative senile cataract patients. Small samples (approximately 50 μL) of intraocular fluid from the aqueous humour of each participant were obtained under topical anesthesia from the anterior chamber of each eye by means of aspiration using a fine 30-gauge needle that was attached to a syringe.

2.2. Multiplex Analysis. All specimens were frozen immediately. Samples were stored at −80°C until they were analyzed. No more than one freeze-thaw cycle was allowed prior to analysis. The protein concentrations in the aqueous humour were measured using multiplex xMAP technology on a Luminex 100 instrument with commercially available panels from Millipore Corporation (Billerica, MA, USA), MILLIPLEX MAP Human Cytokine/Chemokine Panel, and MILLIPLEX MAP TGFβ-1. The procedures were performed according to the manufacturer's instructions, and the control samples that were provided within the kits were assayed in each analysis. The xMAP technology that was applied is a combination of immunoanalysis and flow cytometry based on bead particles that can be distinguished by internal dyes, as described, for example, by Kellar and Iannone [7]. In our study, the levels of EGF, IL-6, VEGF, TNF-α, IL-8, IP-10, MCP-1, PDGF AA, TGFβ-1, fractalkine, PDGF AB/BB, IL-10, IFN-γ, FGF-2, CNTF, BDNF, and RANTES were studied.

2.3. Statistical Methods. A descriptive statistic was calculated for each of the markers. The results under the calibration curve ranges were stated as the value of the lowest calibration point. The Mann-Whitney U test (independent samples) and Kruskal-Wallis test were used to compare marker levels between groups. Borderline significance was determined to be reflected by P values ranging from 0.05 to 0.0001, and significance was reflected by P values below 0.0001. MedCalc 11.2 statistics software was used for analysis.

3. Results

The median, lower, and upper quartile values for all of the markers within each group are listed in Table 1. When comparing the groups, significantly higher levels of IL-6, IL-8, IP-10, PDGF AA, and VEGF were found among PDR patients compared with patients in the control group. The concentrations of TGFβ-1 were higher in PDR patients compared with the control group. Patients in group 3 (those with neovascular glaucoma that was refractory to treatment) had higher levels of IL-6, TGFβ-1, and VEGF compared with patients in PDR group 1 and PDR group 2 (the nonneovascular glaucoma groups). The differences in concentrations were all of borderline significance (see Tables 1 and 2). No significant differences in marker levels were found between PDR group 1 (with no complications) and PDR group 2 (with repeated vitreous bleeding). No differences between groups were found in the levels of BDNF, CNTF, EGF, and MCP-1. See Table 2 for the results of the group comparisons. Boxplots of the VEGF concentrations in each of the groups are provided in Figure 1, and boxplots of the markers for which levels in control eyes differed significantly from levels in the eyes of patients in PDR group 1 are shown in Figure 2. Because the vast majority of patients had intraocular fluid concentrations of fractalkine, PDGFAB/BB, IL-10, IFN-γ, TNF-α, FGF-2, and RANTES that were below the detection limit of the panels that were used, the results from assays for these markers are not presented. Although the concentration of TGFβ-1 was below the detection limit in the control group,

TABLE 1: Descriptive statistics. Median values and 5th and 95th percentile values in pg/mL for all markers and groups are shown. Proliferative diabetic retinopathy (PDR) patients were divided into groups. Group 1: PDR patients with no need for repeated surgical intervention; group 2: PDR patients with repeated vitreous bleeding, which is a less serious complication of PDR; group 3: PDR patients with refractory neovascular glaucoma, which is a serious complication of PDR; group 0: control group.

	Groups							
	0		1		2		3	
	Median	5–95 P	Median	5–95 P	Median	5–95 P	Median	5–95 P
BDNF	12.00	12.00–59.67	12.00	12.00–49.37	12.00	12.00–103.23	30.00	12.00–81.43
CNTF	122.00	122.00–2667.92	393.19	122.00–1787.45	276.19	122.00–573.63	388.29	197.96–578.61
EGF	24.88	13.893–115.99	36.22	14.02–133.31	96.47	4.23–120.42	37.48	3.95–114.20
IL-6	3.20	3.200–196.312	37.19	3.992–4577.38	25.22	3.37–299.13	384.74	22.63–9982.69
IL-8	3.20	3.20–15.49	25.28	13.21–184.62	27.96	13.84–53.67	33.76	20.04–96.37
IP-10	105.92	12.93–307.68	460.68	159.49–2237.28	365.35	150.90–758.61	874.06	463.94–1698.36
MCP-1	962.59	3.20–2931.63	2772.21	353.18–3249.45	2336.77	2020.39–2653.15	661.23	3.20–2881.94
PDGFAA	111.26	5.85–212.85	227.96	104.57–756.34	208.36	151.58–344.62	192.66	79.91–316.61
TGFβ-1	49.00	49.00–49.00	49.00	49.00–220.41	49.00	49.00–84.71	414.40	119.85–955.58
VEGF	69.85	16.00–200.63	211.62	48.10–1990.98	187.96	4.28–523.25	352.82	132.84–7052.89

BDNF: brain-derived neurotrophic factor; CNTF: ciliary neurotrophic factor; EGF: epidermal growth factor; IL: interleukin; IP-10: γ-interferon inducible protein 10; MCP-1: monocyte chemoattractant protein 1; PDGF AA: platelet-derived growth factor AA; TGFβ-1: transforming growth factor beta 1; VEGF: vascular endothelial growth factor.
P: percentile.

TABLE 2: Comparison of biomarker levels between groups. P values are listed.

	Kruskal-Wallis	Mann-Whitney U 0×1	Mann-Whitney U 1×2	Mann-Whitney U 2×3	Mann-Whitney U 1×3
BDNF	NS	NS	NS	NS	NS
CNTF	NS	NS	NS	NS	NS
EGF	NS	NS	NS	NS	NS
IL-6	<0.0001	<0.0001	NS	0.0088	0.0096
IL-8	<0.0001	<0.0001	NS	NS	NS
IP-10	<0.0001	<0.0001	NS	NS	NS
MCP-1	NS	NS	NS	NS	NS
PDGFAA	<0.0001	<0.0001	NS	NS	NS
TGFβ-1	<0.0001	0.0027	NS	0.0037	0.0017
VEGF	<0.0001	<0.0001	NS	0.0265	0.0454

BDNF: brain-derived neurotrophic factor; CNTF: ciliary neurotrophic factor; EGF: epidermal growth factor; IL: interleukin; IP-10: γ-interferon inducible protein 10; MCP1: monocyte chemoattractant protein 1; PDGF AA: platelet-derived growth factor AA; TGFβ-1: transforming growth factor beta 1; VEGF: vascular endothelial growth factor.
NS: nonsignificant.

TGFβ-1 levels in some of the PDR patients were measureable; thus, the results are presented.

4. Discussion

Biomarkers in disease detection and management have become important tools in modern clinical medicine, and their application to retinal disease should be no exception. Because multiplex analysis based on xMAP technology allows for the analysis of tens of analytes in a small sample volume (10–50 μL), this is a potent technology for introducing laboratory medicine into ophthalmology.

In this study, we have confirmed that the patients with PDR have higher intraocular concentrations of proangiogenic, antiangiogenic, and inflammatory cytokines compared with nonPDR patients. Intraocular levels of IL-6, IL-8, IP-10, PDGF AA, TGFβ-1, and VEGF were increased in patients with PDR. Today, many studies compare the intraocular concentrations of various cytokines in PDR patients versus patients who do not have PDR. Maier et al. found that mean cytokine levels of IP-10, MCP-1, and VEGF in the vitreous humour were significantly higher compared to those of normal controls [8]. Murugeswari et al. documented that levels of IL-6, IL-8, MCP-1, and VEGF in the vitreous were

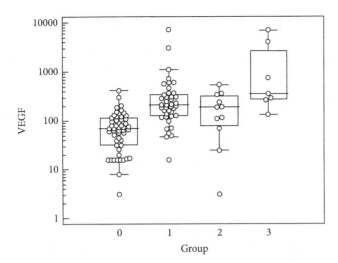

FIGURE 1: Vascular endothelial growth factor levels for each group. Group 1: proliferative diabetic retinopathy (PDR) patients with no need for repeated surgical intervention; group 2: PDR patients with repeated vitreous bleeding, which is a less serious complication of PDR; group 3: PDR patients with refractory neovascular glaucoma, which is a serious complication of PDR; group 0: control group.

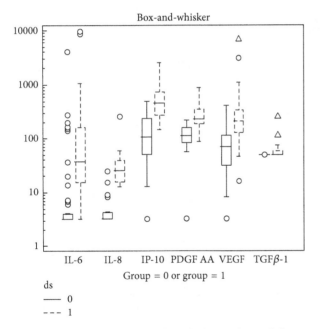

FIGURE 2: Levels of biomarkers for which significant differences between the levels in control group 0 and those in proliferative diabetic retinopathy group 1 were found. IL: interleukin; IP-10: γ-interferon inducible protein 10; PDGF AA: platelet-derived growth factor AA; VEGF: vascular endothelial growth factor; TGFβ-1: transforming growth factor beta 1.

significantly higher in PDR patients compared with levels in macular hole patients. Conversely, the vitreous level of PEDF was significantly reduced in patients with PDR [9]. Yoshimura et al. performed a comprehensive analysis of mediators in the vitreous fluids in PDR patients and in patients with other ocular diseases, and they found elevated levels of VEGF, MCP-1, IL-8, and IL-6 compared with control patients [10]. We found similar results in this study, but we have not demonstrated that the concentration of MCP-1 increases in patients with PDR. However, we have shown that higher intraocular concentrations of PDGF AA and nonmeasurable values of PDGF AB/BB can be seen in PDR patients. Contrary to our result, Freyberger et al. published results showing that PDGF AB levels are elevated in patients with PDR [11].

In a clinical environment, it is essential to further stratify the PDR patients; however, only a few studies that compare the levels of biomarkers in PDR patients with differing disease severities exist. Funatsu et al. divided PDR patients into subgroups based on disease progression and regression. The vitreous levels of VEGF and IL-6 were significantly higher in the eyes of patients in the progression group than they were in eyes with PDR regression. Multivariate logistic regression analysis showed that higher vitreous levels of VEGF were associated with the progression of PDR following vitreous surgery. A high vitreous level of VEGF was identified as a significant risk factor in determining the outcome of vitreous surgery in patients with PDR [12]. Freyberger et al. studied 23 patients with PDR, four of whom had rubeosis iridis, which is an indicator of very high vasoproliferative activity. Significantly elevated concentrations of PDGF AB were found among individuals with PDR; even higher levels were found in conjunction with rubeosis iridis [11]. In our study, patients with neovascular glaucoma that was refractory to treatment showed higher levels of IL-6, TGFβ-1, and VEGF than other PDR patients, which implies that the levels of these three factors are correlated with the severity of PDR. No differences in biomarker levels were found between patients who belonged to group 2 (those with repeated vitreous bleeding) and those who belonged to group 1 (those who had no complications).

The novel multiplex technology that we proposed not only saves time, labor, and costs of immunoanalysis, but it also rapidly reduces the sample volume requirements compared to a traditional immunoanalysis method (single ELISA) while allowing the full comparability of all studied parameters. The last two points are critical when entering laboratory measurements into the diagnostic and risk assessment process in ophthalmology. One limitation of xMAP technology could be that it is limited in its ability to detect some factors. In the present study, we were not able to detect fractalkine, PDGF AB/BB, IL-10, IFN-γ, TNF-α, FGF-2, and RANTES in the aqueous humour. Similarly, Yoshimura et al. found that the intraocular concentrations of IL-1β, IL-2, IL-4, IL-5, IL-10, IL-17, IFN-γ, TNF-α, eotaxin, MIP-1α, RANTES, EGF, and FGF-2 were lower than the detection level [10].

We have chosen three works as examples of studies that have shown the potency of xMAP technology in ophthalmology. Curnow et al. measured a panel of cytokines in the aqueous humour, and from the spectra of cytokines that they studied, they used random forest analysis to show that only IL-6, IL-8, MCP-1, IL-13, IL-2, and TNF-α are required to distinguish between noninflammatory control and idiopathic uveitis with 100% classification accuracy [13]. Funding et al. used xMAP technology to simultaneously quantify and compare the concentrations of 17 immune mediators in aqueous humour samples from patients with corneal rejection and patients with a noninflammatory condition in the anterior chamber. Their results underscore both the complex immunological interactions of the rejection process and the need for multiplex laboratory measurements based on small sample volumes [14]. Rusnak et al. measured the levels of 12 cytokines in the aqueous humour in 27 eyes that were undergoing vitrectomies for retinal detachment with various degrees of severity of proliferative vitreoretinopathy. According to this study MCP-1 and VEGF may participate in pathogenesis of retinal detachment and proliferative vitreoretinopathy [15].

Sohn et al. have shown that multiplex measurements of cytokine and growth factor concentrations also enable treatment monitoring. After intravitreal injections of 2 antiangiogenic drugs (triamcinolone and bevacizumab), the clinical effects and differences in biomarker levels in the aqueous humour were monitored. A more effective treatment modality was linked to decreases in the concentrations of IL-6, IP-10, MCP-1, PDGF AA, and VEGF compared with those resulting from a less effective treatment; the latter treatment was only connected with a decrease in the concentration of VEGF [16].

The Sohn et al. study [16], in conjunction with our findings in patients with neovascular glaucoma refractory to treatment, shows that biomarkers have a strong potential for use in patient stratification and in determining personalized medical needs. Tailored treatments are necessary due to the introduction and costs of novel treatment. The vast majority of novel types of therapy are based on the inhibition of VEGF. A number of anti-VEGF agents have been introduced into clinical use and are widely used for the treatment of many ocular diseases, but the widespread use of these agents raises new questions. It has been proposed that anti-VEGF agents may have negative effects on retinal cells. Animal studies have shown that systemic neutralization of VEGF with soluble VEGF receptors results in a reduction of the thicknesses of both the inner and the outer nuclear layers in adult mouse retinas. These results indicate that endogenous VEGF plays an important role in the maintenance and function of neuronal cells in the adult retina and suggest that anti-VEGF therapies should be administered with caution [17]. Because of the risks associated with using anti-VEGF therapies, it is absolutely necessary to select patients who can benefit from anti-VEGF treatment despite the risk of adverse effects. In our study, we have shown that certain complications, such as neovascular glaucoma that is refractory to conventional treatment, are correlated with high concentrations of certain biomarkers; in the future, we can use these to justify more aggressive therapies. Our findings suggest that patients could be selected for repeat intravitreal injections of VEGF inhibitors, corticosteroids, more aggressive panretinal laser photocoagulation, cyclocryodestruction, or cyclophotodestruction on the basis of biomarker concentrations. Another study that shows that measuring protein concentrations in the aqueous humour has potential future benefits for treatment monitoring was conducted by Campochiaro et al.; they measured concentrations of VEGF, IL-6, IL-1 beta, tumor necrosis factor, and ranibizumab [18].

Another problem in patients who have been treated with anti-VEGF therapies is determining the concentration of VEGF. The determination of the VEGF concentration is influenced by treatment with anti-VEGF inhibitors via direct interaction in the immunoanalysis, which we verified in our laboratory (data not presented). The interaction requires an adjustment to the approach to determining the intraocular concentrations of VEGF in these patients; the half-life of anti-VEGF therapies in the eye was established as being 9.8 days [19]. Only patients who had never received anti-VEGF treatment or, in advanced cases, had received their most recent administrations of anti-VEGF therapy more than two months prior to aqueous humour sampling for this study were included. With the expansion of anti-VEGF therapy, it is clear that multifactor monitoring, that is, introducing other biomarkers in addition to VEGF, is important. Both our study and others show that there are several possible candidate biomarkers. As more PDR biomarkers are identified, a panel of them has the potential to be effective for identifying high-risk individuals, monitoring disease progression, and evaluating the efficacy of therapeutic interventions.

In conclusion, the results of our study suggest that the concentrations of IL-6, TGFβ-1, and VEGF correlate with the severity of PDR. In future, assessment of PDR biomarkers in intraocular fluid could be effective method for treatment monitoring and early detection of PDR progression.

Consent

Each participant signed informed consent approved by the Institutional Review Board.

Conflict of Interests

The authors declare that there is no conflict of interests regarding the publication of this paper.

Acknowledgment

This study was supported by the government granting agency IGA MZ NS10251-3.

References

[1] E. Adeghate, P. Schattner, and E. Dunn, "An update on the etiology and epidemiology of diabetes mellitus," *Annals of the New York Academy of Sciences*, vol. 1084, pp. 1–29, 2006.

[2] R. Klein and B. Klein, The Beaver Dam Eye Study, 1987–2010, http://www.bdeyestudy.org/.

[3] B. E. K. Klein, "Overview of epidemiologic studies of diabetic retinopathy," *Ophthalmic Epidemiology*, vol. 14, no. 4, pp. 179–183, 2007.

[4] R. Simó, E. Carrasco, M. García-Ramírez, and C. Hernández, "Angiogenic and antiangiogenic factors in proliferative diabetic retinopathy," *Current Diabetes Reviews*, vol. 2, no. 1, pp. 71–98, 2006.

[5] R. F. Gariano and T. W. Gardner, "Retinal angiogenesis in development and disease," *Nature*, vol. 438, no. 7070, pp. 960–966, 2005.

[6] R. F. Spaide, "Peripheral areas of nonperfusion in treated central retinal vein occlusion as imaged by wide-field fluorescein angiography," *Retina*, vol. 31, no. 5, pp. 829–837, 2011.

[7] K. L. Kellar and M. A. Iannone, "Multiplexed microsphere-based flow cytometric assays," *Experimental Hematology*, vol. 30, no. 11, pp. 1227–1237, 2002.

[8] R. Maier, M. Weger, E.-M. Haller-Schober et al., "Multiplex bead analysis of vitreous and serum concentrations of inflammatory and proangiogenic factors in diabetic patients," *Molecular Vision*, vol. 14, pp. 637–643, 2008.

[9] P. Murugeswari, D. Shukla, A. Rajendran, R. Kim, P. Namperumalsamy, and V. Muthukkaruppan, "Proinflammatory cytokines and angiogenic and anti-angiogenic factors in vitreous of patients with proliferative diabetic retinopathy and eales' disease," *Retina*, vol. 28, no. 6, pp. 817–824, 2008.

[10] T. Yoshimura, K.-H. Sonoda, M. Sugahara et al., "Comprehensive analysis of inflammatory immune mediators in vitreoretinal diseases," *PLoS ONE*, vol. 4, no. 12, Article ID e8158, 2009.

[11] H. Freyberger, M. Bröcker, H. Yakut et al., "Increased levels of platelet-derived growth factor in vitreous fluid of patients with proliferative diabetic retinopathy," *Experimental and Clinical Endocrinology & Diabetes*, vol. 108, no. 2, pp. 106–109, 2000.

[12] H. Funatsu, H. Yamashita, T. Mimura, H. Noma, S. Nakamura, and S. Hori, "Risk evaluation of outcome of vitreous surgery based on vitreous levels of cytokines," *Eye*, vol. 21, no. 3, pp. 377–382, 2007.

[13] S. J. Curnow, F. Falciani, O. M. Durrani et al., "Multiplex bead immunoassay analysis of aqueous humor reveals distinct cytokine profiles in uveitis," *Investigative Ophthalmology and Visual Science*, vol. 46, no. 11, pp. 4251–4259, 2005.

[14] M. Funding, T. K. Hansen, J. Gjedsted, and N. Ehlers, "Simultaneous quantification of 17 immune mediators in aqueous humour from patients with corneal rejection," *Acta Ophthalmologica Scandinavica*, vol. 84, no. 6, pp. 759–765, 2006.

[15] S. Rusnak, J. Vrzalova, L. Hecová, M. Kozova, O. Topolcan, and R. Ricarova, "Defining the seriousness of proliferative vitreoretinopathy by aspiration of cytokines from the anterior chamber," *Biomarkers in Medicine*, vol. 7, no. 5, pp. 759–767, 2013.

[16] H. J. Sohn, D. H. Han, I. T. Kim et al., "Changes in aqueous concentrations of various cytokines after intravitreal triamcinolone versus bevacizumab for diabetic macular edema," *American Journal of Ophthalmology*, vol. 152, no. 4, pp. 686–694, 2011.

[17] M. Saint-Geniez, A. S. R. Maharaj, T. E. Walshe et al., "Endogenous VEGF is required for visual function: evidence for a survival role on Müller cells and photoreceptors," *PLoS ONE*, vol. 3, no. 11, Article ID e3554, 2008.

[18] P. A. Campochiaro, D. F. Choy, D. V. Do et al., "Monitoring ocular drug therapy by analysis of aqueous samples," *Ophthalmology*, vol. 116, no. 11, pp. 2158–2164, 2009.

[19] T. U. Krohne, N. Eter, F. G. Holz, and C. H. Meyer, "Intraocular pharmacokinetics of bevacizumab after a single intravitreal injection in humans," *The American Journal of Ophthalmology*, vol. 146, no. 4, pp. 508–512, 2008.

Local Relationship between Global-Flash Multifocal Electroretinogram Optic Nerve Head Components and Visual Field Defects in Patients with Glaucoma

Chan Hee Moon,[1] Jungwoo Han,[2] Young-Hoon Ohn,[2] and Tae Kwann Park[2]

[1]Department of Ophthalmology, Seoul St. Mary's Hospital, The Catholic University of Korea College of Medicine, Seoul 06591, Republic of Korea
[2]Department of Ophthalmology, Soonchunhyang University College of Medicine, Bucheon Hospital, Bucheon 14584, Republic of Korea

Correspondence should be addressed to Tae Kwann Park; tkpark@schmc.ac.kr

Academic Editor: Patrik Schatz

Purpose. To investigate the local relationship between quantified global-flash multifocal electroretinogram (mfERG) optic nerve head component (ONHC) and visual field defects in patients with glaucoma. *Methods.* Thirty-nine patients with glaucoma and 30 normal controls were enrolled. The ONHC amplitude was measured from the baseline to the peak of the second positive deflection of the induced component. The ONHC amplitude was normalized by dividing ONHC amplitude by the average of seven largest ONHC amplitudes. The ONHC amplitude ratio map and ONHC deficiency map were constructed. The local relationship between the ONHC measurements and visual field defects was evaluated by calculating the overlap between the ONHC deficiency maps and visual field defect plots. *Results.* The mean ONHC amplitude measurements of patients with glaucoma (6.01 ± 1.91 nV/deg^2) were significantly lower than those of the normal controls (10.29 ± 0.94 nV/deg^2) ($P < 0.001$). The average overlap between the ONHC deficiency map and visual field defect plot was 71.4%. The highest overlap (75.0%) was between the ONHC ratios less than 0.5 and the total deviations less than 5%. *Conclusions.* The ONHC amplitude was reduced in patients with glaucoma compared to that in normal controls. Loss of the ONHC amplitude from the global-flash mfERG showed a high local agreement with visual field defects in patients with glaucoma.

1. Introduction

The multifocal electroretinogram (mfERG) technique was developed to provide a topographic measure of retinal activity. It provides objective, noninvasive measures of retinal function loss [1, 2]. The mfERG has been demonstrated to be a valuable test to detect and monitor outer retinal disorders, as well as some inner retinal diseases, such as diabetic retinopathy [3]. However, the responses in conventional mfERGs originate largely from the outer retina and capture relatively little information from the ganglion cells [4]. When the mfERG technique was applied to the study of glaucoma, conventional stimulation was not sensitive enough to detect early stages of glaucoma, which mainly affects retinal ganglion cells and their axons. Although the photopic negative response from the multifocal ERG and second-order kernel responses have been suggested for sensitive detection of inner retinal dysfunction, there is no definite correlation between those responses and visual field defects in glaucoma [5, 6].

Global-flash is a recently introduced modification of the mfERG stimulation paradigms [7–10]. In global-flash protocols, at least one global-flash frame is inserted in the *m*-sequence. Direct component (DC) and induced component (IC) waveforms are then obtained. The DC is the response to the focal flash and is analogous to the conventional mfERG response. The IC is the response to the global flash and reflects the recovery response from the preceding focal flash and is believed to be generated by the inner retina [11]. The IC component is enlarged in the global-flash protocol and the underlying ONHC is responsible for the nasotemporal asymmetry. The ONHC is a component of the electroretinogram that originates from optic nerve fibers and retinal ganglion cell axons at the optic nerve head. It is identified by its implicit time course, which increases with distance along the stimulated area from the optic disc; this is defined as nasotemporal asymmetry. This increase is due to the relatively slow propagation of action potentials along unmyelinated retinal ganglion cell axons [12, 13].

Recently, several glaucoma studies reported their results with the global-flash paradigms and ONHC. Luo et al. noted that losses of nasotemporal asymmetry and low-frequency component power occurred in the global-flash mfERG signals from eyes of nonhuman primates with experimental glaucoma [7, 8]. Fortune et al. demonstrated selective loss of an oscillatory feature in the IC response in patients with glaucoma and suggested that this effect may be due in part to a loss of the ONHC [9]. However, there are no previous studies that quantified the ONHC deficiency in the global-flash response or examined local correlation with visual field defects in human eyes.

In the present study, we quantified the ONHC by measuring the amplitude of the second positive deflection of the IC response waveform, which demonstrates nasotemporal asymmetry. Then, the local relationship between the quantified ONHC and visual field defects obtained by standard automated perimetry (SAP) was investigated.

2. Materials and Methods

2.1. Subjects. The present study enrolled 39 patients with primary open angle glaucoma (POAG) and 30 age-matched healthy subjects. This study was approved by the Institutional Review Board of Soonchunhyang University Hospital, Bucheon, and conformed to the tenets of the Declaration of Helsinki. Informed consent was obtained from all patients and normal control subjects.

The diagnosis of POAG was based on the presence of a glaucomatous optic disc associated with visual field defects measured by SAP and an open angle confirmed by gonioscopy. The glaucomatous optic disc was determined by a cup/disc ratio of at least 0.5 with typical glaucomatous changes including localized neuroretinal rim thinning. According to the diagnostic criterion for minimal abnormality in the visual field, a visual field defect was determined to be glaucomatous when it met one of three criteria [14]: (1) the pattern deviation plot showed a cluster of three or more nonedge points that had lower sensitivities than 5% of that of the normal population ($P < 0.05$) and one of the points had a sensitivity level that was less than 1% of the population ($P < 0.01$); (2) the value of the corrected pattern standard deviation was less than that of 5% of the normal visual field ($P < 0.05$); or (3) the Glaucoma Hemifield Test showed that the field was outside the normal limits. All patients had a history of a highest measured central corneal thickness adjusted intraocular pressure (IOP) above 21 mm Hg and controlled IOP at the time of testing. The adjusted IOP was calculated by using the following compensation formula; adjusted IOP = measured IOP + (550 − CCT) × 0.040 [15].

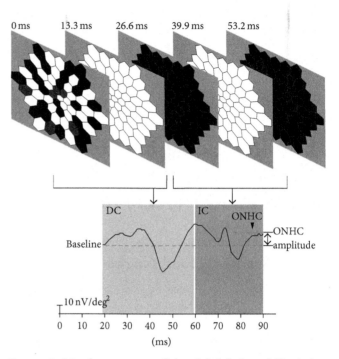

FIGURE 1: Stimulus sequence of the global-flash multifocal electroretinogram and the resulting response. The global-flash protocol contained a standard m-sequence step, followed by a global flash, then a dark frame, another global flash, and lastly a dark frame. The interval for each frame was 13.33 ms. The amplitude from the baseline to the peak of the second positive deflection in IC response epoch which selected from 60–90 ms was recorded as the ONHC amplitude.

The age-matched controls had no history of chronic ocular or systemic disease and no other pathologic features in a complete ophthalmic examination.

2.2. mfERG Recordings. The mfERGs were recorded with the VERIS Science 6.4.1 (Visual Evoked Response Imaging System; Electro-Diagnostic Imaging Inc., Redwood City, CA). Pupils were fully dilated with a topical application of 1% tropicamide and 2.5% phenylephrine hydrochloride. Burian-Allen bipolar contact lens electrodes (Hansen Ophthalmic Development Labs, Iowa City, IA) were used, with the ground electrode placed on the earlobe. The stimulus matrix consisted of 61 hexagonal elements. The size of the hexagons was scaled with eccentricity to elicit approximately equal amplitude responses at all locations. At a viewing distance of 27 cm, the radius of the stimulus array subtended approximately 30°. Fixation stability was monitored with a built-in infrared camera. The global-flash protocol contained a standard m-sequence step, followed by a global flash, then a dark frame, another global flash, and lastly a dark frame (Figure 1) [7, 8]. The interval for each frame was 13.33 ms. The recording was taken in a room with luminance of 100 cd/m^2. The maximum luminance of the m-sequence and global-flash frames was 200 cd/m^2, and the dark frames of both stimuli were 15 cd/m^2. The background luminance of each frame was 55 cd/m^2. The duration of the data acquisition was about 8 minutes, divided into 16 segments of 30 seconds each. Signals

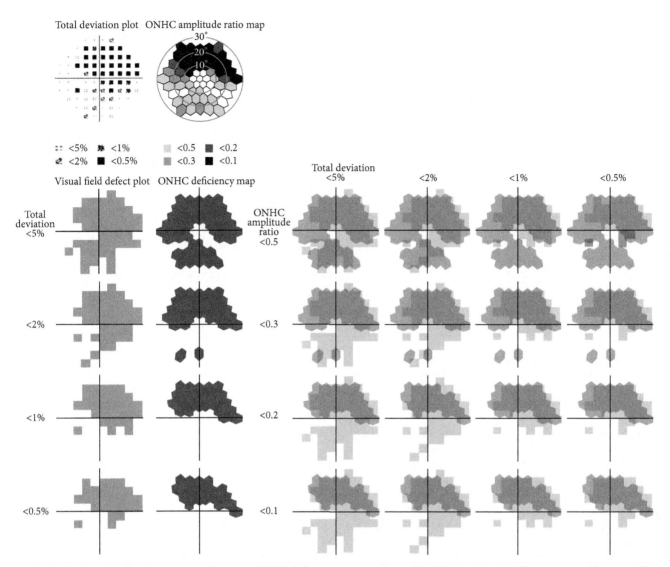

FIGURE 2: Calculations of overlapping rates between ONHC deficiency maps and visual field defect plots at different stages of functional loss. Areas of visual field defects were extracted from the total deviation plots in each of the four stages: visual sensitivities lower than 5%; lower than 2%; lower than 1%; and lower than 0.5%. ONHC deficiency maps were extracted from the ONHC ratio maps in each of the four stages: ONHC ratio lower than 0.5; lower than 0.3; lower than 0.2; and lower than 0.1. Four visual field defect plots and four ONHC deficiency maps were overlapped for each comparison and the spatial agreement between the ONHC deficiencies and visual field defects was evaluated by calculating rate of overlapping area.

were amplified with a gain of 50,000 and band pass filtered from 10–300 Hz (A Grass PS22, Grass-Telefactor; Astro-Med Inc., West Warwick, RI).

2.3. *Quantification of ONHC.* The response epoch comprising the IC was selected, 60–90 ms. The amplitude from the baseline to the peak of the second positive deflection was recorded as the ONHC amplitude, at 61 hexagons. The amplitude of the initial DC response at 20 ms was set as the baseline (Figure 1). The ONHC ratio was calculated to normalize the responses by dividing the measured ONHC amplitudes by the average of the seven largest ONHC amplitude measurements among the 61 hexagons. Seven hexagonal elements were selected from within ring 3 and most were chosen from rings 1 and 2. ONHC deficiency was defined as an ONHC ratio less than 0.5. ONHC deficiency was divided into four stages: between 0.5 and 0.3; between 0.3 and 0.2; between 0.2 and 0.1; and less than 0.1. ONHC ratio maps were constructed using gray scale according to the calculated values. Then, ONHC deficiency maps were extracted from the ONHC ratio maps (Figure 2).

2.4. *Automated Perimetry.* Automated perimetry was conducted using the Central 30-2 Swedish Interactive Threshold Algorithm (SITA) with a Humphrey visual field Analyzer II (Carl Zeiss Meditec, Dublin, CA) and a Goldmann size III stimulus on a 31.5-apostilb background. Areas of visual field defects were extracted from the total deviation (TD) plots in

TABLE 1: Demographic characteristics.

Variable	Normal	Glaucoma	P value
Number	30	39	
Age	49.25 ± 12.80	50.83 ± 13.70	0.858
Sex ratio (M/F)	0.60	0.85	0.235
MD (dB)	−0.08 ± 0.39	−8.44 ± 5.07	<0.001
PSD (dB)	1.43 ± 0.27	8.72 ± 4.69	<0.001
Average ONHC amplitude (nV/deg^2)	10.29 ± 0.94	6.01 ± 1.91	<0.001
Average of seven largest ONHC amplitudes (nV/deg^2)	16.91 ± 2.99	14.60 ± 4.01	0.104

TABLE 2: ONHC amplitude measurements and calculated ONHC ratio.

	Normal		Glaucoma	
	ONHC amplitude (nV/deg^2)	ONHC ratio	ONHC amplitude (nV/deg^2)	ONHC ratio
Ring 1	16.90 ± 2.99	0.95 ± 0.25	14.33 ± 4.25	0.98 ± 0.21
Ring 2	12.27 ± 5.07	0.67 ± 0.32	7.57 ± 5.12	0.52 ± 0.31
Ring 3	10.69 ± 3.72	0.60 ± 0.29	6.49 ± 5.24	0.43 ± 0.32
Ring 4	8.04 ± 3.26	0.43 ± 0.38	3.98 ± 3.32	0.28 ± 0.22

each of the four stages: visual sensitivities lower than those of 5% of the normal population; lower than 2%; lower than 1%; and lower than 0.5% (Figure 2).

2.5. Evaluation of Local Relationship between ONHC Deficiency and Visual Field Defect. 61 hexagonal arrays of mfERGs and total deviation plots of SAP, both covering central 30 degrees of the visual field each, were matched in the same image size. Next, four visual field defect plots and four ONHC deficiency maps were overlapped for each comparison (Figure 2). The local relationship between the ONHC deficiencies and visual field defects was evaluated by the overlap. The overlap between an ONHC deficiency map and visual field defect plot was calculated as follows: [(intersection area between the ONHC deficiency map and visual field defect plot) × 2]/(sum of the area of ONHC deficiency and visual field defect plot), (% presentation). Image processing and area measuring were conducted using imaging software (ImageJ 1.43u, Wayne Rasband, National Institutes of Health, available at http://rsb.info.nih.gov/ij/index.html).

2.6. Statistical Analysis. An independent t-test was performed to compare both the averages of the seven largest ONHC amplitudes between patients with glaucoma and normal controls. Differences in overlap between the visual field defects and ONHC deficiencies across various stages were evaluated by one-way analysis of variance (ANOVA) using a post hoc Bonferroni test. Statistical analysis was conducted using SPSS Statistics Version 21 (IBM Corporation, Somers, NY). All tests were two tailed and $P < 0.05$ was considered statistically significant.

3. Results

3.1. General Characteristics. The average age of the patients with glaucoma was 50.83±13.70 years, and it was 49.25±12.80 years for the normal controls. The mean deviation (MD) was −8.44 ± 5.07 in patients with glaucoma and −0.08 ± 0.39 for normal controls ($P < 0.001$). Pattern standard deviation (PSD) was 8.72 ± 4.69 in patients with glaucoma and 1.43 ± 0.27 in normal controls ($P < 0.001$) (Table 1).

3.2. ONHC Measurement in Normal and Glaucoma Groups. The mean ONHC amplitude from the 61 hexagons was 6.01 ± 1.91 nV/deg^2 in patients with glaucoma and 10.29 ± 0.94 nV/deg^2 in normal controls. The difference was significant ($P < 0.001$). However, the average of the seven largest ONHC amplitudes was 14.6 ± 4.01 nV/deg^2 in patients with glaucoma and 16.91 ± 2.99 nV/deg^2 in normal controls. The difference was not significant ($P = 0.104$) (Table 1). Cut-off values of ONHC amplitude of $p < 5\%$, $p < 2\%$, $p < 1\%$, and $p < 0.5\%$ were 1.73, 0.94, 0.62, and 0.44 nV/deg^2, respectively. Cut-off values of ONHC ratio of $p < 5\%$, $p < 2\%$, $p < 1\%$, and $p < 0.5\%$ were 0.10, 0.63, 0.62, and 0.55, respectively, on 30 healthy volunteers. ONHC amplitude measurements and calculated ONHC ratio were demonstrated in Table 2.

3.3. Local Relationship between ONHC Deficiencies and Visual Field Defects. The ONHC ratios less than 0.5 showed the highest local agreement with the total deviation of visual sensitivities less than 5%. The overlap was 75.0 ± 14.21%. The ONHC ratios <0.3 highly correlated with both TD <5% and <2%. The overlaps were 70.2 ± 12.22% for the less than 5% group and 68.8 ± 11.77% for the less than 2% group. The difference of overlap between the TD <5% group and the <2% group was not significant ($P = 0.139$). The ONHC ratio <0.2 showed high agreement with both TD <2% and <1%. Overlaps were 72.3 ± 13.60% and 68.1 ± 13.54%. The difference of agreement rates between TD <2% and <1% was not significant ($P = 0.094$). The ONHC ratio <0.1 showed the best agreement with TD <0.5%. The overlap was 68.2 ± 12.77% (Table 3, Figure 3).

TABLE 3: Overlap between total deviation and optic nerve head component ratios.

Total deviation	Optic nerve head component ratio			
	<0.5	<0.3	<0.2	<0.1
<5%	75.0 ± 14.21	70.2 ± 12.22	56.1 ± 14.23	54.7 ± 12.00
P value	<0.001	0.139	<0.001	0.877
<2%	68.0 ± 12.92	68.8 ± 11.77	72.3 ± 13.60	54.8 ± 13.41
P value	<0.001	<0.001	0.094	<0.001
<1%	60.1 ± 15.12	57.8 ± 13.31	68.1 ± 13.54	62.5 ± 11.93
P value	<0.001	0.005	<0.001	0.001
<0.5%	53.1 ± 13.85	53.4 ± 13.35	62.4 ± 13.87	68.2 ± 12.77

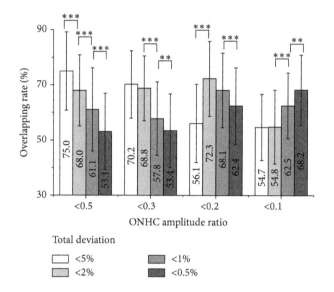

FIGURE 3: Overlapping rates between total deviation and optic nerve head component ratios. $^{**}P < 0.01$, $^{***}P < 0.001$.

4. Discussion

In the present study, we measured ONHC amplitudes obtained from global-flash mfERGs and investigated the local relationship between the ONHC amplitudes and visual field defects in patients with glaucoma. The ONHC is identified by its implicit time course, which increases with distance along the stimulated area from the optic disc which is called nasotemporal asymmetry [12, 13]. It has been reported that pharmacological suppression of inner retinal activity by intravitreal injection of tetrodotoxin (TTX, a blocker of sodium-channel dependent action potentials) reduced or eliminated the nasotemporal asymmetry in fast flicker mfERGs [16–18]. The nasotemporal asymmetry is augmented by the global-flash protocol [8, 19]. There are different ways of inserting the global flash in the m-sequence, and the aim is to enhance the adaptive effect of the retina to obtain the inner retinal contribution [20]. The IC of the global-flash mfERG response waveform resembles higher order kernels of the fast flicker mfERG (in terms of interflash interaction) and is believed to be generated by the inner retina [11, 21]. The ONHC can be refined by extracting the signal with the Sutter and Bears time-domain algorithm [12]; however, application of this multistep mathematical algorithm to extract the component is somewhat complicated in practical use. In this study, we quantified the ONHC by directly measuring the amplitude of the second positive deflection of the IC response waveform that comprised the nasotemporal asymmetry. The amplitude of the second positive deflection of the IC is representative of ONHC activity. The reduction of the second positive deflection of the IC response waveform with the global-flash paradigm implies a loss of the nasotemporal asymmetry (Figure 4); this loss of nasotemporal asymmetry reflects the loss of the ONHC. Therefore, the reduction of the second positive deflection of the IC response can demonstrate a loss of ONHC.

The mean ONHC amplitude measurements from the patients with glaucoma were significantly lower than that of normal controls. This result is in keeping with previous studies of experimental glaucoma, which showed a decrease of nasotemporal asymmetry after intravitreal TTX injections [16–18]. However, the average of the seven largest ONHC amplitudes between patients with glaucoma and normal controls was not significantly different, though normal controls have slightly higher values. This result may be due to the moderate disease severity of the enrolled patients and the characteristics of glaucomatous visual field loss. The average MD of glaucoma patients was −8.44. All of the glaucoma patients had preserved central 5 to 10 degrees of visual field sensitivity. Central 10 degrees of the visual field correspond to rings 1-2 of mfERG, and rings 1-2 are composed of seven hexagonal elements. Therefore, we use the average value of seven hexagonal elements as reference for normalization in each subject. Relative central visual field conservation and preserved central mfERG responses were responsible for the similar large ONHC amplitudes values between patients with glaucoma and normal controls.

Loss of the ONHC amplitude showed a high local agreement with visual field defects. The average overlap between the ONHC deficiency map and the visual field defect plot was 71.42% across the different stages of functional loss. The highest agreement was between the ONHC ratio <0.5 and TD <5%; the ONHC ratio <0.2 and TD <2% and 1%; and the ONHC ratio <0.1 and TD <0.5%. The ONHC ratio <0.3 showed high agreement with TD <5% and 2%. However, the overlaps were smaller than that of the ONHC ratio <0.5 and TD <5% (70.2% versus 75.0%) and the ONHC ratio <0.2 in

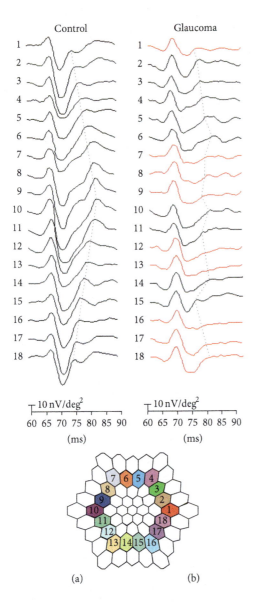

FIGURE 4: Induced component waveforms in normal controls and patients with glaucoma. IC of normal controls (a) shows intact second positive deflection waveform and nasotemporal asymmetry. IC of patients with glaucoma (b) shows reduced second positive deflection in some waveforms (red line) and disrupted nasotemporal asymmetry. Dot line indicates optic nerve head components.

TD <2% (68.8% versus 72.3%). When one has fixed area and the other has changed, the overlap necessarily demonstrates a negative quadric curve (Figure 5). When one area is fixed and the other area becomes larger, the intersection area increases but the overlap decreases. In contrast, when one area is fixed and the other area becomes smaller, the intersection area decreases and the overlap subsequently decreases. The vertex value is given when the two other areas completely overlap more in size. Therefore, when estimating the quadric curve of the overlap between the ONHC ratios less than 0.3 and visual field defects, the vertex value is presumed to be a total deviation of 3 or 4% (Figure 5). Namely, the ONHC ratio less than 0.3 may show the best agreement with a total deviation less than 3 or 4%.

There were a number of limitations to this study. The 61-hexagon stimulus array was scaled to obtain equal amplitude responses. The array used for the perimetry was not scaled, and hence hexagons at different locations contained different numbers of visual field test points. For this reason, we compared the total area of the visual field defects and ONHC deficiencies to reduce the inaccuracy of the one to one correspondence, rather than compare the hexagon elements and visual field test points by matched pairs.

Patients with visual field defects are more likely to have electrophysiological abnormalities than patients with preperimetric glaucoma. Further investigations are required for evaluating the usefulness of ONHC amplitude from the global-flash mfERG in patients with preperimetric glaucoma.

The ONHC amplitude measurements varied considerably from person to person; therefore, a normal value was not established. In the present study, ONHC ratios were used for analysis to reduce the interpersonal variation. This study enrolled the patients with mild to moderate glaucoma and subjects had preserved central visual field sensitivity and good mfERGs response. The averages of the seven largest ONHC amplitudes between glaucoma patients and normal controls were not significantly different. However, if the mfERG responses from every hexagonal element were proportionally reduced in advanced glaucoma, the normalization using an intraindividual ratio format would not provide any useful information. In such a case, normalization using a normal range value obtained from controls of large population will be needed.

The main way for evaluating functional loss of visual field in glaucoma is a perimetry. Perimetry is based on psychophysics and is a subjective measurement. Although perimetry is an excellent tool, there is always a need for determining the functional loss with objective method. Electroretinogram, involving mfERG, is one of the objective tools. However, conventional mfERG mostly reflects outer retinal function and is not suitable for early detection of glaucoma. In this study, we used global-flash mfERG protocols, which are more targeted at the inner retinal function. Even more, we directly measured the second positive deflection amplitude of the IC as ONHC for easier practical use and evidenced a significant agreement between ONHC amplitude loss and visual field defect in SAP. We imply that ONHC amplitude can be used as objective tool for evaluating functional loss in glaucoma, with further investigations.

5. Conclusions

The ONHC amplitude was reduced in patients with glaucoma compared to normal controls. Loss of global-flash mfERG ONHC amplitudes showed a high local agreement with visual field defects obtained by SAP in patients with glaucoma. The ONHC amplitude measurements from global-flash mfERG serve as an objective method to evaluate local functional loss in patients with glaucoma. The overlap was greatest when the largest range of severity for the deviation and amplitude reductions were compared.

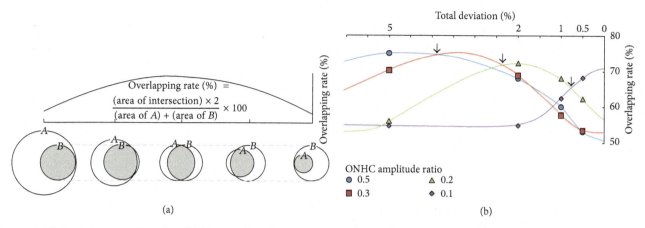

Figure 5: (a) Quadric curve of overlap. (b) Estimated overlap curve between total deviation and optic nerve head component ratios. When one area is fixed and the other area changes, the overlapping rate values necessarily demonstrate a negative quadric curve (a). The highest correspondence was between ONHC ratios <0.5 and TD <5%, ONHC ratio <0.3 and TD <3 or 4%, ONHC ratio <0.2 and TD <2 and 1%, and ONHC ratio <0.1 and TD <0.5% (b).

Conflict of Interests

The authors declare that there is no conflict of interests regarding the publication of this paper.

Acknowledgments

This work was supported by grants from the Basic Science Research Program through the National Research Foundation of Korea (NRF) as funded by the ministry of Education, Science, and Technology (Grant no. 2013R1A1A2009899; Seoul, South Korea) and partially by the Soonchunhyang University Research Fund.

References

[1] E. E. Sutter and D. Tran, "The field topography of ERG components in man—I. The photopic luminance response," *Vision Research*, vol. 32, no. 3, pp. 433–446, 1992.

[2] M. A. Bearse Jr. and E. E. Sutter, "Imaging localized retinal dysfunction with the multifocal electroretinogram," *Journal of the Optical Society of America A: Optics, Image Science, and Vision*, vol. 13, no. 3, pp. 634–640, 1996.

[3] T. Y. Y. Lai, W.-M. Chan, R. Y. K. Lai, J. W. S. Ngai, H. Li, and D. S. C. Lam, "The clinical applications of multifocal electroretinography: a systematic review," *Survey of Ophthalmology*, vol. 52, no. 1, pp. 61–96, 2007.

[4] D. C. Hood, J. G. Odel, C. S. Chen, and B. J. Winn, "The multifocal electroretinogram," *Journal of Neuro-Ophthalmology*, vol. 23, no. 3, pp. 225–235, 2003.

[5] U. Kretschmann, M. Bock, R. Gockeln, and E. Zrenner, "Clinical applications of multifocal electroretinography," *Documenta Ophthalmologica*, vol. 100, no. 2, pp. 99–113, 2000.

[6] M. Kaneko, S. Machida, Y. Hoshi, and D. Kurosaka, "Alterations of photopic negative response of multifocal electroretinogram in patients with glaucoma," *Current Eye Research*, vol. 40, no. 1, pp. 77–86, 2015.

[7] X. Luo, N. B. Patel, L. P. Rajagopalan, R. S. Harwerth, and L. J. Frishman, "Relation between macular retinal ganglion cell/inner plexiform layer thickness and multifocal electroretinogram measures in experimental glaucoma," *Investigative Ophthalmology and Visual Science*, vol. 55, no. 7, pp. 4512–4524, 2014.

[8] X. Luo, N. B. Patel, R. S. Harwerth, and L. J. Frishman, "Loss of the low-frequency component of the global-flash multifocal electroretinogram in primate eyes with experimental glaucoma," *Investigative Ophthalmology & Visual Science*, vol. 52, no. 6, pp. 3792–3804, 2011.

[9] B. Fortune, M. A. Bearse Jr., G. A. Cioffi, and C. A. Johnson, "Selective loss of an oscillatory component from temporal retinal multifocal ERG responses in glaucoma," *Investigative Ophthalmology & Visual Science*, vol. 43, no. 8, pp. 2638–2647, 2002.

[10] P. H. W. Chu, H. H. L. Chan, and B. Brown, "Glaucoma detection is facilitated by luminance modulation of the global flash multifocal electroretinogram," *Investigative Ophthalmology and Visual Science*, vol. 47, no. 3, pp. 929–937, 2006.

[11] Y. Shimada, Y. Li, M. A. Bearse Jr., E. E. Sutter, and W. Fung, "Assessment of early retinal changes in diabetes using a new multifocal ERG protocol," *British Journal of Ophthalmology*, vol. 85, no. 4, pp. 414–419, 2001.

[12] E. E. Sutter and M. A. Bearse Jr., "The optic nerve head component of the human ERG," *Vision Research*, vol. 39, no. 3, pp. 419–436, 1999.

[13] D. C. Hood, M. A. Bearse Jr., E. E. Sutter, S. Viswanathan, and L. J. Frishman, "The optic nerve head component of the monkey's (*Macaca mulatta*) multifocal electroretinogram (mERG)," *Vision Research*, vol. 41, no. 16, pp. 2029–2041, 2001.

[14] D. R. Anderson, *Automated Static Perimetry*, Mosby, St. Louis, Mo, USA, 2nd edition, 1999.

[15] M. Kohlhaas, A. G. Boehm, E. Spoerl, A. Pürsten, H. J. Grein, and L. E. Pillunat, "Effect of central corneal thickness, corneal curvature, and axial length on applanation tonometry," *Archives of Ophthalmology*, vol. 124, no. 4, pp. 471–476, 2006.

[16] D. C. Hood, L. J. Frishman, S. Viswanathan, J. G. Robson, and J. Ahmed, "Evidence for a ganglion cell contribution to the primate electroretinogram (ERG): effects of TTX on the

multifocal ERG in macaque," *Visual Neuroscience*, vol. 16, no. 3, pp. 411–416, 1999.

[17] D. C. Hood, V. Greenstein, L. Frishman et al., "Identifying inner retinal contributions to the human multifocal ERG," *Vision Research*, vol. 39, no. 13, pp. 2285–2291, 1999.

[18] L. J. Frishman, S. Saszik, R. S. Harwerth et al., "Effects of experimental glaucoma in macaques on the multifocal ERG. Multifocal ERG in laser-induced glaucoma," *Documenta Ophthalmologica*, vol. 100, no. 2, pp. 231–251, 2000.

[19] J. M. Miguel-Jiménez, L. Boquete, S. Ortega, J. M. Rodríguez-Ascariz, and R. Blanco, "Glaucoma detection by wavelet-based analysis of the global flash multifocal electroretinogram," *Medical Engineering and Physics*, vol. 32, no. 6, pp. 617–622, 2010.

[20] H. H.-L. Chan, Y. Ng, and P. H. Chu, "Applications of the multifocal electroretinogram in the detection of glaucoma," *Clinical & Experimental Optometry*, vol. 94, pp. 247–258, 2011.

[21] P. H. W. Chu, H. H. L. Chan, Y.-F. Ng et al., "Porcine global flash multifocal electroretinogram: possible mechanisms for the glaucomatous changes in contrast response function," *Vision Research*, vol. 48, no. 16, pp. 1726–1734, 2008.

Effect of Storage Temperature on Key Functions of Cultured Retinal Pigment Epithelial Cells

Lara Pasovic,[1,2] Jon Roger Eidet,[1] Berit S. Brusletto,[1] Torstein Lyberg,[1] and Tor P. Utheim[1,3]

[1]Department of Medical Biochemistry, Oslo University Hospital, Kirkeveien 166, P.O. Box 4956, Nydalen, 0424 Oslo, Norway
[2]Faculty of Medicine, University of Oslo, Sognsvannsveien 9, 0372 Oslo, Norway
[3]Department of Oral Biology, Faculty of Dentistry, University of Oslo, Sognsvannsveien 10, P.O. Box 1052, Blindern, 0316 Oslo, Norway

Correspondence should be addressed to Lara Pasovic; larapasovic@gmail.com

Academic Editor: Manuel Vidal-Sanz

Purpose. Replacement of the diseased retinal pigment epithelium (RPE) with cells capable of performing the specialized functions of the RPE is the aim of cell replacement therapy for treatment of macular degenerative diseases. A storage method for RPE is likely to become a prerequisite for the establishment of such treatment. Herein, we analyze the effect of storage temperature on key functions of cultured RPE cells. *Methods.* Cultured ARPE-19 cells were stored in Minimum Essential Medium at 4°C, 16°C, and 37°C for seven days. Total RNA was isolated and the gene expression profile was determined using DNA microarrays. Comparison of the microarray expression values with qRT-PCR analysis of selected genes validated the results. *Results.* Expression levels of several key genes involved in phagocytosis, pigment synthesis, the visual cycle, adherens, and tight junctions, and glucose and ion transport were maintained close to control levels in cultures stored at 4°C and 16°C. Cultures stored at 37°C displayed regulational changes in a larger subset of genes related to phagocytosis, adherens, and tight junctions. *Conclusion.* RPE cultures stored at 4°C and 16°C for one week are capable of maintaining the expression levels of genes important for key RPE functions close to control levels.

1. Introduction

The retinal pigment epithelium (RPE) is a highly specialized tissue. Situated between the neuroretina and choroid, it performs several functions that are crucial for supporting sight. Among the most important are phagocytosis of shed photoreceptor (PR) outer segments, regeneration of the visual cycle pigment rhodopsin, transportation of glucose and nutrients from the choroid to the distal part of the neuroretina, and transportation of excess fluid in the opposite direction [1, 2]. Malfunction of the RPE, implying a disrupted ability to perform these tasks, is a direct cause of prevalent retinal diseases like age-related macular degeneration (AMD) [3, 4] and a consequence of inherited disorders like Stargardt disease [5].

A promising approach for treatment of these diseases is the transplantation of tissue engineered RPE [6–10]. However, for the prospect of tissue engineering to become a widespread treatment option, it is necessary to ensure cell availability during short-term storage and transportation of RPE cells. In the process of establishing such a protocol, our research group has demonstrated that storage temperature has a crucial impact on the viability and morphology of cultured RPE cells [11]. ARPE-19 cultures stored at 16°C displayed the greatest number of viable cells compared to cells stored at eight other temperatures (4°C, 8°C, 12°C, 20°C, 24°C, 28°C, 32°C, and 37°C) after seven days of storage [11].

Having established the potential effect of storage temperature on cell viability, we herein aim to investigate the effect of storage temperature on the gene expression associated with many highly specialized functions of the RPE, using microarray technology. Increased knowledge of the effects of storage on cultured ARPE-19 cells is imperative for future use of RPE transplantation in treatment of eye diseases affecting millions of people worldwide [12].

2. Materials and Methods

2.1. Cell Culture Media and Reagents. Adult retinal pigment epithelial cells (ARPE-19) were purchased from the American

Type Culture Collection (ATCC) (Manassas, VA). Dulbecco's Modified Eagle's Medium (DMEM), Nutrient Mixture F12, fetal bovine serum (FBS), trypsin-EDTA, phosphate-buffered saline (PBS), 4-(2-hydroxyethyl)-1-piperazineethanesulfonic acid (HEPES), sodium bicarbonate, gentamycin, penicillin, and streptomycin were from Sigma-Aldrich (St. Louis, MO). Minimum Essential Medium (MEM) was purchased from Invitrogen (Carlsbad, CA). Nunclon T25 and T75 flasks, pipettes, and other routine plastics were purchased from VWR (West Chester, PA). The miRNeasy Mini Kit containing the QIAzol Lysis Reagent was obtained from Qiagen (Venlo, Netherlands).

2.2. Cell Culture and Storage. RPE cells from the ARPE-19 cell line were cultured under standard conditions in 95% air and 5% CO_2 at 37°C in DMEM/F12 medium containing 10% FBS, 50 units/mL penicillin, and 50 μg/mL streptomycin. All ARPE-19 cells were from passage 4 and lower after acquisition from the vendor. Upon reaching confluence, the cells were seeded (5000 cells/cm^2) in Nunclon T25 and T75 flasks. The culture medium was changed after two days, and confluent cultures were obtained on the third day. Three cultures were immediately processed for mRNA amplification and used as controls, while nine cultures were prepared for storage. The cells were rinsed with PBS, and the culture medium was replaced by storage medium consisting of MEM, 25 mM HEPES, 22.3 mM sodium bicarbonate, and 50 μg/mL gentamycin, hereafter referred to as MEM. The cultures were then placed in storage containers maintaining a stable temperature of either 4°C, 16°C, or 37°C and stored for seven days. The configuration and design of the custom-made storage containers have been explained earlier [11].

2.3. RNA Extraction and Microarray Hybridization. Cultured ARPE-19 cells that had been stored for seven days at 4°C, 16°C, and 37°C, as well as control cultures that had not been stored, were rinsed with PBS and directly lysed with QIAzol Lysis Reagent. 150 ng of total RNA was subjected to GeneChip HT One-Cycle cDNA Synthesis Kit and GeneChip HT IVT Labeling Kit, following the manufacturer's protocol for whole genome gene expression analysis (Affymetrix, Santa Clara, CA, USA). Microarray analyses were performed using the Affymetrix GeneChip Human Gene 1.0 ST Arrays (Affymetrix, Santa Clara, CA), which contains approximately 28,000 gene transcripts. Biotinylated and fragmented single stranded cDNAs were hybridized to the GeneChips. The arrays were washed and stained using FS-450 fluidics station (Affymetrix). Signal intensities were detected by Hewlett Packard Gene Array Scanner 3000 7G (Hewlett Packard, Palo Alto, CA, USA).

The scanned images were processed using the AGCC (Affymetrix GeneChip Command Console) software and the CEL files were imported into Partek Genomics Suite software (Partek, Inc. MO, USA). The Robust Multichip Analysis (RMA) algorithm was applied for generation of signal values and normalization. Gene transcripts with maximal signal values of less than 32 across all arrays were removed to filter for low and nonexpressed genes, reducing the number of gene transcripts to 17,684. For expression comparisons of different groups, profiles were compared using a 1-way ANOVA model. The results were expressed as fold changes (FC) and P values.

2.4. Microarray Data Analysis. Gene networks and canonical pathways representing key genes were identified using Ingenuity Pathways Analysis (IPA) (http://www.ingenuity.com/). Briefly, the data set containing gene identifiers and corresponding fold changes and P values was uploaded into the web-delivered application and each gene identifier was mapped into its corresponding gene object in the Ingenuity Pathways Knowledge Base (IPKB). The functional analysis identified the biological functions and/or diseases that were most significant to the data sets. Fisher's exact test was performed to calculate a P value determining the probability that each biological function and/or disease assigned to the data set was due to chance alone. The data sets were mined for significant pathways with the IPA library of canonical pathways and networks were generated by using IPA as graphical representations of the molecular relationships between genes and gene products.

The presentation of the microarray data was divided into two manuscripts: the present and another addressing the genes not presented herein. This was done to allow for a more profound discussion of our findings.

2.5. Validation by PCR. The differential gene expression data were validated for selected transcripts (TYRP1, DSC1, and GLUT12) using TaqMan Gene Expression Assays and the Applied Biosystems ViiA 7 real-time PCR system (Applied Biosystems, Life Technologies). Briefly, 200 ng of total RNA was reverse transcribed using qScript cDNA Super Mix (Quanta Biosciences) following the manufacturer's instructions. After completion of cDNA synthesis, 1/10th of the first strand reaction was used for PCR amplification. A total of 9 μL of diluted cDNA (diluted in H_2O), 1 μL of selected primer/probes TaqMan Gene Expression Assays (Life Technologies), and 10 μL TaqMan Universal Master Mix (Life Technologies) were used following the manufacturer's instructions. Transducin-like enhancer of split 1 (TLE1) was used as endogenous control due to low coefficient of variation (CV) (0.444) in the Affymetrix study. Each gene was run in duplicates. TaqMan Gene Expression Assays (Life Technology) used assays detecting TYRP1 (Hs00167051_m1), DSC1 (Hs00245189_m1), GLUT12 (Hs01547015_m1), and TLE1 (Hs00270768_m1).

P values were calculated using Student's t-test in Microsoft Excel using delta Ct values. Normalized target gene expression levels (FC) were calculated using the formula: $2^{-\Delta\Delta Ct}$.

3. Results

3.1. Analysis of Retinal Pigment Epithelial Cell Functions. In order to elucidate the expression patterns of genes critical to important RPE functions, we investigated the expression levels of individual genes associated with distinctive cellular properties (i.e., phagocytosis, pigment synthesis, visual cycle,

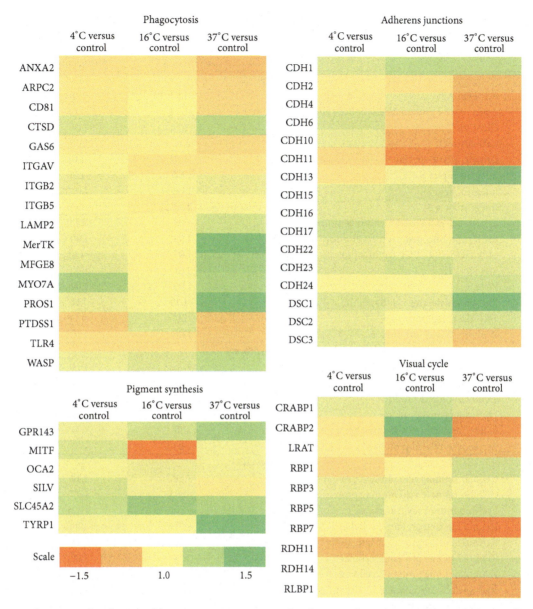

FIGURE 1: Heat map diagrams of a selection of the most important genes related to RPE phagocytosis, pigment synthesis, adherens junctions, and visual cycle, respectively. The color scale illustrates the relative expression level of mRNAs: green color represents a high expression level and orange color represents a low expression level.

adherens and tight junctions, and glucose and ion transport). Only significantly regulated genes are mentioned, namely, those displaying a P value below 0.05. Results are presented in Table 1 and Figures 1-2.

Phagocytosis. Phagocytosis of photoreceptor (PR) outer segments is a crucial function of the RPE, and the components of its phagocytic machinery have been thoroughly described [13]. Compared to control cells, cells that had been stored at 4°C and 16°C showed no difference in levels of expression for any of the 16 identified genes important for phagocytic functions. Cells that had been stored at 37°C displayed significant changes in gene regulation of several genes; however, only the engulfment-related gene PROS1 displayed a fold change of more than 1.5.

Pigment Synthesis. Production of melanin pigment by the RPE has two important functions in vivo: photoprotection, due to the antioxidant effect of melanin, and prevention of internal reflection of light from the sclera back to the retina [14]. Of six identified genes related to pigment synthesis, SLC45A2 showed a 1.4-fold increase and MITF a 2.3-fold decrease in expression at 16°C compared to controls. TYRP1 showed a notable 3.6-fold upregulation at 37°C compared to control cells. At 4°C there were no significant differences in expression levels.

TABLE 1: Expression of genes involved in key functions of the RPE at different temperatures compared to controls.

Gene symbol	Gene description	Fold change		
		4°C versus C	16°C versus C	37°C versus C
Phagocytosis				
ANXA2	Annexin A2	−1.07	−1.06	−1.21
ARPC2	Actin related protein 2/3 complex, subunit 2, 34 kDa	−1.04	−1.01	**−1.10**
CD81	CD81 molecule	−1.04	1.01	−1.10
CTSD	Cathepsin D	1.11	1.05	**1.23**
GAS6	Growth arrest-specific 6	−1.03	−1.01	−1.09
ITGAV	Integrin, alpha V	1.02	−1.05	−1.05
ITGB2	Integrin, beta 2	1.06	1.03	1.06
ITGB5	Integrin, beta 5	1.01	−1.01	1.01
LAMP2	Lysosomal-associated membrane protein 2	1.03	−1.00	**1.13**
MerTK	MER protooncogene, tyrosine kinase	1.04	1.00	1.73
MFGE8	Milk fat globule-EGF factor 8 protein	1.07	−1.01	1.32
MYO7A	Myosin VIIa	1.31	1.02	1.28
PROS1	Protein S	1.06	1.02	**1.73**
PTDSS1	Phosphatidylserine synthase 1	**−1.15**	1.11	**−1.18**
TLR4	Toll-like receptor 4	−1.07	−1.08	−1.15
WASP	Wiskott-Aldrich syndrome	1.06	1.10	**1.23**
Pigment synthesis				
GPR143	G protein-coupled receptor 143	1.05	1.14	1.33
MITF	Microphthalmia-associated transcription factor	1.12	**−2.35**	1.03
OCA2	Oculocutaneous albinism II	1.03	1.05	1.03
PMEL	Premelanosome protein	1.12	1.03	−1.02
SLC45A2	Solute carrier family 45, member 2	1.18	**1.37**	1.28
TYRP1	Tyrosinase-related protein 1	1.03	1.02	**3.62**
Visual cycle				
CRABP1	Cellular retinoic acid binding protein 1	1.08	**1.14**	1.11
CRABP2	Cellular retinoic acid binding protein 2	−1.03	1.77	−1.40
LRAT	Lecithin retinol acyltransferase	−1.01	−1.21	−1.23
RBP1	Retinol binding protein 1, cellular	−1.09	−1.00	1.15
RBP3	Retinol binding protein 3, interstitial	1.05	1.06	1.03
RBP5	Retinol binding protein 5, cellular	1.13	1.03	1.14
RBP7	Retinol binding protein 7, cellular	1.01	1.04	**−1.60**
RDH11	Retinol dehydrogenase 11	**−1.19**	1.00	1.06
RDH14	Retinol dehydrogenase 14	1.03	−1.09	1.15
RLBP1	Retinaldehyde binding protein 1	−1.00	1.21	−1.31
Adherens junctions				
CDH1	Cadherin 1, type 1, E-cadherin (epithelial)	1.11	1.22	1.21
CDH2	Cadherin 2, type 1, N-cadherin (neuronal)	−1.02	−1.07	−1.23
CDH4	Cadherin 4, type 1, R-cadherin (retinal)	−1.02	1.07	−1.35
CDH6	Cadherin 6, type 2, K-cadherin (fetal kidney)	1.12	−1.12	**−3.04**
CDH10	Cadherin 10, type 2 (T2-cadherin)	1.06	−1.27	**−1.73**
CDH11	Cadherin 11, type 2, OB-cadherin (osteoblast)	−1.08	−1.43	**−2.16**
CDH13	Cadherin 13	−1.05	1.03	**2.02**
CDH15	Cadherin 15	1.08	1.12	1.05
CDH16	Cadherin 16, KSP-cadherin	1.08	1.09	1.07
CDH17	Cadherin 17, LI cadherin (liver-intestine)	1.14	−1.02	1.35
CDH22	Cadherin 22, type 2	1.06	1.02	1.04
CDH23	Cadherin-related 23	1.09	**1.14**	1.08
CDH24	Cadherin 24, type 2	1.01	1.01	1.13
DSC1	Desmocollin 1	1.11	1.08	**8.34**
DSC2	Desmocollin 2	1.06	1.01	1.11
DSC3	Desmocollin 3	1.09	−1.04	**−1.17**

TABLE 1: Continued.

Gene symbol	Gene description	Fold change		
		4°C versus C	16°C versus C	37°C versus C
Tight junctions				
ACTB	Actin, beta	−1.05	−1.02	**−1.18**
CALM1	Calmodulin 1 (phosphorylase kinase, delta)	−1.04	**1.09**	**−1.18**
CLDN3	Claudin 3	1.14	−1.01	**−1.16**
CLDN9	Claudin 9	−1.02	1.08	**1.21**
CLDN11	Claudin 11	−1.11	1.07	**−2.91**
CLDN15	Claudin 15	1.04	−1.07	**1.28**
CLDN18	Claudin 18	1.12	**1.22**	1.12
CLDN19	Claudin 19	1.13	1.12	1.15
CLDN23	Claudin 23	1.13	**1.18**	1.14
CRB3	Crumbs family member 3	**1.17**	**1.17**	1.15
CTNNA	Catenin (cadherin-associated protein), alpha 1	−1.03	−1.03	1.03
F11R	F11 receptor	−1.02	1.04	**−1.52**
JAM3	Junctional adhesion molecule 3	−1.08	1.01	**−1.18**
MAGI1	Membrane associated guanylate kinase, WW and PDZ domain containing 1	1.03	**−1.50**	−1.08
MAGI3	Membrane associated guanylate kinase, WW and PDZ domain containing 3	−1.04	**−1.82**	**−1.33**
MPDZ	Multiple PDZ domain protein	1.09	**−1.29**	1.01
MYO7A	Myosin VIIA	1.31	1.02	1.28
OCLN	Occludin	1.09	−1.15	1.49
PTEN	Phosphatase and tensin homolog	1.02	−1.01	**−1.14**
RAB3B	RAB3B, member RAS oncogene family	−1.15	1.08	**−2.19**
TJP1	Tight junction protein 1	1.02	−1.10	−1.02
TJP2	Tight junction protein 2	−1.01	1.25	**−1.40**
TJP3	Tight junction protein 3	1.06	1.08	1.04
Glucose transport				
SLC2A1	Solute carrier family 2 (facilitated glucose transporter), member 1	1.04	−1.01	1.05
SLC2A3	Solute carrier family 2 (facilitated glucose transporter), member 3	1.11	**2.00**	1.13
SLC2A4	Solute carrier family 2 (facilitated glucose transporter), member 4	1.05	1.12	1.05
SLC2A5	Solute carrier family 2 (facilitated glucose transporter), member 5	1.10	1.16	1.13
SLC2A6	Solute carrier family 2 (facilitated glucose transporter), member 6	−1.11	1.03	−1.06
SLC2A8	Solute carrier family 2 (facilitated glucose transporter), member 8	1.01	**1.21**	**1.21**
SLC2A10	Solute carrier family 2 (facilitated glucose transporter), member 10	1.07	1.13	1.14
SLC2A11	Solute carrier family 2 (facilitated glucose transporter), member 11	1.08	−1.01	1.07
SLC2A12	Solute carrier family 2 (facilitated glucose transporter), member 12	−1.08	−1.39	**−2.69**
SLC2A13	Solute carrier family 2 (facilitated glucose transporter), member 13	1.01	−1.05	−1.08
SLC2A14	Solute carrier family 2 (facilitated glucose transporter), member 14	1.08	**1.58**	1.07
Na-K-ATPase				
ATP1A1	ATPase, Na^+/K^+ transporting, alpha 1 polypeptide	−1.04	−1.03	**1.21**
ATP1A2	ATPase, Na^+/K^+ transporting, alpha 2 polypeptide	1.08	1.06	1.22
ATP1A3	ATPase, Na^+/K^+ transporting, alpha 3 polypeptide	−1.01	**1.38**	1.17
ATP1B1	ATPase, Na^+/K^+ transporting, beta 1 polypeptide	1.01	1.12	−1.01
ATP1B2	ATPase, Na^+/K^+ transporting, beta 2 polypeptide	1.10	**1.17**	1.09
ATP1B3	ATPase, Na^+/K^+ transporting, beta 3 polypeptide	−1.16	1.10	**1.49**

P values < 0.05 are marked in bold font.

Visual Cycle. The RPE serves a crucial function in the visual cycle by reisomerizing all-trans-retinal to 11-cis-retinal, and defects in key proteins of the cycle can in themselves lead to various retinal diseases [1, 15]. Most of the identified visual cycle genes were maintained at expression levels similar to controls. RLBP1 and RBP7 expression was decreased 1.3-fold and 1.6-fold, respectively, in cells stored at 37°C, while RDH11 was decreased 1.2-fold in cells stored at 4°C. In cultures stored at 16°C, CRABP2 (RBP6) expression was increased 1.8-fold.

Adherens Junctions. Adherens junctions link actin filaments between epithelial cells and provide a strong mechanical attachment in cellular monolayers. Cadherins form homodimers with cadherins of adjacent cells and are pivotal for

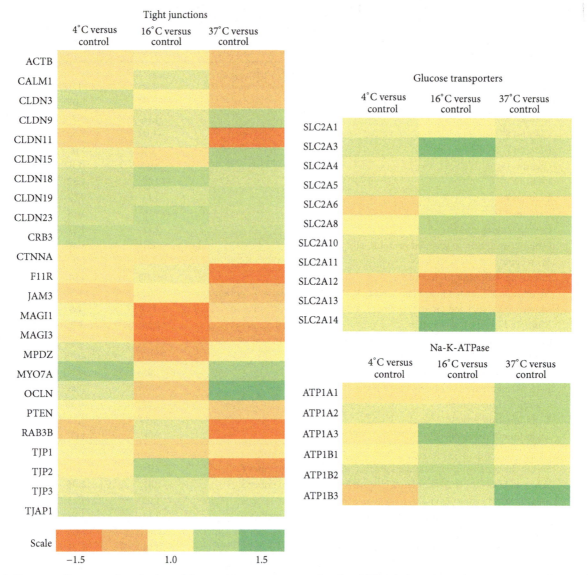

FIGURE 2: Heat map diagrams of a selection of the most important genes related to RPE tight junctions, glucose transportation, and Na-K-ATPase, respectively. The color scale illustrates the relative expression level of mRNAs: green color represents a high expression level and orange color represents a low expression level.

the integrity of the junction [16]. A total of 13 different cadherins were identified in our data set, and their expression levels were unchanged in cells stored at 4°C and 16°C compared to the control. At 37°C, cadherins 6, 10, and 11 were downregulated 3.0-fold, 1.7-fold, and 2.2-fold, respectively, while DSC1 and CDH13 were upregulated 8.3-fold and 2.0-fold, respectively, compared to control cells.

Tight Junctions. Tight junctions of the RPE regulate cell polarity, proliferation, and paracellular diffusion, and they are constituents of the blood-retinal barrier [17]. Of the 23 identified genes involved in the tight junction complex, seven were differentially expressed in cells stored at 16°C, but only the downregulation of MAGI1 and MAGI3 exceeded a fold change of 1.5. A total of 14 genes were differentially expressed at 37°C, of which CLDN11, F11R, and RAB3B were downregulated more than 1.5-fold. CRB3 was increased 1.2-fold in cells stored at 4°C.

Glucose Transport. The RPE is critical for supplying the inner part of the retina with glucose, and the maintenance and regulation of GLUT channels are essential for this function [18, 19]. In cells that had been stored at 16°C, we found an increased expression of three of a total of 11 glucose transporter isoforms identified in our material. GLUT3 was increased 2-fold, GLUT8 1.2-fold, and GLUT14 1.6-fold. In cells stored at 37°C, there was a 1.2-fold increase in expression of GLUT8 and a 2.7-fold decrease of GLUT12. No changes in expression were detected at 4°C.

Ion Transport. The Na-K-ATPase establishes and maintains electrochemical gradients across the plasma membrane [20],

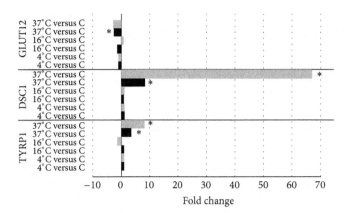

FIGURE 3: Validation of microarray expression results by qRT-PCR. Selected mRNAs (TYRP1, DSC1, and GLUT12) were differentially expressed in cultured RPE cells stored at different temperatures (4°C, 16°C, or 37°C) compared to control cells that had not been stored. Black bars indicate microarray expression values and grey bars represent PCR verification values. $^{*}P < 0.01$.

thereby providing the energy for transepithelial transport [15]. Of six identified genes involved in the Na-K-ATPase, ATP1A3 and ATP1B2 were upregulated 1.4-fold and 1.2-fold at 16°C storage, respectively. ATP1A1 and ATP1B3 were upregulated 1.2-fold and 1.5-fold, respectively, at 37°C storage. There were no significant changes at 4°C compared to controls.

3.2. PCR Validation of Key Genes. Relative quantification of a few key genes (TYRP1, DSC1, and GLUT12) was performed with real-time PCR (Figure 3). The expression of TYRP1 was significantly upregulated to 8.2-fold at 37°C compared to controls. In comparison, the microarray data showed a 3.6-fold upregulation of this gene at 37°C. DSC1 expression was significantly and considerably upregulated in the 37°C group compared to controls, with a 67.0-fold upregulation. This is higher than the corresponding microarray data, which yielded an 8.3-fold upregulation at this temperature. PCR analysis of GLUT12 expression showed a similar downregulation compared to microarray results (3.0-fold and 2.7-fold, resp.). However, results were nonsignificant in the PCR group (P value = 0.068). PCR validation showed that expression of TYRP1, DSC1, and GLUT12 was not significantly regulated in the 4°C and 16°C culture groups, which is in line with the microarray data.

4. Discussion

In this study, we investigated the effect of storage temperature on important cellular functions of ARPE-19 cells by comparing the expression levels of genes associated with phagocytosis, pigment synthesis, visual cycle, adherens and tight junctions, and glucose and ion transport.

The ARPE-19 cell line is recognized for displaying significant functional differentiation and forming polarized epithelial monolayers and tight junctions with barrier properties [21, 22]. However, the cell line does not mirror all the functions and characteristics of native RPE [23–25]. Some studies have demonstrated a relatively lower expression of some RPE-specific transcripts in ARPE-19 cells compared to native RPE cells [26], while others have not [27]. Native RPE exhibits considerable regional variation, and thus any culture models will be inherently heterogeneous [23, 28, 29]. Cells and cell lines in culture can exceed the normal variation described in RPE in vivo [23, 30–32]. Gene expression by cultured RPE cells is substrate dependent [33], and ARPE-19 grown on plastic displays the phenotype closest to native RPE, capable of yielding a functional profile of differentially expressed genes [34]. The global expression profile of ARPE-19 cells can also be directed towards that of primary RPE cells by withdrawing serum [24]. In the present study, cells were cultured and stored on plastic, and the storage medium contained no xenobiotic components.

Phagocytosis of shed photoreceptor outer segments is vital to photoreceptor repair and represents one of the most critical functions of the RPE [1, 35]. We found no changes in expression of phagocytosis-associated genes after storage at 4°C and 16°C compared to control cells (Table 1). Two receptor ligand pairs are recognized for exhibiting key roles in the molecular machinery of RPE phagocytosis. These include the receptor tyrosine kinase MerTK and its secreted ligands Gas6 and Protein S, as well as the integrin receptor $\alpha V\beta 5$ and its secreted ligand MFG-E8 [36]. ARPE-19 cells are capable of phagocytosing photoreceptor outer segments [37–39], but some differences exist compared to primary cultures. Both require the integrin receptor $\alpha v\beta 5$ for the binding and internalization of outer segments [21, 37], the main difference being observed at the level of promoter strength, yielding much higher transcriptional activity in ARPE-19 [40]. With the exception of Protein S, expression of all of these important genes was maintained during storage at all temperatures. Although the differences in expression of the remaining phagocytosis associated genes were modest, these results may indicate a slightly disrupted phagocytic ability in cells stored at 37°C.

The expression of genes associated with pigment synthesis in the RPE was also evaluated due to its many functions, including protection from oxidative stress [41–43]. Four genes have been described as key contributors in the melanin biosynthesis pathway: TYR, TYRP1, TYRP2, and P gene (OCA2) [44]. Smith-Thomas et al. [14] found that primary human RPE cells failed to express TYRP2 and that a very low percentage of the cells expressed TYRP1, but only if cultured for more than 3 weeks. Lu et al. [44] found that human RPE cultured under standard conditions failed to express any of the four key genes mentioned above. However, we were able to detect both OCA2 and TYRP1 in all culture groups, as well as several other genes related to pigment synthesis (Table 1).

Upon transduction of light energy into electrical impulses in the PR, 11-cis-retinal is converted to all-trans-retinal, which is cycled to the RPE for reisomerization [15]. A string of proteins contributes in the visual cycle, and the expression levels of critically important proteins such as cellular retinol binding protein 1 (RBP1, also known as CRBP1), lecithin retinol acyltransferase (LRAT), cellular retinaldehyde binding protein 1 (RLBP1, also referred to as CRALBP), and cellular retinol binding protein 5 (RBP5) were maintained at control levels during storage at all three temperatures. This indicates that the visual cycle can be preserved under the storage conditions used in this study.

Cell-cell adhesion is important for maintaining the correct RPE phenotype [45, 46]. Cultures stored at 4°C and 16°C did not differ from controls in regard to expression of adherens junction genes. Cultures stored at 37°C, however, showed a differential regulation of five adherens junction genes, among them an 8.3-fold upregulation of DSC1 and a change in expression of several cadherins. These changes might indicate a slight perturbance of adherens junction properties after 37°C storage. This group also showed the largest expression changes of tight junction genes, mostly downregulation. This might indicate a loss of integrity of the intercellular junction in cells stored at 37°C compared to control cells. The classic tight junction proteins ZO-1 and occludin did not display any changes in expression levels after storage at any of the three temperatures.

In a previous study, we demonstrated that the number of viable ARPE-19 cells at 4°C storage dropped to less than 4% compared to the control group [11]. In the present study, we find few differences between the 4°C group and the control. This seemingly contradictory finding can have at least two explanations. First, the cultures stored at 4°C contain a large number of dead and dying cells, which have a tendency to detach and be washed away during preparations, thereby not being included in the analysis. Second, temperature has a crucial effect on the adhesive abilities of several cell types [47–50] and adhesion seems to be severely affected during 4°C storage, resulting in the loss of otherwise viable and well-functioning cells from the monolayer. Unpublished data from our research group demonstrates improved viability following storage at 4°C by implementing a radical change in the culture protocol in order to improve cell adhesion. This finding supports our hypothesis that cellular adhesion is severely affected at low storage temperatures.

We also assessed the expression of glucose and ion transporters. Several GLUT proteins were identified in our material, with GLUT1 expression being dominant (Table 1). This is in line with existing gene expression studies on native RPE [18, 51, 52]. Expression of GLUT1 was maintained at control levels during storage at all temperatures. Given the dominant role of this transporter in RPE cells, the maintenance of its expression in all storage groups indicates a preservation of glucose transport function after storage. In an earlier study by Takagi et al. [52], the addition of FBS to the culture medium was shown to increase the expression of GLUT1 in human RPE cells. Based on this observation, one might anticipate a downregulation of this isoform when replacing the FBS-containing growth medium with a xenobiotic-free storage medium. However, that was not the case in our cultures. Expression of GLUT3 was increased 2-fold after storage at 16°C. GLUT3 is highly effective, displaying both a higher affinity and a fivefold greater transport capacity for glucose than other isoforms including GLUT1 [53]. Its expression has been identified in several cell types characterized by very specific and high metabolic demand, such as neurons and placental trophoblasts [53–55]. Its expression in neurons increases in an activity-related manner to meet an increased demand [53]. We speculate whether this strategy is utilized by ARPE-19 cells stored at 16°C and if it contributes to preserving a larger number of viable cells compared to other temperatures where GLUT3 expression remains unchanged.

Active transport of Na^+ across the apical membrane of RPE cells creates a high Na^+ concentration in the subretinal space, which is crucial for the photoreceptor dark current and for transport of solutes through symporters and antiporters of the RPE [17]. Three isoforms of each of the Na-K-ATPase α and β subunits were identified, and most were expressed close to control levels in all storage groups. The same isoforms were identified in a recent study on native RPE [51].

5. Conclusion

When comparing the expression levels of genes involved in important RPE functions, it is evident that cells stored at 37°C display expression changes in a larger number of genes than cells stored at 4°C and 16°C. In conclusion, the findings of this study show that cells stored at 4°C and 16°C are capable of maintaining expression levels of genes important for key RPE functions close to the control levels.

Conflict of Interests

The authors declare no conflict of interests.

Acknowledgments

The study has received funding from the Norwegian Research Council, the South-Eastern Norway Regional Health Authority, and the Norwegian Association of the Blind and Partially Sighted. The authors wish to thank Dr. Dong Feng Chen, Schepens Eye Research Institute, Harvard Medical School, for excellent help and support.

References

[1] J. R. Sparrrow, D. Hicks, and C. P. Hamel, "The retinal pigment epithelium in health and disease," *Current Molecular Medicine*, vol. 10, no. 9, pp. 802–823, 2010.

[2] M. F. Marmor, "Control of subretinal fluid: experimental and clinical studies," *Eye*, vol. 4, no. 1, pp. 340–344, 1990.

[3] P. T. V. M. de Jong, "Age-related macular degeneration," *The New England Journal of Medicine*, vol. 355, no. 14, pp. 1474–1485, 2006.

[4] A.-J. F. Carr, M. J. K. Smart, C. M. Ramsden, M. B. Powner, L. da Cruz, and P. J. Coffey, "Development of human embryonic stem cell therapies for age-related macular degeneration," *Trends in Neurosciences*, vol. 36, no. 7, pp. 385–395, 2013.

[5] S. Walia and G. A. Fishman, "Natural history of phenotypic changes in Stargardt macular dystrophy," *Ophthalmic Genetics*, vol. 30, no. 2, pp. 63–68, 2009.

[6] C. M. Sheridan, S. Mason, D. M. Pattwell, D. Kent, I. Grierson, and R. Williams, "Replacement of the RPE monolayer," *Eye*, vol. 23, no. 10, pp. 1910–1915, 2009.

[7] N. Yaji, M. Yamato, J. Yang, T. Okano, and S. Hori, "Transplantation of tissue-engineered retinal pigment epithelial cell sheets in a rabbit model," *Biomaterials*, vol. 30, no. 5, pp. 797–803, 2009.

[8] R. D. Lund, P. Adamson, Y. Sauvé et al., "Subretinal transplantation of genetically modified human cell lines attenuates loss of visual function in dystrophic rats," *Proceedings of the National Academy of Sciences of the United States of America*, vol. 98, no. 17, pp. 9942–9947, 2001.

[9] P. J. Coffey, S. Girman, S. M. Wang et al., "Long-term preservation of cortically dependent visual function in RCS rats by transplantation," *Nature Neuroscience*, vol. 5, no. 1, pp. 53–56, 2002.

[10] L. da Cruz, F. K. Chen, A. Ahmado, J. Greenwood, and P. Coffey, "RPE transplantation and its role in retinal disease," *Progress in Retinal and Eye Research*, vol. 26, no. 6, pp. 598–635, 2007.

[11] L. Pasovic, T. P. Utheim, R. Maria et al., "Optimization of storage temperature for cultured ARPE-19 cells," *Journal of Ophthalmology*, vol. 2013, Article ID 216359, 11 pages, 2013.

[12] A. Chopdar, U. Chakravarthy, and D. Verma, "Age related macular degeneration," *British Medical Journal*, vol. 326, no. 7387, pp. 485–488, 2003.

[13] B. M. Kevany and K. Palczewski, "Phagocytosis of retinal rod and cone photoreceptors," *Physiology*, vol. 25, no. 1, pp. 8–15, 2010.

[14] L. Smith-Thomas, P. Richardson, A. J. Thody et al., "Human ocular melanocytes and retinal pigment epithelial cells differ in their melanogenic properties in vivo and in vitro," *Current Eye Research*, vol. 15, no. 11, pp. 1079–1091, 1996.

[15] O. Strauss, "The retinal pigment epithelium in visual function," *Physiological Reviews*, vol. 85, no. 3, pp. 845–881, 2005.

[16] M. Kaida, F. Cao, C. M. B. Skumatz, P. E. Irving, and J. M. Burke, "Time at confluence for human RPE cells: effects on the adherens junction and in vitro wound closure," *Investigative Ophthalmology and Visual Science*, vol. 41, no. 10, pp. 3215–3224, 2000.

[17] L. J. Rizzolo, "Development and role of tight junctions in the retinal pigment epithelium," *International Review of Cytology*, vol. 258, pp. 195–234, 2007.

[18] Y. Ban and L. J. Rizzolo, "Regulation of glucose transporters during development of the retinal pigment epithelium," *Developmental Brain Research*, vol. 121, no. 1, pp. 89–95, 2000.

[19] P. D. Senanayake, A. Calabro, J. G. Hu et al., "Glucose utilization by the retinal pigment epithelium: evidence for rapid uptake and storage in glycogen, followed by glycogen utilization," *Experimental Eye Research*, vol. 83, no. 2, pp. 235–246, 2006.

[20] K. Geering, "Subunit assembly and functional maturation of Na,K-ATPase," *Journal of Membrane Biology*, vol. 115, no. 2, pp. 109–121, 1990.

[21] K. C. Dunn, A. E. Aotaki-Keen, F. R. Putkey, and L. M. Hjelmeland, "ARPE-19, a human retinal pigment epithelial cell line with differentiated properties," *Experimental Eye Research*, vol. 62, no. 2, pp. 155–169, 1996.

[22] K. C. Dunn, A. D. Marmorstein, V. L. Bonilha, E. Rodriguez-Boulan, F. Giordano, and L. M. Hjelmeland, "Use of the ARPE-19 cell line as a model of RPE polarity: basolateral secretion of FGF5," *Investigative Ophthalmology and Visual Science*, vol. 39, no. 13, pp. 2744–2749, 1998.

[23] Y. Luo, Y. Zhuo, M. Fukuhara, and L. J. Rizzolo, "Effects of culture conditions on heterogeneity and the apical junctional complex of the ARPE-19 cell line," *Investigative Ophthalmology and Visual Science*, vol. 47, no. 8, pp. 3644–3655, 2006.

[24] J. Tian, K. Ishibashi, S. Honda, S. A. Boylan, L. M. Hjelmeland, and J. T. Handa, "The expression of native and cultured human retinal pigment epithelial cells grown in different culture conditions," *British Journal of Ophthalmology*, vol. 89, no. 11, pp. 1510–1517, 2005.

[25] P. Geisen, J. R. McColm, B. M. King, and M. E. Hartnett, "Characterization of barrier properties and inducible VEGF expression of several types of retinal pigment epithelium in medium-term culture," *Current Eye Research*, vol. 31, no. 9, pp. 739–748, 2006.

[26] N. V. Strunnikova, A. Maminishkis, J. J. Barb et al., "Transcriptome analysis and molecular signature of human retinal pigment epithelium," *Human Molecular Genetics*, vol. 19, no. 12, Article ID ddq129, pp. 2468–2486, 2010.

[27] H. Cai and L. V. Del Priore, "Gene expression profile of cultured adult compared to immortalized human retinal pigment epithelium," *Molecular Vision*, vol. 12, pp. 1–14, 2006.

[28] J. M. Burke, F. Cao, and P. E. Irving, "High levels of E-/P-cadherin: correlation with decreased apical polarity of Na/K ATPase in bovine RPE cells in situ," *Investigative Ophthalmology and Visual Science*, vol. 41, no. 7, pp. 1945–1952, 2000.

[29] J. M. Burke and L. M. Hjelmeland, "Mosaicism of the retinal pigment epithelium: seeing the small picture," *Molecular Interventions*, vol. 5, no. 4, pp. 241–249, 2005.

[30] A. Ando, M. Ueda, M. Uyama, Y. Masu, T. Okumura, and S. Ito, "Heterogeneity in ornithine cytotoxicity of bovine retinal pigment epithelial cells in primary culture," *Experimental Eye Research*, vol. 70, no. 1, pp. 89–96, 2000.

[31] B. S. Mckay and J. M. Burke, "Separation of phenotypically distinct subpopulations of cultured human retinal pigment epithelial cells," *Experimental Cell Research*, vol. 213, no. 1, pp. 85–92, 1994.

[32] D. M. Albert, M. O. M. Tso, and A. S. Rabson, "In vitro growth of pure cultures of retinal pigment epithelium," *Archives of Ophthalmology*, vol. 88, no. 1, pp. 63–69, 1972.

[33] R. K. Sharma, W. E. Orr, A. D. Schmitt, and D. A. Johnson, "A functional profile of gene expression in ARPE-19 cells," *BMC Ophthalmology*, vol. 5, article 25, 2005.

[34] J. Tian, K. Ishibashi, and J. T. Handa, "The expression of native and cultured RPE grown on different matrices," *Physiological Genomics*, vol. 17, no. 2, pp. 170–182, 2004.

[35] S. Binder, B. V. Stanzel, I. Krebs, and C. Glittenberg, "Transplantation of the RPE in AMD," *Progress in Retinal and Eye Research*, vol. 26, no. 5, pp. 516–554, 2007.

[36] F. Mazzoni, H. Safa, and S. C. Finnemann, "Understanding photoreceptor outer segment phagocytosis: use and utility of RPE cells in culture," *Experimental Eye Research*, vol. 126, pp. 51–60, 2014.

[37] S. C. Finnemann, V. L. Bonilha, A. D. Marmorstein, and E. Rodriguez-Boulan, "Phagocytosis of rod outer segments by retinal pigment epithelial cells requires $\alpha v\beta 5$ integrin for binding but not for internalization," *Proceedings of the National Academy of Sciences of the United States of America*, vol. 94, no. 24, pp. 12932–12937, 1997.

[38] E. U. Irschick, R. Sgonc, G. Böck et al., "Retinal pigment epithelial phagocytosis and metabolism differ from those of macrophages," *Ophthalmic Research*, vol. 36, no. 4, pp. 200–210, 2004.

[39] E. U. Irschick, G. Haas, M. Geiger et al., "Phagocytosis of human retinal pigment epithelial cells: evidence of a diurnal rhythm, involvement of the cytoskeleton and interference of antiviral drugs," *Ophthalmic Research*, vol. 38, no. 3, pp. 164–174, 2006.

[40] S. Proulx, S. Landreville, S. L. Guérin, and C. Salesse, "Integrin $\alpha 5$ expression by the ARPE-19 cell line: comparison with

primary RPE cultures and effect of growth medium on the α5 gene promoter strength," *Experimental Eye Research*, vol. 79, no. 2, pp. 157–165, 2004.

[41] S. Memoli, A. Napolitano, M. D'Ischia, G. Misuraca, A. Palumbo, and G. Prota, "Diffusible melanin-related metabolites are potent inhibitors of lipid peroxidation," *Biochimica et Biophysica Acta—Lipids and Lipid Metabolism*, vol. 1346, no. 1, pp. 61–68, 1997.

[42] Z. Wang, J. Dillon, and E. R. Gaillard, "Antioxidant properties of melanin in retinal pigment epithelial cells," *Photochemistry and Photobiology*, vol. 82, no. 2, pp. 474–479, 2006.

[43] U. Schraermeyer and K. Heimann, "Current understanding on the role of retinal pigment epithelium and its pigmentation," *Pigment Cell Research*, vol. 12, no. 4, pp. 219–236, 1999.

[44] F. Lu, D. Yan, X. Zhou, D.-N. Hu, and J. Qu, "Expression of melanin-related genes in cultured adult human retinal pigment epithelium and uveal melanoma cells," *Molecular Vision*, vol. 13, pp. 2066–2072, 2007.

[45] W. K. Jin, H. K. Kyung, P. Burrola, T. W. Mak, and G. Lemke, "Retinal degeneration triggered by inactivation of PTEN in the retinal pigment epithelium," *Genes & Development*, vol. 22, no. 22, pp. 3147–3157, 2008.

[46] S. Tamiya, L. Liu, and H. J. Kaplan, "Epithelial-mesenchymal transition and proliferation of retinal pigment epithelial cells initiated upon loss of cell-cell contact," *Investigative Ophthalmology and Visual Science*, vol. 51, no. 5, pp. 2755–2763, 2010.

[47] F. Rico, C. Chu, M. H. Abdulreda, Y. Qin, and V. T. Moy, "Temperature modulation of integrin-mediated cell adhesion," *Biophysical Journal*, vol. 99, no. 5, pp. 1387–1396, 2010.

[48] G. Sagvolden, I. Giaever, E. O. Pettersen, and J. Feder, "Cell adhesion force microscopy," *Proceedings of the National Academy of Sciences of the United States of America*, vol. 96, no. 2, pp. 471–476, 1999.

[49] E. B. Lomakina and R. E. Waugh, "Micromechanical tests of adhesion dynamics between neutrophils and immobilized ICAM-1," *Biophysical Journal*, vol. 86, no. 2, pp. 1223–1233, 2004.

[50] R. L. Juliano and E. Gagalang, "The adhesion of Chinese hamster cells. I. Effects of temperature, metabolic inhibitors and proteolytic dissection of cell surface macromolecules," *Journal of Cellular Physiology*, vol. 92, no. 2, pp. 209–220, 1977.

[51] Z. Zhang, Y. Zhang, H. Xiao, X. Liang, D. Sun, and S. Peng, "A gene expression profile of the developing human retinal pigment epithelium," *Molecular Vision*, vol. 18, pp. 2961–2975, 2012.

[52] H. Takagi, H. Tanihara, Y. Seino, and N. Yoshimura, "Characterization of glucose transporter in cultured human retinal pigment epithelial cells: gene expression and effect of growth factors," *Investigative Ophthalmology and Visual Science*, vol. 35, no. 1, pp. 170–177, 1994.

[53] I. A. Simpson, D. Dwyer, D. Malide, K. H. Moley, A. Travis, and S. J. Vannucci, "The facilitative glucose transporter GLUT3: 20 years of distinction," *American Journal of Physiology—Endocrinology and Metabolism*, vol. 295, no. 2, pp. E242–E253, 2008.

[54] D. Z. Gerhart, M. A. Broderius, N. D. Borson, and L. R. Drewes, "Neurons and microvessels express the brain glucose transporter protein GLUT3," *Proceedings of the National Academy of Sciences of the United States of America*, vol. 89, no. 2, pp. 733–737, 1992.

[55] M. Pantaleon, M. B. Harvey, W. S. Pascoe, D. E. James, and P. L. Kaye, "Glucose transporter GLUT3: ontogeny, targeting, and role in the mouse blastocyst," *Proceedings of the National Academy of Sciences of the United States of America*, vol. 94, no. 8, pp. 3795–3800, 1997.

Choroidal Thickness in Patients with Mild Cognitive Impairment and Alzheimer's Type Dementia

Mehmet Bulut,[1] Aylin Yaman,[2] Muhammet Kazim Erol,[1] Fatma Kurtuluş,[2] Devrim Toslak,[1] Berna Doğan,[1] Deniz Turgut Çoban,[1] and Ebru Kaya Başar[3]

[1]*Antalya Training and Research Hospital, Ophthalmology Department, 07050 Antalya, Turkey*
[2]*Antalya Training and Research Hospital, Neurology Department, 07050 Antalya, Turkey*
[3]*Department of Animal Science Biometry and Genetics Unit, Faculty of Agriculture, Akdeniz University, 07070 Antalya, Turkey*

Correspondence should be addressed to Muhammet Kazim Erol; muhammetkazimerol@gmail.com

Academic Editor: Jesús Pintor

Aim. To asses both choroidal thickness differences among Alzheimer's type dementia (ATD) patients, mild cognitive impairment (MCI) patients, and healthy control (C) subjects and choroidal thickness relationships with cognitive performance. *Methods.* A total of 246 eyes of 123 people (41 ATD, 38 MCI, and 44 healthy C subjects) were included in this study. Complete ophthalmological and neurological examination was performed in all subjects. Choroidal thicknesses (CT) were measured at seven locations: the fovea, 500-1500-3000 μm temporal and 500-1500-3000 μm nasal to the fovea by enhanced depth imaging optical coherence tomography (EDI-OCT). Detailed neurological examination including mini mental state examination (MMSE) test which evaluates the cognitive function was applied to all participants. *Results.* The ages and genders of all participants were similar in all groups. Compared with healthy C subjects, the CT measurements at all regions were significantly thinner both in patients with ATD and in patients with MCI than in healthy C subjects ($p < 0.05$). The MMSE scores were significantly different among ATD patients, MCI patients, and healthy C subjects. They were 19.3 ± 1.8, 24.8 ± 0.9, and 27.6 ± 1.2 in ATD, MCI, and healthy controls, respectively ($p < 0.001$). There were also significant correlation between MMSE score and choroidal thickness at each location ($p < 0.05$). *Conclusions.* CT was reduced in ATD patients and MCI patients. Since vascular structures were affected in ATD patients and MCI patients, they had thin CT. Besides CT was correlated with degree of cognitive impairment. Therefore CT may be a new biomarker in diagnosis and follow-up of MCI and ATD patients.

1. Introduction

Alzheimer's type dementia disease (ATD) is the most frequent form of dementia and is characterized by cognitive deficits including progressive memory disturbance, higher cortical functions, executive functions, and other components of cognition [1]. Mild cognitive impairment (MCI) is a recently described syndrome in which patients experience subjective and objective memory deficits or have impairment of other cognitive abilities other than memory. They may yield abnormal scores on memory tests, but their activities of daily living and occupational functions are not affected. MCI represents a clinical condition in which the risk of developing dementia is increased and is accepted as a transitional stage between "healthy" and "dementia" [2]. As human life expectancy continues to increase, the prevalence of ATD and MCI is expected to increase along with the need to treat patients with these diseases [3].

Although ATD is primarily a disease of the brain characterized by cognitive abnormalities, it is also associated with impairments in visual function, including impairments in color perception, depth perception, contrast sensitivity, and visual field [4]. The retina is an extension of the brain that is, like other regions of the brain, derived from the neural tube [5]. Recent reports suggest that degenerative diseases of the retina, including age-related macular degeneration and glaucoma, share common features with ATD. Indeed, ATD, age-related macular degeneration, and glaucoma are all complex, multifactorial forms of degeneration of central nervous system tissue in which age is the primary risk factor

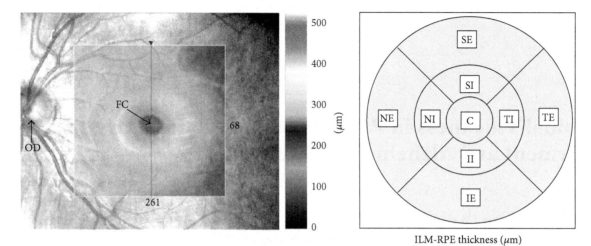

FIGURE 1: The map was divided into nine ETDRS macular fields. C: central field; SI: superior internal field; TI: temporal internal field; II: inferior internal field; NI: nasal internal field; SE: superior external field; TE: temporal external field; IE: inferior external field; NE: nasal external field.

and is characterized by protein-aggregate deposition and similar mechanisms for induction of cell injury [6–8].

Clinical studies have indicated that vascular changes play an important role early in ATD pathogenesis, though cerebral amyloid beta (Aβ) plaques and neurodegeneration are the main hallmarks of the disease [9, 10]. Interestingly, both retinal and choroidal vascular Aβ deposits have been observed in animal models of ATD [11]. Although previous studies have reported that choroidal thickness (CT) decreases in ATD patients, none has reported observance of changes in CT in MCI patients [3, 12]. To fill this research gap, this study measured CT in MCI and ATD patients using enhanced depth imaging optical coherence tomography (EDI-OCT) and compared their CT values to those of healthy controls.

2. Materials and Methods

The study was approved by the local ethics committee of the site at which it was conducted and performed in accordance with the ethical standards outlined in the Declaration of Helsinki. Informed consent was obtained by all participating subjects prior to their inclusion in the study. 41 Alzheimer's type dementia (ATD) patients, 38 MCI patients, and 44 cognitively healthy age-matched volunteers were enrolled in this study.

The criterion for inclusion for the ATD patients was fulfillment of the National Institute of Neurological and Communicative Disorders and Stroke and the Alzheimer's Disease and Related Disorders Association (NINCDS-ADRDA) criteria. The criteria for inclusion of MCI patients were the absence of other neurological diseases except cognitive impairment or ophthalmologic diseases, the reporting of memory complaints, and an abnormal score on delayed memory recall tests (i.e., two or three missing words), which is a part of mini mental state examination test (MMSE). All the ATD and MCI patients were evaluated by an experienced neurologist. Detailed neurological and mental state examinations and dementia screening tests were completed, supportive laboratory tests were performed, and all the patients were diagnosed clinically as ATD or MCI. Orientation, attention, memory, language, and shape copying are evaluated with MMSE test. Maximum points are 30. For Turkish society the study for validity and reliability was done by Güngen and his associates in 2002 and the cut-off value was determined as 23/24 [13]. This test is considered reliable for identifying the degree of mild dementia. The criterion for inclusion of control subjects was the absence of cognitive impairment and other neurological or ophthalmologic diseases. None of the subjects in the control group had subjective memory complaints. These healthy subjects in the control group also were screened for dementia and underwent a neurological examination by the same neurologist. The exclusion criteria for all groups of patients were having a history or showing evidence of other neurologic or psychiatric disorders, other types of dementia except ATD, retinal disease (i.e., macular degeneration), glaucoma, ocular trauma, ocular surgery, ocular inflammation refractive errors outside −5 to +3 D, diabetes mellitus, systemic arterial hypertension, cardiovascular disease, or other serious chronic systemic diseases, and currently being a smoker.

All subjects underwent optical coherence tomography (OCT) measurement, a complete ophthalmic examination that included assessment of visual acuity and intraocular pressure, slit lamp biomicroscopy, visual field examination, and axial length measurement with optical biometry (Lenstar LS 900, Haag-Streit AG, Köniz, Switzerland).

Spectral-domain OCT (SD-OCT) imaging was performed using the Cirrus HD OCT system (Cirrus Carl Zeiss Meditec Inc., Dublin, CA, USA) using the macular cube 512 × 128 protocol, according to which retinal thickness was quantitatively measured in each of the nine regions (Figure 1). EDI-CT was performed by two technicians blind to the patients' diagnoses using the Cirrus HD-OCT Model 5000 (Carl Zeiss Meditec Inc., Dublin, CA, USA). Choroidal thickness imaging was performed by the same independent technician using EDI-OCT following a previously described technique [14]. The participants were asked not to consume caffeine for at least 12 h before examination. Three consecutive

TABLE 1: Demographic and clinical characteristics of the study subjects.

	ATD patients ($n = 82$ eyes)	MCI patients ($n = 76$ eyes)	Control subjects ($n = 88$ eyes)	p value
Age	73.34 ± 7.0	71.68 ± 7.4	70.65 ± 7.5	0.874
Sex (M/F)	20/21	19/19	21/23	0.752
IOP	14.9 ± 2.7	15.3 ± 2.6	15.2 ± 2.4	0.783
AXL	22.95 ± 1.9	23.02 ± 1.9	23.1 ± 2.1	0.678
MMSE score	19.39 ± 18	24.84 ± 0.9	27.64 ± 1.2	**<0.001**

ATD: Alzheimer's type disease; MCI: mild cognitive impairment; AXL: axial length; IOP: intraocular pressure; and MMSE: mini mental state examination.

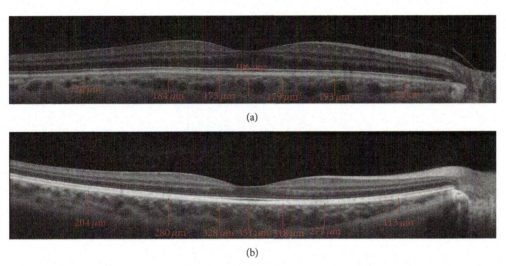

FIGURE 2: This figure shows that choroidal thickness measurement at each location in both a healthy individual (b) and a patient with ATD (a).

measurements of CT at each localization were performed over three days and the average values were calculated. All scans were required to have a signal strength of at least 6/10 to be included in the data analysis. Two technicians blind to the patients' diagnoses measured the perpendicular choroidal thickness from the outer edge of the hyperreflective retinal pigment epithelium to the inner sclera at seven locations: at the fovea; at 500, 1500, and 3000 microns temporal to the fovea; and at 500, 1500, and 3000 microns nasal to the fovea (Figure 2). Three consecutive measurements were taken at each location and the average value was calculated.

The data obtained from the eyes were used for the statistical analysis. One-way analysis of variance analysis (ANOVA) with Bonferroni correction and Spearman correlation analysis were performed using SPSS ver. 20 (SPSS Inc., Chicago, IL, USA). Descriptive statistics were presented in terms of the mean ± standard deviation. p value less than 0.05 was accepted as significant.

3. Results

Table 1 shows the demographic and clinical characteristics of the patients. As can be observed, no significant differences were found among the three groups regarding age, sex, intraocular pressure, and axial length measurements. Tables 2, 3, and 4 and Figure 3 show the results of the data analysis. Table 2 shows that significant differences were found among the three groups regarding CT at each location, with the

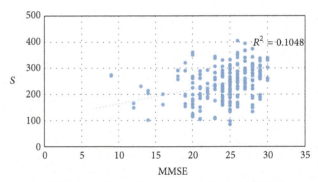

FIGURE 3: This figure shows that correlation between MMSE scores and subfoveal choroidal thickness.

ATD and MCI patients found to have the lowest CT values and the control subjects found to have the highest CT value. Table 3 and Figure 3 show that a significant correlation was also found between MMSE score and CT at each location. Although the macular thickness values of the ATD patients were lower than that of the MCI patients and control subjects at each location, the differences among these values were not found to be statistically significant (Table 4).

4. Discussion

Recent research reflects an increased effort to identify a new visual biomarker that can be used to diagnose ATD patients

TABLE 2: Relationship of choroidal thickness with Alzheimer's type dementia (ATD) and mild cognitive impairment (MCI).

Choroidal thickness (μm)	ATD (n = 82) Mean thickness (SD)	MCI (n = 76) Mean thickness (SD)	Controls (n = 88) Mean thickness (SD)	*p value	ATD versus controls Mean difference (SE)	†p value	MCI versus controls Mean difference (SE)	†p value	ATD versus MCI Mean difference (SE)	†p value
Subfoveal	215.6 ± 64.5	228.7 ± 52.9	272.7 ± 60.1	<0.001	−57.1 (9.4)	<0.001	−44.0 (9.6)	<0.001	−13.1 (9.9)	0.187
Temporal 0.5 mm	200.4 ± 60.0	211.0 ± 49.9	250.2 ± 55.3	<0.001	−49.7 (8.7)	<0.001	−39.2 (8.9)	<0.001	−10.5 (9.2)	0.253
Nasal 0.5 mm	194.9 ± 63.4	204.7 ± 53.6	244.2 ± 60.5	<0.001	−49.3 (9.4)	<0.001	−39.5 (9.6)	<0.001	−9.7 (9.8)	0.324
Temporal 1.5 mm	192.5 ± 59.3	198.3 ± 47.9	239.0 ± 53.4	<0.001	−46.5 (8.5)	<0.001	−40.7 (8.6)	<0.001	−5.7 (8.9)	0.519
Nasal 1.5 mm	171.3 ± 64.3	182.7 ± 59.7	216.6 ± 68.4	<0.001	−45.3 (10.2)	<0.001	−33.9 (10.4)	0.001	−11.3 (10.7)	0.289
Temporal 3 mm	172.1 ± 50.1	174.4 ± 48.0	210.2 ± 43.9	<0.001	−38.1 (7.4)	<0.001	−35.8 (7.6)	<0.001	−2.2 (7.8)	0.772
Nasal 3 mm	116.5 ± 39.2	120.0 ± 48.3	141.7 ± 52.8	0.002	−21.7 (7.5)	0.004	−25.2 (7.6)	0.001	3.5 (7.9)	0.657

SD: standard deviation, SE: standard error, * p value represents comparison among three groups, and † p value represents the pairwise comparison between two groups.
ANOVA.
Post hoc Bonferroni test.

TABLE 3: Correlation between MMSE score and choroidal thickness at each location.

Choroidal region	p value	r value
Subfoveal	<0.001	0.324
Temporal 0.5 mm	<0.001	0.318
Nasal 0.5 mm	<0.001	0.298
Temporal 1.5 mm	<0.001	0.285
Nasal 1.5 mm	<0.001	0.281
Temporal 3 mm	<0.001	0.255
Nasal 3 mm	0.013	0.164

Results obtained by Spearman correlation test.

early in the disease process and then to follow the disease process. As MCI patients are considered to have an early form of ATD, it is believed that identification of such a biomarker would assist in their diagnosis and treatment as well. In our attempt to identify such a biomarker, we observed thinning of CT at all localizations in the sample of ATD and MCI patients that we studied. As one of the most vascularized tissues of the body, the choroid functions to provide oxygen and nutrition to the external retinal tissue. Thus, thinning of choroidal tissue in ATD and MCI patients may be related to hypoperfusion and changes due to atrophy, along with the thinning associated with aging [15].

Our findings support previous observation of CT thinning in ATD patients in several recent studies [3, 12]. To our knowledge, the current study was the first in which the thinning of choroidal tissue was observed in MCI patients as well as ATD patients. Accumulation of Aβ and development of neurofibrillary tangles (NFTs) are responsible for the pathogenesis of ATD. Both of these substances first cause neurotoxicity, neuronal and synaptic loss, and vascular angiopathy [4]. In previous studies a relationship between vascular changes and the neurodegenerative process in the clinical risk and progression of ATD was discovered [16, 17]. In accordance with the knowledge that cerebral vascular damage in ATD patients plays a vital role in the disease pathogenesis, it was also observed that cerebral amyloid angiopathy resulted from cerebral arterioles and accumulation of Aβ in the capillaries [18–20]. It has been also observed that accumulation of soluble Aβ causes an increase in vascular resistance of the brain cortex in mice as well as cerebral hypoperfusion and vasoconstriction [21]. It is believed that all these cerebral vascular changes cause oxidative stress and neurotoxicity before clinical dementia starts [18–21].

Both Aβ accumulation and NFTs are found in many parts of the visual system in ATD patients, including the retina [22, 23]. In a mouse model of ATD, Aβ deposits were found in the retina, specifically in the retinal ganglion cells (RGCs), consistent with the pathology observed in the brain [24]. Several researchers have also observed accumulation of Aβ in choroidal vascular tissue in normal aging mice as well as in a mouse model of ATD. Based on their findings, these researchers suggest that like the development of angiopathy in the brain is due to the accumulation of Aβ, it can cause angiopathy in the choroid and, consequently, atrophy [24, 25].

OCT studies seeking to identify a new visual biomarker for early diagnosis and with which to follow the progression of disease in AD and MCI patients have primarily focused on retinal nerve fiber layer (RNFL) and retinal ganglion cell layer (RGCL) thickness. Thinning of RNFL and RGCL thickness is determined in relation to the neurodegenerative period that plays a role in pathogenesis [26–29]. However, few studies have examined the role of CT in this process. To our knowledge, only two previous studies observed lower CT values in AD patients compared with healthy controls [3, 12]. Our study was the first to identify not only a significant decrease in CT values in ATD patients at all locations compared to healthy control subjects, a finding consistent with previous studies, but also a significant decrease in CT values in MCI patients compared with healthy controls.

As MCI has a similar pathogenesis as ATD and is accepted as the early phase of ATD, it was not surprising that we obtained similar findings in the ATD and MCI patients. Based on our findings, we hypothesize that the thinning of choroidal thickness in both ATD and MCI patients is related to the toxicity caused by Aβ accumulation. As previously discussed, Aβ accumulation can cause angiopathy of the cerebral vascular tissue in ATD patients, which leads to causing atrophy. As choroidal tissue is mostly vascular tissue and ATD and MCI have a similar pathogenesis, the accumulation of Aβ may cause angiopathy in a similar way in both AD and MCI patients. This angiopathy will in turn cause atrophy of choroidal tissue, reflected in a reduction in CT values.

In our study, we separately observed a significantly positive correlation between the CT values at all localizations and the MMSE scores, which assess cognitive state. In contrast, Bayhan et al. found no correlation between CT values and MMSE score in their study. Although we observed a decrease in the macular thickness values in AD and MCI patients compared to healthy controls, the differences in the values among these groups were not statistically significant. Previous findings regarding these values are mixed; while some observed thinning in macular thickness in AD patients, others observed no thinning [12, 26, 28].

Our study faced an important limitation that should be considered when evaluating the findings. This limitation was our measurement of CT manually using EDI-OCT, which we believe that it can cause errors in measurement. To help overcome this limitation, we designed the study so that two technicians blind to the patients' diagnoses performed the measurements. We then used the mean values of three different measurements at each localization taken over three days in the data analysis. We believe that the ability to automatically perform CT measurement using new software in the swept source- (SS-) OCT format will greatly decrease measurement error, and hence more fully overcome this limitation, in the future.

In conclusion, we observed that CT values at all locations decrease in both ATD and MCI patients compared to those of healthy controls and identified a positive correlation between MMSE score and CT value. Based on our findings, we propose measurement of CT value using noninvasive, easily performed methods, such as SD-OCT, and use of this value as a new biomarker for early diagnosis of AD and MCI patients,

TABLE 4: Comparison of macular thickness among the study groups.

Macular thickness (μm)	ATD ($n = 82$) Mean thickness (SD)	MCI ($n = 76$) Mean thickness (SD)	Controls ($n = 88$) Mean thickness (SD)	*p value
Average	271.3 ± 15.6	275.8 ± 13.6	276.5 ± 14.0	0.070
C	248.2 ± 26.7	252.5 ± 29.5	254.6 ± 27.1	0.337
SE	274.0 ± 15.2	274.0 ± 20.4	275.6 ± 15.9	0.802
NE	289.6 ± 15.0	291.9 ± 19.6	293.7 ± 15.6	0.320
IE	262.1 ± 19.6	264.3 ± 18.7	265.4 ± 15.0	0.481
TE	257.5 ± 17.8	258.9 ± 17.1	261.0 ± 15.4	0.450
SI	310.1 ± 38.3	318.3 ± 22.0	319.2 ± 19.3	0.081
NI	315.8 ± 17.8	320.2 ± 21.9	321.3 ± 18.7	0.178
II	312.6 ± 20.3	315.4 ± 21.2	317.4 ± 19.2	0.324
TI	303.6 ± 19.0	308.4 ± 21.3	309.3 ± 19.1	0.159

Results obtained by one-way ANOVA test. ATD: Alzheimer's type disease; MCI: mild cognitive impairment; SD: standard deviation, C: central field; SI: superior internal field; TI: temporal internal field; II: inferior internal field; NI: nasal internal field; SE: superior external field; TE: temporal external field; IE: inferior external field; and NE: nasal external field.
*p value represents comparison among the three groups.

follow-up of progression, and evaluation of the efficiency of new-generation medicines used in their treatment.

Disclosure

None of the authors has a financial and proprietary interest in any material or method mentioned and there is no public or private support. Study has not been presented in anywhere before.

Conflict of Interests

The authors declare that there is no conflict of interests regarding the publication of this paper.

References

[1] C. Paquet, M. Boissonnot, F. Roger, P. Dighiero, R. Gil, and J. Hugon, "Abnormal retinal thickness in patients with mild cognitive impairment and Alzheimer's disease," *Neuroscience Letters*, vol. 420, no. 2, pp. 97–99, 2007.

[2] R. C. Petersen, R. Doody, A. Kurz et al., "Current concepts in mild cognitive impairment," *Archives of Neurology*, vol. 58, no. 12, pp. 1985–1992, 2001.

[3] H. A. Bayhan, S. A. Bayhan, A. Celikbilek, N. Tanik, and C. Gürdal, "Evaluation of the chorioretinal thickness changes in Alzheimer's disease using spectral-domain optical coherence tomography," *Clinical & Experimental Ophthalmology*, vol. 43, no. 2, pp. 145–151, 2015.

[4] R. Tzekov and M. Mullan, "Vision function abnormalities in Alzheimer disease," *Survey of Ophthalmology*, vol. 59, no. 4, pp. 414–433, 2014.

[5] F. Müller and R. O'Rahilly, "The development of the human brain from a closed neural tube at stage 13," *Anatomy and Embryology*, vol. 177, no. 3, pp. 203–224, 1988.

[6] K. Kaarniranta, A. Salminen, A. Haapasalo, H. Soininen, and M. Hiltunen, "Age-related macular degeneration (AMD): Alzheimer's disease in the eye?" *Journal of Alzheimer's Disease*, vol. 24, no. 4, pp. 615–631, 2011.

[7] J. M. Sivak, "The aging eye: common degenerative mechanisms between the Alzheimer's brain and retinal disease," *Investigative Ophthalmology and Visual Science*, vol. 54, no. 1, pp. 871–880, 2013.

[8] J. A. Ghiso, "Alzheimer's disease and glaucoma: mechanistic similarities and differences," *Journal of Glaucoma*, vol. 22, no. 5, pp. S36–S38, 2013.

[9] R. E. Tanzi, R. D. Moir, and S. L. Wagner, "Clearance of Alzheimer's Aβ peptide: the many roads to perdition," *Neuron*, vol. 43, no. 5, pp. 605–608, 2004.

[10] B. V. Zlokovic, "Clearing amyloid through the blood-brain barrier," *Journal of Neurochemistry*, vol. 89, no. 4, pp. 807–811, 2004.

[11] Y. Tsai, B. Lu, A. V. Ljubimov et al., "Ocular changes in TgF344-AD rat model of Alzheimer's disease," *Investigative Ophthalmology & Visual Science*, vol. 55, no. 1, pp. 523–534, 2014.

[12] M. Gharbiya, A. Trebbastoni, F. Parisi et al., "Choroidal thinning as a new finding in Alzheimer's Disease: evidence from enhanced depth imaging spectral domain optical coherence tomography," *Journal of Alzheimer's Disease*, vol. 40, no. 4, pp. 907–917, 2014.

[13] C. Güngen, T. Ertan, E. Eker, R. Yasar, and F. Engin, "Reliability and validity of the standardized mini mental state examination in the diagnosis of mild dementia in Turkish population," *Türk Psikiyatri Dergisi*, vol. 13, no. 4, pp. 273–281, 2002.

[14] S. K. Vance, Y. Imamura, and K. B. Freund, "The effects of sildenafil citrate on choroidal thickness as determined by enhanced depth imaging optical coherence tomography," *Retina*, vol. 31, no. 2, pp. 332–335, 2011.

[15] R. S. Ramrattan, T. L. van der Schaft, C. M. Mooy, W. C. de Bruijn, P. G. H. Mulder, and P. T. V. M. de Jong, "Morphometric analysis of Bruch's membrane, the choriocapillaris, and the choroid in aging," *Investigative Ophthalmology and Visual Science*, vol. 35, no. 6, pp. 2857–2864, 1994.

[16] J. C. de La Torre, "Is Alzheimer's disease a neurodegenerative or a vascular disorder? Data, dogma, and dialectics," *The Lancet Neurology*, vol. 3, no. 3, pp. 184–190, 2004.

[17] T. Takano, X. Han, R. Deane, B. Zlokovic, and M. Nedergaard, "Two-photon imaging of astrocytic Ca^{2+} signaling and the microvasculature in experimental mice models of Alzheimer's

disease," *Annals of the New York Academy of Sciences*, vol. 1097, pp. 40–50, 2007.

[18] R. N. Kalaria, "The role of cerebral ischemia in Alzheimer's disease," *Neurobiology of Aging*, vol. 21, no. 2, pp. 321–330, 2000.

[19] J. C. De la Torre, "Alzheimer disease as a vascular disorder: nosological evidence," *Stroke*, vol. 33, no. 4, pp. 1152–1162, 2002.

[20] D. R. Thal, W. S. T. Griffin, R. A. I. de Vos, and E. Ghebremedhin, "Cerebral amyloid angiopathy and its relationship to Alzheimer's disease," *Acta Neuropathologica*, vol. 115, no. 6, pp. 599–609, 2008.

[21] Z. Suo, J. Humphrey, A. Kundtz et al., "Soluble Alzheimers β-amyloid constricts the cerebral vasculature in vivo," *Neuroscience Letters*, vol. 257, no. 2, pp. 77–80, 1998.

[22] M. Koronyo-Hamaoui, Y. Koronyo, A. V. Ljubimov et al., "Identification of amyloid plaques in retinas from Alzheimer's patients and noninvasive in vivo optical imaging of retinal plaques in a mouse model," *NeuroImage*, vol. 54, supplement 1, pp. S204–S217, 2011.

[23] M. Parnell, L. Guo, M. Abdi, and M. F. Cordeiro, "Ocular manifestations of Alzheimer's disease in animal models," *International Journal of Alzheimer's Disease*, vol. 2012, Article ID 786494, 13 pages, 2012.

[24] A. Ning, J. Cui, E. To, K. H. Ashe, and J. Matsubara, "Amyloid-β deposits lead to retinal degeneration in a mouse model of Alzheimer disease," *Investigative Ophthalmology & Visual Science*, vol. 49, no. 11, pp. 5136–5143, 2008.

[25] J. H. Kam, E. Lenassi, and G. Jeffery, "Viewing ageing eyes: diverse sites of amyloid beta accumulation in the ageing mouse retina and the up-regulation of macrophages," *PLoS ONE*, vol. 5, no. 10, Article ID e13127, 2010.

[26] E. Marziani, S. Pomati, P. Ramolfo et al., "Evaluation of retinal nerve fiber layer and ganglion cell layer thickness in Alzheimer's disease using spectral-domain optical coherence tomography," *Investigative Ophthalmology and Visual Science*, vol. 54, no. 9, pp. 5953–5958, 2013.

[27] C. Y. Cheung, Y. T. Ong, S. Hilal et al., "Retinal ganglion cell analysis using high-definition optical coherence tomography in patients with mild cognitive impairment and Alzheimer's disease," *Journal of Alzheimer's Disease*, vol. 45, no. 1, pp. 45–56, 2015.

[28] L. Gao, Y. Liu, X. Li, Q. Bai, and P. Liu, "Abnormal retinal nerve fiber layer thickness and macula lutea in patients with mild cognitive impairment and Alzheimer's disease," *Archives of Gerontology and Geriatrics*, vol. 60, no. 1, pp. 162–167, 2015.

[29] E. O. Oktem, E. Derle, S. Kibaroglu, C. Oktem, I. Akkoyun, and U. Can, "The relationship between the degree of cognitive impairment and retinal nerve fiber layer thickness," *Neurological Sciences*, vol. 36, no. 7, pp. 1141–1146, 2015.

Comparison of Two Botulinum Neurotoxin A Injection Patterns with or without the Medial Lower Eyelid in the Treatment of Blepharospasm

Hui Yang, Jing Lu, Xiujuan Zhao, Xiaohu Ding, Zhonghao Wang, Xiaoyu Cai, Yan Luo, and Lin Lu

State Key Laboratory of Ophthalmology, Zhongshan Ophthalmic Center, Sun Yat-sen University, Guangzhou 510060, China

Correspondence should be addressed to Lin Lu; lulin888@126.com

Academic Editor: Jesús Pintor

The aim of this study was to evaluate the efficacy of two botulinum toxin A (BoNT-A) injection patterns with or without the medial lower eyelid (MLE) in treating benign essential blepharospasm (BEB) and influencing lacrimal drainage. Two different injection patterns of BoNT-A were randomly applied to 98 eyes of 49 BEB patients: MLE Group received a full injection pattern of 5 sites and non-MLE Group received a MLE waived injection pattern of 4 sites. Tear breakup time (BUT), Schirmer I test, lagophthalmos height, and lower lid tear meniscus height (TMH) were measured and Jankovic Rating Scale (JRS) was surveyed before injection and at 1 week, 1 month, and 3 months after injection. The symptom of BEB was relieved in both groups as suggested by JRS scores at all time points after injection, and MLE Group came up with a better JRS score at 3 months. The increases of Schirmer I test value and TMH in MLE Group were higher than those in non-MLE Group at 1 week after injection. This study shows that the MLE-involved full injection pattern is a better choice for patients with BEB. It has longer-lasting effects in relieving BEB symptoms and better efficacy in reducing lacrimal drainage. Clinical Trials registration number is NCT02327728.

1. Introduction

Benign essential blepharospasm (BEB) is a condition of bilateral orbicularis oculi dystonia with unknown etiology, which leads to intermittent or complete involuntary eyelid closure and vision impairment [1]. Common manifestations of BEB include dry eyes, photophobia, unpleasant sensations, eyelid fluttering, and increased frequency of blinking [2]. The dysfunction might lie in the basal ganglia [3] or might be related to the impairment in corticosensory processing and a loss of inhibition of the blink reflex [4].

Botulinum neurotoxin A (BoNT-A) injection is a well-established treatment for blepharospasm and was firstly used to treat blepharospasm in 1985 [5]. The treatment efficacy lasts 3-4 months in most patients but can vary from a few weeks to more than 6 months [6]. BoNT-A injection can induce different side effects such as blurred vision, diplopia, lagophthalmos, eyelid ptosis, and increased lacrimation [7]. Injection into the pretarsal, rather than the preseptal portion of the orbicularis oculi, is more effective for treatment of BEB [8]. Also in patients with resistant blepharospasm, the pretarsal portion of the orbicularis oculi should be involved [9]. Universally used injection sites include the lateral upper and lower eyelid margins, the medial upper eyelid margin, and the lateral canthi, while additional sites differ greatly depending on patients' symptoms and the ophthalmologists' experience [8, 10–13].

However, whether the medial lower eyelid (MLE) should be involved in the treatment of patients with BEB remains unclear. Our previous study, which used a MLE-involved injection pattern, showed alleviation of dry eye symptoms via BoNT-A injection [14], while a study elsewhere, which used an injection pattern that avoided MLE, showed ineffectiveness of BoNT-A injection in treating dry eye symptoms [15]. Yet, since the injection sites of these two studies were quite different, it was impossible to make comparison and determine the effect of the MLE injection site on lacrimal drainage. Since the manifestations of BEB include dry eye, it

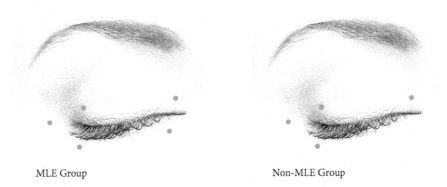

Figure 1: Injection sites in the MLE Group and the non-MLE Group for patients with BEB.

would be of great benefit if we could improve ocular surface lubrication while treating the blepharospasm. Therefore, the aim of this study was to compare the efficacy of two BoNT-A injection patterns—with or without the MLE injection—in treating BEB and reducing lacrimal drainage.

2. Methods

2.1. Subjects. During February 2013 to December 2014 period, a total of 49 patients (13 males and 36 females; age range: 38–78 years, mean 59 years) with bilateral BEB were enrolled. The BEB symptoms should have lasted for at least 6 months prior to the baseline visit. Patients who had previously received injections of BoNT-A had to have a 24-week washout since the last injection. Exclusion criteria included blepharospasm of known etiology (caused by medication, injury, or so on), history of surgical intervention for BEB (myectomy or neurectomy), current ophthalmologic infection, and apraxia of eyelid opening associated with levator palpebrae dysfunction.

The study was approved by the Institutional Review Board of Zhongshan Ophthalmic Center, Sun Yat-Sen University (approval number 2013MEKY019), and was carried out in accordance with the tenets of the Declaration of Helsinki. Informed consent for the study was obtained from each patient at the time of enrollment.

2.2. Treatment. To prepare injections, 100 U of BoNT-A (Botox, Allergan, Inc., Irvine, California, USA) was diluted in 2 mL saline for a final concentration of 5 U/0.1 mL; dosage per injection was 2.5 U/site. A 32-gauge needle was used and injections were angled away from the center of the eyelid to reduce the risk of levator muscle infiltration.

Each patient received 9 sites of injection (Figure 1). Right and left sides were assigned to MLE Group or non-MLE Group using a randomized digital chart. Eyes in MLE Group received a full injection pattern of 5 sites (the medial upper and lower eyelid margins, the lateral upper and lower eyelid margins, and the lateral canthi), for a total dosage of 12.5 U. Non-MLE Group eyes received a MLE waived injection pattern of 4 sites (same sites as MLE Group but excluding the MLE margin), for a total dosage of 10 U.

2.3. Assessments. Ocular examinations, including spasm frequency and severity, tear breakup time (BUT), Schirmer I test, lagophthalmos height, and lower lid tear meniscus height (TMH), were performed before treatment (baseline) and at 1 week, 1 month, and 3 months after injection. At each evaluation point, patients also completed a subjective questionnaire of Jankovic Rating Scale (JRS).

Tear BUT was measured as the interval between the last complete blink and the appearance of the first corneal dry spot. After one drop of fluorescein was applied to the inferior fornix, the patient was instructed to perform a complete blink and then gaze straight ahead. The mean value of three consecutive measurements was recorded. Tear BUT less than 5 sec was considered pathological.

Schirmer I test was performed with anesthesia (0.5% proxymetacaine; Alcaine, Alcon, Fort Worth, TX, USA), using a commercially available 35 mm paper strip placed on the inferior fornix between the lateral third and the middle third of the eyelid. Results were recorded in millimeters (mm) of wetting distance after 5 min; a distance less than 5 mm was considered abnormal, indicating an aqueous-deficient state.

Lower lid TMH was measured by commercial optical coherence tomography (VisanteTM OCT, version 1.0.12.1896, Carl Zeiss Meditec Inc.), from the lower eyelid-meniscus junction to the cornea-meniscus junction at the middle of the lower lid.

The JRS evaluates the severity and frequency of blepharospasm using a rating scale of symptoms from 0 to 4 [16].

2.4. Statistical Analysis. Data were analyzed using IBM SPSS Statistics version 20.0 (IBM Corporation, New York, USA). A level of $p < 0.05$ was considered statistically significant. Differences in Schirmer I test results between the two groups at each time point were analyzed with paired t-tests, while differences in tear BUT, TMH, lagophthalmos height, and JRS ratings at each time point were analyzed with Wilcoxon rank

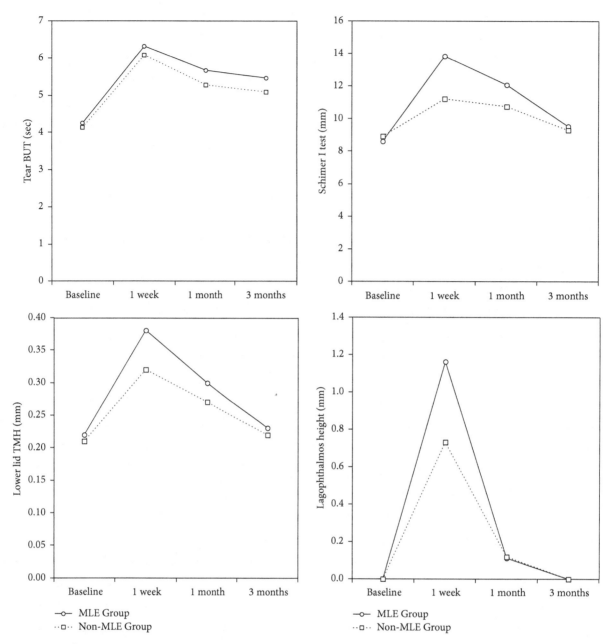

FIGURE 2: Changes in objective parameters of the MLE Group and the non-MLE Group before and after BoNT-A injection.

tests. Friedman and Kendall were used to make multiple comparisons between different time points for each parameter.

3. Results

Parameters at baseline, 1 week, 1 month, and 3 months after BoNT-A injection for each treatment group are shown in Table 1. Changes in parameters over 3 months are illustrated in Figures 2 and 3. All results in this section are given as mean and standard deviation (M ± SD).

Tear BUT, Schirmer I test value, and the lower lid TMH of the MLE Group increased significantly at Week 1 ($p = 0.008$, 0.000, 0.000, resp.) and Month 1 ($p = 0.034$, 0.014, 0.001, resp.) after injection. However, for the non-MLE Group, none of the follow-up tear BUT were statistically different from the baseline; Schirmer I test value increased at Week 1 only ($p = 0.034$); the lower lid TMH increased at Week 1 ($p = 0.000$) and Month 1 ($p = 0.003$). When comparing the two groups, the improvement in tear BUT at all time points showed no significant difference between the two groups; the increase of Schirmer I test value of the MLE Group was higher than that of the non-MLE Group at Week 1 and Month 1; the increase of the lower lid TMH of the MLE Group was more than that of the non-MLE Group at Week 1.

For both groups, the lagophthalmos height increased significantly at Week 1 ($p = 0.000$ for both groups) and returned back to baseline at Months 1 and 3. In comparison, the lagophthalmos height of the MLE Group increased more

TABLE 1: Between-group comparisons of ocular surface parameters and subjective symptoms in the MLE Group and the non-MLE Group before and after BoNT-A injection.

		Baseline (M (SD))$_0$	One week (M (SD))$_{1w}$	(M (SD))$_{1w-0}$	One month (M (SD))$_{1m}$	(M (SD))$_{1m-0}$	Three months (M (SD))$_{3m}$	(M (SD))$_{3m-0}$
Tear BUT, s	MLE	4.26 (2.83)	6.32 (3.57)	2.06 (4.33)	5.68 (3.00)	1.41 (3.61)	5.47 (3.20)	1.21 (2.65)
	Non-MLE	4.15 (2.71)	6.09 (4.20)	1.94 (4.76)	5.29 (2.69)	1.15 (3.53)	5.09 (2.21)	0.94 (2.35)
	Difference (95% CI)	0.12 (−0.31 to 0.55)		0.12 (−0.76 to 1.03)		0.26 (−0.33 to 0.86)		0.26 (−0.68 to 1.21)
	p value	0.608		0.747		0.409		0.807
Schirmer I test, mm	MLE	8.59 (5.09)	13.82 (6.45)	5.24 (4.92)	12.09 (5.94)	3.50 (4.32)	9.53 (4.35)	0.94 (3.27)
	Non-MLE	8.91 (4.68)	11.21 (6.00)	2.29 (4.19)	10.76 (5.27)	1.85 (4.09)	9.32 (4.05)	0.41 (2.63)
	Difference (95% CI)	−0.32 (−1.46 to 0.81)		2.94 (1.41 to 4.47)		1.65 (0.20 to 3.10)		0.53 (−0.65 to 1.71)
	p value	0.566		0.000*		0.027*		0.369
Lower lid TMH, mm	MLE	0.22 (0.13)	0.38 (0.17)	0.16 (0.17)	0.30 (0.14)	0.08 (0.12)	0.23 (0.13)	0.01 (0.07)
	Non-MLE	0.21 (0.09)	0.32 (0.14)	0.11 (0.13)	0.27 (0.12)	0.06 (0.11)	0.22 (0.09)	0.01 (0.06)
	Difference (95% CI)	0.01 (−0.02 to 0.04)		0.05 (0.01 to 0.10)		0.01 (−0.02 to 0.04)		0.00 (−0.02 to 0.02)
	p value	0.660		0.012*		0.336		0.535
Lagophthalmos height, mm	MLE	0	1.16 (0.95)	1.16 (0.95)	0.11 (0.38)	0.11 (0.38)	0	0
	Non-MLE	0	0.73 (0.81)	0.73 (0.81)	0.12 (0.39)	0.12 (0.39)	0	0
	Difference (95% CI)			0.44 (0.20 to 0.67)		−0.01 (−0.06 to 0.04)		
	p value			0.001*		0.655		
JRS score, points	MLE	7.70 (0.92)	1.82 (1.55)	−5.89 (1.65)	0.24 (0.83)	−7.45 (1.18)	0.88 (1.52)	−6.82 (1.65)
	Non-MLE	7.70 (0.92)	1.94 (1.48)	−5.76 (1.56)	0.30 (0.88)	−7.39 (1.20)	1.88 (1.60)	−5.82 (1.78)
	Difference (95% CI)			−0.12 (−0.29 to 0.05)		−0.06 (−0.18 to 0.06)		−1.00 (−1.35 to −0.65)
	p value			0.157		0.317		0.000*

*$p < 0.05$.

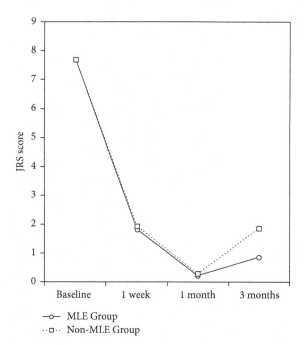

FIGURE 3: Changes in JRS score of the MLE Group and the non-MLE Group before and after BoNT-A injection.

than that of the non-MLE Group at Week 1. For both groups, no ectropion, ptosis, or fluorescein staining of the cornea related to lagophthalmos was recorded, and no complaints of epiphora or diplopia were reported.

Compared to the baseline, mean posttreatment JRS scores decreased over time. There was no significant difference in JRS scores between groups at Week 1 and Month 1, but at Month 3, the MLE Group had a lower score than the non-MLE Group.

4. Discussion

In this study, we firstly evaluated whether the MLE site should be involved in injection of BoNT-A in treating BEB. We investigated the effects of two BoNT-A injection patterns—with or without the MLE on subjective symptoms of BEB and objective condition of the ocular surface. As suggested by JRS scores, BEB symptoms of both groups were alleviated at Week 1 and Month 1 after injection, but patients in the MLE Group had fewer complaints about blepharospasm at Month 3. This may be because an additional BoNT-A injection in the MLE chemodenervated the pretarsal orbicularis oculi, which is particularly involved in spontaneous blinking [17], more evenly. Thus, the full injection pattern had its efficacy waned at a slower rate and relieved BEB symptoms for a longer duration.

In addition, both injection patterns in this study reduced lacrimal drainage, but the full injection pattern had more noticeable effect. The lacrimal drainage may be reduced by two mechanisms, with the first being blink rate reduction. With each blink draining approximately $2\,\mu L$ of tears, the lacrimal drainage capacity is significantly influenced by the blink rate [18]. Therefore, less blink rate may result in less lacrimal drainage and better lubrication of the ocular surface. Second, lower eyelid laxity may play a role in lacrimal drainage reduction. Since BoNT-A injected into the MLE can paralyze the orbicularis oculi pars lacrimalis muscle, the lower eyelids and the ends of the lacrimal canals are loosened, leading to dysfunction of the lacrimal pump [19]. These explain why, in our study, eyes in the full injection pattern group had higher value of Schirmer test and TMH, while in other studies, BoNT-A injection patterns without the MLE resulted in unchanged [13] or even decreased [15] Schirmer test value.

In our study, the adverse effects of the two different BoNT-A injection patterns were also evaluated. Although some patients in both groups temporarily experienced mild lagophthalmos at 1 week after injection, no other complications such as diplopia, ptosis, epiphora, ectropion, or corneal exposure were observed. The limited adverse events in our study may be owing to the low BoNT-A dose we used, since the incidence of adverse events was dose related [7].

Although there have been several studies about the influence of BoNT-A injection on lacrimal drainage, none of them focused on the MLE injection site. In Dae Il Park's study [20], they studied the effect of BoNT-A on tear production and drainage in patients with BEB, but they did not discuss the role the MLE plays in this effect. In another study of ocular surface alterations after BoNT-A injection [21], variable injection patterns were used according to the region of contractions. Both of them emphasized the effect of BoNT-A on ocular surface condition, but they put no effort in illustrating the effect of injection sites. In Sven Sahlin's studies [19, 22], they compared two BoNT-A injection patterns with or without the upper medial lid injection in patients with dry eyes. However, the study subjects (patients with BEB) and injection sites (MLE) investigated in our study were totally different. Therefore, to the best of our knowledge, our study is the first to explore the role of the MLE in treating BEB and influencing lacrimal drainage.

In conclusion, both BoNT-A injection patterns were effective in relieving blepharospasm, but the full injection pattern involving the MLE had better efficacy at Month 3. The full injection pattern also reduced lacrimal drainage more significantly, though the influence disappeared at Month 3. Therefore, we propose that the full injection pattern, rather than the medial lower lid waived pattern, be a better choice for treating BEB.

Disclosure

The funding organizations had no role in the design or conduct of the study.

Conflict of Interests

The authors declare that there is no conflict of interests regarding the publication of this paper.

Authors' Contribution

Hui Yang made the design of the study; Hui Yang, Xiujuan Zhao, Xiaohu Ding, Zhonghao Wang, and Xiaoyu Cai conducted the study; data collection was done by Jing Lu, Xiujuan Zhao, and Xiaohu Ding, Hui Yang, Jing Lu, and Lin Lu managed the study; data analysis was done by Jing Lu and Hui Yang and data interpretation by Jing Lu, Hui Yang, and Yan Luo; Hui Yang, Jing Lu, Yan Luo, and Lin Lu prepared the study; review was done by Hui Yang, Yan Luo, Jing Lu, and Lin Lu; and Hui Yang, Yan Luo, and Lin Lu approved the manuscript.

Acknowledgments

This work was supported by grants from the National Basic Research Development Program of China (973 Program: 2013CB967000), the Natural Science Foundation of Guangdong Province, China (S2012010008439, Hui Yang), and the National Natural Science Foundation of China (81170863, Lin Lu).

References

[1] J. Jankovic and J. Orman, "Blepharospasm: demographic and clinical survey of 250 patients," *Annals of Ophthalmology*, vol. 16, no. 4, pp. 371–376, 1984.

[2] J. Jankovic, W. E. Havins, and R. B. Wilkins, "Blinking and blepharospasm. Mechanism, diagnosis, and management," *The Journal of the American Medical Association*, vol. 248, no. 23, pp. 3160–3164, 1982.

[3] M. Fiorio, M. Tinazzi, A. Scontrini et al., "Tactile temporal discrimination in patients with blepharospasm," *Journal of Neurology, Neurosurgery and Psychiatry*, vol. 79, no. 7, pp. 796–798, 2008.

[4] T. Fayers, S. R. Shaw, S. C. Hau, and D. G. Ezra, "Changes in corneal aesthesiometry and the sub-basal nerve plexus in benign essential blepharospasm," *British Journal of Ophthalmology*, vol. 99, no. 11, pp. 1509–1513, 2015.

[5] A. B. Scott, R. A. Kennedy, and H. A. Stubbs, "Botulinum A toxin injection as a treatment for blepharospasm," *Archives of Ophthalmology*, vol. 103, no. 3, pp. 347–350, 1985.

[6] J. J. Dutton and A. M. Fowler, "Botulinum toxin in ophthalmology," *Survey of Ophthalmology*, vol. 52, no. 1, pp. 13–31, 2007.

[7] D. Truong, C. Comella, H. H. Fernandez, and W. G. Ondo, "Efficacy and safety of purified botulinum toxin type A (Dysport) for the treatment of benign essential blepharospasm: a randomized, placebo-controlled, phase II trial," *Parkinsonism and Related Disorders*, vol. 14, no. 5, pp. 407–414, 2008.

[8] R. Çakmur, V. Ozturk, F. Uzunel, B. Donmez, and F. Idiman, "Comparison of preseptal and pretarsal injections of botulinum toxin in the treatment of blepharospasm and hemifacial spasm," *Journal of Neurology*, vol. 249, no. 1, pp. 64–68, 2002.

[9] M. Esposito, A. Fasano, C. Crisci, R. Dubbioso, R. Iodice, and L. Santoro, "The combined treatment with orbital and pretarsal botulinum toxin injections in the management of poorly responsive blepharospasm," *Neurological Sciences*, vol. 35, no. 3, pp. 397–400, 2014.

[10] J. Price, S. Farish, H. Taylor, and J. O'Day, "Blepharospasm and hemifacial spasm. Randomized trial to determine the most appropriate location for botulinum toxin injections," *Ophthalmology*, vol. 104, no. 5, pp. 865–868, 1997.

[11] H. Iwashige, Y. Nemeto, H. Takahashi, and T. Maruo, "Botulinum toxin type A purified neurotoxin complex for the treatment of blepharospasm: a dose-response study measuring eyelid force," *Japanese Journal of Ophthalmology*, vol. 39, no. 4, pp. 424–431, 1995.

[12] R. L. Levy, D. Berman, M. Parikh, and N. R. Miller, "Supramaximal doses of botulinum toxin for refractory blepharospasm," *Ophthalmology*, vol. 113, no. 9, pp. 1665–1668, 2006.

[13] P. G. Costa, I. P. Cardoso, F. P. Saraiva, A. C. P. Raiza, L. K. Tanaka, and S. Matayoshi, "Lacrimal film evaluation of patients with facial dystonia during botulinum toxin type A treatment," *Arquivos Brasileiros de Oftalmologia*, vol. 69, no. 3, pp. 319–322, 2006.

[14] R. Lu, R. Huang, K. Li et al., "The influence of benign essential blepharospasm on dry eye disease and ocular inflammation," *American Journal of Ophthalmology*, vol. 157, no. 3, pp. 591–597.e2, 2014.

[15] J. Horwath-Winter, J. Bergloeff, I. Floegel, E.-M. Haller-Schober, and O. Schmut, "Botulinum toxin A treatment in patients suffering from blepharospasm and dry eye," *British Journal of Ophthalmology*, vol. 87, no. 1, pp. 54–56, 2003.

[16] J. Jankovic and J. Orman, "Botulinum A toxin for cranial-cervical dystonia: a double-blind, placebo-controlled study," *Neurology*, vol. 37, no. 4, pp. 616–623, 1987.

[17] G. Gordon, "Observations upon the movements of the eyelids," *The British Journal of Ophthalmology*, vol. 35, no. 6, pp. 339–351, 1951.

[18] S. Sahlin and E. Chen, "Gravity, blink rate, and lacrimal drainage capacity," *American Journal of Ophthalmology*, vol. 124, no. 6, pp. 758–764, 1997.

[19] S. Sahlin and R. Linderoth, "Eyelid botulinum toxin injections for the dry eye," *Developments in Ophthalmology*, vol. 41, pp. 187–192, 2008.

[20] D. I. Park, H. M. Shin, S. Y. Lee, and H. Lew, "Tear production and drainage after botulinum toxin A injection in patients with essential blepharospasm," *Acta Ophthalmologica*, vol. 91, no. 2, pp. e108–e112, 2013.

[21] S. Kocabeyoglu, H. T. Sekeroglu, M. C. Mocan, E. Muz, M. Irkec, and A. S. Sanac, "Ocular surface alterations in blepharospasm patients treated with botulinum toxin A injection," *European Journal of Ophthalmology*, vol. 24, no. 6, pp. 830–834, 2014.

[22] S. Sahlin, E. Chen, T. Kaugesaar, H. Almqvist, K. Kjellberg, and G. Lennerstrand, "Effect of eyelid botulinum toxin injection on lacrimal drainage," *American Journal of Ophthalmology*, vol. 129, no. 4, pp. 481–486, 2000.

Outcomes of 23-Gauge Vitrectomy Combined with Phacoemulsification, Panretinal Photocoagulation, and Trabeculectomy without Use of Anti-VEGF Agents for Neovascular Glaucoma with Vitreous Hemorrhage

Hua Yan

Department of Ophthalmology, Tianjin Medical University General Hospital, No. 154, Anshan Road, Tianjin 300052, China

Correspondence should be addressed to Hua Yan; zyyyanhua@tmu.edu.cn

Academic Editor: Antonio Ferreras

Purpose. To evaluate the outcomes of 23-gauge vitrectomy combined with phacoemulsification, PRP and trabeculectomy without use of anti-VEGF-agents for NVG. *Methods*. Eighteen eyes of 18 patients with NVG underwent 23-gauge vitrectomy combined with phacoemulsification, PRP and trabeculectomy without use of anti-VEGF agents. The preoperative BCVA ranged from light perception to 0.2. The preoperative IOP ranged from 38 mmHg to 64 mmHg with a mean of 54 ± 8 mmHg. The average follow-up time was 14.5 ± 3 months with a range from 11 to 24 months. *Results*. The postoperative VA increased in 14 eyes and was stable in 4 eyes at the final follow-up. The mean IOP was 12 ± 3 mmHg at postoperative day 1. The mean IOP was 15 ± 2 mmHg, 16 ± 3 mmHg, 23 ± 5 mmHg, 28 ± 4 mmHg, 22 ± 5 mmHg, 17 ± 3 mmHg, and 19 ± 4 mmHg at postoperative days 2 and 3, 1, 2, 3, and 12 weeks, and 1 year postoperatively, respectively, with a range from 10 to 30 mmHg at the final follow-up time point of one year. The IOP was significantly lower than the preoperative one 12 weeks postoperatively ($p < 0.05$). *Conclusion*. 23-gauge vitrectomy combined with phacoemulsification, PRP, and trabeculectomy without use of anti-VEGF-agents is a safe and effective method in treating NVG.

1. Introduction

Neovascular glaucoma (NVG) complicated by vitreous hemorrhage (VH) is commonly caused by retinal ischemia secondary to central retinal vein occlusion (CRVO), branch retinal vein occlusion (BRVO), and/or proliferative diabetic retinopathy (PDR) [1–3]. Vision can be severely affected by NVG, which often causes permanent damage to the optic nerve secondary to high intraocular pressures associated with angle closure. Ischemic neovascular vessels can form and occlude the angle. Hypoxia caused by CRVO, BRVO, and PDR induces production and release of vascular endothelial growth factor (VEGF) and inflammatory mediators. These neovascular vessels are leaky and fragile and can cause VH and NVG and are also associated with leakage of inflammatory molecules which can cause macular edema.

NVG is one of the most recalcitrant glaucoma types to treatment and has one of the worst outcomes of the many types of glaucoma. NVG often needs surgical treatment because medical treatment of elevated IOP is often inadequate. The standard of early treatment once NVG occurs is panretinal photocoagulation (PRP), which destroys ischemic retina and decreases the production of proangiogenic factors such as VEGF. PRP can prevent ischemic retina from progressing to NVG. Glaucoma drainage implants, trabeculectomy with mitomycin C, cyclocryotherapy, or diode laser coagulation of the ciliary body is another treatment option available for the treatment of recalcitrant and end-stage NVG [4–6]. Pars plana vitrectomy (PPV) combined with glaucoma drainage implantation can produce good control of intraocular pressure (IOP) in NVG patients with PDR [7, 8].

Antivascular endothelial growth factor (anti-VEGF) molecules have been used for many ocular diseases, including NVG. A number of studies have evaluated the use of anti-VEGF agents as stand-alone or adjunctive treatment for NVG [9]. Adjunctive anti-VEGF treatment promotes the surgical success rate for NVG. IOP lowering surgery combined with PRP or intravitreal injection of anti-VEGF antibodies aids in regression of neovascularization and stabilization of vision [10, 11].

The optimal approaches to treating NVG with VH are to provide patients with an individualized management plan according to etiology, stage of disease, and visual potential among other factors. PPV combined with PRP can reduce the occurrence of NVG and increases visual acuity (VA) in CRVO with VH [12]. In this retrospective study, we investigated the long term surgical outcomes, including VA and IOP of NVG eyes complicated with VH, after treatment with 23-gauge vitrectomy combined with phacoemulsification, PRP, and trabeculectomy without use of anti-VEGF agents. We suggest that this is an effective method for the treatment of NVG induced by retinal vessel occlusion and PDR.

2. Patients and Methods

2.1. Patients. The study was approved by Tianjin Medical University General Hospital Medical Ethics Committee and complies with the Declaration of Helsinki, including current revisions, and with the Good Clinical Practice guidelines. The procedures followed were in accordance with institutional guidelines; all the subjects provided their written informed consent for sampling according to the Declaration of Helsinki. All the subjects were recruited from the ophthalmology department of Tianjin General Hospital.

Eighteen eyes of 18 consecutive patients who had NVG and VH underwent 23-gauge vitrectomy combined with phacoemulsification, PRP, and trabeculectomy without use of anti-VEGF agents from January 2012 to June 2014. Ten patients were males, and 8 were females. The age ranged from 58 to 76 years with a mean of 62 ± 6 years. Three patients were with hypertension, 7 patients were with diabetes mellitus complicated with hypertension, and 8 patients were with diabetes mellitus complicated with renal failure. Eight eyes had a history of CRVO, 6 eyes had PDR complicated with BRVO, and 4 eyes had PDR alone (Table 1). The rubeosis iridis conditions were present in 18 NVG eyes preoperatively (Figure 1). The preoperative VA ranged from light perception to 0.2. The preoperative IOP ranged from 38 to 64 mmHg with a mean of 54 ± 8 mmHg. The average follow-up was 14.5 ± 3 months with a range from 12 to 24 months.

Eyes with a prior history of intravitreal injection of steroids or anti-VEGF agents, VH without retinal vessels occlusion and PDR, ocular trauma, ocular tumors, and corneal opacity precluding PRP, or cataract extraction before NVG was diagnosed were excluded.

2.2. Pre- and Postoperative Examinations. Pre- and postoperative examinations included VA, slit-lamp examination, gonioscopy, indirect ophthalmoscopy, IOP, and B-scan.

2.3. Surgical Procedures. We performed 23-gauge PPV using a three-port technique in all patients. The eye received retrobulbar and peribulbar 2% lidocaine for anesthesia, and the eye was then prepared for a standard three-port 23-gauge vitrectomy. After the infusion cannula was placed, the cataract was extracted by phacoemulsification through a clear corneal incision approach. The posterior capsule was preserved in 10 eyes and was completely resected in 8 eyes. During PPV, posterior hyaloid separation was induced by suction using the vitreous cutter over the optic nerve head in eyes without posterior vitreous detachment. In each case, the meticulous shaving of the vitreous base under a wide-angle viewing system with assisted sclera depression was performed to remove as much residual blood as possible. After the VH was completely removed, any fibrovascular tissue present was removed using the microvitrector tip. Hemostasis was maintained by raising the IOP through the infusion fluid or by using endodiathermy intraoperatively.

PRP was performed in all eyes, and subsequent peripheral retinal cryotherapy was given only in severe NVG eyes during the surgery. A 4×3 mm lamellar sclera flap was created in the superior region to the limbal border, and then a mitomycin C trabeculectomy was performed. Postoperative examinations were completed at 1, 2, and 3 days, 1, 2, 3, and 12 weeks, and 1 year after the surgery. Intraocular lenses were implanted in 3 eyes 3 months after the combined surgery. No supplemental PRP was given in the postoperative period.

Paired Student's t-test was used to analyze changes in pre- and postoperative IOP.

3. Results

After the combined surgery, the conjunctival incisions healed well, and the conjunctival flap was formed significantly. Corneas were clear, and iridectomies were patent. Rubeosis iridis has regressed in all eyes 1 week postoperatively (Figure 1). At the final follow-up postoperatively, rubeosis iridis disappeared in the iris and conjunctiva filtering bleb was flat.

3.1. VA. The postoperative VA increased in 14 eyes with the BCVA ranging from 0.02 to 0.4 and was stable relative to the preoperative vision in 4 eyes at the final follow-up. The change trend of BCVA pre- and postoperatively was demonstrated in Figure 2. The BCVA significantly increased within three months postoperatively compared with the preoperative BCVA ($p < 0.05$) and then remained stable ($p > 0.05$).

3.2. IOP. The mean IOP was 12 ± 3 mmHg, 15 ± 2 mmHg, 16 ± 3 mmHg, 23 ± 5 mmHg, 28 ± 4 mmHg, 22 ± 5 mmHg, 17 ± 3 mmHg, and 19 ± 4 mmHg at 1, 2, and 3 days, 1, 2, 3, and 12 weeks, and 1 year, postoperatively. The IOP ranged from 10 to 30 mmHg 1 year postoperatively. The IOP was significantly lower at three months compared to the preoperative baseline IOP ($p < 0.05$) and then remained stable to the final follow-up ($p > 0.05$) (Figure 3). IOP was not in normal range in 8 eyes 1 month postoperatively, and 2% carteolol hydrochloride was used twice a day for 1 month in 5 eyes and combined with brinzolamide 3 times a day for 1 month in 3 eyes for making IOP to normal range.

3.3. Postoperative Complications. Postoperative complications mainly included fibrosis exudates in the anterior chamber (7 eyes), temporary IOP elevation at 2 weeks

TABLE 1: Clinical data of patients with NVG.

Case number	Sex	Age (y)	Systemic disease	Diagnosis	Previous treatment	BCVA Preop.	BCVA Postop.	IOP (mmHg) Preop.	IOP (mmHg) Postop.	Complications	Follow-up (months)
1	M	76	Hypertension	CRVO	B + C	0.02	0.08	58	21	Fibrosis exudates in AC	16
2	M	61	DM + hypertension	CRVO	B + C, partial laser	0.04	0.04	53	22	None	17
3	F	58	DM + RF	PDR + BRVO	B + C	LP	0.02	60	30	Fibrosis exudates in AC	12
4	F	62	DM + hypertension	CRVO	B + C, partial laser	HM	0.04	58	20	None	15
5	M	59	DM + RF	PDR + BRVO	B + C	CF	0.04	59	18	Temporary IOP elevation	14
6	F	61	DM + RF	PDR	B + C	0.08	0.1	48	17	None	17
7	M	63	DM + hypertension	CRVO	B + C	0.06	0.1	61	19	Fibrosis exudates in AC	12
8	M	63	DM + RF	PDR	B + C, partial laser	0.1	0.3	40	15	Fibrosis exudates in AC	13
9	F	59	DM + RF	PDR + BRVO	B + C	0.08	0.08	39	16	None	12
10	M	58	DM + hypertension	CRVO	B + C, partial laser	0.04	0.06	56	21	Fibrosis exudates in AC	12
11	F	60	DM + hypertension	PDR + BRVO	B + C	HM	0.02	58	19	SCH	24
12	F	63	DM + hypertension	PDR + BRVO	B + C	HM	0.08	57	18	None	13
13	M	59	DM + RF	PDR	B + C, partial laser	0.02	0.02	56	20	Fibrosis exudates in AC	17
14	M	71	Hypertension	CRVO	B + C	0.02	0.04	54	18	Fibrosis exudates in AC	12
15	F	63	DM + RF	PDR + BRVO	B + C	LP	0.04	64	19	Temporary IOP elevation	16
16	M	58	DM + hypertension	CRVO	B + C	CF	0.06	55	17	None	14
17	M	63	DM + RF	PDR	B + C	0.04	0.04	54	18	None	13
18	F	65	Hypertension	CRVO	B + C, partial laser	0.2	0.4	38	10	None	13

F = female; M = male; DM = diabetes mellitus; RF = renal failure; BCVA = best corrected visual acuity; AC = anterior chamber; SCH = suprachoroidal hemorrhage; B = brinzolamide; C = 2% carteolol hydrochloride.

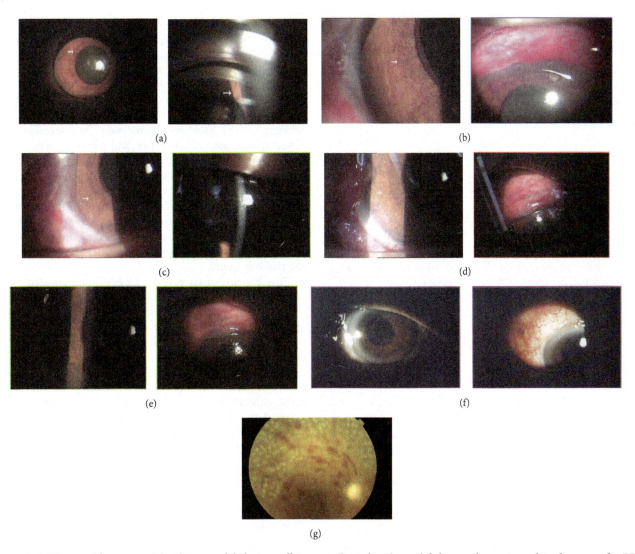

FIGURE 1: A 63-year-old woman with a history of diabetes mellitus complicated with renal failure underwent combined surgery for PDR complicated with NVG. The preoperative VA was LP and increased to 0.04 postoperatively, with IOP decreasing from 64 mmHg preoperatively to 19 mmHg at the final follow-up postoperatively. Rubeosis iridis was present in the iris preoperatively and regressed 1 week postoperatively. At the final follow-up postoperatively, rubeosis iridis disappeared in the iris and conjunctiva filtering bleb was flat. (a) Rubeosis iridis (white arrow) was present in the iris preoperatively, and new vessels (white arrow) were seen at the anterior chamber angle by gonioscopy. IOP was 64 mmHg. (b) Rubeosis iridis (white arrow) was still present in the iris 1 day postoperatively, and conjunctiva filtering bleb was formed. IOP was 16 mmHg. (c) Rubeosis iridis (white arrow) was significantly decreased in the iris 2 days postoperatively, and cornea was clear. IOP was 15 mmHg. (d) Rubeosis iridis (white arrow) was not significant in the iris 3 days postoperatively, and conjunctiva filtering bleb was obvious. IOP was 15 mmHg. (e) Rubeosis iridis regressed in the iris 1 week postoperatively, and conjunctiva filtering bleb was stable. IOP was 15 mmHg. (f) Rubeosis iridis disappeared in the iris at the final follow-up postoperatively, and conjunctiva filtering bleb was flat. IOP was 19 mmHg. (g) Intraoperative PRP for treatment of PDR complicated with BRVO in patients with NVG and optic nerve atrophy 1 week postoperatively.

postoperatively (2 eyes), and postoperative suprachoroidal hemorrhage (1 eye).

4. Discussion

A cyclodestructive method or glaucoma drainage surgery is frequently the final option for treatment of severe NVG, but the postoperative VA rarely increases, and IOP is sometimes poorly controlled after aggressive treatment [4, 5]. We treated NVG using 23-gauge vitrectomy combined with phacoemulsification, PRP, and trabeculectomy without use of anti-VEGF agents and obtained predictable results.

NVG develops secondary to extensive ischemic retinal changes, such as occurring with PDR and CRVO. In CRVO, when the retinal vein is occluded, the ischemic retina releases VEGF and inflammatory cytokines into the vitreous cavity, posterior chamber, anterior chamber, and anterior chamber angle [13]. The VEGF in the anterior chamber stimulates neovascularization of the iris and the angle, restricts aqueous outflow, and results eventually in the development of NVG.

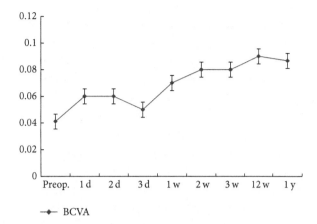

FIGURE 2: The chart clearly demonstrates the change trend of BCVA pre- and postoperatively. The BCVA significantly increased within three months postoperatively compared with the preoperative BCVA ($p < 0.05$) and then remained stable ($p > 0.05$).

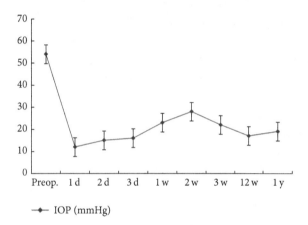

FIGURE 3: The chart clearly demonstrates the change trend of IOP pre- and postoperatively. The IOP was significantly lower within three months postoperatively compared with the preoperative baseline IOP ($p < 0.05$) and then remained stable ($p > 0.05$).

Wakabayashi et al. [14] reported high intraocular VEGF level at the time of primary vitrectomy in patients with PDR, which was identified as a significant risk factor for postoperative early VH. Goto et al. [15] reported that the risk factors for NVG after vitrectomy in eyes with PDR are independently associated with male sex, younger age, higher baseline IOP, preoperative neovascularization in the angle, and NVG in the fellow's eye.

In this study, 8 patients had hypertension complicated with CRVO, 6 patient had hypertension complicated with BRVO, and 4 patients had PDR. The 4 patients with PDR were also complicated with either CRVO or BRVO. PDR in these 4 patients was not very severe. Therefore, the main reason resulting in NVG was either CRVO or BRVO. In our experience, NVG caused by CRVO or BRVO occurs more quickly than by diabetic retinopathy. In patients with CRVO or BRVO, the observation of IOP, rubeosis irides, and retinal neovascularization should be emphasized, and PRP should be performed for decreasing the risk of developing NVG.

Phacoemulsification, vitrectomy, PRP, and trabeculectomy were adopted to treat NVG complicated with VH according to the different treatment mechanisms. Phacoemulsification to remove a cataract can improve the view so vitrectomy and PRP can be performed more easily. In patients without a posterior capsule preserved after phacoemulsification, the postoperative IOP may be lowered significantly because of the free communication of aqueous humor between the anterior chamber and vitreous cavity. However, postoperative suprachoroidal hemorrhage occasionally occurred because of sudden decrease of postoperative IOP or simultaneously ocular trauma. In this study, 1 eye without posterior capsule preservation developed suprachoroidal hemorrhage because of ocular trauma 3 days postoperatively and were treated with drainage of suprachoroidal hemorrhage through sclerotomies and placement of 30% C3F8 into the vitreous cavity.

The benefits of vitrectomy for NVG complicated by VH are as follows: (1) vitrectomy removes VH and clears the vitreous cavity which can increase VA, (2) vitrectomy removes and may reduce the expression of VEGF, which is a vital factor for neovascularization, (3) vitrectomy to remove VH can prevent hemolytic or ghost cell glaucoma, and (4) PRP can be performed completely and easily after PPV. In NVG with VH, performing complete PRP is often difficult even in cases with minimal VH.

PRP, the standard of care for treating NVG in ischemic CRVO and PDR, decreases oxygen consumption and production of VEGF and aids in the regression of rubeosis irides. In patients with previous partial retinal laser treatment, additional laser photocoagulation can be performed intraoperatively because it is conducted under anesthesia and patient feels no or minimal pain which allows for more complete PRP along with the greater peripheral retinal view for additional PRP. Rubeosis iridis does not regress immediately after PRP, and effect on IOP can be minimal or delayed after PRP. Therefore, in patients with open angle NVG, trabeculectomy is effective in decreasing the IOP temporarily as, in patients with angle closure NVG, trabeculectomy is used to decrease the IOP for a longer term.

In recent years, anti-VEGF agents have been widely applied for the treatment of ischemic retinopathy, including retinal vessel occlusion and PDR. Anti-VEGF agents used in PDR can reduce intra- and postoperative hemorrhage associated with the surgical removal of VH. Although very little information about the role of anti-VEGF treatment in NVG complicated with VH exists, trabeculectomy combined with injection of anti-VEGF agents into the vitreous body for NVG has been documented. However, the long term effect of decreasing the IOP does not appear to be significant compared with trabeculectomy alone. Anti-VEGF agents can cause temporary regression of iris neovascularization, but the long term use for anti-VEGF agents for NVG is not as clear as it is for age-related macular degeneration. Additionally, long term use of anti-VEGF agents for NVG can be very expensive.

Other protocols for treatment of NVG have been described. Bartz-Schmidt et al. [16] treated NVG with vitrectomy combined with PRP, direct laser coagulation of ciliary processes, and silicone oil tamponade. The IOP normalized in 59% of eyes at 6 months postoperatively and in 72% of eyes after 1 year. Chuang et al. [12] reported 56 eyes with CRVO complicated by VH which underwent PPV combined with PRP, and the most important result was a lower incidence of NVG development and VA improvement. Kinoshita et al. [17] reported PPV combined with lensectomy with anterior capsule preservation, endophotocoagulation, and silicon oil tamponade for NVG. The IOP decreased from 29 ± 19 mmHg to 17 ± 6 mmHg 1 year postoperatively with a success rate of 69.2%. Luttrull and Avery [18] reported the treatment of NVG with vitrectomy combined with pars plana glaucoma drainage implant, and all patients had normal IOPs 1 year postoperatively. Wallsh et al. [7] reported pars plana placement of Ahmed valved glaucoma drainage implants in combination with PPV in the treatment of NVG. The IOP decreased from 37.6 mmHg to 13.8 mmHg. Jeong et al. [8] reported pars plana Ahmed GDI placement combined with 23-gauge vitrectomy for NVG in DR, and IOP decreased from 35.9 ± 6.3 mmHg to 13.3 ± 3.2 mmHg at the last visit. Control of IOP was achieved in all patients, but 91% needed antiglaucoma medications. Sevim et al. [19] reported the effect of intravitreal bevacizumab injection before Ahmed glaucoma valve implantation in NVG and the surgical success rate was 79%. In this study, the IOP was normal in 71.4% during postoperative follow-up, and the neovascularization of the iris disappeared in all eyes. Preoperative use of bevacizumab may be to have a better result when our combined surgery is not practical or feasible [20].

In conclusion, vitrectomy combined with phacoemulsification, PRP, and trabeculectomy without use of anti-VEGF agents is a safe and effective method in treating NVG complicated with VH. In some cases, loss of VA was decreased. This combined surgery may be considered as a first treatment option for NVG complicated VH, and the long term effects of the combined surgery should be investigated.

Conflict of Interests

The author has stated that he does not have a significant financial interest or other relationships with any product manufacturer or provider of services discussed in this paper. The author also does not discuss the use of off-label products, which includes unlabeled, unapproved, or noninvestigative products or devices.

References

[1] T.-S. An and S.-I. Kwon, "Neovascular glaucoma due to branch retinal vein occlusion combined with branch retinal artery occlusion," *Korean Journal of Ophthalmology*, vol. 27, no. 1, pp. 64–67, 2013.

[2] C. K. Chan, M. S. Ip, P. C. Vanveldhuisen et al., "SCORE study report #11: incidences of neovascular events in eyes with retinal vein occlusion," *Ophthalmology*, vol. 118, no. 7, pp. 1364–1372, 2011.

[3] G. H. Bresnick, G. De Venecia, F. L. Myers, J. A. Harris, and M. D. Davis, "Retinal ischemia in diabetic retinopathy," *Archives of Ophthalmology*, vol. 93, no. 12, pp. 1300–1310, 1975.

[4] A. Tzamalis, D.-T. Pham, and C. Wirbelauer, "Diode laser cyclophotocoagulation versus cyclocryotherapy in the treatment of refractory glaucoma," *European Journal of Ophthalmology*, vol. 21, no. 5, pp. 589–596, 2011.

[5] Y. Takihara, M. Inatani, M. Fukushima, K. Iwao, M. Iwao, and H. Tanihara, "Trabeculectomy with mitomycin C for neovascular glaucoma: prognostic factors for surgical failure," *American Journal of Ophthalmology*, vol. 147, no. 5, pp. 912.e1–918.e1, 2009.

[6] A. W. Fong, G. A. Lee, P. O'Rourke, and R. Thomas, "Management of neovascular glaucoma with transscleral cyclophotocoagulation with diode laser alone versus combination transscleral cyclophotocoagulation with diode laser and intravitreal bevacizumab," *Clinical and Experimental Ophthalmology*, vol. 39, no. 4, pp. 318–323, 2011.

[7] J. O. Wallsh, R. P. Gallemore, M. Taban, C. Hu, and B. Sharareh, "Pars plana Ahmed valve and vitrectomy in patients with glaucoma associated with posterior segment disease," *Retina*, vol. 33, no. 10, pp. 2059–2068, 2013.

[8] H. S. Jeong, D. H. Nam, H. J. Paik, and D. Y. Lee, "Pars plana Ahmed implantation combined with 23-gauge vitrectomy for refractory neovascular glaucoma in diabetic retinopathy," *Korean Journal of Ophthalmology*, vol. 26, no. 2, pp. 92–96, 2012.

[9] K. Kimoto and T. Kubota, "Anti-VEGF agents for ocular angiogenesis and vascular permeability," *Journal of Ophthalmology*, vol. 2012, Article ID 852183, 11 pages, 2012.

[10] Y. Takihara, M. Inatani, T. Kawaji et al., "Combined intravitreal bevacizumab and trabeculectomy with mitomycin C versus trabeculectomy with mitomycin C alone for neovascular glaucoma," *Journal of Glaucoma*, vol. 20, no. 3, pp. 196–201, 2011.

[11] A. A. Alkawas, E. A. Shahien, and A. M. Hussein, "Management of neovascular glaucoma with panretinal photocoagulation, intravitreal bevacizumab, and subsequent trabeculectomy with mitomycin C," *Journal of Glaucoma*, vol. 19, no. 9, pp. 622–626, 2010.

[12] L.-H. Chuang, N.-K. Wang, Y.-P. Chen et al., "Vitrectomy and panretinal photocoagulation reduces the occurrence of neovascular glaucoma in central retinal vein occlusion with vitreous hemorrhage," *Retina*, vol. 33, no. 4, pp. 798–802, 2013.

[13] L. P. Aiello, R. L. Avery, P. G. Arrigg et al., "Vascular endothelial growth factor in ocular fluid of patients with diabetic retinopathy and other retinal disorders," *The New England Journal of Medicine*, vol. 331, no. 22, pp. 1480–1487, 1994.

[14] Y. Wakabayashi, Y. Usui, Y. Okunuki et al., "Intraocular VEGF level as a risk factor for postoperative complications after vitrectomy for proliferative diabetic retinopathy," *Investigative Ophthalmology & Visual Science*, vol. 53, no. 10, pp. 6403–6410, 2012.

[15] A. Goto, M. Inatani, T. Inoue et al., "Frequency and risk factors for neovascular glaucoma after vitrectomy in eyes with proliferative diabetic retinopathy," *Journal of Glaucoma*, vol. 22, no. 7, pp. 572–576, 2013.

[16] K. U. Bartz-Schmidt, G. Thumann, A. Psichias, G. K. Krieglstein, and K. Heimann, "Pars plana vitrectomy, endolaser coagulation of the retina and the ciliary body combined with silicone oil endotamponade in the treatment of uncontrolled neovascular glaucoma," *Graefe's Archive for Clinical and Experimental Ophthalmology*, vol. 237, no. 12, pp. 969–975, 1999.

[17] N. Kinoshita, A. Ota, F. Toyoda, H. Yamagami, and A. Kakehashi, "Surgical results of pars plana vitrectomy combined with pars plana lensectomy with anterior capsule preservation,

endophotocoagulation, and silicon oil tamponade for neovascular glaucoma," *Clinical Ophthalmology*, vol. 5, no. 1, pp. 1777–1781, 2011.

[18] J. K. Luttrull and R. L. Avery, "Pars plana implant and vitrectomy for treatment of neovascular glaucoma," *Retina*, vol. 15, no. 5, pp. 379–387, 1995.

[19] M. S. Sevim, I. B. Buttanri, S. Kugu, D. Serin, and S. Sevim, "Effect of intravitreal bevacizumab injection before ahmed glaucoma valve implantation in neovascular glaucoma," *Ophthalmologica*, vol. 229, no. 2, pp. 94–100, 2013.

[20] E. Vandewalle, L. A. Pinto, T. Van Bergen et al., "Intracameral bevacizumab as an adjunct to trabeculectomy: a 1-year prospective, randomised study," *British Journal of Ophthalmology*, vol. 98, no. 1, pp. 73–78, 2014.

Evaluation of Dry Eye and Meibomian Gland Dysfunction in Teenagers with Myopia through Noninvasive Keratograph

Xiu Wang,[1] Xiaoxiao Lu,[1] Jun Yang,[1] Ruihua Wei,[1] Liyuan Yang,[1] Shaozhen Zhao,[1] and Xilian Wang[2]

[1]Tianjin Medical University Eye Hospital, Fukang Road No. 251, Nankai District, Tianjin 300384, China
[2]Tianjin Beichen Hospital, Beiyi Road No. 7, Beichen District, Tianjin 300400, China

Correspondence should be addressed to Ruihua Wei; weirhua2009@126.com

Academic Editor: Chuanqing Ding

Purpose. This study aims to evaluate dry eye and ocular surface conditions of myopic teenagers by using questionnaire and clinical examinations. *Methods.* A total of 496 eyes from 248 myopic teenagers (7–18 years old) were studied. We administered Ocular Surface Disease Index (OSDI) questionnaire, slit-lamp examination, and Keratograph 5M. The patients were divided into 2 groups based on OSDI dry eye standard, and their ocular surfaces and meibomian gland conditions were evaluated. *Results.* The tear meniscus heights of the dry eye and normal groups were in normal range. Corneal fluorescein scores were significantly higher whereas noninvasive break-up time was dramatically shorter in the dry eye group than in the normal group. All three meibomian gland dysfunction parameters (i.e., meibomian gland orifice scores, meibomian gland secretion scores, and meibomian gland dropout scores) of the dry eye group were significantly higher than those of the normal group ($P < 0.0001$). *Conclusions.* The prevalence of dry eye in myopic teenagers is 18.95%. Meibomian gland dysfunction plays an important role in dry eye in myopic teenagers. The Keratograph 5M appears to provide an effective noninvasive method for assessing ocular surface situation of myopic teenagers.

1. Introduction

Dry eye disease is defined by the Report of the Definition and Classification Subcommittee of the International Dry Eye WorkShop as a multifactorial disease of tears and ocular surface, which results in symptoms of discomfort, visual disturbance, and tear film instability, with potential damage to the ocular surface [1]. Dry eye is a common ocular surface disease that often occurs in the elderly [2]. More than 20% of people in 30–40-year-olds have dry eye, and the prevalence of dry eye in people over 70 years old is as high as 36.1% [3]. Currently, with the increasing popularity of computers, video games, and smartphones in the younger generation, the incidence of myopia in teenagers is increasing annually, with a growing number of myopic teenagers exhibiting frequent blinking, sensitivity to light, and other dry eye ocular discomfort [4]. Dry eye is of an increasingly important clinical significance in myopic adolescents as it affects their quality of life. Diagnosis of dry eye currently relies on break-up time (BUT) and Schirmer's tests. However, BUT speed is different for different people. Moreover, fluorescein sodium affects the tear film's stability. BUT and Schirmer's tests are both invasive examinations. Adolescents are more difficult to evaluate than adults for ocular surface dysfunction because of poorer compliance with the procedure. Thus the traditional diagnostic methods for identifying dry eye in adolescents are less definitive since children are more sensitive to the procedure than adults. Accordingly, the data reproducibility is more variable making it more difficult to identify the disease signs in an adolescent population. Accordingly, reported dry eye incidence in myopics is underdiagnosed. Given the lower prevalence of dry eye disease in children, the diagnosis of dry eye is often overlooked by many ophthalmologists [5]. Previous studies have confirmed that Keratograph 5M (Oculus, Wetzlar, Germany) noninvasively measures noninvasive break-up time (NIBUT), tear meniscus height, and meibography with low irritability [6–10]. Therefore, in this study, we used Keratograph 5M combined with slit-lamp examination and dry eye questionnaire to give myopic adolescents a series of dry eye-related inspections and assessments and to determine the prevalence of dry eye and ocular surface conditions among myopic adolescents.

2. Materials and Methods

2.1. Materials. A total of 248 consecutive patients (average age 12.26 ± 1.86 years, range 7–18 years; 132 female, 116 male, male to female ratio = 1 : 1.14) who went to Tianjin Medical University Eye Hospital myopia clinic from January to June in 2014 with no systemic or ocular treatment, contact lens wear, keratitis, ocular allergic disease, any other ocular surface disease, glaucoma, active and chronic uveitis, or previous ocular surgery or injury were recruited in this prospective study.

Written informed consent was obtained from the parents of the patients. The study was approved by the Institutional Review Board of the Tianjin Medical University Eye Hospital and performed in accordance with the tenets of the Declaration of Helsinki.

2.2. Methods. This study was a prospective study, and all inspections were performed by the same experienced examiner.

2.2.1. Questionnaire Regarding Dry Eye. Before clinical examination, each patient completed an Ocular Surface Disease Index (OSDI) questionnaire for assessment of ocular surface symptoms and the severity of dry eye. This questionnaire [11] included questions regarding the frequency of dry eye symptoms experienced in the previous week (light sensitivity, gritty sensation, painful or sore eyes, blurred vision, and poor vision), vision-related daily activities (reading, watching TV, working on computers, and driving at night), and environmental triggers (wind, air conditioning, and low humidity). Each answer was scored on a 5-point scale (all of the time: 4, most of the time: 3, half of the time: 2, some of the time: 1, and none of the time: 0), and the OSDI score was calculated as follows: {(sum of scores × 25)/total number of questions}. Thus, the total OSDI score ranged from 0 to 100. A higher OSDI score represented greater disability. Answering was completed with the assistance of one doctor, and the completion time was controlled within 4–6 min. Currently, no uniform national standards have been established for the diagnosis of dry eye, and the diagnostic criteria are inconsistent worldwide. Based on their OSDI scores, the patients were categorized as having a normal ocular surface (0–12 points) or as having mild (13–22 points), moderate (23–32 points), or severe (33–100 points) ocular surface disease [12]. The study population was divided into normal and dry eye groups, which included those with mild dry eye, moderate dry eye, and severe dry eye. The two groups were compared to assess their ocular surface conditions.

2.2.2. Keratograph 5M: Noninvasive Measurement for Ocular Surface. Keratograph 5M inspection items include noninvasive tear film break-up time, noninvasive tear meniscus height, and meibography. The tests were first measured in the right eye and then the left eye. Three measurements were taken, and the average of results was considered in the statistics.

Keratograph 5M was used to grade the right eyelid using the following meibomian gland dropout degrees as meiboscore [13]: Grade 0: no loss of meibomian gland; Grade 1: loss of < 1/3 of the whole gland area; Grade 2: loss of 1/3-2/3 of the whole gland area; and Grade 3: loss of > 2/3 of the whole gland area. The meiboscore of each eye was calculated as the sum of the scores from both upper and lower eyelids, making the total meiboscore per eye in a range of 0–6.

2.2.3. Slit-Lamp Examination of the Anterior Segment. The following examinations were carried out sequentially using a slit-lamp: meibomian gland orifices, meibomian gland lipid secretion, and corneal fluorescein staining scores.

The quality of the meibomian gland orifices was scored semiquantitatively in the central eight glands of the lower right eyelid as follows: Grade 0 is normal, that is, no obstruction of orifice and being covered with a thin and smooth fluid; Grade 1 is obstruction of one or two meibomian gland orifices or secretions or occlusion; Grade 2 is obstruction of two or three meibomian gland orifices with thick fluid; Grade 3 is obstruction or narrowing of almost half of the meibomian gland orifices; Grade 4 is obstruction or narrowing of more than half of the meibomian gland orifices with sticky secretions.

The quality of the meibum was scored semiquantitatively in the central eight glands of the lower right eyelid as follows (0–24 points in total) [14]: Grade 0: clear fluid; Grade 1: cloudy fluid; Grade 2: cloudy, particulate fluid; and Grade 3: inspissated, toothpaste-like fluid.

Corneal fluorescein staining was graded from 0 to 12, which was a sum of the scores of corneal four quadrants scored individually as 0 (no staining), 1 (mild staining with a few scattered dots of stains), 2 (moderate staining between 1 and 3), and 3 (severe staining with confluent stains or corneal filaments) [15].

2.3. Statistical Analysis. Statistical analysis was performed using SPSS version 19.0. All variables were expressed as the mean ± standard deviation. Indexes were analyzed using nonparametric Mann-Whitney U test, and the intergroup data were compared using Shapiro-Wilk test. Spearman correlation analysis was used to estimate the correlations between various factors. Categorical variables were compared between the groups using the chi-square test. The confidence interval was set at 95%, and probability values of $P < 0.05$ were considered statically significant.

3. Results

3.1. Dry Eye Detection Rate. A total of 248 subjects (496 eyes, average age 12.26 ± 1.86 years) were recruited for the study. A total of 116 males (average age 11.9 ± 2.55 years) and 132 females (average age 12.2 ± 2.45 years) participated.

OSDI screened out 201 normal people (81.05%), 23 mild dry eye people (9.27%), 15 moderate dry eye people (6.05%),

TABLE 1: Comparison of general condition and ocular surface parameters between the dry eye group and the normal group.

Group	Dry eye	Normal	P
Age (year)	12.45 ± 1.54	11.75 ± 1.95	0.051
Sex ratio (male/female)	25/22	98/103	0.175
OSDI	27.02 ± 14.35	7.29 ± 3.36	<0.001
Tear meniscus height (mm)	0.23 ± 0.03	0.22 ± 0.03	0.214
NIBUT (s)	6.32 ± 2.49	13.14 ± 3.67	<0.001
Corneal fluorescein scores	3.51 ± 1.67	1.23 ± 2.32	<0.0001

TABLE 2: Comparison of meibomian gland functional indexes between the dry eye group and the normal group.

Group	Dry eye	Normal	P
Meibomian gland orifice scores	1.82 ± 0.53	0.51 ± 0.62	<0.0001
Meibomian gland secretion scores	1.35 ± 0.59	0.41 ± 0.35	<0.0001
Meibomian gland dropout scores	3.21 ± 1.02	0.61 ± 0.65	<0.0001

and 9 severe dry eye people (3.63%). Based on the OSDI dry eye standard, 47 (18.95%) dry eye populations were detected. The right eyes of the 47 dry eye patients were included in the dry eye group (25 males and 22 females) and the right eyes of 201 normal eye patients were included in the normal group (98 males and 103 females). Statistical comparison of the two groups was then carried out.

3.2. Comparison of General Condition and Ocular Statistical Indexes between the Dry Eye Group and the Normal Group. Table 1 shows that no significant differences in age, gender, and tear meniscus height were found between the dry eye and the normal groups. Tear meniscus height was normal for both groups (>0.20 mm), with 0.23 ± 0.03 mm in the dry eye group and 0.22 ± 0.03 mm in the normal group.

The average score of OSDI of the dry eye group was 27.02 ± 14.35, and the average score of corneal fluorescein in the dry eye group was 3.51 ± 1.67. The average score of corneal fluorescein in the normal group was 7.29 ± 3.36 and the average score of corneal fluorescein in the normal group was 1.23 ± 2.32. These two indicators were significantly higher in the dry eye group than in the normal group ($P < 0.001$). The average of NIBUT in the dry eye group was 6.32 ± 2.49 and was significantly lower than that of the normal group, which was 13.14 ± 3.67 ($P < 0.001$).

3.3. Comparison of Meibomian Gland Indexes between the Dry Eye Group and the Normal Group. In contrast with the normal group, the meibomian gland orifice scores, meibomian gland secretion scores, and meibomian gland dropout scores were significantly higher in the dry eye group ($P < 0.0001$) (Table 2).

3.4. Correlation Analyses between Scores of Complaining of Dry Eye and Ocular Surface Analysis Indicators. A highly

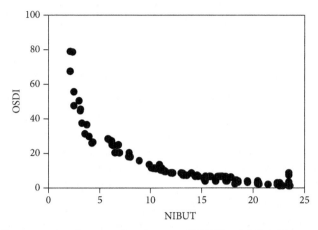

FIGURE 1: Correlation analysis between NIBUT and OSDI. Negative correlation was found between NIBUT and OSDI in the two groups.

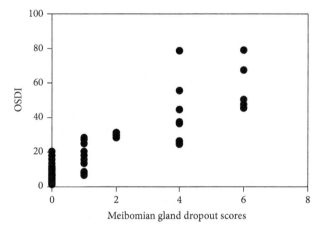

FIGURE 2: Correlation analysis between meibomian gland dropout scores and OSDI. Positive correlation was found between meibomian gland dropout scores and OSDI in the two groups.

significant inverse correlation was observed between the value of OSDI and NIBUT ($r_s = -0.982$, $P = 0.000$) (Figure 1). Moreover, a highly significant correlation was observed between the value of OSDI and meibomian gland dropout scores ($r_s = 0.838$, $P = 0.000$) (Figure 2).

4. Discussion

Recent studies showed that dry eye is a major clinical problem affecting quality of life [4] as it reduces the immunity of ocular surface, causes eye symptoms in children, leads to visual fluctuations during the day, and affects visual clarity in the daytime. Moreover, dry eye can reduce learning efficiency in children. Dry eye is widely believed to be a type of disease whose incidence increases with age [5], and thus scholars have conducted much dry eye research for the elderly. The ability of children to express eye symptoms are worse than adults, or some children may be able to express it clearly but dry eye examinations are difficult. Moreover, allergic conjunctivitis has a higher prevalence in children, and many children who have this condition also suffer from dry eye, making dry eye diagnosis more difficult [16]. Thus, the dry eye incidence in children was underestimated by many scholars. In this study, we use Keratograph 5M combined with slit-lamp examination and dry eye questionnaire to give myopic adolescents a series of dry eye-related inspections and assessments. Dry eye incidence in children was found to be 18.95% which is lower than that in adults but still not significant. Undiagnosed dry eye can lead to fragile ocular surface environment, irreversible eye damage, and increased possibility of corneal ulcers and scars [5]. Accurate diagnosis, systemic treatment, and etiological control can improve eye health and ensure good visual quality in young people.

Keratograph 5M is an objective, comprehensive, and noninvasive dry eye diagnostic device that can detect NIBUT, noninvasive tear meniscus height, and meibomian gland dropout. Keratograph 5M exhibits high accuracy in the dry eye diagnosis in adults [17]. The current study shows that Keratograph 5M has a good implementation even in children, and it can be combined with questionnaire to facilitate clinical diagnosis of dry eye in children. OSDI, NIBUT, and meibomian gland dropout are correlated to dry eye in adolescents, which means that aggravated dry eye symptoms are associated with worse unstable tear film and increased meibomian gland dropout. The lower prevalence of dry eye disease in children relative to adults, limitations of diagnosis, lower degree of the subjective assessment of symptoms in children, and the lack of clinician attention reduce dry eye awareness.

The meibomian glands are the main source of lipids for human tear film. The lipid layer of the tear film slows evaporation of the aqueous of tear film, preserves a clear optical surface, and forms a barrier to protect the eye from microbial agents and organic matter [18]. The meibomian gland plays a more important role than aqueous tear volume in determining the severity of ocular discomfort and dry eye conditions [19]. Lipid-deficient dry eye caused by meibomian gland dysfunction (MGD) has increasingly drawn ophthalmologists' attention. MGD is a chronic, diffuse abnormality of the meibomian glands, commonly characterized by terminal duct obstruction or qualitative/quantitative changes in the glandular secretions. MGD may result in alteration of the tear film, symptoms of eye irritation, clinically apparent inflammation, and ocular surface disease [20]. MGD could reduce tear film stability and cause ocular complaints, inflammation, and other ocular surface disorders [21]. The mean values of tear meniscus height in the dry eye and the normal groups were both in the normal range, whereas NIBUT in the dry eye group was shorter than that of the normal group, which suggests that the dry eye group has normal tear volume but relatively unstable tear film relative to the normal group. The dry eye group of myopic teenagers has a high corneal staining score, more abnormality of meibomian gland orifices and meibomian gland lipid secretions, and more meibomian gland dropouts, causing serious MGD. This result is similar to that of previous studies where lack of meibomian gland is also accompanied by damaged meibomian gland function [7]. This result implies that the common type of dry eye among myopic teenagers is lipid abnormalities of dry eye (i.e.,

evaporative dry eye). Currently, the clinical evaluation of dry eye is mainly based on BUT and Schirmer tests, whereas the evaluation of meibomian gland function and lipid layer is deficiency. Keratograph 5M, which has a high compatibility in children, has been found to provide early diagnostic and therapeutic values in children for the diagnosis of meibomian gland function and tear film stability. Combined with the questionnaire, the ratio of failure diagnosis of dry eye in children can be reduced.

Currently, the main correction methods of juvenile myopia are frame glasses, contact lens, and orthokeratology (ortho-k). The effectiveness of overnight orthokeratology in flattening the cornea and temporarily reducing myopia has been widely documented [22]. Parents increasingly choose night-wear ortho-k to control myopia of their children. Given that ortho-k is placed on the cornea for the whole night, the ocular surface condition of adolescents with refractive errors should be fully assessed. When considering adolescent ortho-k treatment, we should also pay attention to the situation of the ocular surface of the patients, especially meibomian gland function and dry eye prevalence, which can help improve the safety of the treatment.

The clinical and epidemiological aspects of dry eye in children have not been as well described as in adults [5]. The prevalence of dry eye disease in children varies greatly depending on which criteria and methods were used in previous research. Reportedly, 9.7% of all children have been diagnosed with dry eye disease [4]. Dry eye disease associated with longtime reading can have many signs and symptoms involved, a lot of which are still not understood. Many Chinese children with arduous learning tasks have experienced these signs and symptoms. Myopia has been associated with strenuous near task as well. Blink rates during near work are decreased leading to improper tear film placement. In this study, only normal myopic adolescents were chosen to analyze dry eye and ocular surface. The results suggest that the prevalence of dry eye in adolescents with myopia is 18.95% higher than other research documents entail. For further study regarding dry eye disease in children expanding the number of patients and the inclusion of emmetropes adolescents should be considered.

Conflict of Interests

None of the authors has conflict of interests related to the paper.

Authors' Contribution

Xiu Wang and Xiaoxiao Lu contributed to the work equally and should be regarded as co-first authors.

Acknowledgments

This work was supported by grants from Tianjin Municipal Science and Technology Commission Grants (11JCYBJC26000, 13JCYBJC23300) and Science and Technology Foundation of Beichen District of Tianjin (BC2014-10).

References

[1] "The definition and classification of dry eye disease: report of the definition and classification subcommittee of the International Dry Eye WorkShop (2007)," *The Ocular Surface*, vol. 5, no. 2, pp. 75–92, 2007.

[2] S. E. Moss, R. Klein, and B. E. K. Klein, "Long-term incidence of dry eye in an older population," *Optometry and Vision Science*, vol. 85, no. 8, pp. 668–674, 2008.

[3] A. Sahai and P. Malik, "Dry eye: prevalence and attributable risk factors in a hospital-based population," *Indian Journal of Ophthalmology*, vol. 53, no. 2, pp. 87–91, 2005.

[4] J. H. Moon, M. Y. Lee, and N. J. Moon, "Association between video display terminal use and dry eye disease in school children," *Journal of Pediatric Ophthalmology and Strabismus*, vol. 51, no. 2, pp. 87–92, 2014.

[5] M. Alves, A. C. Dias, and E. M. Rocha, "Dry eye in childhood: epidemiological and clinical aspects," *Ocular Surface*, vol. 6, no. 1, pp. 44–51, 2008.

[6] Y. Jiang, H. Ye, J. Xu, and Y. Lu, "Noninvasive Keratograph assessment of tear film break-up time and location in patients with age-related cataracts and dry eye syndrome," *Journal of International Medical Research*, vol. 42, no. 2, pp. 494–502, 2014.

[7] D. Finis, P. Ackermann, N. Pischel et al., "Evaluation of meibomian gland dysfunction and local distribution of meibomian gland atrophy by non-contact infrared meibography," *Current Eye Research*, vol. 40, no. 10, pp. 982–989, 2015.

[8] S. Koh, C. Ikeda, S. Watanabe et al., "Effect of non-invasive tear stability assessment on tear meniscus height," *Acta Ophthalmologica*, vol. 93, no. 2, pp. e135–e139, 2015.

[9] W. Ngo, S. Srinivasan, M. Schulze, and L. Jones, "Repeatability of grading meibomian gland dropout using two infrared systems," *Optometry and Vision Science*, vol. 91, no. 6, pp. 658–667, 2014.

[10] N. Best, L. Drury, and J. S. Wolffsohn, "Clinical evaluation of the Oculus Keratograph," *Contact Lens and Anterior Eye*, vol. 35, no. 4, pp. 171–174, 2012.

[11] F. Özcura, S. Aydin, and M. R. Helvaci, "Ocular surface disease index for the diagnosis of dry eye syndrome," *Ocular Immunology and Inflammation*, vol. 15, no. 5, pp. 389–393, 2007.

[12] K. L. Miller, J. G. Walt, D. R. Mink et al., "Minimal clinically important difference for the ocular surface disease index," *Archives of Ophthalmology*, vol. 128, no. 1, pp. 94–101, 2010.

[13] R. Arita, K. Itoh, S. Maeda et al., "Proposed diagnostic criteria for obstructive meibomian gland dysfunction," *Ophthalmology*, vol. 116, no. 11, pp. 2058–2063.e1, 2009.

[14] A. Tomlinson, A. J. Bron, D. R. Korb et al., "The international workshop on meibomian gland dysfunction: report of the diagnosis subcommittee," *Investigative Ophthalmology & Visual Science*, vol. 52, no. 4, pp. 2006–2049, 2011.

[15] A. A. Afonso, D. Monroy, M. E. Stern, W. J. Feuer, S. C. G. Tseng, and S. C. Pflugfelder, "Correlation of tear fluorescein clearance and Schirmer test scores with ocular irritation symptoms," *Ophthalmology*, vol. 106, no. 4, pp. 803–810, 1999.

[16] M. M. Hom, A. L. Nguyen, and L. Bielory, "Allergic conjunctivitis and dry eye syndrome," *Annals of Allergy, Asthma and Immunology*, vol. 108, no. 3, pp. 163–166, 2012.

[17] S. Srinivasan, K. Menzies, L. Sorbara, and L. Jones, "Infrared imaging of meibomian gland structure using a novel keratograph," *Optometry and Vision Science*, vol. 89, no. 5, pp. 788–794, 2012.

[18] K. B. Green-Church, I. Butovich, M. Willcox et al., "The international workshop on meibomian gland dysfunction: report of the subcommittee on tear film lipids and lipid-protein interactions in health and disease," *Investigative Ophthalmology and Visual Science*, vol. 52, no. 4, pp. 1979–1993, 2011.

[19] H. Wu, Y. Wang, N. Dong et al., "Meibomian gland dysfunction determines the severity of the dry eye conditions in visual display terminal workers," *PLoS ONE*, vol. 9, no. 8, Article ID e105575, 2014.

[20] K. K. Nichols, G. N. Foulks, A. J. Bron et al., "The international workshop on meibomian gland dysfunction: executive summary," *Investigative Ophthalmology & Visual Science*, vol. 52, no. 4, pp. 1922–1929, 2011.

[21] G. Geerling, J. Tauber, C. Baudouin et al., "The international workshop on meibomian gland dysfunction: report of the subcommittee on management and treatment of meibomian gland dysfunction," *Investigative Ophthalmology and Visual Science*, vol. 52, no. 4, pp. 2050–2064, 2011.

[22] C. Maldonado-Codina, S. Efron, P. Morgan, T. Hough, and N. Efron, "Empirical versus trial set fitting systems for accelerated orthokeratology," *Eye & Contact Lens*, vol. 31, no. 4, pp. 137–147, 2005.

Analysis of the Retinal Nerve Fiber Layer in Retinitis Pigmentosa Using Optic Coherence Tomography

Medine Aslı Yıldırım,[1] Burak Erden,[2] Mehmet Tetikoğlu,[3] Özlem Kuru,[4] and Mustafa Elçioğlu[2]

[1]Department of Ophthalmology, Bahcelievler State Hospital, 34180 Istanbul, Turkey
[2]Department of Ophthalmology, Okmeydanı Education and Research Hospital, 34384 Istanbul, Turkey
[3]Department of Ophthalmology, Dumlupinar University School of Medicine, 43270 Kutahya, Turkey
[4]Department of Ophthalmology, Mus State Hospital, 49000 Mus, Turkey

Correspondence should be addressed to Medine Aslı Yıldırım; asocan84@hotmail.com

Academic Editor: Suphi Taneri

Aim. To evaluate the peripapillary retinal nerve fiber layer (RNFL) changes in retinitis pigmentosa (RP) patients using spectral domain optic coherence tomography (Sd-OCT). *Methods.* We retrospectively examined medical records of forty-four eyes of twenty-two RP patients. The results were also compared with those of previously reported forty-four eyes of twenty-two normal subjects (controls). Records of average and four quadrants peripapillary RNFL thickness measurements using Sd-OCT were assessed. *Results.* In RP patients the mean RNFL thickness was $97.57 \pm 3.21\,\mu$m. The RNFL in the superior, temporal, nasal, and inferior quadrants was $119.18 \pm 4.47\,\mu$m, $84.68 \pm 2.31\,\mu$m, $75.09 \pm 3.34\,\mu$m, and $113.88 \pm 4.25\,\mu$m, respectively. While the thinning of RNFL was predominantly observed in the inferior quadrant, the thickening was mostly noted in temporal quadrant. The differences between mean, superior, and nasal quadrant RNFL thicknesses were not statistically significant when compared with control group. The RP patients had thinner inferior quadrant and thicker temporal quadrant than control group ($p < 0.05$). *Conclusion.* Sd-OCT is highly sensitive and effective instrument to detect RNFL changes in RP patients. RNFL measurements can provide information about the progression of retinitis pigmentosa and may provide prognostic indices for future treatment modalities.

1. Introduction

Retinitis pigmentosa (RP) is a genetically heterogeneous disease characterised by progressive retinal photoreceptor degeneration [1, 2]. The worldwide population affected has been estimated to be over one million individuals, whereas the frequency is approximately 1/4000 [3, 4].

Although RP has several mutations and genetical patterns, the symptoms and histopathological findings are similar [5]. Common symptoms are nyctalopia, impairment of visual acuity, and restriction of peripheral visual field. Characteristic findings by fundus examination include peripheral pigmented bone spicule-like lesions, retinal arteriolar attenuation, and optic disc pallor [6]. Diagnosis is often made through a combination of clinical investigation, visual field exams, and electrodiagnostic methods such as electroretinography (ERG) [5].

Various histopathological studies of RP have demonstrated a reduction of rod and cone cells and thinning of the outer photoreceptor layer. Secondary to the outer retinal thinning, the inner retinal structure degenerates through suspected transneuronal damage, vascular compromise, or axonal compression [7–9]. Previously published reports by Newman et al. demonstrated that patients of various retinal hereditary dystrophies, including RP, had ophthalmoscopically evident retinal nerve fiber defects [10].

The optic coherence tomography (OCT) is a noninvasive diagnostic tool for rapid scanning and imaging of the retinal structures with high axial resolution of almost $5\,\mu$m, especially in spectral domain models. The OCT scans give the clinician crucial information about the retinal nerve fiber layer (RNFL), retinal pigment epithelium complex, and the junction of inner and outer segments of photoreceptors (IS-OS line). The new therapeutic modalities in RP, such as gene therapy [11–14] or retinal stem cell transplantation [15, 16], are limited because they only improve the outer retinal layers. The outcome of new therapies must focus on the pretreatment status of the inner retinal layers as well as the outer layers making OCT a useful technique in the treatment prediction for such RP patients. In this study, we aimed to examine the peripapillary RNFL thickness and documented the changes in a group of RP patients.

2. Methods

Medical records of forty-four eyes of twenty-two RP patients who were followed up in Okmeydanı Training and Research Hospital, Department of Retina, and forty-four eyes of twenty-two healthy subjects (control) were enrolled into this study. The diagnosis in all cases was made by retinal specialists using the following criteria: clinical history, fundus examination, visual field defects, and reduced amplitudes in ERG.

The exclusion criteria used in our study were high refractive errors (±6 diopters sphere; ±3 diopters cylinder), low degree of central fixation, significant media opacities (e.g., posterior subcapsular cataract), diabetic retinopathy, glaucoma, or cystoid macular edema.

All cases underwent a complete ocular examination, including best-corrected visual acuity (BCVA) using Snellen chart, slit lamp biomicroscopic examination, dilated fundus examination, and intraocular pressure measurement with Goldmann applanation.

Average and four quadrants peripapillary RNFL thickness values which were scanned by spectral-domain OCT (Cirrus, Carl Zeiss Meditec, Inc., software 5.1.1.6) made by the same operator were analyzed. The scans only with signal strength > 5 were included in this study. Any RNFL layer thickness greater than 95th percentile was defined as thickening, whereas thickness lower than the 5th percentile was determined as thinning (Figure 1). Statistical analysis of the data was determined with the SPSS 19.0 software.

3. Results

The mean age of the RP patients was 37.09 ± 2.55 years (range 18–75) and the mean age of control group was 39 ± 1.70 years (range 18–54). The mean age, sex, and intraocular pressure of the two groups did not differ significantly. In the RP patients the peripapillary RNFL was evaluated and the mean thickness was observed to be $97.57 \pm 3.2\,\mu m$. RNFL thickness in the 4 quadrants (superior, temporal, nasal, and inferior) was shown to be $119.18 \pm 4.47\,\mu m$, $84.68 \pm 2.31\,\mu m$, 75.09 ± 3.34, and $113.88 \pm 4.25\,\mu m$, respectively.

In 20 of the total 44 eyes (45%), RNFL thinning was found in at least one quadrant. In two eyes (4%) thinning was determined in 3 quadrants, in 11 cases (25%) in 2 quadrants, and in 7 eyes (15%) in only one quadrant. Regarding the RNFL thinning of quadrants, the thinning was diagnosed in 12 cases (27%) in superior quadrant, in 9 eyes (20%) in the nasal quadrant, and in 14 eyes (32%) in inferior quadrant. Temporal quadrant thinning was not found in any of the patients.

In 21 (48%) patients, thickening of the RNFL was found in at least one quadrant. Five eyes (11%) showed thickening in 3 quadrants, 2 (4%) eyes in 2 quadrants, and 14 (31%) eyes in only one quadrant. Five patients (11%) had thickness in the superior quadrant, 8 patients (18%) were in the nasal, 19 eyes (43%) were in the temporal, and only 1 patient (2%) was in the inferior quadrant. In 8 patients, all 4 quadrants were found within the normal values. In 5 patients there was thinning and thickening of the RNFL layer in different quadrants.

The thinning of the RNFL was most commonly observed in the inferior and moderately in the nasal and superior quadrants. Temporal RNFL thinning was not determined in any patient, whereas the temporal region was the most commonly thickened RNFL area followed by the nasal, the superior, and finally the inferior quadrant.

In control group the average RNFL thickness was $99.95 \pm 1.38\,\mu m$. In the quadrant evaluation, the RNFL thickness in the superior, temporal, nasal, and inferior quadrants was $123.13 \pm 2.96\,\mu m$, $66.75 \pm 2.02\,\mu m$, $75.20 \pm 1.44\,\mu m$, and $130.54 \pm 1.72\,\mu m$, respectively. There was no significant difference in average, superior, and nasal thickness between two groups ($p = 0.497; 0.463; 0.975$, resp.). The RP patients had thinner inferior quadrant and thicker temporal quadrant than control group. This difference was statistically significant ($p = 0.01, p = 0.00$). Distribution of RNFL thickness between RP patients and control group is shown in Figure 2.

4. Discussion

In RP, the photoreceptor layer progressively degenerates, followed by global changes within the inner retinal structure. In particular, the RNFL develops thinning or thickening secondary to photoreceptor cell loss. Morphometric and histological studies reported ganglion cell reduction in RP compared to the normal population [10, 17, 18]. Other reports suggested that vascular compromise or direct genetic effect on the ganglion cells was the reason for inner retinal layer reduction [18, 19].

Regarding the in vivo studies, Walia et al. reported using time-domain and Fourier-domain OCT to define RNFL thinning in 40% and 38% of RP patients [20, 21]. A similar result was reported by Anastasakis et al. [22] which showed RNFL thinning in 38% of studied eyes, whereas Oishi et al. [23] found no significant difference between normal population and RP patient RNFL thickness using time-domain OCT. In our study, 45% of eyes showed RNFL thinning, similar to Walia and Anastasakis' study results. In the previously mentioned studies, the RNFL thickening was found in 40% and 42% of study cohorts, respectively. In our study we found that 48% of the studied eyes had peripapillary RNFL thickening, mostly in temporal quadrant. The exact mechanism underlying this RNFL thickening is not clear but it may result from glial tissue proliferation (which is secondary to the nerve fiber layer atrophy) or edema of the remnant RNFL

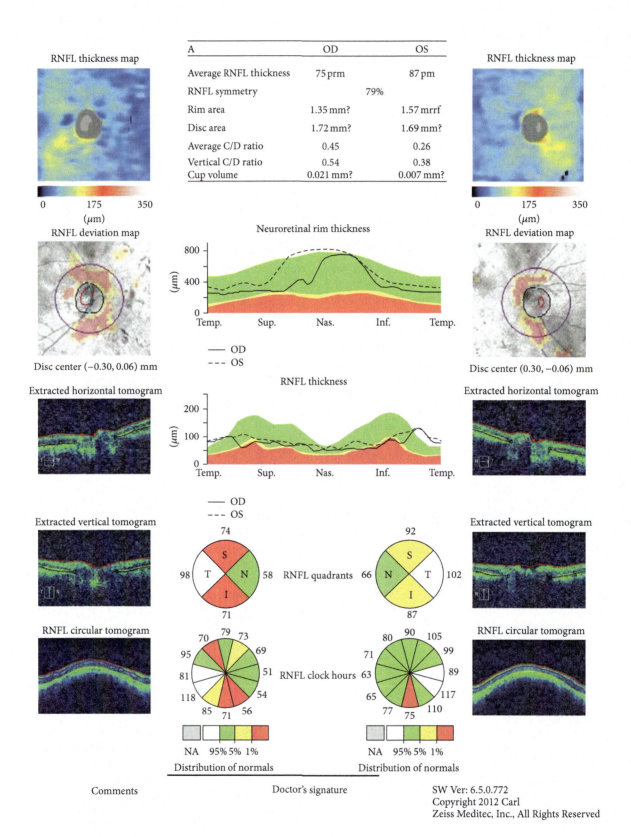

Figure 1: Retinal nerve fiber layer analysis in patients with retinitis pigmentosa.

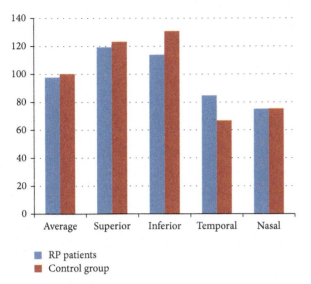

Figure 2: Distribution of RNFL thickness between RP patients and control group.

[23, 24]. In fact, Hood et al. measured RNFL thickness in RP patients from peripheral retina and macular regions with Fourier-domain OCT and manual segmentation software. They found that the RNFL was significantly thicker, especially in the horizontal meridian compared to the normal values [25]. In the same study, it was also suggested that the thickening might be a mechanical dysfunction, where the RNFL stretches to fill the empty space left by the photoreceptor degeneration. The peripapillary RNFL changes in the four quadrants vary between several studies. In histopathological examination of RP patients, Flannery et al. [26] found that the highest ratio of the photoreceptor loss was encountered in the inferonasal region, which may facilitate the RNFL thinning in this region. Walia et al. reported in their studies [20, 21] that the nasal quadrant was the most thinned, followed by inferior and superior quadrants. Anastasakis et al. [22]. observed the quadrants' thinning sequence as inferior (most common) followed by the nasal and superior regions. In both Xue's et al. [27] and Hood's et al. [25] studies, the only thinning quadrant was the nasal area. Xue et al. [27] found that all quadrants in their RP patient study were significantly thicker than the normal population, except the nasal quadrant, which was surprisingly thinner than the normal control group values. In our studies, the mostly thinned quadrant was the inferior followed by the superior and the nasal quadrants. Regarding the thickening of the RNFL, in several studies [20–22, 24, 27], the most commonly thickened quadrant was the temporal. Interestingly, no reports have observed thinning in temporal peripapillary area. Similar to these reports, we found that the temporal quadrant was the most commonly thickened region with no observed RNFL thinning. This might be due to the retinal glial proliferation, which is most strongly seen between the temporal arcades [28].

Considering future therapeutic approaches, understanding the mechanism and progression of retinal degeneration in RP will be crucial to predicting proper patient treatment. High resolution Sd-OCT scans will be extremely helpful for the clinician in both aspects. Further studies might enhance our clinical evaluation of such patients.

Conflict of Interests

The authors declare that there is no conflict of interests.

References

[1] M.-N. Delyfer, T. Léveillard, S. Mohand-Saïd, D. Hicks, S. Picaud, and J.-A. Sahel, "Inherited retinal degenerations: therapeutic prospects," *Biology of the Cell*, vol. 96, no. 4, pp. 261–269, 2004.

[2] Y. Wen, M. Klein, D. C. Hood, and D. G. Birch, "Relationships among multifocal electroretinogram amplitude, visual field sensitivity, and SD-OCT receptor layer thicknesses in patients with retinitis pigmentosa," *Investigative Ophthalmology & Visual Science*, vol. 53, no. 2, pp. 833–840, 2012.

[3] D. T. Hartong, E. L. Berson, and T. P. Dryja, "Retinitis pigmentosa," *The Lancet*, vol. 368, no. 9549, pp. 1795–1809, 2006.

[4] R. Vámos, E. Tátrai, J. Németh, G. E. Holder, D. C. DeBuc, and G. M. Somfai, "The structure and function of the macula in patients with advanced retinitis pigmentosa," *Investigative Ophthalmology and Visual Science*, vol. 52, no. 11, pp. 8425–8432, 2011.

[5] Y. Mitamura, S. Mitamura-Aizawa, T. Nagasawa, T. Katome, H. Eguchi, and T. Naito, "Diagnostic imaging in patients with retinitis pigmentosa," *Journal of Medical Investigation*, vol. 59, no. 1-2, pp. 1–11, 2012.

[6] S. Chang, L. Vaccarella, S. Olatunji, C. Cebulla, and J. Christoforidis, "Diagnostic challenges in retinitis pigmentosa: genotypic multiplicity and phenotypic variability," *Current Genomics*, vol. 12, no. 4, pp. 267–275, 2011.

[7] R. B. Szamier, E. L. Berson, R. Klein, and S. Meyers, "Sex-linked retinitis pigmentosa: ultrastructure of photoreceptors and pigment epithelium," *Investigative Ophthalmology and Visual Science*, vol. 18, no. 2, pp. 145–160, 1979.

[8] A. H. Milam, Z.-Y. Li, and R. N. Fariss, "Histopathology of the human retina in retinitis pigmentosa," *Progress in Retinal and Eye Research*, vol. 17, no. 2, pp. 175–205, 1998.

[9] R. N. Fariss, Z.-Y. Li, and A. H. Milam, "Abnormalities in rod photoreceptors, amacrine cells, and horizontal cells in human retinas with retinitis pigmentosa," *The American Journal of Ophthalmology*, vol. 129, no. 2, pp. 215–223, 2000.

[10] N. M. Newman, R. A. Stevens, and J. R. Heckenlively, "Nerve fibre layer loss in diseases of the outer retinal layer," *British Journal of Ophthalmology*, vol. 71, no. 1, pp. 21–26, 1987.

[11] J. Bennett, T. Tanabe, D. Sun et al., "Photoreceptor cell rescue in retinal degeneration (rd) mice by in vivo gene therapy," *Nature Medicine*, vol. 2, no. 6, pp. 649–654, 1996.

[12] C. Jomary, J. Grist, J. Milbrandt, M. J. Neal, and S. E. Jones, "Epitope-tagged recombinant AAV vectors for expressing neurturin and its receptor in retinal cells," *Molecular Vision*, vol. 7, pp. 36–41, 2001.

[13] R. Kumar-Singh and D. B. Farber, "Encapsidated adenovirus mini-chromosome-mediated delivery of genes to the retina: application to the rescue of photoreceptor degeneration," *Human Molecular Genetics*, vol. 7, no. 12, pp. 1893–1900, 1998.

[14] G. M. Acland, G. D. Aguirre, J. Ray et al., "Gene therapy restores vision in a canine model of childhood blindness," *Nature Genetics*, vol. 28, no. 1, pp. 92–95, 2001.

[15] D. M. Chacko, J. A. Rogers, J. E. Turner, and I. Ahmad, "Survival and differentiation of cultured retinal progenitors transplanted in the subretinal space of the rat," *Biochemical and Biophysical Research Communications*, vol. 268, no. 3, pp. 842–846, 2000.

[16] M. Tomita, T. Mori, K. Maruyama et al., "A comparison of neural differentiation and retinal transplantation with bone marrow-derived cells and retinal progenitor cells," *Stem Cells*, vol. 24, no. 10, pp. 2270–2278, 2006.

[17] J. L. Stone, W. E. Barlow, M. S. Humayun, E. de Juan Jr., and A. H. Milam, "Morphometric analysis of macular photoreceptors and ganglion cells in retinas with retinitis pigmentosa," *Archives of Ophthalmology*, vol. 110, no. 11, pp. 1634–1639, 1992.

[18] Z.-Y. Li, D. E. Possin, and A. H. Milam, "Histopathology of bone spicule pigmentation in retinitis pigmentosa," *Ophthalmology*, vol. 102, no. 5, pp. 805–816, 1995.

[19] M. S. Humayun, M. Prince, E. de Juan Jr. et al., "Morphometric analysis of the extramacular retina from postmortem eyes with retinitis pigmentosa," *Investigative Ophthalmology and Visual Science*, vol. 40, no. 1, pp. 143–148, 1999.

[20] S. Walia, G. A. Fishman, D. P. Edward, and M. Lindeman, "Retinal nerve fiber layer defects in RP patients," *Investigative Ophthalmology and Visual Science*, vol. 48, no. 10, pp. 4748–4752, 2007.

[21] S. Walia and G. A. Fishman, "Retinal nerve fiber layer analysis in RP patients using fourier-domain OCT," *Investigative Ophthalmology and Visual Science*, vol. 49, no. 8, pp. 3525–3528, 2008.

[22] A. Anastasakis, M. A. Genead, J. J. McAnany, and G. A. Fishman, "Evaluation of retinal nerve fiber layer thickness in patients with retinitis pigmentosa using spectral-domain optical coherence tomography," *Retina*, vol. 32, no. 2, pp. 358–363, 2012.

[23] A. Oishi, A. Otani, M. Sasahara et al., "Retinal nerve fiber layer thickness in patients with retinitis pigmentosa," *Eye*, vol. 23, no. 3, pp. 561–566, 2009.

[24] Q. Huang, V. Chowdhury, and M. T. Coroneo, "Evaluation of patient suitability for a retinal prosthesis using structural and functional tests of inner retinal integrity," *Journal of Neural Engineering*, vol. 6, no. 3, Article ID 035010, 2009.

[25] D. C. Hood, C. E. Lin, M. A. Lazow, K. G. Locke, X. Zhang, and D. G. Birch, "Thickness of receptor and post-receptor retinal layers in patients with retinitis pigmentosa measured with frequency-domain optical coherence tomography," *Investigative Ophthalmology and Visual Science*, vol. 50, no. 5, pp. 2328–2336, 2009.

[26] J. G. Flannery, D. B. Farber, A. C. Bird, and D. Bok, "Degenerative changes in a retina affected with autosomal dominant retinitis pigmentosa," *Investigative Ophthalmology and Visual Science*, vol. 30, no. 2, pp. 191–211, 1989.

[27] K. Xue, M. Wang, J. Chen, X. Huang, and G. Xu, "Retinal nerve fiber layer analysis with scanning laser polarimetry and RTVue-OCT in patients of retinitis pigmentosa," *Ophthalmologica*, vol. 229, no. 1, pp. 38–42, 2013.

[28] S. Gartner and P. Henkind, "Pathology of retinitis pigmentosa," *Ophthalmology*, vol. 89, no. 12, pp. 1425–1432, 1982.

Size of the Optic Nerve Head and Its Relationship with the Thickness of the Macular Ganglion Cell Complex and Peripapillary Retinal Nerve Fiber Layer in Patients with Primary Open Angle Glaucoma

Nobuko Enomoto, Ayako Anraku, Kyoko Ishida, Asuka Takeyama, Fumihiko Yagi, and Goji Tomita

Department of Ophthalmology, Toho University, Ohashi Medical Center, 2-17-5 Ohashi, Meguro-ku 153-8515, Japan

Correspondence should be addressed to Nobuko Enomoto; nobuko.enomoto@med.toho-u.ac.jp

Academic Editor: Gianmarco Vizzeri

Purpose. To evaluate the relationships among the optic nerve head (ONH) area, macular ganglion cell complex (mGCC) thickness, circumpapillary retinal nerve fiber layer (cpRNFL) thickness, and visual field defects in patients with primary open angle glaucoma (POAG). *Methods.* This retrospective study included 90 eyes of 90 patients with POAG. The ONH area, rim area, mGCC thickness, and cpRNFL thickness were measured using optical coherence tomography. Mean deviation (MD) was measured using standard automated perimetry. The relationships among clinical factors including age, refraction, the ONH area, the rim area, the mGCC thickness, the cpRNFL thickness, and MD were evaluated using correlation coefficients and multiple regression analyses. *Results.* The significant correlation of the ONH area with refraction ($r = 0.362$, $P < 0.001$), the mGCC thickness ($r = 0.225$, $P = 0.033$), and the cpRNFL thickness ($r = 0.253$, $P = 0.016$) was found. Multiple regression analysis showed that the ONH area, rim area, and MD were selected as significant contributing factors to explain the mGCC thickness and cpRNFL thickness. No factor was selected to explain MD. *Conclusions.* The ONH area, in other words, the disc size itself may affect the mGCC thickness and cpRNFL thickness in POAG patients.

1. Introduction

Glaucomatous optic neuropathy is characterized by the progressive loss of retinal ganglion cells and their respective axons, which comprise the retinal nerve fiber layer (RNFL) [1]. With regard to the evaluation of glaucoma, optical coherence tomography (OCT) provides reproducible quantitative measurements of RNFL around the optic nerve head (ONH) [2] and in the macular region [3–7]. RNFL assessment is important because RNFL often precedes functional changes detected by perimetry [8–17].

Conversely, the ONH size is not constant among individuals, with an interindividual variability of approximately 1 : 7 in a normal Caucasian population [18]. The African-American population has a relatively high incidence of glaucoma [19]. The ONH size is reportedly a possible risk factor for glaucomatous optic nerve damage [20–24]. However, several groups have reported no difference in susceptibility between patients with a large disc and those with a small disc [25–30]. Therefore, the relationship between ONH size and glaucomatous optic nerve damage remains controversial. Furthermore, the influence of the ONH size on circumpapillary RNFL (cpRNFL) thickness is not fully understood. Several studies have found that the cpRNFL thickness measured at a fixed diameter is positively correlated with the optic disc area [31, 32]. The implication was that the number of nerve fibers in cpRNFL depends on the disc area and that it might be possible to decrease the variations in the measured cpRNFL thickness if the scan diameter was adjusted according to the disc diameter, although this possibility was not supported by Huang et al. [33] in normal healthy subjects. To the best of our knowledge, there are no published clinical reports evaluating the relationship between the ONH size and the macular ganglion cell complex (mGCC) thickness in eyes with primary open angle glaucoma (POAG). The aim of the present study was to evaluate the relationships among the ONH area, mGCC thickness, and cpRNFL thickness measured using spectral-domain OCT (SD-OCT) and visual field defects in patients with POAG.

2. Materials and Methods

2.1. Study Participants. This retrospective study was performed in adherence with the guidelines of the Declaration of Helsinki and was approved by the Institutional Review Board (number 13-29) of Toho University, Ohashi Medical Center, Tokyo, Japan. Because of the retrospective nature of this study, the requirement for written informed consent was waived.

We retrospectively reviewed the medical records of 90 eyes of 90 patients with POAG, including normal tension glaucoma (NTG). The patients underwent SD-OCT for measurement of the ONH area, rim area, mGCC thickness, and cpRNFL thickness and standard automated perimetry (SAP) within a 3-month period at our outpatient clinic between May 2008 and September 2012. SAP was performed using the Humphrey Field Analyzer (Humphrey-Zeiss Systems, Dublin, CA, USA) with the 30-2 Swedish Interactive Threshold Algorithm (SITA). The visual field tests were considered reliable when the fixation losses were <20% and the false-positive and false-negative rates were <25%. The mean deviation (MD) was used to assess the severity of visual field loss.

All subjects underwent complete ophthalmological examination and assessment of medical and family histories. The ophthalmological procedures included visual acuity testing with refraction, slit-lamp biomicroscopy, gonioscopy, Goldmann applanation tonometry for the measurement of intraocular pressure (IOP), and dilated stereoscopic fundus examination. The diagnostic criteria for POAG used in this study included the following: normal open anterior chamber angles on slit-lamp biomicroscopy and gonioscopy, presence of a glaucomatous ONH on stereoscopy with corresponding visual field defects, a best-corrected visual acuity of at least 20/25, refractive errors in the spherical equivalent (SE) not exceeding −6 or +3 diopters, and a cylindrical correction of less than 3 diopters. A visual field defect was defined as the presence of three or more significant ($P < 0.05$), contiguous nonedge points with at least one point at $P < 0.01$ level in the pattern deviation plot, along with grading outside the normal limits on the Glaucoma Hemifield test (GHT). Exclusion criteria included the following: a history of intraocular surgery, the presence of intraocular diseases such as diabetic retinopathy or age-related macular degeneration that affect image quality or visual field test results, and a history of systemic diseases such as intracranial disease and/or a history of steroid use, both of which affect IOP and visual field test results. When both eyes were eligible for the study, one eye was randomly selected.

2.2. SD-OCT. SD-OCT was performed using the RTVue-100 system (software version 4.0, Optovue Inc., Fremont, CA, USA) to measure the cpRNFL thickness and mGCC thickness. SD-OCT uses a scanning laser diode that emits a beam with a wavelength of 840 ± 10 nm and provides images of ocular microstructures. For all participants, measurements were obtained from both regions on the same day.

In this study, the GCC scanning protocol was used for measuring the mGCC thickness. This protocol includes one horizontal scan and 15 vertical scans that cover 7 mm^2 region. To achieve the best possible coverage within the temporal region, the GCC protocol centered the scan 1 mm temporal to the center of the fovea. During the total scanning period, 15,000 data points were captured within 0.6 s. The GCC scan creates a 6 mm map, which corresponds to approximately 20° on the visual field map.

The ONH protocol used in this study was designed to measure the cpRNFL thickness and ONH parameters. The total time required to acquire a single scan was 0.55 s. Using the SD-OCT-generated fundus image (video baseline protocol), we were able to manually trace the ONH contour. Using the ONH scanning protocol software, the RNFL thickness was automatically measured at a 3.45 mm diameter around the center of the optic disc. A total of 775 A-scans were obtained under this condition. The ONH scan ring did not pass over peripapillary atrophy. The cpRNFL thickness parameter was designed to evaluate the mean thickness in 360° area. In addition, the ONH protocol includes 12 radial scans measuring 3.4 mm in length (452 A-scans each) and six concentric ring scans measuring 2.5–4.0 mm (587–775 A-scans each), all of which are centered around the optic disc contour line automated by the three-dimensional topographic image protocol. The areas between the A-scans were interpolated and various parameters generated to describe the optic disc. The ONH area and rim area were obtained as disc parameters. Measurements were obtained by a well-trained operator. Data with signal strength index (SSI) values of <30 were excluded.

2.3. Statistical Analysis. In this study, the following factors were included for analysis: age, refraction, the ONH area, the rim area, the mGCC thickness, the cpRNFL thickness, and MD. Spearman's rank correlation coefficient was used to evaluate the relationship of the ONH area with other factors. Multiple regression analysis was used to evaluate the relationship of the mGCC thickness or cpRNFL thickness with age, refraction, the rim area, MD, and the ONH area, as well as the relationship of MD with the mGCC thickness, the cpRNFL thickness, age, refraction, the rim area, and the ONH area. All statistical analyses were performed using SPSS statistical software (version 20.0, SPSS Inc., Chicago, IL, USA). Data are expressed as means ± standard deviations (SDs), and a P value of < 0.05 was considered statistically significant.

3. Results

In the present study, we assessed 90 patients with POAG, including 66 patients (73.3%) with NTG. Table 1 shows the background characteristics of all patients. Most of the

TABLE 1: Demographics of the study participants ($n = 90$).

Variable	Total ($n = 90$)
Sex (male/female)	39/51
Age (years)	60.75 ± 11.45 (28–82)
Type (POAG/NTG) (eyes)	24/66
Refractive error (D)	−2.71 ± 2.41 (−5.9–2.3)
ONH area (mm^2)	2.27 ± 0.47 (1.23–3.73)
Rim area (mm^2)	0.66 ± 0.31 (0.09–1.79)
mGCC thickness (μm)	77.75 ± 8.34 (58.5–98.7)
cpRNFL thickness (μm)	81.79 ± 8.95 (61.15–99.98)
MD (dB)	−3.71 ± 3.03 (−11.31–1.45)

Mean ± standard deviation (range).
POAG: primary open angle glaucoma, NTG: normal tension glaucoma, D: diopter, ONH: optic nerve head, mGCC: macular ganglion cell complex, cpRNFL: circumpapillary retinal nerve fiber layer, and MD: mean deviation.

TABLE 2: Correlations of the ONH area with other factors.

	r	P value
Age	0.173	0.102
Ref.	0.362	**<0.001**
Rim area	−0.089	0.406
mGCC thickness	0.225	**0.033**
cpRNFL thickness	0.253	**0.016**
MD	0.139	0.192

r: Spearman's rank correlation coefficient.
ONH: optic nerve head, Ref.: refractive errors in the spherical equivalent, mGCC: macular ganglion cell complex, cpRNFL: circumpapillary retinal nerve fiber layer, and MD: mean deviation.

TABLE 3: Multiple regression analysis for the relationship between the mGCC thickness and other factors.

	Slope	SE	β	95% CI	P value
Age	−0.113	0.072	−0.155	−0.256, 0.030	0.120
Ref.	0.314	0.361	0.091	−0.403, 1.031	0.386
ONH area	4.283	1.698	0.241	0.907, 7.659	**0.014**
Rim area	10.329	2.525	0.386	5.309, 15.350	**<0.001**
MD	0.569	0.261	0.207	0.051, 1.087	**0.032**

mGCC: macular ganglion cell complex, SE: standard error, β: standardized partial regression coefficient, CI: confidence interval, Ref.: refractive errors in the spherical equivalent, ONH: optic nerve head, and MD: mean deviation.

TABLE 4: Multiple regression analysis for the relationship between the cpRNFL thickness and other factors.

	Slope	SE	β	95% CI	P value
Age	−0.127	0.075	−0.162	−0.276, 0.023	0.096
Ref.	0.688	0.377	0.185	−0.061, 1.438	0.071
ONH area	4.394	1.774	0.231	0.865, 7.922	**0.015**
Rim area	11.079	2.639	0.386	5.832, 16.327	**<0.001**
MD	0.658	0.272	0.223	0.117, 1.200	**0.019**

cpRNFL: circumpapillary retinal nerve fiber layer, SE: standard error, β: standardized partial regression coefficient, CI: confidence interval, Ref.: refractive errors in the spherical equivalent, ONH: optic nerve head, and MD: mean deviation.

TABLE 5: Multiple regression analysis for the relationship between MD and other factors.

	Slope	SE	β	95% CI	P value
Age	0.001	0.003	0.003	−0.058, 0.060	0.980
Ref.	<0.001	0.148	<0.001	−0.294, 0.295	0.997
ONH area	0.065	0.720	0.010	−1.368, 1.498	0.929
Rim area	1.415	1.150	0.145	−0.872, 3.703	0.222
mGCC thickness	0.063	0.047	0.174	−0.029, 0.156	0.178
cpRNFL thickness	0.075	0.044	0.221	−0.013, 0.163	0.094

MD: mean deviation, SE: standard error, β: standardized partial regression coefficient, CI: confidence interval, Ref.: refractive errors in the spherical equivalent, ONH: optic nerve head, mGCC: macular ganglion cell complex, and cpRNFL: circumpapillary retinal nerve fiber layer.

patients had an early stage of glaucoma. The averages of MD were −3.71 ± 3.03 dB.

Table 2 shows Spearman's rank correlation coefficients between the ONH area and age, refraction, the rim area, the mGCC thickness, the cpRNFL thickness, and MD. Three factors were significantly correlated with the ONH area: refraction ($r = 0.362$, $P < 0.001$), the mGCC thickness ($r = 0.225$, $P = 0.033$), and the cpRNFL thickness ($r = 0.253$, $P = 0.016$).

Tables 3 and 4 show the results of multiple regression analysis, wherein the mGCC thickness or cpRNFL thickness was used as the dependent variable and age, refraction, the ONH area, the rim area, and MD were used as explanatory variables. Consequently, the ONH area (slope = 4.283 μm/mm^2, a standard partial regression coefficient (β) = 0.241, 95% confidence interval (CI) = 0.907 to 7.659, and $P = 0.014$), the rim area (slope = 10.329 μm/mm^2, β = 0.386, 95% CI = 5.309 to 15.350, and $P < 0.001$), and MD (slope = 0.569 μm/dB, β = 0.207, 95% CI = 0.051 to 1.087, and $P = 0.032$) were selected as significant contributing factors to explain the mGCC thickness. Similarly, the ONH area (slope = 4.394 μm/mm^2, β = 0.231, 95% CI = 0.865 to 7.922, and $P = 0.015$), the rim area (slope = 11.079 μm/mm^2, β = 0.386, 95% CI = 5.832 to 16.327, and $P < 0.001$), and MD (slope = 0.658 μm/dB, β = 0.223, 95% CI = 0.117 to 1.200, and $P = 0.019$) were selected as significant contributing factors to explain the cpRNFL thickness.

Table 5 shows the results of multiple regression analysis, wherein MD was used as the dependent variable and age, refraction, the ONH area, the rim area, the mGCC thickness, and the cpRNFL thickness were used as explanatory variables. Consequently, no factor was selected to explain MD.

4. Discussion

In the present study, the ONH area was significantly correlated with refraction, the mGCC thickness, and the cpRNFL thickness. With regard to significant correlation between the ONH area and refraction, we acknowledge that this finding was a consequence of the lack of correction for refraction magnification, which is characteristic of the RTVue-100 system. A previous study reported that refraction was correlated with the cpRNFL thickness and mGCC thickness [34] and that RNFL thickness and ONH parameters including disc size measured by SD-OCT are subject to influence from the axial length in normal eyes [35].

The present study, which does not measure the axial length, included 90 patients, with 49 eyes exhibiting refractive errors of less than −3 diopters. Therefore, it is expected that eyes with an axial length longer than the standard were predominant. Accordingly, the fact that a significantly positive correlation was observed between the disc size and refraction indicates the possibility of influence from the axial length, as shown in previous studies [34, 35]. In the future, it is necessary to consider influence of refraction and axial length when we will evaluate the parameters measured using SD-OCT.

With regard to the relationship between the ONH area and the mGCC thickness or cpRNFL thickness, several studies evaluated the mGCC thickness and cpRNFL thickness and reported that the ONH area affects the ability to detect glaucoma [36, 37]. Significant correlations between the rim area and the mGCC thickness and between MD and the mGCC thickness have been also reported [38, 39]. However, no study has ever mentioned a correlation between the ONH area and mGCC thickness. According to Table 3, we found a significant correlation between the mGCC thickness and the ONH area, the rim area, and MD using multiple regression analysis. Although the underlying reason remains unclear, our study suggests that the smaller ONH area, the thinner mGCC thickness.

Similarly, as shown in Table 4, we found a significant correlation between the cpRNFL thickness and the ONH area, the rim area, and MD using multiple regression analysis. Several studies have reported the correlation between the ONH area and the cpRNFL thickness [31, 32, 35]. Savini et al. [31] found a positive correlation between the optic disc size and the 360° RNFL thickness, both of which were measured using OCT. Histological studies also reported a positive correlation between the disc size and number of nerve fibers [40, 41]. However, Huang et al. [33] reported no significant association between the RNFL thickness and the optic disc area. The authors stated that previous publications showing such an association may have been biased by the effects of the axial length on fundus image magnification. Several other investigators found that the cpRNFL thickness was correlated with the axial length and refractive error [35, 42–44]. In the present study, even though patients with high myopia were excluded, a significant correlation was still observed between the ONH area and cpRNFL thickness using multiple regression analysis. Considering the findings of former studies and our results, the ONH area may be related to the cpRNFL thickness.

On the other hand, multiple regression analyses using the mGCC thickness and cpRNFL thickness as objective variables showed corresponding coefficients of determination (R^2) values of 0.297 (Table 3) and 0.333 (Table 4), respectively. This indicates that the strength of the association was not necessarily high. However, the fact that the disc area was shown as a significant variable in multiple regression analyses including all available factors proves that the disc area itself may affect the mGCC thickness and cpRNFL thickness.

This study also examined the effects of the ONH area, rim area, mGCC thickness, and cpRNFL thickness on visual field defects; no factor was identified as a significant contributing factor to explain MD (Table 5). This result supported those of a meta-analysis [45] that concluded that the ONH area was not an independent risk factor for glaucoma. Previous studies reported significant correlation between the mGCC thickness, cpRNFL thickness, and MD [39, 46]. In most former studies, the enrolled subjects suffered from glaucoma with a mean MD value of less than −7.0 dB from SAP. In contrast, our subjects' mean MD value was −3.7 dB. This means that the subjects in our current study had glaucoma with relatively earlier stages than those in former studies, and these factors may not be well correlated with the visual field defects. Moreover, it was reported that GCC thickness was most useful parameter to evaluate structure and function within the central 10° of macula in glaucoma [47]. Therefore we should further investigate by adding the SITA 10-2 program to visual field tests in future studies.

The strength of the present study was that it revealed, for the first time to our knowledge, the relationship between the disc size and the mGCC thickness. The study also has several limitations. First, because of the retrospective study design, there may be a possible bias in the selection of subjects. Second, we did not have data for the normal subjects for comparison. Third, the magnification was not adjusted for the axial length or refraction. Fourth, it remains unclear whether our findings will be beneficial for glaucoma practice in the future.

In conclusion, the results of the present study suggest that the ONH area is significantly positive correlated with the mGCC thickness and cpRNFL thickness. Furthermore, the ONH area is selected as significant contributing factor to explain the mGCC thickness and cpRNFL thicknesses. Therefore, the disc size itself may affect the mGCC thickness and cpRNFL thickness in eyes with POAG. Further studies are required to provide further evidence supporting our findings and confirm the magnitude of the influence of the disc area on the mGCC thickness and cpRNFL thickness.

Conflict of Interests

The authors report no conflict of interests.

Acknowledgment

The authors thank Yuji Nishiwaki, M.D., Ph.D., for assistance with statistical analyses.

References

[1] R. D. Fechtner and R. N. Weinreb, "Mechanisms of optic nerve damage in primary open angle glaucoma," *Survey of Ophthalmology*, vol. 39, no. 1, pp. 23–42, 1994.

[2] J. E. DeLeón-Ortega, S. N. Arthur, G. McGwin Jr., A. Xie, B. E. Monheit, and C. A. Girkin, "Discrimination between glaucomatous and nonglaucomatous eyes using quantitative imaging devices and subjective optic nerve head assessment," *Investigative Ophthalmology and Visual Science*, vol. 47, no. 8, pp. 3374–3380, 2006.

[3] J. S. Schuman, M. R. Hee, C. A. Puliafito et al., "Quantification of nerve fiber layer thickness in normal and glaucomatous eyes using optical coherence tomography: a pilot study," *Archives of Ophthalmology*, vol. 113, no. 5, pp. 586–596, 1995.

[4] J. S. Schuman, T. Pedut-Kloizman, E. Hertzmark et al., "Reproducibility of nerve fiber layer thickness measurements using optical coherence tomography," *Ophthalmology*, vol. 103, no. 11, pp. 1889–1898, 1996.

[5] E. Z. Blumenthal, J. M. Williams, R. N. Weinreb, C. A. Girkin, C. C. Berry, and L. M. Zangwill, "Reproducibility of nerve fiber layer thickness measurements by use of optical coherence tomography," *Ophthalmology*, vol. 107, no. 12, pp. 2278–2282, 2000.

[6] L. A. Paunescu, J. S. Schuman, L. L. Price et al., "Reproducibility of nerve fiber thickness, macular thickness, and optic nerve head measurements using StratusOCT," *Investigative Ophthalmology and Visual Science*, vol. 45, no. 6, pp. 1716–1724, 2004.

[7] P. Carpineto, M. Ciancaglini, E. Zuppardi, G. Falconio, E. Doronzo, and L. Mastropasqua, "Reliability of nerve fiber layer thickness measurements using optical coherence tomography in normal and glaucomatous eyes," *Ophthalmology*, vol. 110, no. 1, pp. 190–195, 2003.

[8] A. Sommer, I. Pollack, and A. E. Maumenee, "Optic disc parameters and onset of glaucomatous field loss, I. Methods and progressive changes in disc morphology," *Archives of Ophthalmology*, vol. 97, no. 8, pp. 1444–1448, 1979.

[9] J. E. Pederson and D. R. Anderson, "The mode of progressive disc cupping in ocular hypertension and glaucoma," *Archives of Ophthalmology*, vol. 98, no. 3, pp. 490–495, 1980.

[10] A. Sommer, H. A. Quigley, A. L. Robin, N. R. Miller, J. Katz, and S. Arkell, "Evaluation of nerve fiber layer assessment," *Archives of Ophthalmology*, vol. 102, no. 12, pp. 1766–1771, 1984.

[11] A. Sommer, J. Katz, H. A. Quigley et al., "Clinically detectable nerve fiber atrophy precedes the onset of glaucomatous field loss," *Archives of Ophthalmology*, vol. 109, no. 1, pp. 77–83, 1991.

[12] H. A. Quigley, J. Katz, R. J. Derick, D. Gilbert, and A. Sommer, "An evaluation of optic disc and nerve fiber layer examinations in monitoring progression of early glaucoma damage," *Ophthalmology*, vol. 99, no. 1, pp. 19–28, 1992.

[13] T. G. Zeyen and J. Caprioli, "Progression of disc and field damage in early glaucoma," *Archives of Ophthalmology*, vol. 111, no. 1, pp. 62–65, 1993.

[14] H. A. Quigley, C. Enger, J. Katz, A. Sommer, R. Scott, and D. Gilbert, "Risk factors for the development of glaucomatous visual field loss in ocular hypertension," *Archives of Ophthalmology*, vol. 112, no. 5, pp. 644–649, 1994.

[15] A. Sommer, N. R. Miller, I. Pollack, A. E. Maumenee, and T. George, "The nerve fiber layer in the diagnosis of glaucoma," *Archives of Ophthalmology*, vol. 95, no. 12, pp. 2149–2156, 1977.

[16] B. C. Chauhan, T. A. McCormick, M. T. Nicolela, and R. P. LeBlanc, "Optic disc and visual field changes in a prospective longitudinal study of patients with glaucoma: Comparison of scanning laser tomography with conventional perimetry and optic disc photography," *Archives of Ophthalmology*, vol. 119, no. 10, pp. 1492–1499, 2001.

[17] M. A. Kass, D. K. Heuer, E. J. Higginbotham et al., "The Ocular Hypertension Treatment Study: a randomized trial determines that topical ocular hypotensive medication delays or prevents the onset of primary open-angle glaucoma," *Archives of Ophthalmology*, vol. 120, no. 6, pp. 701–713, 829–830, 2002.

[18] J. B. Jonas, W. M. Budde, and S. Panda-Jonas, "Ophthalmoscopic evaluation of the optic nerve head," *Survey of Ophthalmology*, vol. 43, no. 4, pp. 293–320, 1999.

[19] M. J. Martin, A. Sommer, E. B. Gold, and E. L. Diamond, "Race and Primary open-angle glaucoma," *American Journal of Ophthalmology*, vol. 99, no. 4, pp. 383–387, 1985.

[20] R. O. W. Burk, K. Rohrschneidern, H. Noack, and H. E. Völcker, "Are large optic nerve heads susceptible to glaucomatous damage at normal intraocular pressure? A three-dimensional study by laser scanning tomography," *Graefe's Archive for Clinical and Experimental Ophthalmology*, vol. 230, no. 6, pp. 552–560, 1992.

[21] G. Tomita, K. Nyman, C. Raitta, and M. Kawamura, "Interocular asymmetry of optic disc size and its relevance to visual field loss in normal-tension glaucoma," *Graefe's Archive for Clinical and Experimental Ophthalmology*, vol. 232, no. 5, pp. 290–296, 1994.

[22] A. Tuulonen and P. J. Airaksinen, "Optic disc size in exfoliative, primary open angle, and low-tension glaucoma," *Archives of Ophthalmology*, vol. 110, no. 2, pp. 211–213, 1992.

[23] P. R. Healey and P. Mitchell, "Optic disk size in open-angle glaucoma: the Blue Mountains Eye Study," *The American Journal of Ophthalmology*, vol. 128, no. 4, pp. 515–517, 1999.

[24] L. Wang, K. F. Damji, R. Munger et al., "Increased disk size in glaucomatous eyes versus normal eyes in the Reykjavik eye study," *American Journal of Ophthalmology*, vol. 135, no. 2, pp. 226–228, 2003.

[25] J. B. Jonas, M. C. Fernandez, and G. O. H. Naumann, "Correlation of the optic disc size to glaucoma susceptibility," *Ophthalmology*, vol. 98, no. 5, pp. 675–680, 1991.

[26] J. B. Jonas, J. Stürmer, K. I. Papastathopoulos, F. Meier-Gibbons, and A. Dichtl, "Optic disc size and optic nerve damage in normal pressure glaucoma," *British Journal of Ophthalmology*, vol. 79, no. 12, pp. 1102–1105, 1995.

[27] L. M. Zangwill, R. N. Weinreb, J. A. Beiser et al., "Baseline topographic optic disc measurements are associated with the development of primary open-angle glaucoma: the Confocal Scanning Laser Ophthalmoscopy Ancillary Study to the Ocular Hypertension Treatment Study," *Archives of Ophthalmology*, vol. 123, no. 9, pp. 1188–1197, 2005.

[28] H. A. Quigley, R. Varma, J. M. Tielsch, J. Katz, A. Sommer, and D. L. Gilbert, "The relationship between optic disc area and open-angle glaucoma: the Baltimore Eye Survey," *Journal of Glaucoma*, vol. 8, no. 6, pp. 347–352, 1999.

[29] J. B. Jonas, L. Xu, L. Zhang, Y. Wang, and Y. Wang, "Optic disk size in chronic glaucoma: the Beijing eye study," *The American Journal of Ophthalmology*, vol. 142, no. 1, pp. 168–170, 2006.

[30] J. B. Jonas, P. Martus, F. K. Horn, A. Jünemann, M. Korth, and W. M. Budde, "Predictive factors of the optic nerve head for development or progression of glaucomatous visual field loss," *Investigative Ophthalmology and Visual Science*, vol. 45, no. 8, pp. 2613–2618, 2004.

[31] G. Savini, M. Zanini, V. Carelli, A. A. Sadun, F. N. Ross-Cisneros, and P. Barboni, "Correlation between retinal nerve

[31] ...fibre layer thickness and optic nerve head size: An optical coherence tomography study," *The British Journal of Ophthalmology*, vol. 89, no. 4, pp. 489–492, 2005.

[32] P. Carpineto, M. Ciancaglini, A. Aharrh-Gnama, D. Cirone, and L. Mastropasqua, "Custom measurement of retinal nerve fiber layer thickness using STRATUS OCT in normal eyes," *European Journal of Ophthalmology*, vol. 15, no. 3, pp. 360–366, 2005.

[33] D. Huang, V. Chopra, A. T.-H. Lu, O. Tan, B. Francis, and R. Varma, "Does optic nerve head size variation affect circumpapillary retinal nerve fiber layer thickness measurement by optical coherence tomography?" *Investigative Ophthalmology and Visual Science*, vol. 53, no. 8, pp. 4990–4997, 2012.

[34] A. Takeyama, Y. Kita, R. Kita, and G. Tomita, "Influence of axial length on ganglion cell complex (GCC) thickness and on GCC thickness to retinal thickness ratios in young adults," *Japanese Journal of Ophthalmology*, vol. 58, no. 1, pp. 86–93, 2014.

[35] G. Savini, P. Barboni, V. Parisi, and M. Carbonelli, "The influence of axial length on retinal nerve fibre layer thickness and optic-disc size measurements by spectral-domain OCT," *The British Journal of Ophthalmology*, vol. 96, no. 1, pp. 57–61, 2012.

[36] H. L. Rao, M. T. Leite, R. N. Weinreb et al., "Effect of disease severity and optic disc size on diagnostic accuracy of RTVue spectral domain optical coherence tomograph in glaucoma," *Investigative Ophthalmology and Visual Science*, vol. 52, no. 3, pp. 1290–1296, 2011.

[37] D. V. Cordeiro, V. C. Lima, D. P. Castro et al., "Influence of optic disc size on the diagnostic performance of macular ganglion cell complex and peripapillary retinal nerve fiber layer analyses in glaucoma," *Clinical Ophthalmology*, vol. 5, no. 1, pp. 1333–1337, 2011.

[38] S. T. Takagi, Y. Kita, A. Takeyama, and G. Tomita, "Macular retinal ganglion cell complex thickness and its relationship to the optic nerve head topography in glaucomatous eyes with hemifield defects," *Journal of Ophthalmology*, vol. 2011, Article ID 914250, 5 pages, 2011.

[39] N. R. Kim, E. S. Lee, G. J. Seong, J. H. Kim, H. G. An, and C. Y. Kim, "Structure-function relationship and diagnostic value of macular ganglion cell complex measurement using Fourier-domain OCT in glaucoma," *Investigative Ophthalmology and Visual Science*, vol. 51, no. 9, pp. 4646–4651, 2010.

[40] J. B. Jonas, A. M. Schmidt, J. A. Muller-Bergh, U. M. Schlotzer-Schrehardt, and G. O. H. Naumann, "Human optic nerve fiber count and optic disc size," *Investigative Ophthalmology and Visual Science*, vol. 33, no. 6, pp. 2012–2018, 1992.

[41] H. A. Quigley, A. L. Coleman, and M. E. Dorman-Pease, "Larger optic nerve heads have more nerve fibers in normal monkey eyes," *Archives of Ophthalmology*, vol. 109, no. 10, pp. 1441–1443, 1991.

[42] N. B. Patel, X. Luo, J. L. Wheat, and R. S. Harwerth, "Retinal nerve fiber layer assessment: area versus thickness measurements from elliptical scans centered on the optic nerve," *Investigative Ophthalmology and Visual Science*, vol. 52, no. 5, pp. 2477–2489, 2011.

[43] F. M. Rauscher, N. Sekhon, W. J. Feuer, and D. L. Budenz, "Myopia affects retinal nerve fiber layer measurements as determined by optical coherence tomography," *Journal of Glaucoma*, vol. 18, no. 7, pp. 501–505, 2009.

[44] S. H. Kang, S. W. Hong, S. K. Im, S. H. Lee, and M. D. Ahn, "Effect of myopia on the thickness of the retinal nerve fiber layer measured by cirrus HD optical coherence tomography," *Investigative Ophthalmology and Visual Science*, vol. 51, no. 8, pp. 4075–4083, 2010.

[45] E. M. Hoffmann, L. M. Zangwill, J. G. Crowston, and R. N. Weinreb, "Optic disk size and glaucoma," *Survey of Ophthalmology*, vol. 52, no. 1, pp. 32–49, 2007.

[46] H. L. Rao, L. M. Zangwill, R. N. Weinreb, M. T. Leite, P. A. Sample, and F. A. Medeiros, "Structure-function relationship in glaucoma using spectral-domain optical coherence tomography," *Archives of Ophthalmology*, vol. 129, no. 7, pp. 864–871, 2011.

[47] S. Ohkubo, T. Higashide, S. Udagawa et al., "Focal relationship between structure and function within the central 10 degrees in glaucoma," *Investigative Ophthalmology and Visual Science*, vol. 55, no. 8, pp. 5269–5277, 2014.

Endothelial Cell Loss after Phacoemulsification according to Different Anterior Chamber Depths

Hyung Bin Hwang, Byul Lyu, Hye Bin Yim, and Na Young Lee

Department of Ophthalmology, Incheon St. Mary's Hospital, College of Medicine, The Catholic University of Korea, 222 Banpo-daero, Seocho-gu, Seoul 137-701, Republic of Korea

Correspondence should be addressed to Na Young Lee; nyny5555@naver.com

Academic Editor: Lisa Toto

Purpose. To compare the loss of corneal endothelial cells after phacoemulsification according to different anterior chamber depths (ACDs). *Methods.* We conducted a prospective study on 135 eyes with senile cataracts. Eyes with nuclear density grades of 2 to 4 were divided into three groups according to ACD: ACD I, 1.5 < ACD ≤ 2.5 mm; ACD II, 2.5 < ACD ≤ 3.5 mm; or ACD III, 3.5 < ACD ≤ 4.5 mm. Intraoperative mean cumulative dissipated energy (CDE) was measured. Clinical examinations included central corneal thickness (CCT) and endothelial cell count (ECC) preoperatively and 2 months postoperatively. *Results.* There were no significant differences in CDE among the ACD groups ($P > 0.05$). Endothelial cell loss was significantly higher in ACD I than in ACD III in grades 3 and 4 cataract density groups 2 months after phacoemulsification ($P < 0.05$). There were also more changes in CCT in all of the cataract density groups in the ACD I group compared to the ACD II and III groups 2 months postoperatively, but the difference was not statistically significant. *Conclusions.* Eyes with shallow ACDs, especially those with relatively hard cataract densities, can be vulnerable to more corneal endothelial cell loss in phacoemulsification surgery.

1. Introduction

Corneal endothelial cells are nonreplicative, and the loss of these cells is only compensated for by the migration, enlargement, and increasing heterogeneity of the cells [1]. Loss of endothelial function by the damage of endothelial cells can lead to increased corneal thickness and decreased corneal transparency because of increased stromal hydration due to compromised pump function [2]. Corneal decompensation is a rare but potentially vision-threatening complication after phacoemulsification surgery. Thus, the evaluation of risk factors for preoperative, intraoperative, and postoperative endothelial cell loss provides important information for the cataract surgeon. Some unfavorable preoperative factors and improper intraoperative procedures can lead to corneal decompensation after phacoemulsification surgery. Several studies have reported that some preoperative and intraoperative parameters influence the risk of endothelial cell loss after phacoemulsification. Specifically, advanced age, hard nucleus density, high ultrasound energy, long phacoemulsification time, the phacoemulsification technique, and large infusion volumes can increase the risk of endothelial cell loss after phacoemulsification [3–6].

Phacoemulsification surgery is performed in a limited, confined space; however, securing adequate surgical space during an operation can decrease the risk of corneal endothelial cell loss as a result of the phacoemulsification procedure. Thus, anatomical and surgical factors, such as adequate anterior chamber depth (ACD), are important for preserving these cells from the mechanical and thermal damage that can occur during the procedure. Some studies have demonstrated that ACD did not affect endothelial cell loss after phacoemulsification surgery using a statistical correlation method [6, 7]. However, these studies did not give careful consideration to other surgical factors, such as cumulative dissipated energy (CDE), ultrasound time (UST), and balanced salt solution (BSS) use as confounding factors. It is well known that UST and ultrasound power are important risk factors for endothelial cell loss after phacoemulsification [3]. Thus, we should control for these factors in evaluating the effects of anatomical factors on endothelial cell loss after phacoemulsification. To the best of our knowledge, no stratified controlled study has compared endothelial cell damage according to different ACDs, controlling for confounding factors such as age, cataract nucleus density, CDE, UST, and BSS use. Thus, we compared corneal endothelial cell loss according to different ACDs in patients with various cataract nucleus densities.

2. Materials and Methods

The present prospective stratified controlled study examined eyes with cataracts that were randomly assigned to have phacoemulsification and posterior chamber intraocular lens (IOL) implantation at St. Mary's Hospital between May 2012 and March 2015. This project was approved by the Ethics Committees of Incheon St. Mary's Hospital, Incheon, Korea. All of the subjects provided written informed consent before participation. The study conformed to the tenets of the Declaration of Helsinki.

We prospectively examined 135 eyes in 135 patients scheduled to undergo phacoemulsification surgery. Specifically, we divided patients into three groups according to ACD: ACD I, 1.5 < ACD ≤ 2.5 mm; ACD II, 2.5 < ACD ≤ 3.5 mm; and ACD III, 3.5 < ACD ≤ 4.5 mm. Each ACD group was further divided into three subgroups according to three cataract densities (nuclear opalescence [NO]2, NO3, and NO4). Then, we recruited 15 eyes of 15 patients equally per subgroup for a total of 135 eyes of 135 patients. We used the Lens Opacities Classification System (LOCS) III for grading the NO of cataracts preoperatively [8]. Exclusion criteria included a history of previous ocular surgery or inflammation, trauma, corneal pathology, ECC less than 2000 cells/mm^2, and intraoperative complications, such as posterior capsule rupture and postoperative complications.

2.1. ACD Measurement. Preoperatively, ACD (mm) was recorded using partial coherence laser interferometry (Zeiss IOL Master; Carl Zeiss AG, Oberkochen, Germany). The IOL Master uses a slit-based measurement method; it measures from the anterior cornea vertex to the anterior lens vertex in calculating ACD. The mechanism is the same as an ultrasound method. Using built-in facilities and programming the IOL Master, five consecutive ACD measurements were recorded and averaged.

2.2. ECC and Central Corneal Thickness. The ECC with central corneal thickness (CCT) was measured using a noncontact specular microscope (Konan Noncon ROBO SP-9000; Konan Medical Corporation, Fair Lawn, NJ, USA) preoperatively and 1 month and 2 months postoperatively. CCT was measured at the central cornea using the built-in Pachy mode of the specular microscope. The center method was used for endothelial cell counting. The specular microscopy system calculated the ECC using a recorded picture of the endothelial cells. While identifying the center of each endothelial cell, the cell density (cells/mm^2) was computed on the basis of 100 identified cells taken from the picture. Endothelial cell loss was calculated by measuring the percentage decrease in endothelial cell density of the central cornea as follows: endothelial cell loss = (preoperative cell count − postoperative cell count)/(preoperative cell count × 100%). One examiner was blinded to which images belonged in which group. At each visit, three photographs were taken for each eye and averaged.

2.3. Surgical Technique. Phacoemulsification was performed by the same surgeon (HBH). Infiniti vision system and 0.9 mm flared 45° ABS Kelman microtip (Alcon Laboratories, Inc., Fort Worth, TX, USA) were used in all of the surgeries. Ozil torsional ultrasound was used, and the torsional amplitude was set at 90% in linear mode. The aspiration flow rate was set at 30 mL/min, and the height of the infusion bottle was set at 90 cm. In all of the cases, a clear corneal incision was made at a temporal corneal site with a 2.85 mm double-beveled incision knife (Diamatrix Ltd., Inc., TX, USA). Then, the ophthalmic viscosurgical device (OVD; Viscoat, Alcon Laboratories, Inc.) was injected into the anterior chamber. A 5 mm continuous curvilinear capsulorhexis was made using the Masket Capsulorhexis Forceps (Katena Inc., Denville, NJ, USA). Hydrodissection and hydrodelineation were performed using a BSS. In all of the cases, the "divide-and-conquer" technique was used for phacoemulsification. That is, four trenches were sculpted, and the nucleus was divided bimanually into four segments, after which the four divided quadrants were emulsified in the capsular bag. Next, 1% sodium hyaluronate (Healon) was injected into the anterior chamber and capsular bag, and a hydrophilic acrylic IOL (Akreos AO MI60; Bausch & Lomb, Rochester, NY, USA) was implanted in the capsular bag. In all of the cases, the IOL was implanted under the protection of an OVD, which was subsequently removed through irrigation and aspiration. The clear corneal wound was sutured with 10-0 nylon only once. After the surgery, 1% prednisolone acetate (Pred Forte, Allergan, Irvine, CA, USA) and 0.3% gatifloxacin (Gatiflo, Handok, Chungbuk, Korea) were applied four times per day for 2 months.

2.4. Intraoperative and Postoperative Measurements. Intraoperative measurements included total BSS volume used, UST, and mean CDE. Postoperative parameters, postoperative CCT and ECC and corrected distance visual acuity (CDVA), were measured at 1 day, 1 month, and 2 months.

2.5. Statistical Analysis. All of the data are expressed as means ± standard deviation (SD). For comparison of preoperative (age, CDVA, CCT, and ECC), intraoperative (UST, CDE, and BSS use), and postoperative measurements (CDVA) in the three ACD groups in the same nuclear opacity subgroups, one-way analysis of variance (ANOVA) was used. For pairwise comparisons, the Bonferroni and Dunnett's T3 tests were used as post hoc analyses. For CCT increase and ECC decrease in the three ACD groups in the same nuclear opacity subgroups, analysis of covariance (ANCOVA) was used. For the analysis, age, UST, CDE, and BSS use were set as factors of covariates. For pairwise comparison, Bonferroni and Dunnett's T3 methods were also used as post hoc analyses. Statistical analyses were conducted using the SPSS software (ver. 19.0 for Windows; SPSS Inc., Chicago, IL, USA). A P value < 0.05 was considered statistically significant.

3. Results

3.1. Overall Characteristics of the Enrolled Patients. In total, 135 eyes of 135 patients were enrolled. Each subgroup of cataract nucleus density included 45 eyes. Table 1 shows the overall characteristics of the enrolled patients in each ACD group. There was no statistically significant difference in age, mean CDVA, mean CCT, or mean ECC among the groups.

3.2. Intraoperative Measurements. Table 2 shows the values of the intraoperative parameters during surgery. BSS use was significantly higher in the NO2 and NO3 groups in the ACD I group than in the ACD II and III groups ($P < 0.05$). However, BSS use showed no statistically significant difference in the NO4 group among the three ACD groups ($P > 0.05$). There was also no statistically significant difference in CDE and UST in the three cataract nucleus densities among the three ACD groups ($P > 0.05$).

3.3. CDVA. There was an equal and significant improvement in logMAR CDVA among the three ACD groups, from the preoperative period to 2 months postoperatively, in the NO2, NO3, and NO4 subgroups. However, there was no statistically significant difference in logMAR CDVA at postoperative 2 months in the three cataract nucleus density subgroups among the three ACD groups ($P > 0.05$; Table 3).

3.4. CCT. In ANCOVA, setting covariates of age, UST, CDE, and BSS use, although there was less increase in the CCT in all cataract nucleus density subgroups in the ACD III group than the ACD I and II groups 2 months postoperatively, the difference was not statistically significant ($P > 0.05$; Figure 1).

3.5. Corneal Endothelial Cell Loss. In ANCOVA, setting covariates of age, UST, CDE, and BSS use, the mean percentage of endothelial cell loss was significantly different among the three ACD groups in the NO3 and NO4 subgroups ($P < 0.05$). According to the Bonferroni and Dunnett's T3 tests, the mean percentage of endothelial cell loss was significantly higher in the ACD I group (6.04 ± 1.51%; mean ECC, 2658.20 ± 233.04 cells/mm^2 preoperatively and 2498.60±232.52 cells/mm^2 2 months postoperatively) than in the ACD III group (4.01±1.53%; mean ECC, 2602.47±207.51 cells/mm^2 preoperatively and 2498.93 ± 214.72 cells/mm^2 2 months postoperatively) in the NO3 subgroup ($P < 0.05$). In addition, the mean percentage of endothelial cell loss was significantly higher in the ACD I group (12.94 ± 3.16%; mean ECC, 2534.53 ± 272.89 cells/mm^2 preoperatively and 2206.93±255.44 cells/mm^2 2 months postoperatively) than in the ACD III group (9.61±2.96%; mean ECC, 2608.53±298.66 cells/mm^2 preoperatively and 2359.67 ± 298.91 cells/mm^2 2 months postoperatively) in the NO4 subgroup ($P < 0.05$).

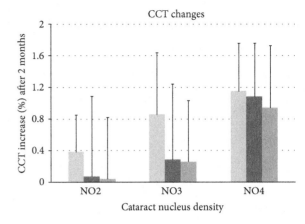

FIGURE 1: Postoperative changes of CCT by cataract nucleus density and ACD groups (no statistical significance in Bonferroni and Dunnett's T3 as post hoc analysis).

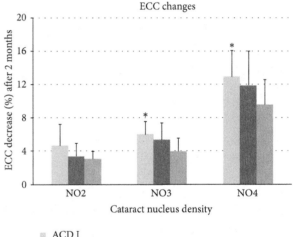

FIGURE 2: Postoperative endothelial cell loss by cataract nucleus density and ACD groups (* = significant in Bonferroni and Dunnett's T3 as post hoc analysis).

Although the percentage of endothelial cell loss was higher in the ACD I group than in the ACD II and III groups in the NO2 subgroup, the difference was not statistically significant (ANCOVA, $P > 0.05$; Figure 2).

4. Discussion

It is inevitable that endothelial cell damage will occur during the phacoemulsification procedure. Many factors for postoperative endothelial cell loss have been evaluated after phacoemulsification, including cataract density, surgery time, phacoemulsification time, and ultrasound power. In addition, IOL contact, instrument-related trauma, incision

TABLE 1: Preoperative clinical characteristics of enrolled patients.

Parameter	ACD I			ACD II			ACD III		
	NO2	NO3	NO4	NO2	NO3	NO4	NO2	NO3	NO4
Mean age (y)	68.60 ± 8.63	70.93 ± 8.46	69.00 ± 8.86	68.73 ± 8.90	71.47 ± 10.25	68.27 ± 9.18	71.67 ± 8.34	69.27 ± 9.35	70.13 ± 7.54
Mean CDVA (logMAR)	0.53 ± 0.15	0.51 ± 0.12	0.56 ± 0.14	0.55 ± 0.17	0.49 ± 0.14	0.52 ± 0.09	0.51 ± 0.15	0.46 ± 0.10	0.52 ± 0.09
Mean CCT (um)	538.00 ± 31.04	551.73 ± 28.28	561.53 ± 31.52	544.13 ± 29.07	543.73 ± 26.87	546.13 ± 28.17	540.73 ± 28.77	540.60 ± 15.27	552.20 ± 24.35
Mean ECC (cells/mm^2)	2608.13 ± 270.18	2658.20 ± 233.04	2534.53 ± 272.89	2700.67 ± 269.16	2646.27 ± 245.07	2532.53 ± 251.90	2710.73 ± 266.66	2602.47 ± 207.51	2608.53 ± 298.66
P value*	>0.05	>0.05	>0.05	>0.05	>0.05	>0.05	>0.05	>0.05	>0.05

Means ± SD.
CDVA = corrected distance visual acuity; CCT = central corneal thickness; ECC = endothelial cell count; NO = nucleus opalescence.
*Comparison of three ACD groups in the same cataract nuclear opacity subgroups (Bonferroni and Dunnett's T3 as post hoc analysis).

TABLE 2: Comparison of UST, CDE, and BSS use among three ACD groups according to cataract nucleus density.

Parameter	Mean ± SD								
	ACD I			ACD II			ACD III		
	NO2	NO3	NO4	NO2	NO3	NO4	NO2	NO3	NO4
UST (s)	44.44 ± 8.15	52.75 ± 8.25	72.70 ± 19.83	44.81 ± 7.91	54.36 ± 12.81	86.01 ± 26.41	39.11 ± 6.50	52.65 ± 9.33	86.83 ± 20.97
CDE	7.99 ± 1.80	10.16 ± 2.18	16.16 ± 5.95	8.06 ± 1.66	10.56 ± 3.10	18.59 ± 6.08	7.87 ± 1.62	9.21 ± 1.13	17.20 ± 5.08
BSS use (mL)	75.03 ± 6.05*	79.74 ± 3.50*	94.29 ± 5.84	67.18 ± 8.68	70.65 ± 6.71	87.77 ± 10.27	70.38 ± 9.89	73.95 ± 10.87	93.17 ± 10.28

UST = ultrasound time; CDE = cumulative dissipated energy; NO = nuclear opalescence.
*$P < 0.05$.

TABLE 3: Preoperative and postoperative logMAR CDVA.

Exam	Mean CDVA ± SD								
	ACD I			ACD II			ACD III		
	NO2	NO3	NO4	NO2	NO3	NO4	NO2	NO3	NO4
Preoperatively	0.53 ± 0.15	0.51 ± 0.12	0.56 ± 0.14	0.55 ± 0.17	0.49 ± 0.14	0.52 ± 0.09	0.51 ± 0.15	0.46 ± 0.10	0.52 ± 0.09
1 d postoperatively	0.19 ± 0.07	0.18 ± 0.07	0.16 ± 0.07	0.21 ± 0.06	0.17 ± 0.07	0.18 ± 0.09	0.19 ± 0.06	0.17 ± 0.07	0.19 ± 0.07
1 mo postoperatively	0.05 ± 0.05	0.07 ± 0.06	0.07 ± 0.08	0.05 ± 0.06	0.09 ± 0.05	0.07 ± 0.07	0.07 ± 0.06	0.04 ± 0.06	0.05 ± 0.06
2 mo postoperatively	0.03 ± 0.05	0.05 ± 0.05	0.05 ± 0.06	0.05 ± 0.05	0.03 ± 0.05	0.06 ± 0.06	0.07 ± 0.06	0.03 ± 0.05	0.04 ± 0.06
P value*	>0.05	>0.05	>0.05	>0.05	>0.05	>0.05	>0.05	>0.05	>0.05

CDVA = corrected distance visual acuity; NO = nuclear opalescence.
*Comparison of three ACD groups in the same cataract nuclear opacity subgroups (Bonferroni and Dunnett's T3 as post hoc analysis).

size, irrigation solution turbulence, type of IOL, and type of OVD can influence corneal endothelial cell loss after phacoemulsification procedures [9–14]. Corneal endothelial cells are not regenerated once they are damaged. Reuschel et al. [15] found a median postoperative endothelial cell loss of 6.9% (4.5–7.9%) 3 months after cataract surgery.

Some studies already examined and proved that ECC decreases with normal aging process [16–19]. A Portuguese study estimated that ECC decreased 5-6% every 10 years [16]. Møller-Pedersen [17] reported 0.3% reduction of ECC every year and Niederer et al. [18] demonstrated 0.5% reduction every year. And Cheng et al. [19] found annual ECC loss reaching even 1%. Because ECC is negatively correlated to increase of age, we controlled the age factor in evaluating the effects of ACD on ECC loss after phacoemulsification in this study. However, phacoemulsification surgery is known to decrease ECC even more. Reuschel et al. [15] reported ECC loss of 4.5–7.9% 3 months after phacoemulsification. Park et al. [20] demonstrated ECC loss of 5.2–9.1% 2 months after phacoemulsification. These values are similar to our results (4.01–12.94%). At 12 months of followup, Storr-Paulsen et al. [5] reported ECC loss of 3.5–5.7% after the phacoemulsification. In this respect, ECC loss seems to continue at least for a year after cataract surgery and would be larger than that of normal aging process. Further study should be done with longer follow-up period considering the age factor.

Corneal endothelial cell damage can induce corneal decompensation after phacoemulsification, especially in high-risk groups. Thus, endothelial cell loss is an important prognostic factor of the outcome of phacoemulsification surgery, and as such it is important to determine the risk factors of corneal endothelial cell loss, including preoperative, intraoperative, and postoperative parameters, for evaluating the prognosis after surgery. Moreover, increased attention is needed during surgery for high-risk groups.

The phacoemulsification surgery is performed in a limited, confined space; however, adequate space during surgery can decrease the risk of corneal endothelial cell damage by the procedure. Thus, an adequate surgical space is important for decreasing endothelial cell damage from the aforementioned risk factors. Within a shallow ACD, surgery can take place closer to the corneal endothelium. Therefore, we hypothesized that a deep ACD would correlate with lower endothelial cell loss during phacoemulsification surgery.

Advanced age, hard nucleus density, high ultrasound energy, long phacoemulsification time, and large infusion volume can increase the risk of endothelial cell loss after phacoemulsification [3, 4, 6]. Thus, we designated age, UST, CDE, and BSS use as confounding factors (covariates) for evaluating the effect of ACD on endothelial cell loss in phacoemulsification and used ANCOVA as a statistics technique. Previous studies used a statistical correlation method to determine that there is no significant relationship between ACD and endothelial cell loss [6, 7]. However, these studies did not control for other factors, such as age, UST, CDE, and BSS use. In contrast, the present study used a stratified and controlled examination, which increases confidence in the results.

The phacoemulsification technique itself can also influence endothelial cell loss. Storr-Paulsen et al. [5] suggested that the divide-and-conquer technique provokes more endothelial cell loss than the phaco chop technique, because the divide-and-conquer method uses more phaco energy, as it cracks the nucleus and facilitates phacoemulsification. Thus, this technique is more suitable for evaluating the effects of ACD on endothelial cell loss.

Moreover, the phaco platform we used has only Ozil torsional mode in order to exclude the effect of conventional longitudinal phaco energy on ECC loss. Also, CDE was calculated based solely on torsional amplitude and torsional time. However, Reuschel et al. [15] demonstrated that there is no significant difference in ECC loss between groups that used torsional phaco and longitudinal phaco. Similarly, Kim et al. [21] reported that torsional phaco showed no significant difference in ECC loss compared to that of longitudinal phaco at postoperative 1 month.

We used the IOL Master to measure ACD. The IOL Master measures ACD using lateral slit illumination of the cornea and crystalline lens, according to the Scheimpflug principle, and a white light-emitting diode (590 nm) as the light source. The lateral slit illumination is 0.7 mm wide and is used at an angle of 30° during ACD measurements. The axial resolution is precisely 10 μm for ACD measurements. The built-in software measures the distance between the anterior corneal surface and the anterior crystalline lens surface. The IOL Master shows good precision and resolution and is highly repeatable and reliable in measuring ACD compared to the other devices and techniques, such as Visante optical coherence tomography (OCT), slit lamp OCT, Pentacam, and Orbscan IIz [22–26].

In the present study, we compared three ACD groups according to nuclear cataract density. We found that shallow ACD could be a risk factor for increasing endothelial cell loss during phacoemulsification. As such, the percentage of corneal endothelial cell loss was higher in the ACD I group than in the ACD III group in eyes with NO3 and NO4 nuclear densities ($P < 0.05$). However, we found no significant difference in postoperative measurements, such as CCT and CDVA, among the three ACD groups in all of the nuclear density subgroups.

There have been some conflicting reports describing the relationship between ACD and endothelial cell loss in phacoemulsification. McCarey et al. [27] demonstrated that surgical instruments could induce more endothelial cell damage, especially in eyes with shallow ACDs. Walkow et al. [6] showed that short axial length could be a risk factor for endothelial cell loss during phacoemulsification, because small confined surgical space in short eyes increases the risk of endothelial touch by surgical instruments and lens fragments. However, the authors could not demonstrate a relationship between ACD and endothelial cell loss. However, O'Brien et al. [3] demonstrated that there was no relationship between ACD or axial length and endothelial cell loss during phacoemulsification, because an adequate surgical space could be obtained using irrigation flow during the operation. In addition, Reuschel et al. [7] reported that ACD was not a risk factor for postoperative endothelial cell loss in their correlation analysis. Jung et al. [28] compared eyes with nanophthalmos and relative anterior microphthalmos with a normal control group in phacoemulsification surgery. They found higher endothelial cell loss of $14.22 \pm 18.45\%$ in nanophthalmic eyes (mean ACD, 1.82 ± 0.31 mm) compared to an ECL of $11.57 \pm 11.34\%$ within relative anterior microphthalmic eyes (ACD, 1.87 ± 0.24 mm) and an endothelial cell loss of $7.61 \pm 8.77\%$ in their normal control eyes (mean, ACD 2.70 ± 1.31 mm). However, their results were not statistically significant. We hypothesized that a shallow ACD would lead to phacoemulsification being performed closer to the endothelium, so that the corneal endothelium could be vulnerable to torsional ultrasound energy, heat energy, movement of lens fragments, and touch by surgical instruments. For this reason, eyes with shallow ACDs are thought to suffer more endothelial cell loss than eyes with deep ACDs.

Our study had some limitations. The enrolled patients were only followed for 2 months. Thus, a long-term study is needed. In addition, our study could not have a blinded design, so other studies with this design are needed. Furthermore, more patients should be enrolled in future studies.

A significant strength of the study is its design, as to the best of our knowledge, this is the first controlled and stratified study to describe the relationship between ACD and corneal endothelial cell loss after phacoemulsification. We demonstrated that a shallow ACD is related to endothelial cell loss in phacoemulsification, especially in patients with relatively hard cataract nuclear densities. Thus, cataract surgeons should pay particular attention to patients with hard cataract nuclear densities and shallow ACDs during phacoemulsification surgery.

Conflict of Interests

The authors report no conflict of interests. The authors alone are responsible for the content and writing of the paper. None of the authors has a financial or proprietary interest in any material or method mentioned.

References

[1] G. O. Waring III, W. M. Bourne, H. F. Edelhauser, and K. R. Kenyon, "The corneal endothelium. Normal and pathologic structure and function," *Ophthalmology*, vol. 89, no. 6, pp. 531–590, 1982.

[2] M. Kohlhaas, O. Stahlhut, J. Tholuck, and G. Richard, "Changes in corneal thickness and endothelial cell density after cataract extraction using phacoemulsification," *Ophthalmologe*, vol. 94, no. 7, pp. 515–518, 1997.

[3] P. D. O'Brien, P. Fitzpatrick, D. J. Kilmartin, and S. Beatty, "Risk factors for endothelial cell loss after phacoemulsification surgery by a junior resident," *Journal of Cataract & Refractive Surgery*, vol. 30, no. 4, pp. 839–843, 2004.

[4] K. Hayashi, H. Hayashi, F. Nakao, and F. Hayashi, "Risk factors for corneal endothelial injury during phacoemulsification," *Journal of Cataract & Refractive Surgery*, vol. 22, no. 8, pp. 1079–1084, 1996.

[5] A. Storr-Paulsen, J. C. Norregaard, S. Ahmed, T. Storr-Paulsen, and T. H. Pedersen, "Endothelial cell damage after cataract surgery: divide-and-conquer versus phaco-chop technique," *Journal of Cataract and Refractive Surgery*, vol. 34, no. 6, pp. 996–1000, 2008.

[6] T. Walkow, N. Anders, and S. Klebe, "Endothelial cell loss after phacoemulsification: relation to preoperative and intraoperative parameters," *Journal of Cataract & Refractive Surgery*, vol. 26, no. 5, pp. 727–732, 2000.

[7] A. Reuschel, H. Bogatsch, N. Oertel, and R. Wiedemann, "Influence of anterior chamber depth, anterior chamber volume, axial length, and lens density on postoperative endothelial cell loss," *Graefe's Archive for Clinical and Experimental Ophthalmology*, vol. 253, no. 5, pp. 745–752, 2015.

[8] L. T. Chylack Jr., J. K. Wolfe, D. M. Singer et al., "The lens opacities classification system III," *Archives of Ophthalmology*, vol. 111, no. 6, pp. 831–836, 1993.

[9] A. Storr-Paulsen, J. C. Nørregaard, G. Farik, and J. Tårnhøj, "The influence of viscoelastic substances on the corneal endothelial cell population during cataract surgery: a prospective study of cohesive and dispersive viscoelastics," *Acta Ophthalmologica Scandinavica*, vol. 85, no. 2, pp. 183–187, 2007.

[10] Y. K. Cho, H. S. Chang, and M. S. Kim, "Risk factors for endothelial cell loss after phacoemulsification: comparison in different anterior chamber depth groups," *Korean Journal of Ophthalmology*, vol. 24, no. 1, pp. 10–15, 2010.

[11] D. Díaz-Valle, J. M. Benítez Del Castillo Sanchez, N. Toledano, A. Castillo, V. Pérez-Torregrosa, and J. García-Sanchez, "Endothelial morphological and functional evaluation after cataract surgery," *European Journal of Ophthalmology*, vol. 6, no. 3, pp. 242–245, 1996.

[12] K. Hayashi, H. Hayashi, F. Nakao, and F. Hayashi, "Corneal endothelial cell loss in phacoemulsification surgery with silicone intraocular lens implantation," *Journal of Cataract & Refractive Surgery*, vol. 22, no. 6, pp. 743–747, 1996.

[13] M. P. Holzer, M. R. Tetz, G. U. Auffarth, R. Welt, and H.-E. Völcker, "Effect of Healon5 and 4 other viscoelastic substances on intraocular pressure and endothelium after cataract surgery," *Journal of Cataract and Refractive Surgery*, vol. 27, no. 2, pp. 213–218, 2001.

[14] E. J. Linebarger, D. R. Hardten, G. K. Shah, and R. L. Lindstrom, "Phacoemulsification and modern cataract surgery," *Survey of Ophthalmology*, vol. 44, no. 2, pp. 123–147, 1999.

[15] A. Reuschel, H. Bogatsch, T. Barth, and R. Wiedemann, "Comparison of endothelial changes and power settings between torsional and longitudinal phacoemulsification," *Journal of Cataract & Refractive Surgery*, vol. 36, no. 11, pp. 1855–1861, 2010.

[16] J. Jorge, A. Queiros, S. C. Peixoto-de-Matos, T. Ferrer-Blasco, and J. M. Gonzalez-Meijome, "Age-related changes of corneal endothelium in normal eyes with a non-contact specular microscope," *Journal of Emmetropia*, vol. 1, no. 2, pp. 132–139, 2010.

[17] T. Møller-Pedersen, "A comparative study of human corneal keratocyte and endothelial cell density during aging," *Cornea*, vol. 16, no. 3, pp. 333–338, 1997.

[18] R. L. Niederer, D. Perumal, T. Sherwin, and C. N. J. McGhee, "Age-related differences in the normal human cornea: a laser scanning *in vivo* confocal microscopy study," *British Journal of Ophthalmology*, vol. 91, no. 9, pp. 1165–1169, 2007.

[19] H. Cheng, P. M. Jacobs, K. McPherson, and M. J. Noble, "Precision of cell density estimates and endothelial cell loss with age," *Archives of Ophthalmology*, vol. 103, no. 10, pp. 1478–1481, 1985.

[20] J. Park, H. R. Yum, M. S. Kim, A. R. Harrison, and E. C. Kim, "Comparison of phaco-chop, divide-and-conquer, and stop-and-chop phaco techniques in microincision coaxial cataract surgery," *Journal of Cataract & Refractive Surgery*, vol. 39, no. 10, pp. 1463–1469, 2013.

[21] D.-H. Kim, W.-R. Wee, J.-H. Lee, and M.-K. Kim, "The comparison between torsional and conventional mode phacoemulsification in moderate and hard cataracts," *Korean Journal of Ophthalmology*, vol. 24, no. 6, pp. 336–340, 2010.

[22] U. A. Dinc, E. Gorgun, B. Oncel, M. N. Yenerel, and L. Alimgil, "Assessment of anterior chamber depth using visante optical coherence tomography, slitlamp optical coherence tomography, IOL Master, Pentacam and Orbscan IIz," *Ophthalmologica*, vol. 224, no. 6, pp. 341–346, 2010.

[23] H. Eleftheriadis, "IOLMaster biometry: refractive results of 100 consecutive cases," *British Journal of Ophthalmology*, vol. 87, no. 8, pp. 960–963, 2003.

[24] R. Connors III, P. Boseman III, and R. J. Olson, "Accuracy and reproducibility of biometry using partial coherence interferometry," *Journal of Cataract & Refractive Surgery*, vol. 28, no. 2, pp. 235–238, 2002.

[25] A. K. C. Lam, R. Chan, and P. C. K. Pang, "The repeatability and accuracy of axial length and anterior chamber depth measurements from the IOLMaster," *Ophthalmic and Physiological Optics*, vol. 21, no. 6, pp. 477–483, 2001.

[26] J. J. Rozema, K. Wouters, D. G. P. Mathysen, and M.-J. Tassignon, "Overview of the repeatability, reproducibility, and agreement of the biometry values provided by various ophthalmic devices," *American Journal of Ophthalmology*, vol. 158, no. 6, pp. 1111–1120.e1, 2014.

[27] B. E. McCarey, F. M. Polack, and W. Marshall, "The phacoemulsification procedure. I. The effect of intraocular irrigating solutions on the corneal endothelium," *Investigative Ophthalmology*, vol. 15, no. 6, pp. 449–457, 1976.

[28] K. I. Jung, J. W. Yang, Y. C. Lee, and S.-Y. Kim, "Cataract surgery in eyes with nanophthalmos and relative anterior microphthalmos," *American Journal of Ophthalmology*, vol. 153, no. 6, pp. 1161–1168, 2012.

Responses of Multipotent Retinal Stem Cells to IL-1β, IL-18, or IL-17

Shida Chen,[1,2] Defen Shen,[1] Nicholas A. Popp,[1] Alexander J. Ogilvy,[3] Jingsheng Tuo,[1] Mones Abu-Asab,[3] Ting Xie,[4,5] and Chi-Chao Chan[1]

[1]*Laboratory of Immunology, National Eye Institute, National Institutes of Health, Bethesda, MD 20892, USA*
[2]*Zhongshan Ophthalmic Center, Sun Yat-sen University, Guangzhou 510060, China*
[3]*Histology Core, National Eye Institute, National Institutes of Health, Bethesda, MD 20892, USA*
[4]*Stowers Institute for Medical Research, Kansas City, MO 64110, USA*
[5]*Department of Anatomy and Cell Biology, University of Kansas School of Medicine, Kansas City, KS 66160, USA*

Correspondence should be addressed to Chi-Chao Chan; chanc@nei.nih.gov

Academic Editor: Naoshi Kondo

Purpose. To investigate how multipotent retinal stem cells (RSCs) isolated from mice respond to the proinflammatory signaling molecules, IL-1β, IL-18, and IL-17A. *Materials and Methods.* RSCs were cultured in a specific culture medium and were treated with these cytokines. Cell viability was detected by MTT assay; ultrastructure was evaluated by transmission electron microscopy; expression of IL-17rc and proapoptotic proteins was detected by immunocytochemistry and expression of *Il-6* and *Il-17a* was detected by quantitative RT-PCR. As a comparison, primary mouse retinal pigment epithelium (RPE) cells were also treated with IL-1β, IL-18, or IL-17A and analyzed for the expression of *Il-6* and *Il-17rc*. *Results.* Treatment with IL-1β, IL-18, or IL-17A decreased RSC viability in a dose-dependent fashion and led to damage in cellular ultrastructure including pyroptotic and/or necroptotic cells. IL-1β and IL-18 could induce proapoptotic protein expression. All treatments induced significantly higher expression of *Il-6* and *Il-17rc* in both cells. However, neither IL-1β nor IL-18 could induce *Il-17a* expression in RSCs. *Conclusions.* IL-1β, IL-18, and IL-17A induce retinal cell death via pyroptosis/necroptosis and apoptosis. They also provoke proinflammatory responses in RSCs. Though IL-1β and IL-18 could not induce *Il-17a* expression in RSCs, they both increase *Il-17rc* expression, which may mediate the effect of *Il-17a*.

1. Introduction

Age-related macular degeneration (AMD) is a progressive disease characterized by the degeneration of retinal pigment epithelium (RPE) and photoreceptor atrophy in the macula [1, 2]. Inflammation, particularly innate immunity, is implicated in AMD pathogenesis [3]. Recently, the inflammasome, a multimeric protein consisting of nod-like receptor (NLR), apoptosis-associated speck-like domain contains a caspase-recruitment domain (ASC), and pro-caspase-1 plays a central role in innate immunity and has been implicated in the pathogenesis of AMD [4, 5]. Activation of the NLRP3 inflammasome results in caspase-1 cleaving pro-IL-1β and pro-IL-18 into their mature proinflammatory forms in macrophages and RPE cells [5, 6]. However, the direct effect of IL-1β and IL-18 on other retinal cells has not been well studied.

In combination with IL-23, IL-1β or IL-18 can induce interleukin-17A (IL-17A) production by Th17 cells, $\gamma\delta$ T cells, and iNKT cells [7–10]. Growing evidence has implicated IL-17A involvement in AMD pathogenesis. Higher levels of IL-17A are found in the serum and macular tissues of the AMD patients when compared to age-matched controls [11, 12]. *In vitro*, IL-17A is cytotoxic to ARPE-19 cells, characterized by the accumulation of cytoplasmic lipids, autophagosome formation, and the presence of cleaved caspase-9 and cleaved caspase-3 [12]. IL-17RC, a member of IL-17R family and the primary receptor for IL-17A, is highly expressed in AMD macular tissues and in ARPE-19 cells [12]. In a study of twins with discordant AMD status, hypomethylation of the IL-17RC promoter was found in those with AMD. This finding was correlated with elevated expression of IL-17RC in peripheral blood cells as well as the macular tissue of AMD patients [13]. However, the direct effect of IL-17A on other cell types remains to be explored.

To test the hypothesis that IL-18 and IL-1β could stimulate IL-17A secretion in retinal cells, we used a mouse-derived multipotent retinal stem cell line (RSCs) as a model. RSCs are cultured stem cells from the mouse retina and can be efficiently differentiated into photoreceptor cells and all major cell types of neural retina under optimized differentiation conditions [14]. Subretinal injection of these differentiated photoreceptors into slowly degenerating rd7 mouse eyes can form new synapses with resident retinal neurons; in fast degenerating rd1 mouse eyes, injection of these cells can restore light response. These findings suggest that human retinal or neuronal stem cells could be useful for treating retinal degeneration in AMD [14]. We stimulated RSCs with IL-1β, IL-18, or IL-17A and characterized the inflammatory and cytotoxic responses.

2. Materials and Methods

2.1. Cell Culture and Stimulation. The RSC line was obtained from primary culture of adult CD-1 mouse neuroretina and cultured as described previously [14]. Briefly, RSCs were cultured in medium for retinal stem cells (RCM) composed of DMEM/F12 (1:1, Sigma, St Louis, MO, USA), insulin-transferrin-selenium-A supplement (Invitrogen, Eugene, OR, USA), 1.0 g/L bovine serum albumin (BSA, Sigma), 1.0 g/L glucose (Sigma), 1.0 g/L lactose (Sigma), 0.045 g/L proline (Sigma), 11.25 μg/mL linoleic acid (Sigma), 5 mM glutamine (Invitrogen), 2 mM nicotinamide (Sigma), 5% knockout serum replacement (Life Technologies, NY, USA), 20 ng/mL epidermal growth factor (EGF, Millipore, Billerica, MA, USA), and 20 ng/mL basic fibroblast growth factor (bFGF, R&D Systems, Minneapolis, MN, USA). Cells were passaged at 90% confluence using Accutase (Sigma). RSCs grown to 70%–80% confluence were treated with 1–100 ng/mL recombinant mouse IL-1β (R&D Systems), recombinant mouse IL-18 (MBL, Woods Hole, MA, USA), or recombinant mouse IL-17 (R&D Systems) for 24 hours.

2.2. Culture of Primary RPE Cells. All procedures using animals adhered to the Association for Research in Vision and Ophthalmology statement for the use of animals and the NEI's Institutional Animal Care and Use Committee approved protocols. Mouse RPE was isolated from retinas of C57/B6J mice at 6–8 weeks of age as described previously [15]. Briefly, mice were euthanized, and their eyes were enucleated. The globes were washed with PBS containing 1% penicillin-streptomycin (Sigma) and then were dissected free of periocular connective tissue. Then, the globe was placed on 2% Dispase II (neutral protease, grade II, Roche, Indianapolis, IN, USA) and incubated at 37°C for 40 min. The globe was transferred to DMEM/F12 media, the anterior segment was removed, and the retina containing the RPE layer was dissected free. The loosely adherent RPE cell layer was gently separated from the retina and transferred to a 15 mL tube containing DMEM/F12, 20% FBS, and 1% L-glutamine-penicillin-streptomycin. Cells were then centrifuged at 1000 rpm for 5 min and resuspended. The RPE suspension was added to 6-well cell culture plates. The medium was changed after 5-6 days and every 2-3 days thereafter. The RPE cells between two and three passages were stimulated with 100 ng/mL recombinant mouse IL-1β (R&D Systems), 10 ng/mL recombinant mouse IL-18 (MBL), or 10 ng/mL recombinant mouse IL-17 (R&D Systems) for 24 hours.

2.3. MTT Assay. The assessment of cell viability was performed using a 3-(4,5-dimethylthiazol-2-yl)-2,5-diphenyl tetrazolium bromide (MTT) assay in RSCs as described previously [15]. Briefly, cells were seeded at 80% confluence to 96-well culture plates. After stimulation with IL-1β, IL-18, or IL-17A for 24 hours, cells were washed with PBS and incubated with 20 μL of 5 mg/mL MTT solution (Sigma) for 4 h at 37°C. The medium was aspirated and 200 μL DMSO was added to each well. Plates were then shaken for 15 min at room temperature. Cell viability was determined by measuring the optical density at 570 nm using an ELISA plate reader (BioTek, Burlington, VT, USA). Cell viability represented the optical density ratio of stimulated cells relative to that of unstimulated cells.

2.4. Transmission Electron Microscopy. For transmission electron microscopy (TEM), cells were fixed in glutaraldehyde (2.5%, PBS buffered) for 24 hours, then suspended in warm low-melting point agarose (1.5%), pelleted down, and refrigerated overnight at 4°C; solidified pellets were rinsed with PBS three times, doubly-fixed with osmium tetroxide, rinsed again three times with PBS, dehydrated in ethanol, and embedded in Spurr's epoxy resin. Ultrathin sections (100 nm) were mounted on 200 lines/inch copper grids, double-stained with uranyl acetate and lead citrate, and viewed with a JEOL JEM-1010 transmission electron microscope.

2.5. Immunocytochemistry. The cells were seeded into 2-well chamber slides, and stimulation was performed at 70% confluence. After stimulation, cells were fixed with acetone, blocked with 1% BSA, and incubated overnight with the following primary antibodies: rabbit anti-mouse FasL (1:100, Santa Cruz, Dallas, Texas, USA); rabbit anti-mouse Fas (1:100, Santa Cruz); rabbit anti-mouse cleaved caspase-3 (1:200, Cell Signaling Technology, Danvers, MA, USA); rabbit anti-mouse cleaved caspase-9 (1:200 Cell Signaling Technology). After washing with PBS, secondary antibodies conjugated to either Alexa-488 or Alexa-555 (1:500, Invitrogen) were added and incubated for 1 h. After rinsing with PBS, cells were counterstained with 40, 6-diamidino-2-phenylindole dihydrochloride (DAPI, 1:1000, Invitrogen) for 5 min. The stained cells were examined under Zeiss 700 Confocal microscope with Zen software.

2.6. RNA Isolation and Quantitative RT-PCR. Total RNA was extracted from RSCs by using an RNeasy Mini Kit (Qiagen, Hilden, Germany), and equal amounts of RNA were synthesized to cDNA with Superscript II RNase H Reverse Transcriptase (Invitrogen) according to the manufacturer's instructions. Quantitative RT-PCR (qRT-PCR) was performed using RT² SYBR Green ROX qPCR Mastermix (Qiagen). cDNA was amplified with primers *β-actin*, *Il-6*, *Il-17rc*, or *Il-17a* (Qiagen) separately for 50 cycles. All data were normalized to the *β-actin* mRNA level. Expression fold-changes were calculated by $2^{-\Delta\Delta CT}$.

2.7. Statistical Analysis. Statistical analyses were performed using SPSS version 17.0 (SPSS, Chicago, IL, USA). Unpaired *t*-tests or analysis of variance (ANOVA) were used to compare the difference among different groups. GraphPad Prism 6 software was used to make the figures. A *p* value <0.05 was considered statistically significant.

3. Results

3.1. Stimulation of the Expression of IL-17RC in RSCs. RSCs cultured in RCM medium maintained spindle-shaped morphology (Figure 1(a)). Because the inflammatory response in RSCs has not yet been characterized, we evaluated expression of Il-17rc, which has been implicated in AMD pathogenesis previously [12, 13]. Indeed, *Il-17rc* mRNA expression was significantly increased in a dose-dependent fashion after stimulation with each cytokine (Figure 1(b)). Further, increased expression of IL-17rc protein was detected after treatment with 100 ng/mL IL-1β, 10 ng/mL IL-18, or 10 ng/mL IL-17A, respectively (Figure 1(c)). Interestingly, *Il-17rc* mRNA expression was also significantly increased in primary cultured mouse RPE cells after stimulation with each cytokine (Figure 1(d)).

3.2. Proapoptotic Effect of IL-1β, IL-18, or IL-17A on RSCs. In order to test whether IL-1β, IL-18, or IL-17A could induce apoptosis in RSCs, cleaved caspase-3, cleaved caspase-9, Fas, and FasL were evaluated by immunohistochemistry. IL-1β (100 ng/mL) or IL-18 (10 ng/mL) induced the expression of all the tested proapoptotic proteins when compared to the untreated cells (Figure 2); however, IL-17A had minimal effect on the cells. Accordingly, the MTT assay results demonstrated lower RSC viability in a dose-dependent manner after the cells were treated with IL-1β and IL-18. Interestingly, RSCs were also less viable after treatment with IL-17A for 24 hours despite little increase in expression of any proapoptotic proteins (Figure 3).

3.3. Ultrastructural Damage in RSCs. To further elucidate the subcellular features of RSCs after treatment with IL-1β, IL-18, or IL-17A, cellular ultrastructure was examined. With treatment of IL-1β (100 ng/mL) or IL-18 (10 ng/mL), the RSCs showed autophagosome formation, mitochondrial degeneration, cytoplasmic vacuoles, and glycogen accumulation (Figure 4). The average number of autophagosomes per cell increased from 1.3 in untreated controls to 9.8, 14.3, and 11 when RSCs were stimulated with IL-1β, IL-18, and Il-17, respectively. A few necroptotic and pyroptotic cells with degradation of cytoplasmic contents and chromatin condensations were also noted. IL-17A (10 ng/mL) had a similar effect as IL-18, but to a lesser extent and without necroptosis (Figure 4).

3.4. Proinflammatory Effect of IL-1β, IL-18, or IL-17A on RSCs. Proinflammatory effects of IL-1β, IL-18, and IL-17A were also explored in RSCs. Surprisingly, only the highest concentration of IL-1β (100 ng/mL) induced significantly higher expression of *Il-6* transcripts in RSCs (Figure 5(a)). Both IL-18 and IL-17A induced high *Il-6* transcripts in a dose-dependent manner (Figures 5(b)-5(c)). Consistent with these findings, IL-1β (100 ng/mL), IL-18 (10 ng/mL), and IL-17A (10 ng/mL) could induce higher expression of *Il-6* mRNA transcripts in primary cultured mouse RPE cells (Figure 5(d)). However, neither IL-1β nor IL-18 could induce detectable *Il-17a* expression from the RSCs (data not shown).

4. Discussion

RSCs can be differentiated into many types of retinal cells, including ganglion cells, bipolar cells, and photoreceptor cells. Differentiated photoreceptors from this stem cell line could effectively integrate into *rd1* or *rd7* mouse retinas, improving vision [14]. Recently, the potential for stem cell therapy in AMD has been highlighted [16, 17]. However, no extensive studies on the inflammatory response of RSCs have been performed previously. In our study, we found that RSCs indeed respond to inflammatory stimuli.

Our TEM finding of necroptosis and pyroptosis in the cells stimulated by the cytokines is unique. In contrast to apoptosis, necroptosis requires the function of RIPK3 [18, 19], which regulates the NLRP3 inflammasome [20, 21]. Pyroptosis is a caspase-dependent form of programmed cell death that differs from apoptosis. It depends on the activation of caspase-1 [22]. NLRP3, ASC, and pro-caspase-1 induce caspase-1 activation and can lead to maturation and secretion of IL-1β and IL-18. This suggests a link between these two cytokines and pyroptosis/necroptosis, which could be novel pathways for cell death in AMD in addition to apoptosis [23]. Further research on the role of RIPK3 and necroptosis in AMD pathogenesis is warranted.

Our findings of releasing proinflammatory cytokines are in parallel with previous studies [4, 12, 24]. We found that IL-1β could induce expression of IL-6 and IL-8 at both the transcript and the protein level in ARPE-19 and human RPE cells, yet this treatment had no effect on cell viability [24]. In our study, IL-1β could also induce *Il-6* expression in primary cultured mouse RPE cells and RSCs. However, IL-1β upregulated proapoptotic protein expression and decreased cell viability in RSCs, suggesting that IL-1β may be more destructive to these cells than to RPE cells. Indeed, the large number of autophagosomes in IL-1β treated RSCs supports this conclusion.

Tarallo and colleagues found that intravitreal injection of recombinant IL-18 could induce RPE degeneration in mice,

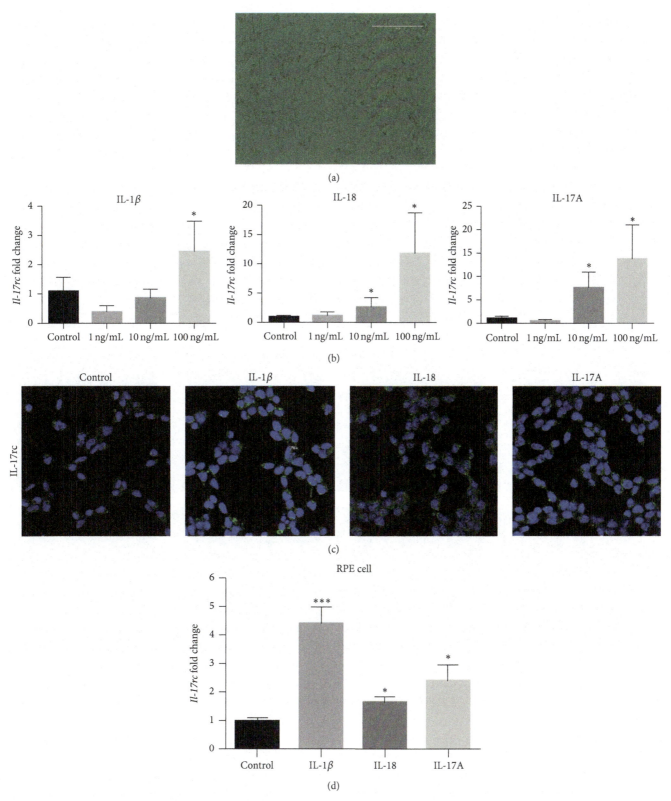

FIGURE 1: Morphology of the RSCs and Il-17rc expression. (a) RSCs are spindle-shaped even after passaging (scale bar: 200 μm). (b) *Il-17rc* mRNA was induced after the stimulation of IL-1β, IL18, or IL-17A in a dose-dependent manner. (c) IL-17rc protein (green) is weakly expressed in nonstimulated RSCs, but more highly expressed after stimulation with IL-1β (100 ng/mL), IL18 (10 ng/mL), or IL-17A (10 ng/mL). The nuclei were stained with DAPI (blue) (scale bar: 20 μm). (d) *Il-17rc* mRNA was induced after the stimulation of 100 ng/mL IL-1β, 10 ng/mL IL-18, or 10 ng/mL IL-17A in primary cultured mouse PRE cells. $^{*}p < 0.05$ compared to control. $^{***}p < 0.001$ compared to control.

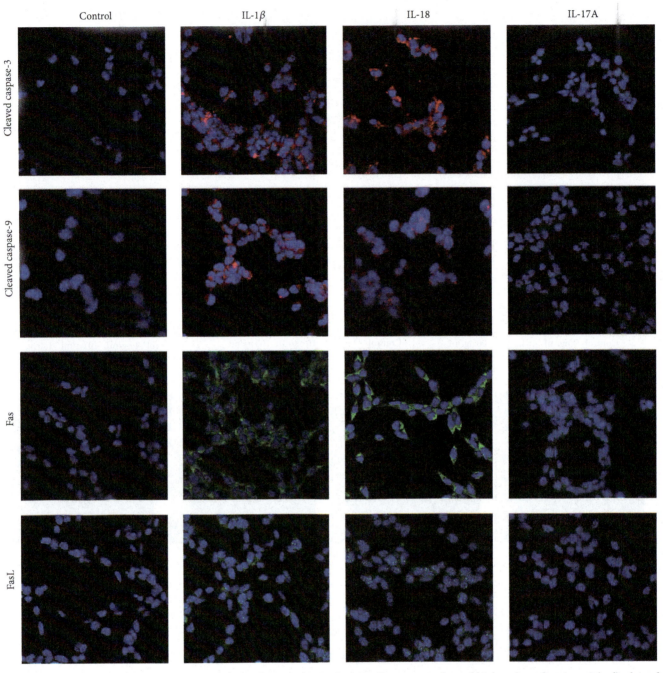

FIGURE 2: Proapoptotic protein expression in RSCs under stimulation. Immunofluorescence showed higher cleaved caspase-3 (red), cleaved caspase-9 (red), Fas (green), and FasL (green) expression in RSCs under stimulation with IL-1β (100 ng/mL) or IL18 (10 ng/mL). IL-17A (10 ng/mL) did not induce these proapoptotic proteins. The nuclei were stained with DAPI (blue) (scale bar: 20 μm).

and IL-18 neutralization protected against pAlu-induced RPE degeneration [4]; however, Doyle and her group reported that IL-18 has a protective role in laser induced choroid neovascularization (CNV), as intravitreally injected IL-18-neutralizing antibodies resulted in increased CNV development in mice [5]. These two seemingly conflicting studies may point to diverging roles of IL-18 in RPE versus the myeloid cells and vascular endothelium. Supporting the hypothesis that IL-18 is damaging to the neuroretina, we found that IL-18 decreased cell viability, induced necroptosis/pyroptosis by ultrastructure (Figure 4), and induced proinflammatory response (*Il-6* production) in RSCs. Furthermore, inflammatory response was similarly upregulated in primary cultured RPE cells. Interestingly, it was found that there are increased level of NLRP3 protein, *IL-1β* and *IL-18* mRNA in the RPE of donor eyes from individuals with geographic atrophy and neovascular AMD [4, 25]. Combined with our findings that both IL-1β and IL-18 could induce RSCs death *in vitro*, this mechanism may to some extent explain neuroretinal (photoreceptor) atrophy in AMD patients.

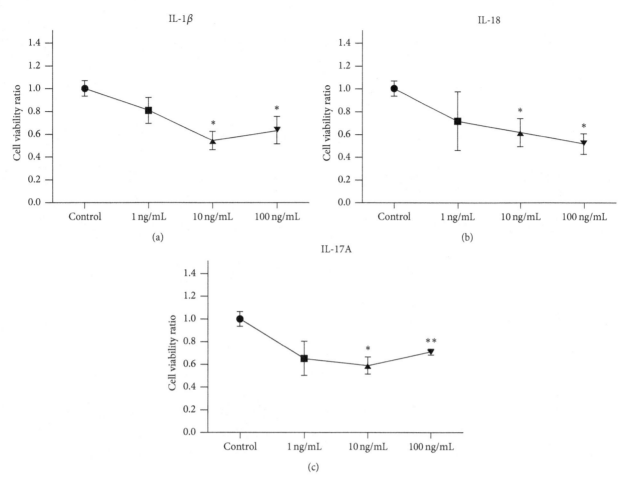

FIGURE 3: RSCs viability was detected with MTT assay. The RSCs were treated with IL-1β (a), IL-18 (b), or IL-17A (c) at different concentrations. $^{*}p < 0.05$; $^{**}p < 0.01$ compared to control.

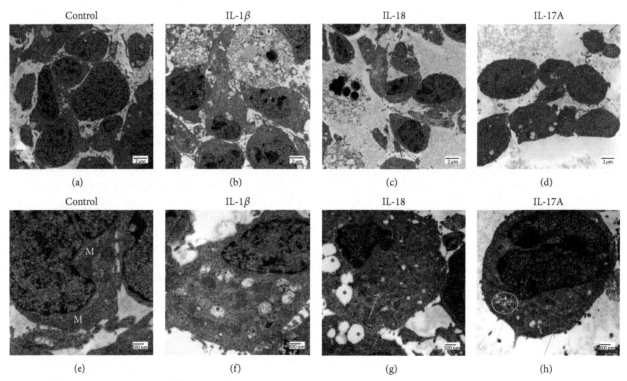

FIGURE 4: RSC ultrastructure change after stimulation. Control ((a), (e)), 100 ng/mL IL-1β ((b), (f)), 10 ng/mL IL-18 ((c), (g)), and 10 ng/mL IL-17A ((d), (h)) (M, mitochondria; black asterisks, cytoplasmic vacuoles; red asterisks, necroptotic cells; blue arrows, degenerated mitochondria; red circle, autophagosome; yellow circle, glycogen deposits).

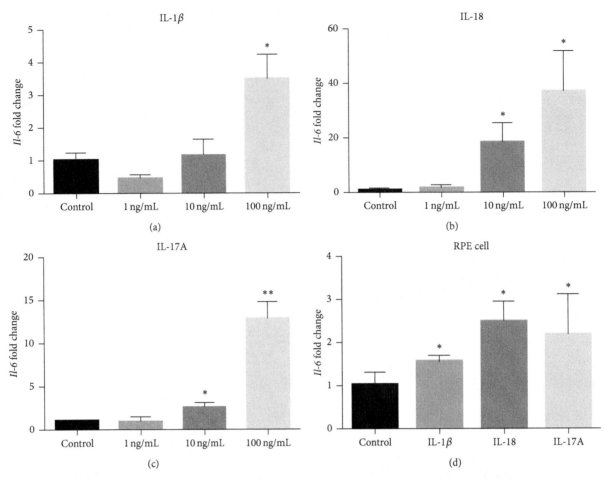

FIGURE 5: Proinflammatory effect of IL-1β, IL-18, or IL-17A. *Il-6* mRNA expression after stimulation with IL-1β (a), IL-18 (b), or IL-17A (c) with different concentrations in RSCs. (d) *Il-6* mRNA was induced after the stimulation of 100 ng/mL IL-1β, 10 ng/mL IL-18, or 10 ng/mL IL-17A in primary cultured mouse PRE cells. The mRNA levels of the *Il-6* were measured by quantitative RT-PCR. $^*p < 0.05$; $^{**}p < 0.01$ compared to control.

IL-17RC serves as an essential subunit of the IL-17 receptor complex and mediates the signal transduction and proinflammatory activities of IL-17A and IL-17F [26], which have been implicated in autoimmune and neurodegenerative diseases [27–29]. Recent research has also implicated the IL-17A/IL-17RC pathway in the pathogenesis of AMD [13, 30]; however, the exact role of IL-17A still remains elusive. In a previous study, we found that IL-17A is cytotoxic to ARPE-19 cells and decreases cell viability. Silencing of IL-17RC could prevent upregulation of cleaved caspase-3 and cleaved caspase-9 and was protective against IL-17A-mediated cell death [12]. In RSCs, IL-17A did not induce measurable proapoptotic proteins but did still decrease cell viability. This may imply that IL-17A-induced effect in RSCs proceeds through pathways other than apoptosis.

One of the most notable roles of IL-17 is its involvement in inducing and mediating proinflammatory response [31]. In synoviocytes, IL-17A could induce IL-6 expression, and knockdown of IL-17RC reversed the effect [32]. Interestingly, we found that not only IL-17A but also IL-1β and IL-18 could induce *Il-6* expression in RSCs and RPE cells. Generally, IL-6 is an important proinflammatory cytokine and has been associated with incidence of early AMD [33]. Furthermore, elevated plasma IL-6 was found in AMD patients with the CC variant in the CFH Y402H polymorphism, indicating a potential role for IL-6 in inflammation-related damage in AMD pathogenesis [34]. It has also been shown that IL-6 can contribute to Th17 cell differentiation from naïve T cells [35]. IL-1β combined with IL-23 can promote IL-17 production in naïve and memory T cells [36, 37]. Thus, IL-6 secretion by RSCs or RPE cells could result in a positive feedback loop through which Th17 and $\gamma\delta$ cells are locally induced. Although neither IL-1β nor IL-18 led to increased expression of *Il-17a* in RSCs, both could independently induce *Il-17rc* expression, which may amplify the effect of IL-17A. Interestingly, primary cultured RPE cells could also express notably higher *Il-17rc* and *Il-6* under the stimulation of IL-1β, IL-18, or IL-17A. These findings may account for a potential mechanism of IL-17A-induced pathogenesis in AMD via IL-6 production.

There are some limitations in this study. First, we only explored the response of RSCs, not the differentiated mature neuroretinal cells to IL-1β, IL-18, and IL-17A; in future studies, we plan to differentiate the RSCs to photoreceptor cells and explore their response to these cytokines, which will be a better model for photoreceptor changes in AMD. Additionally, this study only evaluates the *in vitro* effects of IL-1β, IL-18, and IL-17A; in the future, we hope to explore the effect of these cytokines *in vivo*.

5. Conclusions

In conclusion, we demonstrated that IL-1β, IL-18, and IL-17A have cytotoxic (necroptosis, pyroptosis, and apoptosis) effect and induce proinflammatory response in RSCs. Inflammasome promotes the maturation of IL-1β and IL-18 via caspase-1 activation. Though IL-1β, IL-18 alone could not induce IL-17A expression in RSCs, they all induce IL-17RC expression, which may mediate the effect of IL-17A.

Conflict of Interests

There is no conflict of interests in this research.

Authors' Contribution

Chi-Chao Chan and Shida Chen were responsible for analysis and interpretation of data and drafted the paper. Chi-Chao Chan, Jingsheng Tuo, and Shida Chen designed the study. Shida Chen, Defen Shen, Nicholas A. Popp, and Alexander J. Ogilvy performed experiments. Mones Abu-Asab and Ting Xie took part in analyzing data and revised the paper. All authors reviewed the paper.

Acknowledgment

This research received the NEI intramural research fund. The authors would like to thank Dr. Chun Gao of the Biological Imaging Core, NEI, who helped them with the confocal experiments.

References

[1] J. L. Dunaief, T. Dentchev, G.-S. Ying, and A. H. Milam, "The role of apoptosis in age-related macular degeneration," *Archives of Ophthalmology*, vol. 120, no. 11, pp. 1435–1442, 2002.

[2] J. Ambati, B. K. Ambati, S. H. Yoo, S. Ianchulev, and A. P. Adamis, "Age-related macular degeneration: etiology, pathogenesis, and therapeutic strategies," *Survey of Ophthalmology*, vol. 48, no. 3, pp. 257–293, 2003.

[3] J. Ambati, J. P. Atkinson, and B. D. Gelfand, "Immunology of age-related macular degeneration," *Nature Reviews Immunology*, vol. 13, no. 6, pp. 438–451, 2013.

[4] V. Tarallo, Y. Hirano, B. D. Gelfand et al., "DICER1 loss and Alu RNA induce age-related macular degeneration via the NLRP3 inflammasome and MyD88," *Cell*, vol. 149, no. 4, pp. 847–859, 2012.

[5] S. L. Doyle, M. Campbell, E. Ozaki et al., "NLRP3 has a protective role in age-related macular degeneration through the induction of IL-18 by drusen components," *Nature Medicine*, vol. 18, no. 5, pp. 791–798, 2012.

[6] O. A. Anderson, A. Finkelstein, and D. T. Shima, "A2E induces IL-1β production in retinal pigment epithelial cells via the NLRP3 inflammasome," *PLoS ONE*, vol. 8, no. 6, Article ID e67263, 2013.

[7] S. J. Lalor, L. S. Dungan, C. E. Sutton, S. A. Basdeo, J. M. Fletcher, and K. H. G. Mills, "Caspase-1-processed cytokines IL-1beta and IL-18 promote IL-17 production by gammadelta and CD4 T cells that mediate autoimmunity," *The Journal of Immunology*, vol. 186, no. 10, pp. 5738–5748, 2011.

[8] L. S. Dungan and K. H. G. Mills, "Caspase-1-processed IL-1 family cytokines play a vital role in driving innate IL-17," *Cytokine*, vol. 56, no. 1, pp. 126–132, 2011.

[9] J.-M. Doisne, V. Soulard, C. Bécourt et al., "Cutting edge: crucial role of IL-1 and IL-23 in the innate IL-17 response of peripheral lymph node NK1.1-invariant NKT cells to bacteria," *The Journal of Immunology*, vol. 186, no. 2, pp. 662–666, 2011.

[10] L. Campillo-Gimenez, M.-C. Cumont, M. Fay et al., "AIDS progression is associated with the emergence of IL-17-producing cells early after simian immunodeficiency virus infection," *The Journal of Immunology*, vol. 184, no. 2, pp. 984–992, 2010.

[11] B. Liu, L. Wei, C. Meyerle et al., "Complement component C5a promotes expression of IL-22 and IL-17 from human T cells and its implication in age-related macular degeneration," *Journal of Translational Medicine*, vol. 9, article 111, 12 pages, 2011.

[12] D. Ardeljan, Y. Wang, S. Park et al., "Interleukin-17 retinotoxicity is prevented by gene transfer of a soluble interleukin-17 receptor acting as a cytokine blocker: implications for age-related macular degeneration," *PLoS ONE*, vol. 9, no. 4, Article ID e95900, 2014.

[13] L. Wei, B. Liu, J. Tuo et al., "Hypomethylation of the IL17RC promoter associates with age-related macular degeneration," *Cell Reports*, vol. 2, no. 5, pp. 1151–1158, 2012.

[14] T. Li, M. Lewallen, S. Chen, W. Yu, N. Zhang, and T. Xie, "Multipotent stem cells isolated from the adult mouse retina are capable of producing functional photoreceptor cells," *Cell Research*, vol. 23, no. 6, pp. 788–802, 2013.

[15] Y. Wang, D. Shen, V. M. Wang et al., "Enhanced apoptosis in retinal pigment epithelium under inflammatory stimuli and oxidative stress," *Apoptosis*, vol. 17, no. 11, pp. 1144–1155, 2012.

[16] A.-J. F. Carr, M. J. K. Smart, C. M. Ramsden, M. B. Powner, L. da Cruz, and P. J. Coffey, "Development of human embryonic stem cell therapies for age-related macular degeneration," *Trends in Neurosciences*, vol. 36, no. 7, pp. 385–395, 2013.

[17] K. Bharti, M. Rao, S. C. Hull et al., "Developing cellular therapies for retinal degenerative diseases," *Investigative Ophthalmology & Visual Science*, vol. 55, no. 2, pp. 1191–1202, 2014.

[18] A. Kaczmarek, P. Vandenabeele, and D. V. Krysko, "Necroptosis: the release of damage-associated molecular patterns and its physiological relevance," *Immunity*, vol. 38, no. 2, pp. 209–223, 2013.

[19] A. Linkermann and D. R. Green, "Necroptosis," *The New England Journal of Medicine*, vol. 370, no. 5, pp. 455–465, 2014.

[20] A. Degterev, Z. Huang, M. Boyce et al., "Chemical inhibitor of nonapoptotic cell death with therapeutic potential for ischemic brain injury," *Nature Chemical Biology*, vol. 1, no. 2, pp. 112–119, 2005.

[21] D. Ofengeim and J. Yuan, "Regulation of RIP1 kinase signalling at the crossroads of inflammation and cell death," *Nature Reviews Molecular Cell Biology*, vol. 14, no. 11, pp. 727–736, 2013.

[22] S. W. G. Tait, G. Ichim, and D. R. Green, "Die another way—non-apoptotic mechanisms of cell death," *Journal of Cell Science*, vol. 127, part 10, pp. 2135–2144, 2014.

[23] C. P. Ardeljan, D. Ardeljan, M. Abu-Asab, and C. C. Chan, "Inflammation and cell death in age-related macular degeneration: an immunopathological and ultrastructural model," *Journal of Clinical Medicine*, vol. 3, no. 4, pp. 1542–1560, 2014.

[24] D. Ling, B. Liu, S. Jawad et al., "The tellurium redox immunomodulating compound AS101 inhibits IL-1beta-activated inflammation in the human retinal pigment epithelium," *The British Journal of Ophthalmology*, vol. 97, no. 7, pp. 934–938, 2013.

[25] W. A. Tseng, T. Thein, K. Kinnunen et al., "NLRP3 inflammasome activation in retinal pigment epithelial cells by lysosomal destabilization: implications for age-related macular degeneration," *Investigative Ophthalmology and Visual Science*, vol. 54, no. 1, pp. 110–120, 2013.

[26] S. H. Chang and C. Dong, "Signaling of interleukin-17 family cytokines in immunity and inflammation," *Cellular Signalling*, vol. 23, no. 7, pp. 1069–1075, 2011.

[27] Y. Hu, F. Shen, N. K. Crellin, and W. Ouyang, "The IL-17 pathway as a major therapeutic target in autoimmune diseases," *Annals of the New York Academy of Sciences*, vol. 1217, no. 1, pp. 60–76, 2011.

[28] R. Gold and F. Lühder, "Interleukin-17—extended features of a key player in multiple sclerosis," *The American Journal of Pathology*, vol. 172, no. 1, pp. 8–10, 2008.

[29] W. T. Hu, A. Chen-Plotkin, M. Grossman et al., "Novel CSF biomarkers for frontotemporal lobar degenerations," *Neurology*, vol. 75, no. 23, pp. 2079–2086, 2010.

[30] C.-C. Chan and D. Ardeljan, "Molecular pathology of macrophages and interleukin-17 in age-related macular degeneration," *Advances in Experimental Medicine and Biology*, vol. 801, pp. 193–198, 2014.

[31] D. V. Jovanovic, J. A. Di Battista, J. Martel-Pelletier et al., "IL-17 stimulates the production and expression of proinflammatory cytokines, IL-beta and TNF-alpha, by human macrophages," *The Journal of Immunology*, vol. 160, no. 7, pp. 3513–3521, 1998.

[32] S. Zrioual, M.-L. Toh, A. Tournadre et al., "IL-17RA and IL-17RC receptors are essential for IL-17A-induced ELR$^+$ CXC chemokine expression in synoviocytes and are overexpressed in rheumatoid blood 1," *The Journal of Immunology*, vol. 180, no. 1, pp. 655–663, 2008.

[33] R. Klein, C. E. Myers, K. J. Cruickshanks et al., "Markers of inflammation, oxidative stress, and endothelial dysfunction and the 20-year cumulative incidence of early age-related macular degeneration: the beaver dam eye study," *JAMA Ophthalmology*, vol. 132, no. 4, pp. 446–455, 2014.

[34] S. Cao, A. Ko, M. Partanen et al., "Relationship between systemic cytokines and complement factor H Y402H polymorphism in patients with dry age-related macular degeneration," *American Journal of Ophthalmology*, vol. 156, no. 6, pp. 1176–1183, 2013.

[35] E. Bettelli, Y. Carrier, W. Gao et al., "Reciprocal developmental pathways for the generation of pathogenic effector TH17 and regulatory T cells," *Nature*, vol. 441, no. 7090, pp. 235–238, 2006.

[36] C. E. Sutton, S. J. Lalor, C. M. Sweeney, C. F. Brereton, E. C. Lavelle, and K. H. G. Mills, "Interleukin-1 and IL-23 induce innate IL-17 production from gammadelta T cells, amplifying Th17 responses and autoimmunity," *Immunity*, vol. 31, no. 2, pp. 331–341, 2009.

[37] C. Sutton, C. Brereton, B. Keogh, K. H. G. Mills, and E. C. Lavelle, "A crucial role for interleukin (IL)-1 in the induction of IL-17-producing T cells that mediate autoimmune encephalomyelitis," *The Journal of Experimental Medicine*, vol. 203, no. 7, pp. 1685–1691, 2006.

Risk Factors for Refractory Diabetic Macular Oedema after Sub-Tenon's Capsule Triamcinolone Acetonide Injection

Toshiyuki Oshitari, Yuta Kitamura, Sakiko Nonomura, Miyuki Arai, Yoko Takatsuna, Eiju Sato, Takayuki Baba, and Shuichi Yamamoto

Department of Ophthalmology and Visual Science, Chiba University Graduate School of Medicine, Inohana 1-8-1, Chuo-ku, Chiba Prefecture, Chiba 260-8670, Japan

Correspondence should be addressed to Toshiyuki Oshitari; tarii@aol.com

Academic Editor: Ciro Costagliola

The purpose of this study is to identify the risk factors for a recurrence or persistence of diabetic macular oedema (DME) after a sub-Tenon's capsule triamcinolone acetonide (STTA) injection. The medical records of 124 patients (124 eyes) treated by STTA were reviewed. The age, sex, HbA1c level, best-corrected visual acuity, central macular thickness, insulin use, pioglitazone use, systemic hypertension, serous retinal detachment, proteinuria, panretinal photocoagulation, microaneurysm photocoagulation (MAPC), subthreshold micropulse diode laser photocoagulation (SMDLP), cataract surgery, and history of vitrectomy were examined by logistic regression analysis. Procedures of MAPC and SMDLP were significantly associated with DME treated with STTA ($P = 0.0315$, $P = 0.04$, resp.). However, a history of vitrectomy was found to have significantly fewer recurrences or persistent DME after STTA ($P = 0.0464$). In conclusion, patients who required combined MAPC or SMDLP with a STTA injection had significantly higher refractoriness to STTA, but postvitrectomy may prevent the recurrence or persistence of DME after STTA injection.

1. Introduction

Diabetic macular oedema (DME) is one of the main causes for reduced visual acuity in patients with diabetes [1]. A recent meta-analysis examined the prevalence of DME in 22,896 diabetic patients and found that 6.81% of diabetic patients had DME [2]. Several prospective, randomized studies showed that intravitreal injections of antivascular endothelial growth factor (VEGF) drugs were effective in reducing macular thickness and improving the visual acuity in patients with DME [3–6]. However, the injections had to be repeated which increased the risk of postintravitreal anti-VEGF endophthalmitis and the medical expenses. For example, in the pooled analysis of the RESOLVE and the RESTORE studies, the incidence of endophthalmitis was 1.4% at 1 year for multiple injections [3].

Growing evidence indicates an association between the intraocular inflammation induced by diabetic stress and the development and progression of DME [7]. Several basic studies demonstrated that steroids upregulate the tight junction proteins, occludin and ZO-1, tighten the retinal blood barrier [8], and reduce the expression of VEGF [9, 10]. Thus, posterior sub-Tenon's capsule injection of triamcinolone acetonide (STTA) [11] and intravitreal injections of triamcinolone acetonide (IVTA) [12] have been used to treat DME.

IVTA has a higher risk of endophthalmitis and elevation of the intraocular pressure than STTA. The Japanese survey of triamcinolone acetonide for ocular diseases reported that the incidence of endophthalmitis by IVTA and STTA was 0.12% and 0.008%, respectively, and that the incidence of glaucoma requiring filtration surgery after IVTA and STTA was 0.56% and 0.26%, respectively [13]. Thus, STTA has a lower risk of endophthalmitis and secondary glaucoma than IVTA.

Our recent study indicated that the short-term effect of STTA for DME is comparable to that of pars plana vitrectomy [14]. However, the benefits of steroid therapies were no longer evident at 6 months [15]. Thus, repeated injections or additional treatments such as laser photocoagulation are usually required for the treatment of DME.

The main purpose of this study was to identify the risk factors that led to a recurrence or persistence of DME after a STTA injection.

2. Methods

The medical records of 124 eyes of 124 patients with DME that had STTA between January 2010 and July 2011 at the Chiba University Hospital were reviewed. All of the procedures conformed to the tenets of the World Medical Association Declaration of Helsinki. A signed informed consent was obtained from all patients regarding the procedures to be performed, and approval for this study was obtained from the Institutional Review Board of Chiba University Graduate School of Medicine.

The definition of a recurrence of DME in this study was an eye which initially had a ≧30% decrease of central macular thickness (CMT) compared with the baseline within 1 year after STTA but then increased by ≧30%. The definition of a persistence of DME was an eye which had <30% decrease of the CMT within 1 year after STTA. Seventy-four patients (59.7%; 42 men, 32 women) had a persistent DME or a recurrence within 1 year. In the eyes with a recurrence, the mean interval until the recurrence was 7.7 ± 3.5 months.

The possible risk factors for a recurrence or persistence of a DME after STTA were the age, sex, glycohemoglobin A1c (HbA1c) level, best-corrected visual acuity (BCVA), CMT, insulin use, pioglitazone use, systemic hypertension, serous retinal detachment (SRD), proteinuria, panretinal photocoagulation (PRP), microaneurysm photocoagulation (MAPC), subthreshold micropulse diode laser photocoagulation (SMDLP), cataract surgery, and history of vitrectomy. All possible risk factors for recurrence or persistence of DME after STTA were determined by logistic regression analysis. A $P < 0.05$ was considered significant.

3. Results

The baselines clinical characteristics of the 124 patients with DME are shown in Table 1. The DME of 50 eyes (40.3%) was improved after the STTA injection without any additional treatments, 52 (41.9%) had a recurrence of DME, and 22 eyes (17.7%) had a persistence of the DME after STTA injection. All of the results of multiple logistic regression analyses of the risk factors for a recurrence or persistence of DME after the STTA injection are shown in Table 2.

At the time of treatment, the mean age was 60.3 ± 13.1 years, mean HbA1c was 6.7 ± 1.2%, mean BCVA was 0.6 ± 0.4 logMAR units, and mean CMT was 539.2 ± 156.7 μm. Thirty-eight patients (30.6%) used insulin, 10 used pioglitazone (8.1%), 55 (44.4%) had hypertension, and 47 (37.9%) had proteinuria. Fifty-five patients (44.4%) underwent PRP and 25 patients (20.2%) underwent cataract surgery. None of these factors was found to be significant risk factors (Tables 1 and 2).

TABLE 1: Baseline clinical characteristics of 124 patients with DME.

Factors	Cases (124 eyes)
Sex, men : women (n)	71 : 53
Mean age (y.o.)	60.3 ± 13.1
Mean HbA1c (%)	6.7 ± 1.2
Hypertension, + : − (n)	55 : 69
Insulin use, + : − (n)	38 : 86
Pioglitazone use, + : − (n)	10 : 114
Proteinuria, + : − (n)	47 : 77
Mean BCVA (logMAR)	0.6 ± 0.4
Mean CMT (μm)	539.2 ± 156.7
SRD, + : − (n)	33 : 91
MAPC, + : − (n)	49 : 75
SMDLP, + : − (n)	13 : 111
PRP, + : − (n)	55 : 69
Vitrectomy, + : − (n)	17 : 107
Cataract surgery, + : − (n)	25 : 99

BCVA: best-corrected visual acuity, CMT: central macular thickness, SRD: serous retinal detachment, MAPC: microaneurysm photocoagulation, SMDLP: subthreshold micropulse diode laser photocoagulation, and PRP: panretinal photocoagulation.

Forty-nine patients (39.5%) underwent MAPC and 13 patients (10.5%) underwent SMDLP combined with the STTA injection. These procedures were found to be significantly associated with a persistence or recurrence of the DME ($P = 0.0315$, $P = 0.04$, resp.; Table 2). On the other hand, 17 patients (13.7%) with a history of PPV had significantly fewer recurrences or persistence of DME after STTA injection ($P = 0.0464$; Table 2).

4. Discussion

The results indicated that 40% of patients with DME were successfully treated with a single STTA injection without any additional treatments for at least 1 year. On the other hand, 60% of DME patients had a recurrence or persistence of DME after a single STTA injection and repeated STTA injections or other treatments were required.

The specific indications for MAPC and SMDLP were not determined but the patients with microaneurysms at the posterior pole underwent STTA combined with MAPC immediately or within one month after the STTA injection. The effect of the STTA injection for DME is rapid, and our results indicate that the CMT was significantly reduced 1 month after the STTA injection [14]. In our hospital, SMDLP was determined to be a better treatment than grid laser photocoagulation for DME [16]. Thus, the refractory DME patients without microaneurysms underwent SMDLP and not grid laser photocoagulation as additional treatment after STTA. Basically, both MAPC and SMDLP tended to be performed for patients with mild to moderate DME with CMT >500 μm in our hospital. Therefore, patients with severe DME with CMT <500 μm underwent STTA first, followed by undergoing MAPC or SMDLP.

TABLE 2: Multiple logistic regression analysis of a recurrence and/or persistence of DME after STTA.

Factors	Recurrence (+)	Recurrence (−)	Odds ratio	95% CI	P value
Sex, men : women (n)	42 : 32	29 : 21	0.718	0.034–0.973	0.4846
Mean age (y.o.)	61.6 ± 13.0	58.5 ± 13.2	1.012	0.978–1.049	0.4883
Mean HbA1c (%)	6.83 ± 1.32	6.59 ± 1.09	1.239	0.833–1.843	0.2906
Hypertension, + : −	38 : 36	17 : 33	1.926	0.760–4.879	0.1669
Insulin use, + : − (n)	24 : 50	14 : 36	1.367	0.525–3.562	0.5218
Pioglitazone use, + : − (n)	8 : 66	2 : 48	2.416	0.373–15.628	0.3544
Proteinuria, + : − (n)	30 : 44	17 : 33	1.103	0.420–2.894	0.8422
Mean BCVA (logMAR)	0.61 ± 0.37	0.52 ± 0.33	2.054	0.523–8.065	0.3022
Mean CMT (μm)	557.2 ± 143.7	512.8 ± 172.2	1.002	0.999–1.005	0.1800
SRD, + : − (n)	22 : 52	11 : 39	1.012	0.370–2.769	0.9821
MAPC, + : − (n)	35 : 39	14 : 36	2.566	1.087–6.058	0.0315
SMDLP, + : − (n)	11 : 63	2 : 48	7.772	1.098–55.004	0.0400
PRP, + : − (n)	33 : 41	22 : 28	0.951	0.390–2.321	0.9124
Vitrectomy, + : − (n)	7 : 67	10 : 40	0.182	0.034–0.973	0.0464
Cataract surgery, + : − (n)	15 : 59	10 : 40	1.355	0.336–5.460	0.6691

BCVA: best-corrected visual acuity, CMT: central macular thickness, SRD: serous retinal detachment, MAPC: microaneurysm photocoagulation, SMDLP: subthreshold micropulse diode laser photocoagulation, and PRP: panretinal photocoagulation.

The results of the logistic regression analysis indicated that both MAPC and SMDLP were risk factors for a recurrence or persistence of DME because these patients tended to have refractory DME and needed to undergo additional treatments. Although patients who underwent MAPC had an enough population size, smaller number of patients underwent SMDLP compared to MAPC. Thus, the result of the logistic regression analysis for SMDLP should be interpreted with caution.

Recently Ribeiro et al. suggested that a high microaneurysm turnover rate (sum of the microaneurysm formation and disappearance rates) was a higher risk for developing clinical significant macular oedema (CSME) over a 2-year period [17]. Haritoglou et al. demonstrated that high microaneurysm formation rate was a predictive marker for progression to CSME for a period of up to 5 years [18]. Taken together, microaneurysm formation is probably a sign of severe diabetic stress including oxidative stress in the macula of diabetic patients, and the requirement of MAPC combined with STTA injections may be necessary to treat the DME. However, these patients may increase diabetic stress including oxidative stress in the macula; further pathological changes such as Müller cell swelling, retinal pigment epithelium (RPE) dysfunction, or blood-retinal barrier dysfunction may be accompanied. Such pathological changes may cause refractoriness of DME after STTA with MAPC.

Although the precise mechanism of the effect of SMDLP is unclear, SMDLP may stimulate and activate RPE and improve to draw out the excessive fluid in the retina. But steroid can affect the function of RPE in diabetic patients. Thus, STTA may not be fitted with SMDLP because of exacerbating RPE function.

Vitrectomized eyes had a significantly lower risk for recurrence or persistence of DME after the STTA injection. One possible reason for this is that vitrectomized eyes have no vitreomacular traction. Another possible reason is that, in vitrectomized eyes, pathological cytokines, such as VEGF or IL-6, can easily diffuse and are not in contact with the macula for a long period. Thus, a STTA injection may be one of the options for treatment of DME developing in vitrectomized eyes but a careful management of the steroid response is needed because glaucoma infiltration surgeries are difficult to perform in vitrectomized eyes.

The HbA1c level is known to be a major risk factor for developing DME [19, 20]. However, in this study, the HbA1c level was not found to be a significant risk factor for recurrence or persistence of DME after a STTA injection from the logistic regression analysis. We have classified the grades of DM control as good control group (HbA1c < 6.5%), moderated control group (6.5% ≦ HbA1c ≦ 8.0%), and poor control group (8.0% < HbA1c) and reevaluated whether the DM control was risk factors for recurrence or persistence of DME after STTA injection. But the DM controls have not been identified as risk factors for recurrence or persistence of DME after STTA injection ($P = 0.2203$). However, 80% of the patients with HbA1c levels >9.0% had a recurrence or persistence of the DME after the STTA injection. Thus, a poor glycemic control seems to increase a risk of recurrence or persistence of DME after STTA injection.

The results of two large cohort studies indicated that glitazone is a risk factor for developing DME [21, 22], and we have reported the first case of DME after pioglitazone use in Japan [23]. However, in this study, pioglitazone was not found to be a risk factor for recurrence or persistence of DME after a STTA injection.

From this study, we tentatively suggest the indication of STTA in the clinical practice. STTA may be selected for treatment of DME without MAs or DME after vitrectomy. DME with MAs may be treated with intravitreal injection of anti-VEGF antibodies. SMDLP may not be fitted with STTA. Further studies are needed to evaluate the additive effect of intravitreal injection of anti-VEGF antibodies with SMDLP for patients with DME.

5. Conclusions

Although this study has a limitation because of its retrospective nature, patients who needed to have combined MAPC and SMDLP with a STTA injection had significantly higher refractoriness to DME. However, vitrectomized eyes may reduce the incidence of recurrence or persistent DME after a STTA injection. Additional prospective studies are needed to confirm the risk factors for a recurrence or persistent DME after a STTA injection.

Conflict of Interests

The authors declare that there is no conflict of interests regarding the publication of this paper.

Acknowledgments

This study was supported by a grant from The Eye Research Foundation for the Aged and Charitable Trust Fund for Ophthalmic Research in Commemoration of Santen Pharmaceutical's Founder and a Grant-in-Aid from the Ministry of Education, Science, Sports, and Culture of the Japanese Government. The authors thank Professor Duco Hamasaki for editing the paper.

References

[1] M. O'Doherty, I. Dooley, and M. Hickey-Dwyer, "Interventions for diabetic macular oedema: a systematic review of the literature," *British Journal of Ophthalmology*, vol. 92, no. 12, pp. 1581–1590, 2008.

[2] J. W. Y. Yau, S. L. Rogers, R. Kawasaki et al., "Global prevalence and major risk factors of diabetic retinopathy," *Diabetes Care*, vol. 35, no. 3, pp. 556–564, 2012.

[3] P. Mitchell, F. Bandello, U. Schmidt-Erfurth et al., "The RESTORE study: ranibizumab monotherapy or combined with laser versus laser monotherapy for diabetic macular edema," *Ophthalmology*, vol. 118, no. 4, pp. 615–625, 2011.

[4] M. J. Elman, H. Qin, and L. P. Aiello, "Intravitreal ranibizumab for diabetic macular edema with prompt versus deferred laser treatment: three-year randomized trial results," *Ophthalmology*, vol. 119, no. 11, pp. 2312–2318, 2012.

[5] M. B. Sultan, D. Zhou, J. Loftus, T. Dombi, and K. S. Ice, "A phase 2/3, multicenter, randomized, double-masked, 2-year trial of pegaptanib sodium for the treatment of diabetic macular edema," *Ophthalmology*, vol. 118, no. 6, pp. 1107–1118, 2011.

[6] D. V. Do, Q. D. Nguyen, D. Boyer et al., "One-year outcomes of the da VINCI study of VEGF trap-eye in eyes with diabetic macular edema," *Ophthalmology*, vol. 119, no. 8, pp. 1658–1665, 2012.

[7] T. S. Kern, "Contributions of inflammatory processes to the development of the early stages of diabetic retinopathy," *Experimental Diabetes Research*, vol. 2007, Article ID 95103, 14 pages, 2007.

[8] E. A. Felinski and D. A. Antonetti, "Glucocorticoid regulation of endothelial cell tight junction gene expression: novel treatments for diabetic retinopathy," *Current Eye Research*, vol. 30, no. 11, pp. 949–957, 2005.

[9] M. Nauck, M. Roth, M. Tamm et al., "Induction of vascular endothelial growth factor by platelet-activating factor and platelet-derived growth factor is downregulated by corticosteroids," *American Journal of Respiratory Cell and Molecular Biology*, vol. 16, no. 4, pp. 398–406, 1997.

[10] J. E. Sears and G. Hoppe, "Triamcinolone acetonide destabilizes VEGF mRNA in Müller cells under continuous cobalt stimulation," *Investigative Ophthalmology & Visual Science*, vol. 46, no. 11, pp. 4336–4341, 2005.

[11] N. Ohguro, A. A. Okada, and Y. Tano, "Trans-Tenon's retrobulbar triamcinolone infusion for diffuse diabetic macular edema," *Graefe's Archive for Clinical and Experimental Ophthalmology*, vol. 242, no. 5, pp. 444–445, 2004.

[12] T. C. Ho and W. W. Lai, "Intravitreal cortisone injection for refractory diffuse diabetic macular edema," *Ophthalmologica*, vol. 220, no. 5, pp. 349–350, 2006.

[13] T. Sakamoto, T. Hida, Y. Tano et al., "Committee for Triamcinolone Acetonide for Ocular Disease in Japan: survey of triamcinolone acetonide for ocular diseases in Japan," *Nihon Ganka Gakkai Zasshi*, vol. 111, no. 12, pp. 936–945, 2007.

[14] S. Nonomura, T. Oshitari, M. Arai et al., "The effect of posterior sub-Tenon's capsule triamcinolone acetonide injection to that of pars plana vitrectomy for diabetic macular edema," *Clinical Ophthalmology*, vol. 8, pp. 825–830, 2014.

[15] H.-P. Qi, S. Bi, S.-Q. Wei, H. Cui, and J.-B. Zhao, "Intravitreal versus subtenon triamcinolone acetonide injection for diabetic macular edema: a systematic review and meta-analysis," *Current Eye Research*, vol. 37, no. 12, pp. 1136–1147, 2012.

[16] Y. Takatsuna, S. Yamamoto, Y. Nakamura, T. Tatsumi, M. Arai, and Y. Mitamura, "Long-term therapeutic efficacy of the subthreshold micropulse diode laser photocoagulation for diabetic macular edema," *Japanese Journal of Ophthalmology*, vol. 55, no. 4, pp. 365–369, 2011.

[17] M. L. Ribeiro, S. G. Nunes, and J. G. Cunha-Vaz, "Microaneurysm turnover at the macula predicts risk of development of clinically significant macular edema in persons with mild nonproliferative diabetic retinopathy," *Diabetes Care*, vol. 36, no. 5, pp. 1254–1259, 2013.

[18] C. Haritoglou, M. Kernt, A. Neubauer et al., "Microaneurysm formation rate as a predictive marker for progression to clinically significant macular edema in nonproliferative diabetic retinopathy," *Retina*, vol. 34, no. 1, pp. 157–164, 2014.

[19] R. Klein, B. E. K. Klein, S. E. Moss, and K. J. Cruickshanks, "The Wisconsin epidemiologic study of diabetic retinopathy. XV. The long-term incidence of macular edema," *Ophthalmology*, vol. 102, no. 1, pp. 7–16, 1995.

[20] T.-H. Chou, P.-C. Wu, J. Z.-C. Kuo, C.-H. Lai, and C.-N. Kuo, "Relationship of diabetic macular oedema with glycosylated haemoglobin," *Eye*, vol. 23, no. 6, pp. 1360–1363, 2009.

[21] D. S. Fong and R. Contreras, "Glitazone use associated with diabetic macular edema," *American Journal of Ophthalmology*, vol. 147, no. 4, pp. 583.e1–586.e1, 2009.

[22] I. Idris, G. Warren, and R. Donnelly, "Association between thiazolidinedione treatment and risk of macular edema among patients with type 2 diabetes," *Archives of Internal Medicine*, vol. 172, no. 13, pp. 1005–1011, 2012.

[23] T. Oshitari, N. Asaumi, M. Watanabe, K. Kumagai, and Y. Mitamura, "Severe macular edema induced by pioglitazone in a patient with diabetic retinopathy: a case study," *Vascular Health and Risk Management*, vol. 4, no. 5, pp. 1137–1140, 2008.

Intraoperative Corneal Thickness Changes during Pulsed Accelerated Corneal Cross-Linking Using Isotonic Riboflavin with HPMC

Ahmed M. Sherif,[1] Nihal A. El-Gheriany,[1] Yehia M. Salah El-Din,[1] Lamiaa S. Aly,[1] Amr A. Osman,[1] Michael A. Grentzelos,[2] and George D. Kymionis[2,3]

[1] Department of Ophthalmology, Faculty of Medicine, Cairo University, Cairo 11519, Egypt
[2] Vardinoyiannion Eye Institute of Crete (VEIC), Faculty of Medicine, University of Crete, Heraklion, 71003 Crete, Greece
[3] Bascom Palmer Eye Institute, University of Miami, Miller School of Medicine, Miami, FL 33136, USA

Correspondence should be addressed to Ahmed M. Sherif; asherif1975@yahoo.com

Academic Editor: Neil Lagali

Purpose. To evaluate corneal thickness changes during pulsed accelerated corneal cross-linking (CXL) for keratoconus using a new isotonic riboflavin formula. *Methods.* In this prospective, interventional, clinical study patients with grades 1-2 keratoconus (Amsler-Krumeich classification) underwent pulsed accelerated (30 mW/cm^2) CXL after application of an isotonic riboflavin solution (0.1%) with HPMC for 10 minutes. Central corneal thickness (CCT) measurements were taken using ultrasound pachymetry before and after epithelial removal, after riboflavin soaking, and immediately after completion of UVA treatment. *Results.* Twenty eyes of 11 patients (4 males, 7 females) were enrolled. Mean patient age was 26 ± 3 (range from 18 to 30 years). No intraoperative or postoperative complications were observed in any of the patients. Mean CCT was 507 ± 35 μm (range: 559–459 μm) before and 475 ± 40 μm (range: 535–420 μm) after epithelial removal ($P < 0.001$). After 10 minutes of riboflavin instillation, there was a statistically significant decrease of CCT by 6.2% from 475±40 μm (range: 535–420 μm) to 446±31 μm (range: 508–400) ($P < 0.005$). There was no other statistically significant change of CCT during UVA irradiation. *Conclusions.* A significant decrease of corneal thickness was demonstrated during the isotonic riboflavin with HPMC application while there was no significant change during the pulsed accelerated UVA irradiation.

1. Introduction

Corneal cross-linking (CXL) is a minimally invasive procedure that combines the use of riboflavin and ultraviolet-A (UVA) irradiation resulting in an increase of the biomechanical stability of the corneal tissue [1, 2]. A preoperative corneal thickness of 400 μm as a minimum safety limit to avoid corneal endothelial damage during CXL has been proposed [3]. However, endothelial failure has been reported very occasionally after CXL resulting in corneal edema postoperatively [4, 5]. The etiology of such problems has not been fully elucidated but may be due to severe stromal thinning intraoperatively which has been reported by several authors [6, 7]. Hence, it has become important to monitor corneal thickness during the procedure.

Accelerated CXL is based on the Bunsen-Roscoe law of reciprocity according to which reducing irradiation time and correspondingly increasing irradiation intensity could achieve the same photochemical effect.

The aim of this study was to evaluate the intraoperative pachymetric changes during CXL using isotonic riboflavin (0.1%) and HPMC (hydroxyl propyl methylcellulose, HPMC; VibeX Rapid, Avedro Inc., Waltham, MS, USA) and pulsed accelerated UVA.

2. Materials and Methods

In this prospective, interventional, clinical study patients with grades 1-2 keratoconus (Amsler-Krumeich classification) were enrolled. All patients underwent pulsed high intensity CXL using the KXL system (Avedro Inc., Waltham, MS, USA) preceded by the application of an isotonic riboflavin (0.1%) and HPMC (hydroxyl propyl methylcellulose, HPMC; VibeX Rapid, Avedro Inc., Waltham, MS, USA) for 10 minutes at Eye Care Center, Maadi, Cairo, Egypt, between August 2014 and February 2015. The study was conducted within the tenets of the Declaration of Helsinki after obtaining the institutional review board approval. A written informed consent was obtained from all patients.

Inclusion criteria were progressive keratoconus (progression was confirmed if there was an increase in the K_{max} on Pentacam maps of 1.00 diopter [D], increase of manifest refraction cylinder of 1.00 D, or increase of manifest refraction spherical equivalent of 0.50 D over the period of one year) and corneal thickness more than 400 μm at the thinnest location. Exclusion criteria were corneal scars or opacities, pregnancy or lactation, active anterior segment pathologic features, previous corneal or anterior segment surgery, systemic connective tissue disease, atopic syndrome, and dry eye syndrome. Preoperative data obtained from the case records included patient age and gender, Pentacam central corneal thickness (CCT) and thinnest corneal thickness (TCT) values, and CCT values obtained by ultrasonic corneal pachymetry (Sonomed 300P PacScan Pachymeter; Escalon Medical Corp.), which takes the mean of 256 measurements in each scan.

2.1. Surgical Technique. Corneal cross-linking (CXL) was conducted under sterile conditions. One drop of pilocarpine 1% eye drops was instilled 15 minutes before the procedure. After topical application of benoxinate hydrochloride 0.4% eye drops (Benox; Eipico Inc., Cairo, Egypt), an eye speculum was placed and CCT was measured just before epithelial removal. The probe tip of the ultrasonic pachymetry was disinfected using alcohol swab and was held perpendicular to the cornea. Three consecutive measurements were obtained at the center of the cornea of each eye; the thinnest measurement is used in the statistical analysis. Then, the central 8 mm of the corneal epithelium was removed mechanically using a blunt spatula. After corneal epithelial removal, CCT was measured. Next, dextran-free riboflavin 0.1% with hydroxyl propyl methylcellulose (HPMC; VibeX Rapid, Avedro Inc., Waltham, MS, USA) was instilled every 2 minutes for 10 minutes after which CCT was remeasured. Pulsed accelerated UVA irradiation was next performed using KXL system (Avedro Inc., Waltham, MS, USA) with 1 sec. on/1 sec. off of UVA irradiation of 30 mW/cm^2 for a total duration of 8 minutes and 40 seconds. A final CCT measurement was obtained immediately after completion of UVA irradiation. A therapeutic contact lens was applied and removed at the 3rd postoperative day after complete reepithelialization.

2.2. Statistical Analysis. Statistical analysis was done using paired *t*-test. Statistical Package for the Social Sciences (SPSS) v.16 was used.

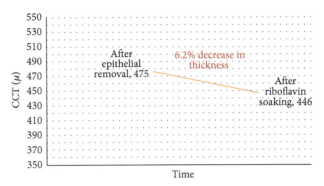

FIGURE 1: CCT changes (in microns) after riboflavin soaking.

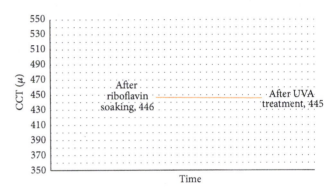

FIGURE 2: CCT changes (in microns) during UVA treatment.

Because both eyes of some patients were used in the study, a nested analysis of variance was used to correct for any correlation between the right and left eyes of the same subject. P value less than 0.05 was considered significant.

3. Results

Twenty eyes of 11 patients were included. Four were males and 7 were females. Mean patient age was 26 ± 3 (range from 18 to 30 years). No intraoperative or postoperative complications were observed in any of the patients.

Mean USP CCT was 506.85 ± 35.4 μm (range: 559–459 μm) before and 474.9 ± 39.75 μm (range: 535–420 μm) after epithelial removal ($P < 0.001$). After 10 minutes of riboflavin installation, there was a statistically significant decrease of CCT by 6.2% (31.95 ± 8.08 μm) from 474.9 ± 39.75 μm (range: 535–420 μm) to 445.7 ± 31.18 μm (range: 508–400 μm) ($P < 0.005$) (Figure 1). There was no statistically significant change of the CCT during UVA irradiation; CCT was 444.65 ± 34.53 μm (range: 521–400 μm) at the end of UVA irradiation ($P = 0.61$) (Figure 2). However, there was a statistically significant decrease by 62.2 ± 34.64 μm in CCT from 506.85 ± 35.4 μm (range: 559–459 μm) before epithelial removal to 444.65 ± 34.53 μm (range: 521–400 μm) at the end of CXL ($P < 0.001$). Results are summarized in Table 1.

TABLE 1: Summary of central epithelial thickness changes.

CCT in microns	Mean	Standard deviation	Maximum	Minimum
Preoperative Pentacam CCT	514.9	±33.12	561	470
Preoperative USP CCT	506.85	±35.4	559	459
USP CCT after epithelial removal	474.9	±39.75	535	420
USP CCT after riboflavin	445.7	±31.18	508	400
USP CCT after UVA	444.65	±34.53	521	400

CCT: central corneal thickness, USP: ultrasound pachymetry, and UVA: ultraviolet.

4. Discussion

Several studies have already reported the intraoperative corneal thickness changes during the CXL procedure using several riboflavin formulas and different UVA settings. Most of the studies evaluated the classic Dresden protocol according to which riboflavin-dextran solution was applied for 30 minutes followed by 30 minutes of UVA 3 mW/cm^2. Thus, Kymionis et al. reported a 20% decrease in CCT after 30 minutes of riboflavin instillation [6]. Mazzotta and Caragiuli observed 32% decrease after 30 minutes of riboflavin-dextran solution instillation; at 10 minutes of the 30-minute instillation procedure the CCT decrease was almost 18% [7]. Hassan et al. showed 23.76% decrease after 15 minutes of riboflavin application [8]. They all reported no corneal thickness changes during UVA treatment [6–8]. However, Tahzib et al. showed stable CCT values after riboflavin solution instillation, which might be attributed to the fact that they removed the eye speculum during riboflavin application [9]. Soeters et al. indicated that avoidance of an eyelid speculum during riboflavin instillation resulted in less CCT reduction [10].

The use of isotonic riboflavin solution without dextran has been suggested to avoid the dehydrating effect of dextran on the corneal stroma. Çinar et al. showed swelling of the cornea instead of corneal thinning after 30 minutes of isotonic riboflavin solution without dextran during CXL procedure [11]. In a comparative study, Oltulu et al. evaluated the corneal thickness changes during CXL performed with isotonic riboflavin solution with and without dextran; the use of riboflavin solution without dextran during CXL caused a steady increase in the corneal thickness during the procedure [12]. Recently, Jain et al. demonstrated no significant decline in the corneal thickness after CXL using isotonic riboflavin with HPMC with accelerated CXL [13].

In this clinical study, an isotonic dextran-free riboflavin formula with HPMC (HPMC; VibeX Rapid, Avedro Inc., Waltham, MS, USA) was used in combination with pulsed accelerated UVA using the KXL system (Avedro Inc., Waltham, MS, USA). The addition of HPMC to 0.1% riboflavin aims to avoid the dehydrating effect of dextran while maintaining adequate concentration of riboflavin into the stroma through its viscosity. After 10 minutes of riboflavin solution instillation, there was a statistically significant decrease of CCT by 6.2% ($31.95 \pm 8.08\ \mu m$) from $475 \pm 40\ \mu m$ (range: 535–420 μm) to $446 \pm 31\ \mu m$ (range: 508–400 μm). There was no other statistically significant change of the CCT during UVA irradiation.

It seems that there was a lesser reduction of CCT in our study compared to previous studies in which riboflavin with dextran was used [7–9]. In the study of Jain et al., no significant difference was found after 20 minutes of isotonic riboflavin with HPMC [13]. However, they did not perform pachymetry measurement at 10 minutes of the 20-minute UVA irradiation process [13]. In our study, we performed a 10-minute riboflavin instillation process and a 6.2% CCT decrease was measured after 10 minutes of isotonic riboflavin with HPMC instillation. In any case, it seems that isotonic riboflavin with HPMC may lead to a significant decrease in the corneal thickness during the instillation process of the CXL procedure, but less than the decrease reported in previous studies using riboflavin-dextran solution [6–8]. Therefore, this riboflavin formula might be actually safer for CXL especially for keratoconic patients with borderline preoperative corneal thickness (near to 400 μm).

Potential limitations of the study included the small sample size, the fact that repeated central corneal thickness, measured by ultrasound pachymetry, is strongly affected by exact centration of the probe on cornea on each measurement, and the fact that the gradient of thickness variation is strong particularly in keratoconic corneas. Taking into consideration that each scan with the Sonomed 300P pachymeter takes the mean of 256 measurements, 3 scans were performed with the thinnest measurement (the lowest mean of 256 measurements) in an attempt to respect the safety aspect during planning or conduction of the procedure.

Pentacam or AS-OCT is much better for corneal thickness assessment than ultrasound pachymetry, especially when a two-dimensional surface is to be analyzed for the thinnest point, but in our study, it was not possible to use the Pentacam intraoperatively for measurements after epithelial removal, after riboflavin, and after UVA exposure as the procedure was performed under aseptic techniques in the operation theater while the Pentacam device is not portable. Repeated transfer of the patient between the operating theater and the investigation unit was judged not feasible due to patient discomfort, the potential risk of contamination, and corneal dehydration.

Preoperative Pentacam CCT values were recorded but were not used instead of the preoperative contact pachymetry CCT values to avoid the bias of using one measurement device preoperatively and another type of measurement device intraoperatively.

In conclusion, a significant corneal pachymetric decrease was demonstrated after 10 minutes of isotonic riboflavin with HPMC instillation during pulsed accelerated CXL. This decrement was less than the reduction observed in previous studies using riboflavin-dextran solution [7–9]. There was no corneal thickness change during pulsed accelerated UVA irradiation. These findings suggest that isotonic riboflavin with HPMC might be useful in CXL treatment of keratoconic patients with thin corneas. Further randomized controlled trials with larger sample sizes are needed to validate these observations.

Conflict of Interests

The authors have no financial or proprietary interests in any materials or methods described herein.

References

[1] G. Wollensak, E. Spoerl, and T. Seiler, "Riboflavin/ultraviolet-A—induced collagen crosslinking for the treatment of keratoconus," *American Journal of Ophthalmology*, vol. 135, no. 5, pp. 620–627, 2003.

[2] G. D. Kymionis, M. A. Grentzelos, D. A. Liakopoulos et al., "Long-term follow-up of corneal collagen cross-linking for keratoconus—the Cretan study," *Cornea*, vol. 33, no. 10, pp. 1071–1079, 2014.

[3] G. Wollensak, "Crosslinking treatment of progressive keratoconus: new hope," *Current Opinion in Ophthalmology*, vol. 17, no. 4, pp. 356–360, 2006.

[4] A. Sharma, J. M. Nottage, K. Mirchia, R. Sharma, K. Mohan, and V. S. Nirankari, "Persistent corneal edema after collagen cross-linking for keratoconus," *American Journal of Ophthalmology*, vol. 154, no. 6, pp. 922.e1–926.e1, 2012.

[5] B. Bagga, S. Pahuja, S. Murthy, and V. S. Sangwan, "Endothelial failure after collagen cross-linking with riboflavin and UV-A: case report with literature review," *Cornea*, vol. 31, no. 10, pp. 1197–1200, 2012.

[6] G. D. Kymionis, G. A. Kounis, D. M. Portaliou et al., "Intraoperative pachymetric measurements during corneal collagen cross-linking with riboflavin and ultraviolet A irradiation," *Ophthalmology*, vol. 116, no. 12, pp. 2336–2339, 2009.

[7] C. Mazzotta and S. Caragiuli, "Intraoperative corneal thickness measurement by optical coherence tomography in keratoconic patients undergoing corneal collagen cross-linking," *American Journal of Ophthalmology*, vol. 157, no. 6, pp. 1156–1162, 2014.

[8] Z. Hassan, L. Modis Jr., E. Szalai, A. Berta, and G. Nemeth, "Intraoperative and postoperative corneal thickness change after collagen crosslinking therapy," *European Journal of Ophthalmology*, vol. 24, no. 2, pp. 179–185, 2013.

[9] N. G. Tahzib, N. Soeters, and A. Van der Lelij, "Pachymetry during cross-linking," *Ophthalmology*, vol. 117, no. 10, pp. 2041–2041.e1, 2010.

[10] N. Soeters, E. van Bussel, R. van der Valk, A. van der Lelij, and N. G. Tahzib, "Effect of the eyelid speculum on pachymetry during corneal collagen crosslinking in keratoconus patients," *Journal of Cataract and Refractive Surgery*, vol. 40, no. 4, pp. 575–581, 2014.

[11] Y. Çinar, A. K. Cingü, A. Şahin, F. M. Türkcü, H. Yüksel, and I. Caca, "Intraoperative corneal thickness measurements during corneal collagen cross-linking with isotonic riboflavin solution without dextran in corneal ectasia," *Cutaneous and Ocular Toxicology*, vol. 33, no. 1, pp. 28–31, 2014.

[12] R. Oltulu, G. Şatirtav, M. Donbaloğlu, H. Kerimoğlu, A. Özkağnici, and A. Karaibrahimoğlu, "Intraoperative corneal thickness monitoring during corneal collagen cross-linking with isotonic riboflavin solution with and without dextran," *Cornea*, vol. 33, no. 11, pp. 1164–1167, 2014.

[13] V. Jain, Z. Gazali, and R. Bidayi, "Isotonic riboflavin and HPMC with accelerated cross-linking protocol," *Cornea*, vol. 33, no. 9, pp. 910–913, 2014.

Acute-Onset Vitreous Hemorrhage of Unknown Origin before Vitrectomy: Causes and Prognosis

Dong Yoon Kim,[1] Soo Geun Joe,[2] Seunghee Baek,[3] June-Gone Kim,[4] Young Hee Yoon,[4] and Joo Yong Lee[4]

[1]*Department of Ophthalmology, College of Medicine, Chungbuk National University, Cheongju, Republic of Korea*
[2]*Department of Ophthalmology, Gangneung Asan Hospital, University of Ulsan, College of Medicine, Gangneung, Republic of Korea*
[3]*Department of Clinical Epidemiology and Biostatistics, Asan Medical Center, University of Ulsan, College of Medicine, Seoul, Republic of Korea*
[4]*Department of Ophthalmology, Asan Medical Center, University of Ulsan, College of Medicine, 88 Olympic-ro 43-gil, Songpa-gu, Seoul 138-736, Republic of Korea*

Correspondence should be addressed to Joo Yong Lee; ophthalmo@amc.seoul.kr

Academic Editor: Zhongfeng Wang

Purpose. To analyze causes and prognosis of acute-onset preoperatively unknown origin vitreous hemorrhage (VH). *Methods.* This study included patients who underwent vitrectomy for acute-onset preoperatively unknown origin VH. The underlying causes of VH, which were identified after vitrectomy, were analyzed. And overall visual prognosis of unknown origin VH was analyzed. Risk scoring system was developed to predict visual prognosis after vitrectomy. *Results.* 169 eyes were included. Among these, retinal vein occlusion (RVO), retinal break, and age-related macular degeneration (AMD) were identified in 74 (43.8%), 50 (29.6%), and 21 (12.4%) patients, respectively. After vitrectomy, logMAR BCVA significantly improved from 1.93 ± 0.59 to 0.47 ± 0.71. However, postoperative BCVA in AMD eyes were significantly poorer than others. Poor visual prognosis after vitrectomy was associated with old age, poor preoperative vision in both eyes, and drusen in the fellow eye. *Conclusions.* RVO, retinal break, and AMD are the most common causes of acute-onset preoperatively unknown origin VH and the most common causes of VH change with age. The visual prognosis of unknown origin VH is relatively good, except among AMD patients. Older patients with poor preoperative BCVA in both eyes and patients with AMD in the fellow eye are at a higher risk of poor visual prognosis following vitrectomy.

1. Introduction

The annual incidence of acute-onset vitreous hemorrhage (VH) in the general population is 7 cases per 100,000 persons [1]. The causes of VH include proliferative diabetic retinopathy (PDR), trauma, retinal break, proliferative retinopathy after retinal vein occlusion (RVO), and posterior vitreous detachment without retinal detachment [2–6]. It is important to determine the underlying cause of acute-onset VH because the natural history and visual prognosis depend on the underlying cause. The visual prognosis of VH caused by retinal break, posterior vitreous detachment, and branch RVO is relatively good [4, 6–10]. However, the visual prognosis of VH secondary to PDR and exudative age-related macular degeneration (AMD) is poor due to recurrent VH, tractional retinal detachment, and submacular hemorrhage [11–14].

VH caused by a retinal break may be less severe and resolve more rapidly. Therefore, upright head position and immobilization of the patient allow blood to settle down in the eye, eventually clearing VH [4, 10, 15]. In cases of VH caused by retinal neovascularization due to diabetic retinopathy or RVO, peripheral laser photocoagulation can regress the abnormal vessels, which may lead to VH.

However, in some cases, it is difficult to determine the underlying cause of acute-onset VH. Lean and Gregor reported that 14% of acute-onset VH eyes were diagnosed on follow-up examination and 4% remained undiagnosed after 1 year [4]. Little is known about the causes and visual prognosis of acute-onset VH of preoperatively unknown origin. Here, we analyzed the causes and overall visual prognosis of acute-onset VH of preoperatively unknown origin. We also analyzed the characteristics of the fellow eye in all patients. In addition, we generated a risk scoring system (RSS) to predict visual prognosis of acute-onset preoperatively unknown origin VH.

2. Materials and Methods

2.1. Study Design and Participants. This retrospective review was conducted on patients who underwent vitrectomy for acute-onset VH of preoperatively unknown origin at Asan Medical Center, Seoul, Republic of Korea, between January 2007 and June 2013. The following inclusion criteria were applied: (1) a history of 3-port pars plana vitrectomy for acute-onset VH, with or without cataract surgery, and (2) the cause of acute-onset VH could not be preoperatively identified because of dense VH which prevented retinal examination. Exclusion criteria included eyes with other ocular diseases that might affect vision, active intraocular inflammation and/or infection, and VH caused by trauma. Patients with more than mild nonproliferative diabetic retinopathy in the fellow eye and those with grades III–IV AMD (AREDS (age-related eye disease study) classification) in the fellow eye were also excluded. This study was approved by the institutional review board of Asan Medical Center and followed the tenets of the Declaration of Helsinki (2014-0358).

2.2. Primary and Secondary Objectives. The primary objective of this study was to analyze the causes of acute-onset VH of preoperatively unknown origin. The secondary objectives of this study were to determine (1) the causes of acute-onset VH of preoperatively unknown origin according to age, (2) the visual prognosis of acute-onset VH of preoperatively unknown origin, (3) differences in the baseline characteristics according to postoperative diagnosis, and (4) characteristics of the fellow eye and (5) to devise an RSS for predicting the visual prognosis of acute-onset VH of preoperatively unknown origin.

2.3. Ophthalmic Examinations. All included patients underwent a complete bilateral ophthalmic examination, including determination of BCVA using the Snellen chart. BCVA results were converted to the logMAR scale. Patients who were only able to count fingers, were only able to detect hand motion, had light perception, or had no light perception were assigned logMAR values 2.0, 2.3, 2.7, and 3.0, respectively [16]. All patients also underwent biomicroscopic examination, dilated fundus examination, and fundus photography of both eyes. Ultrasonography was performed on all eyes with VH of preoperatively unknown origin.

2.4. Identification of Causes of Acute-Onset VH of Preoperatively Unknown Origin. The postoperative diagnosis of acute-onset VH of preoperatively unknown origin was identified by thorough review of each patient's medical records. We divided all included patients according to age ($\leq$60, 60–70, and >70 years), and the causes of VH were analyzed according to age.

2.5. Surgical Procedures. Vitrectomy was performed by well-experienced retinal surgeons (Joo Yong Lee, June-Gone Kim, and Young Hee Yoon). A 20-gauge, 23-gauge, and 25-gauge vitrectomy system was used to perform 3-port vitrectomy. Cataracts were extracted by phacoemulsification if the crystalline lens had significant opacity. After resolving the VH, which obscured retinal inspection, we attempted to determine the cause of VH and recorded the underlying cause of VH as an operative note. After completing vitrectomy, eyes with retinal break received perfluoropropane (C_3F_8) gas tamponade. For complicated cases, such as those with severe tractional retinal detachment or multiple retinal breaks, silicone oil tamponade was performed. The silicone oil was removed 6 months later.

2.6. Statistical Analysis. One-way ANOVA and the Bonferroni post test were used to analyze the visual prognosis of VH according to the postoperative diagnosis. According to the postoperative diagnosis, the clinical characteristics were analyzed using one-way ANOVA with the Bonferroni post test and Pearson Chi-square test. Finally, to develop an RSS for predicting visual prognosis of acute-onset VH of preoperatively unknown origin, multivariate logistic regression modeling was performed. Risk factors were selected using backward elimination from the full logistic model. Model discrimination was estimated using C-tatistic (or AUC), and calibration was assessed by determining agreement between the predicted and recorded prognosis of acute-onset VH of preoperatively unknown origin. We ran an internal validation of discrimination (C-statistic) to produce optimism-corrected values of the C-statistic by using bootstrapping with 500 replications of individuals that were sampled with replacement [17]. After considering the internally validated variables, we developed a scoring system using the model parameter estimates described by Sullivan et al. [18]. ROC curves from the original model and scoring system are presented. SPSS (version 21.0; SPSS, Inc., Chicago, IL) and R 3.0.2 (free software that can be downloaded at http://www.r-project.org/) with package "boot" and "pROC" were used to perform the statistical analyses.

3. Results

In total, 2031 eyes in 2031 patients underwent vitrectomy for VH at Asan Medical Center between January 2007 and June 2013. Among these 2031 patients, the underlying cause of VH was not identified in 169 eyes in 169 patients (8.3%), and these patients therefore satisfied the inclusion criteria for enrollment.

3.1. Primary Objective. The postoperative diagnoses of acute-onset VH of preoperatively unknown origin are listed in Table 1. RVO (74 eyes, 43.8%) was the most common cause.

TABLE 1: Causes of acute-onset vitreous hemorrhage (VH) of preoperatively unknown origin.

Underlying causes of VH	Eyes, n (%)
Retinal vein occlusion	74 (43.8%)
Central retinal vein occlusion (CRVO)	0/74 (0.0%)
Branch retinal vein occlusion (BRVO)	74/74 (100.0%)
BRVO with foveal involvement	10/74 (13.5%)
Vitreous hemorrhage with retinal break	50 (29.6%)
Age-related macular degeneration	21 (12.4%)
Macroaneurysm	8 (4.7%)
Eales disease	3 (1.8%)
Coats' disease	1 (0.6%)
Idiopathic	12 (7.1%)
Total	169 (100%)

All RVO eyes had branch retinal vein occlusion (BRVO). There were no cases of central or hemiretinal vein occlusion. Among the 74 eyes with BRVO, foveal involvement was only found in 10 eyes (13.5%). Fifty (29.6%), 21 (12.4%), and 8 (4.7%) eyes were diagnosed with retinal break, wet age-related macular degeneration (wAMD), or retinal arterial macroaneurysm, respectively, as the cause of preoperatively unknown VH. In 12 eyes (7.1%), we could not identify any retinal pathology even after vitrectomy.

3.2. Secondary Objectives. The causes of acute-onset VH of preoperatively unknown origin according to age are shown in Figure 1. We divided all included patients according to age (≤60, 60–70, and >70 years). In patients aged ≤60 years, retinal break was the most common cause of acute-onset VH of preoperatively unknown origin; however, the proportion of patients with retinal break declined with age. By contrast, the proportion of patients with wAMD increased with age. Among patients aged >60 years, RVO was the most common cause of acute-onset VH of preoperatively unknown origin. Visual prognoses according to postoperative diagnosis are shown in Figure 2. After vitrectomy, logMAR BCVA improved from 1.93 ± 0.59 to 0.47 ± 0.71. Preoperative logMAR BCVA significantly differed according to the postoperative diagnosis. The preoperative logMAR BCVA values of the wAMD patients were significantly poorer than those of other patients (wAMD, 2.37 ± 0.36; RVO, 1.87 ± 0.58; retinal break, 1.97 ± 0.57; $p = 0.001$). The postoperative logMAR BCVA values of the wAMD patients were also significantly worse than those of other patients (wAMD, 1.65 ± 0.88; RVO, 0.30 ± 0.43; retinal break, 0.21 ± 0.40; $p < 0.001$). Visual acuity changes after vitrectomy according to postoperative diagnosis are shown in Figure 2. BCVA significantly improved after vitrectomy among the RVO, retinal break, and idiopathic patients. However, vision did not improve after vitrectomy in wAMD patients.

The clinical characteristics of VH according to postoperative diagnoses are listed in Table 2. Mean age significantly differed according to the postoperative diagnosis. The mean age of the wAMD patients was significantly higher than that of the patients with RVO or retinal break (wAMD, 73.29 ± 8.30

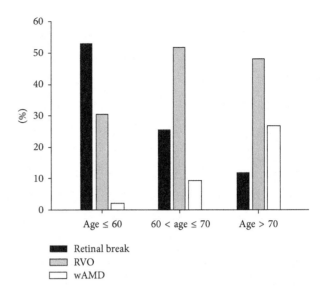

FIGURE 1: Causes of acute-onset vitreous hemorrhage of unknown origin according to age. Among patients aged ≤60 years, retinal break was the main cause of acute-onset VH of preoperatively unknown origin. Moreover, the proportion of cases of acute-onset VH of preoperatively unknown origin that was due to retinal break declined with age. In contrast to retinal break, the proportion of vitreous hemorrhage due to wAMD increased with age. Among patients aged >60 years, RVO was the most common cause of acute-onset VH of preoperatively unknown origin. RVO, retinal vein occlusion; wAMD, wet age-related macular degeneration.

years; RVO, 65.36 ± 9.82 years; retinal break, 58.50 ± 11.78 years; $p = 0.001$). Systemic hypertension was more frequently associated with RVO and wAMD patients. The characteristics of the fellow eyes among patients with acute-onset VH of preoperatively unknown origin are shown in Table 3. The logMAR BCVA values of the fellow eyes in wAMD patients were also significantly lower than in other patients (wAMD, 0.44 ± 0.45; RVO, 0.17 ± 0.38; retinal break, 0.05 ± 0.09; $p < 0.001$). Drusen was more significant in the fellow eyes of wAMD patients than in those of patients with RVO or retinal break (RVO, 6.8%; wAMD, 71.4%; retinal break, 2.0%; $p < 0.001$).

The RSSs used to predict poor visual outcomes after vitrectomy among patients with acute-onset preoperatively unknown origin VH are shown in Table 4, and the risk scores of the included acute-onset VH of preoperatively unknown origin patients are shown in Table 5. The multivariate logistic regression model shows that old age, poor preoperative visual acuity in both the affected and fellow eyes, and drusen in the fellow eye were significantly associated with a poor visual prognosis after vitrectomy. The AUC of the scoring system was 0.907 (95% confidence interval [CI] = 0.853–0.948). Internal validation was investigated using the bootstrap validation algorithm. The optimism-corrected AUC was 0.898, which indicates the reliability of the RSS (Figure 3). In this RSS model, the maximal summation of risk score was −25. Therefore, to prevent obtaining a negative integer for the risk score, we added 25 to each estimated risk score.

TABLE 2: Clinical characteristics of acute-onset vitreous hemorrhage (VH) of preoperatively unknown origin.

	All	RVO	wAMD	Retinal break	Other	p
Number of eyes	169	77	21	50	24	0.001
Age (y)	63.64 ± 12.37	65.36 ± 9.82	73.29 ± 8.30	58.50 ± 11.78	60.63 ± 17.14	<0.001*
Sex (male/female)	83/86	33/41	11/10	31/19	8/16	0.216†
Right/left	88/81	38/36	9/12	29/21	12/12	0.093†
Follow-up duration (mo.)	13.24 ± 14.52	11.34 ± 11.59	15.62 ± 19.19	15.56 ± 17.00	12.21 ± 12.49	0.360*
Gauge of surgery						0.098†
20-gauge	19/169 (11.2%)	10/74 (13.5%)	5/21 (23.8%)	3/50 (6.0%)	1/24 (4.2%)	
23/25-gauge	150/169 (88.8%)	64/74 (86.5%)	16/21 (76.2%)	47/50 (94.0%)	23/24 (95.8%)	
Tamponade						<0.001†
No tamponade	56/169 (33.1%)	34/74 (45.9%)	4/21 (19.0%)	9/50 (18.0%)	9/24 (37.5%)	
Air	55/169 (32.5%)	32/74 (43.2%)	1/21 (4.8%)	13/50 (26.0%)	9/24 (37.5%)	
C_3F_8	24/169 (14.2%)	3/74 (4.1%)	1/21 (4.8%)	19/50 (38.0%)	1/24 (4.2%)	
Silicone oil	34/169 (20.1%)	5/74 (6.8%)	15/21 (71.4%)	9/50 (18.0%)	5/24 (20.8%)	
Systemic disease						
Hypertension	92/169 (54.4%)	48/74 (64.9%)	13/21 (61.9%)	17/50 (34.0%)	14/24 (54.4%)	0.006†
Duration (y)	8.44 ± 7.85	8.55 ± 8.46	6.92 ± 5.39	6.90 ± 5.52	11.57 ± 9.76	0.329*
Diabetes	20/169 (11.8%)	9/74 (12.2%)	2/21 (9.5%)	7/50 (14/0%)	2/24 (8.3%)	0.891†
Duration (y)	9.56 ± 8.46	7.56 ± 4.95	6.50 ± 4.95	12.71 ± 4.45	13.44 ± 9.50	0.658*
Anticoagulant	51/169 (30.2%)	34/74 (45.9%)	3/21 (14.3%)	8/50 (16.0%)	6/24 (25.0%)	0.001†

RVO, retinal vein occlusion; wAMD, wet age-related macular degeneration.
*According to one-way ANOVA with the Bonferroni post test.
†According to the Chi-square test.

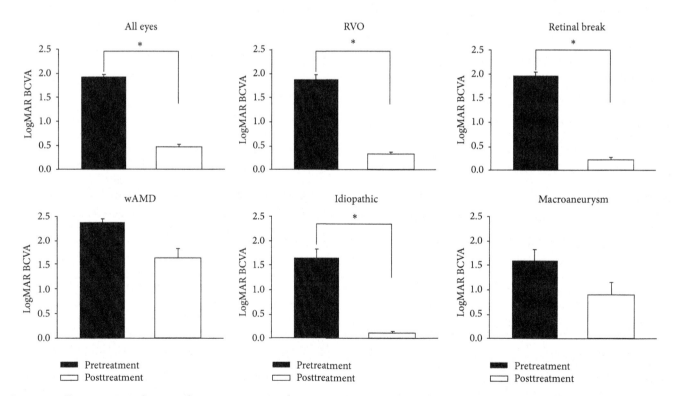

FIGURE 2: Changes in visual acuity after vitrectomy according to postoperative diagnosis. In the retinal vein occlusion, retinal break, and idiopathic groups, BCVA significantly improved after vitrectomy. However, visual improvement was not seen after vitrectomy among patients with wet age-related macular degeneration.

TABLE 3: Findings in the fellow eye of acute-onset vitreous hemorrhage (VH) of preoperatively unknown origin.

	All	RVO	wAMD	Retinal break	p
LogMAR BCVA	0.19 ± 0.46	0.17 ± 0.38	0.44 ± 0.45	0.05 ± 0.09	<0.001*
Fundus finding					
Normal	131/169 (77.5%)	61/74 (82.4%)	4/21 (19.0%)	45/50 (90.0%)	<0.001†
Drusen	21/169 (12.4%)	5/74 (6.8%)	15/21 (71.4%)	1/50 (2.0%)	<0.001†
Retinal break	5/169 (3.0%)	0/74 (0.0%)	0/21 (0.0%)	4/50 (8.0%)	0.020
RVO	1/169 (0.6%)	3/74 (4.1%)	1/21 (4.8%)	0/50 (0.0%)	0.334
Others	8/169 (4.7%)	5/74 (6.8%)	1/21 (4.8%)	0/50 (0.0%)	0.177

BCVA, best-corrected visual acuity; RVO, retinal vein occlusion; wAMD, wet age-related macular degeneration; AMD, age-related macular degeneration.
*According to one-way ANOVA with the Bonferroni post test.
†According to the Chi-square test.

TABLE 4: Risk scoring system used to predict poor visual outcomes after vitrectomy in patients with acute-onset vitreous hemorrhage (VH) of preoperatively unknown origin.

Categories	Reference value (W)	Beta	Beta($W - W_{ref}$)	Point = beta($W - W_{ref}$)/B [Clarify]	Score
Age					
24–40	33.5 (W_{ref})		0	0	0
40–49	44.5		−0.043	−1.0000854	−1
50–59	54.5	−0.004	−0.082	−1.9092539	−2
60–69	64.5		−0.121	−2.8184224	−3
>70	78.5		−0.176	−4.0912583	−4
Preoperative LogMAR BCVA in affected eye					
0–0.5	0.25 (W_{ref})		0	0	0
0.5–1.0	0.75		−0.056	−1.3076873	−1
1.0–1.5	1.25	−0.112	−0.112	−2.6153746	−3
1.5–2.0	1.75		−0.169	−3.9230619	−4
2.0–2.5	2.25		−0.225	−5.2307491	−5
2.5–3.0	2.75		−0.281	−6.5384364	−7
Preoperative LogMAR BCVA in the fellow eye					
0–0.5	0.25 (W_{ref})		0	0	0
0.5–1.0	0.75		−0.048101477	−1.118639	−1
1.0–1.5	1.25	−0.096	−0.096202955	−2.237278	−2
1.5–2.0	1.75		−0.144304432	−3.355917	−3
2.0–2.5	2.25		−0.19240591	−4.474556	−4
2.5–3.0	2.75		−0.240507387	−5.5931951	−6
Drusen in the fellow eye					
no	0 (W_{ref})	−0.358	0	0	0
yes	1		−0.358	−8.3255814	−8

BCVA, best-corrected visual acuity.
W: reference value.
Beta: beta coefficients used in the logistic regression model.
B: number of regression units that correspond to 1 point. We let $B = 0.043$ reflect the increase in risk associated with 10-year increases in age.

4. Discussion

The etiology of VH is diverse, and the cause of VH is identified at the initial visit in 32–79% of eyes with VH [4, 6]. Most cases of acute-onset VH are caused by PDR, trauma, retinal break, proliferative retinopathy after RVO, or posterior vitreous detachment without retinal detachment [2–6]. However, it is often difficult to determine the underlying causes of acute-onset VH because dense VH obscures retinal examination. Lean et al. reported that no diagnosis was made at initial presentation in 21.0% of VH eyes, and Lindgren et al. reported that the underlying disease could not be determined in 68% of VH eyes [2, 4, 6, 19, 20]. Little is known about the causes and visual prognosis of preoperatively unknown origin VH. Therefore, in this study, we analyzed the causes and visual prognosis of acute-onset VH of preoperatively unknown origin.

We excluded VH cases that were associated with PDR. Diabetic retinopathy was assumed to be the cause of acute-onset VH of preoperatively unknown origin if the patient

TABLE 5: Risk scores of study patients with acute-onset vitreous hemorrhage (VH) of preoperatively unknown origin.

Score*	Estimated chance having good vision	All included patients	
		Snellen visual acuity < 20/200 after vitrectomy (no.)	Snellen visual acuity ≥ 20/200 after vitrectomy (no.)
0	0.448		
1	0.459		
2	0.470	1	0
3	0.480		
4	0.491	1	0
5	0.502	1	0
6	0.512	2	2
7	0.523	1	1
8	0.534	3	4
9	0.545	1	2
10	0.555	2	1
11	0.566		
12	0.576	2	1
13	0.587	0	1
14	0.597	1	2
15	0.608	2	4
16	0.618	6	17
17	0.628	1	37
18	0.638	0	29
19	0.648	0	19
20	0.657	0	9
21	0.667	0	5
22	0.677	0	6
23	0.686	0	3
24	0.695	0	2
25	0.704		
Total		24	145

*Estimated risk score after 25 was added to prevent a negative integer as the risk score.

had a medical history of diabetes and fellow eye findings of PDR or severe nonproliferative diabetic retinopathy (NPDR). Therefore, patients with more than mild NPDR in the fellow eye were excluded. After excluding diabetic retinopathy, BRVO was the most common cause of acute-onset VH of preoperatively unknown origin VH (74 eyes [43.8%]).

According to previously published studies, except for PDR, retinal break is the most common cause of acute-onset VH [2, 4, 6, 19, 20]. Unlike previous studies, retinal break was the second most common cause of acute-onset VH of preoperatively unknown origin. This discrepancy between results can be explained by the characteristics of VH caused by retinal breaks. VH caused by a retinal break might be less severe and clear more rapidly [10]. Therefore, retinal breaks that lead to acute-onset VH can be found without vitrectomy. As a result, although retinal break may be the most common cause of acute-onset VH, the proportion of cases for which retinal break is the cause of acute-onset VH of preoperatively unknown origin was relatively small.

In the current study, we analyzed the visual prognosis after vitrectomy of acute-onset VH of preoperatively unknown origin. The overall visual prognosis of unknown origin VH was relatively good. Following vitrectomy, the logMAR BCVA improved from 1.93 ± 0.59 to 0.47 ± 0.71. However, the visual prognosis differed according to the underlying cause of preoperatively unknown origin VH. The preoperative and postoperative logMAR BCVA values of wAMD patients were significantly worse than those of patients with retinal break or RVO.

We believe that these differences in visual prognosis according to cause resulted from the different rates of foveal involvement. In our present study, only 10 cases (13.5%) of RVO involved the fovea and caused VH. In cases of RVO involving the fovea, patients were already diagnosed with RVO before the formation of retinal neovascularization, which eventually leads to VH. Therefore, the rate of foveal involvement was relatively small as a cause of acute-onset VH of preoperatively unknown origin. Because of the lower rate

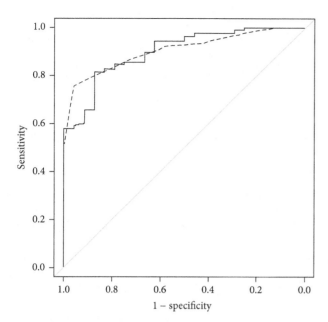

FIGURE 3: ROC curves of the scoring system used to predict the visual prognosis of acute-onset VH of preoperatively unknown origin. The solid line shows the ROC curves of four variables (age, baseline BCVA of the affected eye, baseline BCVA of the unaffected eye, and age-related macular changes in the fellow eyes), which were significantly associated with poor visual acuity following vitrectomy. The dashed line shows the ROC curve of the scoring system. The AUC of the scoring system was 0.907 (95% CI = 0.853–0.948).

of foveal involvement, the visual prognosis of RVO as cause of acute-onset VH of preoperatively unknown origin was relatively good. By contrast, among wAMD patients with acute-onset VH of preoperatively unknown origin, the visual prognosis was poor due to subretinal disciform scar formation.

We also developed an RSS to predict the visual prognosis of unknown origin VH. Our multivariate logistic regression model showed that (1) old age, (2) poor preoperative visual acuity in the affected eye, (3) poor preoperative visual acuity in the fellow eye, and (4) drusen in the fellow eye are significantly associated with poor visual prognosis after vitrectomy. The sensitivity and specificity values of this scoring system were 0.88 and 0.71, respectively. With this simple RSS, we could predict the visual prognosis of acute-onset preoperatively unknown origin VH following vitrectomy. Because of the retrospective nature of this study, we could not validate the accuracy of this RSS. We therefore plan to conduct a future prospective study to validate this system.

To the best of our knowledge, this is the first study to analyze the causes and visual prognosis of acute-onset VH of preoperatively unknown origin. However, our analyses had limitations that are inherent to its retrospective design. In addition, this study was conducted at a single tertiary referring center, which might have caused some selection bias. The sample size of this study was also relatively small, which may have limited the statistical strength of the analysis. Therefore, future studies that examine a larger number of patients are needed to confirm the causes and visual prognosis of acute-onset VH.

In conclusion, the first, second, and third most common causes of acute-onset VH of preoperatively unknown origin were RVO, retinal break, and wAMD, respectively. In addition, the most common cause of acute-onset VH of preoperatively unknown origin changed according to patient age. The visual prognosis of unknown origin VH was relatively good, except among AMD patients. After considering age, preoperative BCVA, and the characteristics of the fellow eye, we predicted visual prognosis of unknown VH. Furthermore, the characteristics of patients with poor visual outcomes following vitrectomy include (1) old age, (2) low preoperative visual acuity in the affected and fellow eyes, and (3) age-related macular changes in the fellow eye. Therefore, in these patients, we expect visual prognosis of acute-onset VH of preoperatively unknown origin to be poor.

Financial Disclosures

All authors certify that they have no affiliations with or involvement in any organization or entity with any financial interest (such as honoraria; educational grants; participation in speakers' bureaus; membership, employment, consultancies, stock ownership, or other equity interest; and expert testimony or patent-licensing arrangements), or nonfinancial interest (such as personal or professional relationships, affiliations, knowledge or beliefs) in the subject matter or materials discussed in this paper.

Conflict of Interests

The authors declare that there is no conflict of interests regarding the publication of this paper.

Authors' Contribution

Dong Yoon Kim, Joo Yong Lee, and June-Gone Kim designed the study. Dong Yoon Kim, Seunghee Baek, and Joo Yong Lee managed the data. Dong Yoon Kim, Joo Yong Lee, Soo Geun Joe, June-Gone Kim, and Joo Yong Lee analyzed, collected, and interpreted the data. Dong Yoon Kim, Seunghee Baek, Joo Yong Lee, Soo Geun Joe, June-Gone Kim, and Joo Yong Lee prepared the paper, performed the statistical analysis, and interpreted the data. Dong Yoon Kim, Joo Yong Lee, Soo Geun Joe, Seunghee Baek, June-Gone Kim, and Joo Yong Lee reviewed and approved the paper.

Acknowledgment

This study was supported by a grant (2014-7206) from the Asan Institute for Life Sciences, Seoul, Republic of Korea.

References

[1] C. W. Spraul and H. E. Grossniklaus, "Vitreous hemorrhage," *Survey of Ophthalmology*, vol. 42, no. 1, pp. 3–39, 1997.

[2] R. L. Winslow and B. C. Taylor, "Spontaneous vitreous hemorrhage: etiology and management," *Southern Medical Journal*, vol. 73, no. 11, pp. 1450–1452, 1980.

[3] M.-R. Dana, M. S. Werner, M. A. G. Viana, and M. J. Shapiro, "Spontaneous and traumatic vitreous hemorrhage," *Ophthalmology*, vol. 100, no. 9, pp. 1377–1383, 1993.

[4] J. S. Lean and Z. Gregor, "The acute vitreous haemorrhage," *British Journal of Ophthalmology*, vol. 64, no. 7, pp. 469–471, 1980.

[5] G. Lindgren and B. Lindblom, "Causes of vitreous hemorrhage," *Current Opinion in Ophthalmology*, vol. 7, no. 3, pp. 13–19, 1996.

[6] G. Lindgren, L. Sjodell, and B. Lindblom, "A prospective study of dense spontaneous vitreous hemorrhage," *American Journal of Ophthalmology*, vol. 119, no. 4, pp. 458–465, 1995.

[7] "Argon laser photocoagulation for macular edema in branch vein occlusion. The Branch Vein Occlusion Study Group," *The American Journal of Ophthalmology*, vol. 98, no. 3, pp. 271–282, 1984.

[8] "Argon laser scatter photocoagulation for prevention of neovascularization and vitreous hemorrhage in branch vein occlusion. A randomized clinical trial. Branch Vein Occlusion Study Group," *Archives of Ophthalmology*, vol. 104, no. 1, pp. 34–41, 1986.

[9] A. Yeshaya and G. Treister, "Pars plana vitrectomy for vitreous hemorrhage and retinal vein occlusion," *Annals of Ophthalmology*, vol. 15, no. 7, pp. 615–617, 1983.

[10] M. H. Seelenfreund, I. Sternberg, I. Hirsch, and B.-Z. Silverstone, "Retinal tears with total vitreous hemorrhage," *American Journal of Ophthalmology*, vol. 95, no. 5, pp. 659–662, 1983.

[11] "Early vitrectomy for severe proliferative diabetic retinopathy in eyes with useful vision. Results of a randomized trial—diabetic retinopathy vitrectomy study report 3. The Diabetic Retinopathy Vitrectomy Study Research Group," *Ophthalmology*, vol. 95, no. 10, pp. 1307–1320, 1988.

[12] "Early vitrectomy for severe vitreous hemorrhage in diabetic retinopathy. Two-year results of a randomized trial. Diabetic Retinopathy Vitrectomy Study report 2. The Diabetic Retinopathy Vitrectomy Study Research Group," *Archives of Ophthalmology*, vol. 103, no. 11, pp. 1644–1652, 1985.

[13] F. El Baba, W. H. Jarrett II, and T. S. Harbin Jr., "Massive hemorrhage complicating age-related macular degeneration. Clinicopathologic correlation and role of anticoagulants," *Ophthalmology*, vol. 93, no. 12, pp. 1581–1592, 1986.

[14] M. Cordido, J. Fernandez-Vigo, J. Fandino, and M. Sanchez-Salorio, "Natural evolution of massive vitreous hemorrhage in diabetic retinopathy," *Retina*, vol. 8, no. 2, pp. 96–101, 1988.

[15] H. Lincoff, I. Kreissig, and M. Wolkstein, "Acute vitreous haemorrhage: a clinical report," *British Journal of Ophthalmology*, vol. 60, no. 6, pp. 454–458, 1976.

[16] C. Lange, N. Feltgen, B. Junker, K. Schulze-Bonsel, and M. Bach, "Resolving the clinical acuity categories 'hand motion' and 'counting fingers' using the Freiburg Visual Acuity Test (FrACT)," *Graefe's Archive for Clinical and Experimental Ophthalmology*, vol. 247, no. 1, pp. 137–142, 2009.

[17] E. W. Steyerberg, F. E. Harrell Jr., G. J. J. M. Borsboom, M. J. C. Eijkemans, Y. Vergouwe, and J. D. F. Habbema, "Internal validation of predictive models: efficiency of some procedures for logistic regression analysis," *Journal of Clinical Epidemiology*, vol. 54, no. 8, pp. 774–781, 2001.

[18] L. M. Sullivan, J. M. Massaro, and R. B. D'Agostino Sr., "Presentation of multivariate data for clinical use: the Framingham Study risk score functions," *Statistics in Medicine*, vol. 23, no. 10, pp. 1631–1660, 2004.

[19] P. H. Morse, A. Aminlari, and H. G. Scheie, "Spontaneous vitreous hemorrhage," *Archives of Ophthalmology*, vol. 92, no. 4, pp. 297–298, 1974.

[20] R. W. Butner and A. R. McPherson, "Spontaneous vitreous hemorrhage," *Annals of Ophthalmology*, vol. 14, no. 3, pp. 268–270, 1982.

Effects of Zeaxanthin on Growth and Invasion of Human Uveal Melanoma in Nude Mouse Model

Xiaoliang L. Xu,[1] Dan-Ning Hu,[2,3] Codrin Iacob,[3] Adrienne Jordan,[3] Sandipkumar Gandhi,[3] Dennis L. Gierhart,[4] and Richard Rosen[2]

[1]Department of Pathology, Memorial Sloan-Kettering Cancer Center, 1275 York Avenue, New York, NY 10021, USA
[2]Department of Ophthalmology, The New York Eye and Ear Infirmary of Mount Sinai, Icahn School of Medicine at Mount Sinai, New York, NY 10003, USA
[3]Department of Pathology, The New York Eye and Ear Infirmary of Mount Sinai, Icahn School of Medicine at Mount Sinai, New York, NY 10003, USA
[4]ZeaVision LLC, Chesterfield, MO 63005, USA

Correspondence should be addressed to Richard Rosen; rrosen@nyee.edu

Academic Editor: Tadeusz Sarna

Uveal melanoma cells were inoculated into the choroid of nude mice and treated with or without intraocular injection of zeaxanthin. After 21 days, mice were sacrificed and the eyes enucleated. Histopathological analysis was performed in hematoxylin and eosin stained frozen sections. Melanoma developed rapidly in the control group (without treatment of zeaxanthin). Tumor-bearing eye mass and tumor mass in the control group were significantly greater than those in zeaxanthin treated group. Melanoma in the controlled eyes occupied a large part of the eye, was epithelioid in morphology, and was with numerous mitotic figures. Scleral perforation and extraocular extension were observed in half of the eyes. Melanomas in zeaxanthin treated eyes were significantly smaller with many necrosis and apoptosis areas and no extraocular extension could be found. Quantitative image analysis revealed that the tumor size was reduced by 56% in eyes treated with low dosages of zeaxanthin and 92% in eyes treatment with high dosages of zeaxanthin, as compared to the controls. This study demonstrated that zeaxanthin significantly inhibits the growth and invasion of human uveal melanoma in nude mice, suggesting that zeaxanthin may be a promising agent to be explored for the prevention and treatment of uveal melanoma.

1. Introduction

Uveal melanoma is the most common malignant intraocular tumor in adults. It accounts for 80% of all noncutaneous melanomas. Up to 50% of uveal melanoma patients die from metastatic disease within 10 years of initial diagnosis and it accounts for 13% of all deaths caused by melanoma [1, 2]. Chemotherapy has had little or no success in both primary and metastatic uveal melanoma [3]. Therefore, it is an urgent necessity to develop more efficient and novel therapeutic agents for improving the survival of uveal melanoma patients.

Zeaxanthin is a nontoxic xanthophyll present in fruits and leafy green vegetables. Zeaxanthin is an antioxidant and can absorb blue light like a yellow filter. It has been used as a nutrition supplement for patients with various ocular diseases [4–9]. In addition to these effects, zeaxanthin may influence the viability and function of cells through various signal pathways or transcription factors [7]. It has been reported that higher intake and higher blood levels of zeaxanthin appear to be associated with a lower risk of occurrence of various cancers [10].

Our previous study demonstrated that zeaxanthin inhibits the proliferation and induces apoptosis of human uveal melanoma cells through intrinsic apoptosis pathway [10]. To our best knowledge, the effects of zeaxanthin on uveal melanoma in experimental animal models have not been reported previously. In the present study, we examined the effects of zeaxanthin on the growth and invasion of human uveal melanoma in an immune-nude mouse model.

2. Materials and Methods

2.1. Experimental Animals. Athymic nude mice were purchased from the Charles River (Kinston, NY) and were incorporated into experiments at 6 weeks of age. This study was approved by the Institutional Animal Care and Use Committee of Memorial Sloan-Kettering Cancer Center. The study complied with the principles of Laboratory Animal Care (NIH publication number 85-23, released in 1985) and also conformed to the ARVO Statement for the Use of Animals in Ophthalmic and Vision Research.

2.2. Uveal Melanoma Cell Line. Melanoma cell line C918 used in this animal study was isolated from a choroidal melanoma patient with liver metastasis at the University of Iowa. This cell line was provided by Dr. Robert Folberg (University of Illinois, Chicago) [10, 11]. C918 cell line is a highly invasive, metastatic, and aggressive melanoma cell line. Melanoma cells in this cell line are epithelioid cells in morphology with round nuclei and prominent nucleoli [10, 11]. Cells were cultured in RPMI 1640 Medium with 10% fetal bovine serum and 1% penicillin/streptomycin (all from Gibco; Grand Island, NY, USA). Cells were trypsinized and resuspended in the above medium and held on ice until inoculation.

2.3. Inoculation of Melanoma Cells and Zeaxanthin Treatment. Mice were randomly divided into three groups, zeaxanthin high dose group (14 eyes) zeaxanthin low dose group (14 eyes), and the control group (not treated with Zeaxanthin, 14 eyes). The methods for inoculation of tumor cells into the posterior segments of the eye have been described previously [12, 13]. Briefly, nude mice were anesthetized by intraperitoneal injection of a ketamine (final concentration; 10 mg/mL) and xylazine (final concentration; 1 mg/mL) mixture (0.01 mL/g mouse weight) and with Alcaine (proparacaine HCL) ocular surface anesthesia. Under a surgical microscope, a 30-gauge sharp needle was used to make two holes through the sclera, one into the intravitreal space to reduce intraocular pressure and one tangentially through the sclera into the subretinal space for injection. Uveal melanoma cells (1×10^6 cells) were injected through the second hole into the choroid and subretinal space using a 1.5 cm, 33-gauge blunt end microinjection needle (7803-05, Hamilton, Reno, NV). After the injection, eyes were covered with ophthalmic bacitracin ointment and buprenorphine was administrated for controlling of pain [12, 13]. Zeaxanthin (supplied by ZeaVision LLC; Chesterfield, MO, USA), solved with DMSO and diluted by PBS, was coinjected with the cellular suspension. The dosages were 114 μg in the low dose group and 570 μg in the high dose group. DMSO at the same levels as zeaxanthin treated group was injected into the eyes in the control group. The mice were kept under sterile conditions in laminar air-flow clean benches at room temperature (25–28°C) and a relative humidity of 55%. Sterile food pellets and water were given. Mice were examined by dissecting microscopy. One week after inoculation of melanoma cells, mice were treated by intravitreous injection of zeaxanthin. Mice were anaesthetized by isoflurane inhalation. Zeaxanthin was solved with DMSO at 50 mM and 57 μg of zeaxanthin was injected into vitreous of mice eyes with 31 G needle in zeaxanthin low group and 114 μg of zeaxanthin in high group. Control groups were injected with 2 μL of DMSO. After 21 days, mice were sacrificed by CO_2 asphyxiation and the eyes enucleated.

2.4. Gross Examination and Measurement of Tumor Mass. Enucleated eyeballs were examined grossly. Extraocular tissue was removed and tumor-bearing eye mass determined. Tumor mass was calculated by the mass of the eye minus the average mass of control uninjected eyes.

2.5. Microscopic Examination and Measurement of Tumor Size. The methods for the fixation of the eye have been reported previously [13]. Briefly, the tumor-bearing eyes were fixed overnight at 4°C in 4% paraformaldehyde in PBS (PFA/PBS), incubated in 30% sucrose/PBS overnight at 4°C, embedded in one-part 30% sucrose/PBS and two-part optimal cutting temperature compound (OCT; Miles Laboratories, Elkhart, IN), frozen, and sectioned at 5 to 7 μm [13]. Slides were fixed with Rapid Fixative (Poly Scientific R&D Corp., Bay Shore, NY). Hematoxylin and eosin (HE) staining was carried out using Leica HE Stainer (Leica Biosystems, Buffalo Grove, IL). HE stained sections were examined by a senior ophthalmic pathologist (CI) and a senior uveal melanoma researcher (DNH) to determine the presence and the extent of melanoma. Microscopic photography of eye section was taken using Olympus BX 41 light microscope (Shinjuku, Tokyo, Japan). Tumor size was determined by using of Adobe Photoshop CS6 [14, 15].

3. Results

3.1. Gross Examination and Tumor Mass. Gross examination revealed that the eyeballs were enlarged in controlled eyes (Figure 1(a)). Half of the eyes had visible extraocular extension of melanoma under stereomicroscope. Most of the zeaxanthin treated eyes were normal in size and were without extraocular extension of melanoma (Figures 1(b) and 1(c)).

Both the eye mass and tumor mass in the eyes of control group were significantly greater than those in eyes of zeaxanthin treated groups (Tables 1 and 2). Furthermore, the eye mass and tumor mass in the eyes of zeaxanthin low group were significantly higher than those in the eyes in zeaxanthin high group (Tables 1 and 2).

3.2. Microscopic Examination. Melanoma grew rapidly in the control eyes (melanoma cells inoculated without zeaxanthin treatment). Microscopic examination confirmed the presence

TABLE 1: Comparison of tumor-bearing eye mass in different groups.

Eye mass	Control	ZL	ZH
Mean (mg, mean ± SD)	21.3 ± 3.5	16.1 ± 3.4	12.4 ± 3.2
Percentage	100%	76%	58%

Control: mice not treated with zeaxanthin; ZL: zeaxanthin low group; ZH: zeaxanthin high group; one-way ANOVA, $p < 0.001$; ZL: control, $p < 0.001$; ZH: control, $p < 0.001$; ZL: ZH, $p < 0.05$.

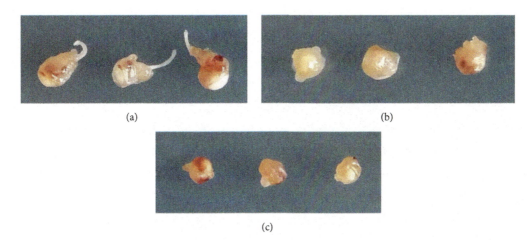

Figure 1: Photographs of enucleated mouse eyes inoculated with human uveal melanoma cells with or without zeaxanthin treatment. Eyes not treated with zeaxanthin (a) show enlargement of the eyeball and with visible extraocular extension of melanoma in some eyes. Eyes treated with zeaxanthin at low dosages (b) or high dosages (c) do not have extraocular extension of melanoma and most of eyeballs are normal in size.

of large melanoma xenografts filling the eyes of most control mice (Figure 2(a)). Half of the eyeballs had definitely scleral perforation and extraocular extension of melanoma cells (Figure 2(a)). Tumor cells in the mouse eye were mostly epithelioid in morphology with few spindle cells. Large nuclei and prominent nucleoli were observed in the tumor cells. Mitoses were common (Figure 3(a)).

Tumors in zeaxanthin low group were smaller than those of the control group (Figure 2(b)). The tumor cells were epithelioid or spindle in morphology with large nuclei and prominent nucleoli. Mitoses were observed occasionally. Necrotic or apoptotic tumor cells were present in part of the eyes. Scleral invasion and extraocular extension of melanoma have not been found in this group.

Tumors in zeaxanthin high group were much smaller than those of the zeaxanthin low group and control group (Figure 2(c)). Patches of definite melanoma cells could be found only in approximately two-thirds of eyes. No miotic figures were present. Necrotic or apoptotic tumor cells could be found in most eyes (Figure 3(b)) and no scleral invasion and extraocular extension of melanoma were present in this group.

3.3. Tumor Size. Tumor size was 1.69 ± 0.95 mm^2 (mean ± standard deviation), 0.74 ± 0.55 mm^2, and 0.13 ± 0.13 mm^2 in the control group, zeaxanthin low group, and zeaxanthin high group, respectively. The difference of tumor size between these three groups was statistically significant ($p < 0.001$). The tumor sizes in the control group were significantly greater than those in both zeaxanthin high and low groups (both $p < 0.0001$), whereas the tumor size in eyes treated with high dosage of zeaxanthin was significantly smaller than that in mice treated with low dose of zeaxanthin ($p < 0.05$). Using the tumor size of control group as 100%, the tumor sizes in zeaxanthin low group and zeaxanthin high group were 43.9% and 7.7%, respectively (Table 3).

Table 2: Comparison of tumor mass in different groups.

Eye mass	Control	ZL	ZH
Mean (mg, mean ± SD)	12.3 ± 3.5	7.1 ± 3.4	3.4 ± 3.2
Percentage	100%	58%	32%

Control: mice not treated with zeaxanthin; ZL: zeaxanthin low group; ZH: zeaxanthin high group; one-way ANOVA, $p < 0.001$; ZL: control, $p < 0.001$; ZH: control, $p < 0.001$; ZL: ZH, $p < 0.05$.

Table 3: Comparison of tumor size in different groups.

Tumor size	Control	ZL	ZH
Mean (mm^2, mean ± SD)	1.70 ± 0.95	0.74 ± 0.55	0.13 ± 0.12
Percentage	100%	44%	7.7%

Control: mice not treated with zeaxanthin; ZL: zeaxanthin low group; ZH: zeaxanthin high group; one-way ANOVA, $p < 0.001$; ZL: control, $p < 0.001$; ZH: control, $p < 0.001$; ZL: ZH, $p < 0.05$.

4. Discussion

Our previous study demonstrated that zeaxanthin significantly inhibits the growth and induces apoptosis of human uveal melanoma cells *in vitro* [10]. However, the results of *in vitro* study may or may not accurately predicate the results obtained from *in vivo* study. For example, it has been reported that interleukin-1 (IL-1) may play a role in promoting uveal melanoma progression. However, inhibiting IL-1 with IL-1ra (an antagonist of IL-1) slows tumor growth only *in vivo* but not *in vitro* [16]. *In vitro* studies test only the direct effects of a medication on the tumor cells. *In vivo* studies test the effects of the medication on the production of various bioactive factors produced by tumor cells or neighbor cells, which in turn may affect the growth and invasion of tumor *in vivo* (paracrine effect), in addition to its direct effects. For example, angiogenesis plays an important role in the growth and progress of uveal melanoma. VEGF is a potent stimulator for angiogenesis. The results of several previous studies suggested that zeaxanthin inhibits the production

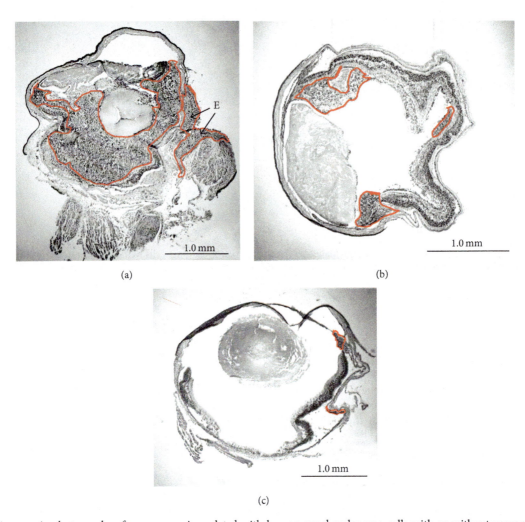

FIGURE 2: Microscopic photographs of mouse eyes inoculated with human uveal melanoma cells with or without zeaxanthin treatment (original magnification ×4). Eyes were enucleated and stained with hematoxylin-eosin in frozen sections. Tumor was marked by red outlines. In the eye not treated with zeaxanthin (control eye), tumor fills large part of the eyeball (a) with scleral perforation and extraocular extension of melanoma (arrow E). Tumor in eye treated with low dosage of zeaxanthin (b) is smaller than that of the control eye. Tumors in eye treated with high dosage of zeaxanthin (c) are much smaller than that of eye treated with low dosage of zeaxanthin and control eye.

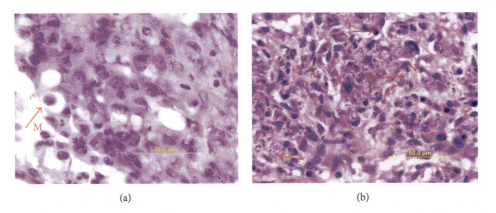

FIGURE 3: Microscopic photographs of mouse eyes inoculated with human uveal melanoma cells with or without zeaxanthin treatment (original magnification ×100). Eyes were stained with hematoxylin-eosin in frozen section and observed under oil lens. Tumor cells in the eye not treated with zeaxanthin are mostly epithelioid in morphology with few spindle cells. Large nuclei and prominent nucleoli were observed in the tumor cells (a). Mitoses are common (arrow M). In eyes treated with high dosage of zeaxanthin, necrotic (arrow N) or apoptotic tumor cells (arrow A) can be observed. No mitotic figures are present (b).

of VEGF by various ocular cells or inflammatory cells [17–21]. This may reduce the angiogenesis and results in the inhibition of the growth of uveal melanoma *in vivo*. *In vivo* studies are an important component of preclinical evaluation of any therapeutic approach to the clinical management of patients with uveal melanoma. For this reason, we designed and carried out the current study for testing the effects of zeaxanthin on the growth and invasion of human uveal melanoma *in vivo* using a nude mouse model.

Numerous animal models have been developed and used in the *in vivo* study of uveal melanoma. The melanoma cells used could be experimental animal melanoma cells (Greene hamster or B16 mouse melanoma cell lines) [22] or human melanoma cells [22–44]. Use of human melanoma cells has the advantage of avoiding the species difference and may more accurately reflect the biological behavior of uveal melanoma in the patients. Tumor cells are antigenic and can induce immune rejection of inoculated tumor graft, especially in transplantation of human tumor cells into experiment animals (xenografts). It has been reported that immune privilege is present in the anterior chamber of the eye, permitting melanoma xenografts to survive if inoculated into the rabbit's anterior chamber [22]. However, since this privilege is incomplete, therefore, in order to grow human melanoma cells in an experiment animal model, it is necessary to use animals incapable of mounting immune rejection to xenograft tumor cells [23–44]. This can be achieved by using immune inhibitory drugs [41–44] or inoculate tumor cells into immune incompetent nude mice [23–40]. The nude mouse is a hairless mutant born without a thymus, which causes a severe defect in cellular immunity, that is, in the transformation process of T lymphocyte precursors to functional T cells. Nude mice have the ability to accept human melanoma cells while preserving many human uveal melanoma characteristics [32]. Therefore, uveal melanoma xenografts in nude mice are a widely used model for studying melanoma growth and response to therapeutic interventions [23–40].

Melanoma cells can be inoculated intraocularly (orthotopic model) [22–31] or subcutaneously (heterotopic model) [32–38]. Tumors transplanted to heterotopic sites may not display biological behavior consistent with the original tumor. The difference of biological behaviors between orthotopic and heterotopic transplantations may be related to the influence of local organ-specific factors. Therefore, the importance of orthotopic, rather than heterotopic, transplantation cannot be overemphasized [24].

The site for intraocular inoculation of melanoma cells could be the anterior part (anterior chamber) [23–25, 29–31, 44] or the posterior part of the eye (vitreous, choroid, subretinal, or suprachoroidal space) [26–28, 30, 45, 46]. Uveal melanoma may arise clinically in the iris (anterior part) or in the ciliary body/choroid (posterior part). Most iris melanomas are relatively benign and only account for approximately 5% of uveal melanoma, which is different from the relatively poor prognosis for patients with melanoma of the ciliary body or choroid [45]. Therefore, we selected the inoculation of melanoma cells into the posterior segment. We ideally inoculated the cells into the choroid; however, in such tiny eyes it is virtually impossible to direct the cells only into the choroid; some cells may enter the suprachoroidal space, subretinal space, or the vitreous [45].

Human uveal melanoma cells used in the present study are the C918 melanoma cell line, which was isolated from a choroidal melanoma patient with liver metastasis. Melanoma cells in this cell line are epithelioid in morphology with round nuclei and prominent nucleoli [10, 11]. The morphologic phenotype of a uveal melanoma provides an important indication of malignancy. The Challender classification scheme categorizes uveal melanoma cellular components as either spindle A, spindle B, or epithelioid. A uveal melanoma predominance of epithelioid components carries significantly greater malignant potential and a shorter patient survival time than melanomas comprised largely spindle cellular elements [47]. C918 cell line is a highly invasive, metastatic, and aggressive melanoma cell line *in vitro* and has been used previously in several animal studies of uveal melanoma [28, 32, 33]. In the present study, melanoma developed rapidly and had potent invasive capacity in mice inoculated with C918 cells and these cells also showed the epithelioid morphology, indicating that this melanoma model reflects the biological behavior of uveal melanoma *in vitro* and in patients with uveal melanoma quite well.

In the present study, melanoma developed in mice without the treatment of zeaxanthin. Melanoma grew rapidly to occupy a large part of the eye and extraocular extension occurred in one-half of the eyes. In zeaxanthin treated groups, zeaxanthin was injected to the posterior part of the eye twice with a total dosage of 171 μg (zeaxanthin low group) or 684 μg (zeaxanthin high group). Zeaxanthin treatment significantly inhibited the growth and invasion of melanoma in nude mice eyes, especially in zeaxanthin high group. Gross examination and histopathological examination found that the tumor mass and size in zeaxanthin treated eyes were significantly less than those in the controls and the extraocular extension only occurred in eyes without the treatment of zeaxanthin. Numerous necrotic or apoptotic tumor cells could be found in eyes treated with zeaxanthin. Quantitative histopathological study demonstrated that the tumor size was reduced by 56% in zeaxanthin low group and 92% in zeaxanthin high group as compared to the control group. All of these results are consistent with those in our previous *in vitro* study which demonstrated the growth inhibition and apoptosis induced effects of zeaxanthin on cultured human uveal melanoma cells.

The dosages used in the animal study have been calculated and compared to the dosages used in the *in vitro* study. In the low dosage group of the animal study, 1×10^6 cells were injected into the eye, and the dosage of zeaxanthin used was 114 μg (first injection) added to 57 μg (second injection); therefore, the total dosage used was 171 μg of zeaxanthin per 1×10^6 cells. The tumor mass in eyes treated with this dosage was 58% of the control (reduced by 42%). In the high dosage group, the total dosages used were 570 μg (first injection) added to 114 μg (second injection); therefore, the total dosage used was 684 μg of zeaxanthin per 1×10^6 cells. The tumor mass in eyes treated with this dosage was 32%

of the control (reduced by 68%). In the *in vitro* study, the ID50 dosage of zeaxanthin in C918 cells was 28.7 μM [10]. In that study, 5×10^3 cells were tested in 96 wells with 200 μL of culture medium containing 28.7 μM zeaxanthin, which equals 3.26 μg of zeaxanthin [10]. Therefore, the dosage of zeaxanthin that can reduce the cell viability to 50% of the control was 3.26 μg zeaxanthin/5×10^3 cells, which equals 652 μg of zeaxanthin per 1×10^6 cells, slightly lower than that used in the high dosage group but greater than in the low dosage group in the animal study. Therefore, the dosages in the animal study are consistent with the dosages used in the *in vitro* study.

It has been reported that zeaxanthin can inhibit the growth and/or induced apoptosis in lymphoma, breast cancer, and neuroblastoma cells *in vitro* [48, 49]. Zeaxanthin had moderate effects in reversing multidrug resistance in mouse lymphoma and human breast cancer cells [48, 50]. Zeaxanthin inhibited the invasion of rat ascites hepatoma cells *in vitro* [51]. Baudelet et al. reported that the extracts of the Glaucophyte *Cyanophora paradoxa* could inhibit the growth of cutaneous melanoma, mammary carcinoma, and lung adenocarcinoma cells *in vitro*. Further analysis indicated that zeaxanthin was one of the three main pigments or derivatives responsible for the cytotoxicity of *Cyanophora paradoxa* fractions in cancer cells [52]. For the experimental animal study, Firdous et al. reported that oral administration of meso-zeaxanthin, another xanthophyll carotenoid, could significantly increase tumor latency period in 3-methylcholanthrene-induced sarcoma in mice. Survival of tumor-bearing mice was significantly increased by meso-zeaxanthin treatment [53]. All of these results are consistent with the results from the present study.

In conclusion, we have demonstrated in the present *in vivo* study that intraocular administration of zeaxanthin significantly inhibits the growth and invasion of human uveal melanoma in nude mice. The results of the present study may be useful for the development of a novel therapeutic approach to the management of uveal melanoma, especially for the combination of zeaxanthin with other aggressive uveal melanoma treatments.

Conflict of Interests

Dr. Dennis L. Gierhart is the chairman of ZeaVision, LLC. Dr. Rosen and Dr. Hu have intellectual property related to malignant tumors and zeaxanthin. None of the other authors have financial interests relevant to the contents of this paper.

Acknowledgments

This work was supported in part by the Bendheim Family Retina Fund, the Wise Family Foundation, the Dennis Gierhart Charitable Gift Fund, and Research to Prevent Blindness.

References

[1] O. Dratviman-Storobinsky, Y. Cohen, S. Frenkel et al., "The role of RASSF1A in uveal melanoma," *Investigative Ophthalmology & Visual Science*, vol. 53, no. 6, pp. 2611–2619, 2012.

[2] E. Kujala, T. Mäkitie, and T. Kivelä, "Very long-term prognosis of patients with malignant uveal melanoma," *Investigative Ophthalmology & Visual Science*, vol. 44, no. 11, pp. 4651–4659, 2003.

[3] J. J. Augsburger, Z. M. Corrêa, and A. H. Shaikh, "Effectiveness of treatments for metastatic uveal melanoma," *American Journal of Ophthalmology*, vol. 148, no. 1, pp. 119–127, 2009.

[4] X. Gong and L. P. Rubin, "Role of macular xanthophylls in prevention of common neovascular retinopathies: retinopathy of prematurity and diabetic retinopathy," *Archives of Biochemistry and Biophysics*, vol. 572, no. 1, pp. 40–48, 2015.

[5] S. S. Ahmed, M. N. Lott, and D. M. Marcus, "The macular xanthophylls," *Survey of Ophthalmology*, vol. 50, no. 2, pp. 183–193, 2005.

[6] "Lutein and zeaxanthin. Monograph," *Alternative Medicine Review*, vol. 10, no. 2, pp. 128–135, 2005.

[7] A. Kijlstra, Y. Tian, E. R. Kelly, and T. T. J. M. Berendschot, "Lutein: more than just a filter for blue light," *Progress in Retinal and Eye Research*, vol. 31, no. 4, pp. 303–315, 2012.

[8] A. J. Whitehead, J. A. Mares, and R. P. Danis, "Macular pigment: a review of current knowledge," *Archives of Ophthalmology*, vol. 124, no. 7, pp. 1038–1045, 2006.

[9] R. A. Bone, J. T. Landrum, L. Fernandez, and S. L. Tarsis, "Analysis of the macular pigment by HPLC: retinal distribution and age study," *Investigative Ophthalmology & Visual Science*, vol. 29, no. 6, pp. 843–849, 1988.

[10] M.-C. Bi, R. Rosen, R.-Y. Zha, S. A. McCormick, E. Song, and D.-N. Hu, "Zeaxanthin induces apoptosis in human uveal melanoma cells through Bcl-2 family proteins and intrinsic apoptosis pathway," *Evidence-Based Complementary and Alternative Medicine*, vol. 2013, Article ID 205082, 12 pages, 2013.

[11] K. J. Daniels, H. C. Boldt, J. A. Martin, L. M. Gardner, M. Meyer, and R. Folberg, "Expression of type VI collagen in uveal melanoma: its role in pattern formation and tumor progression," *Laboratory Investigation*, vol. 75, no. 1, pp. 55–66, 1996.

[12] X. L. Xu, H. P. Singh, L. Wang et al., "Rb suppresses human cone-precursor derived retinoblastoma tumours," *Nature*, vol. 514, no. 7522, pp. 385–388, 2014.

[13] X. L. Xu, Y. Fang, T. C. Lee et al., "Retinoblastoma has properties of a cone precursor tumor and depends upon cone-specific MDM2 signaling," *Cell*, vol. 137, no. 6, pp. 1018–1031, 2009.

[14] Y. Choi and S. R. Eo, "Two-dimensional analysis of palpebral opening in blepharoptosis: visual iris-pupil complex percentage by digital Photography," *Annals of Plastic Surgery*, vol. 72, no. 4, pp. 375–380, 2014.

[15] K. P. Egan, T. A. Brennan, and R. J. Pignolo, "Bone histomorphometry using free and commonly available software," *Histopathology*, vol. 61, no. 6, pp. 1168–1173, 2012.

[16] P. L. Triozzi, W. Aldrich, and A. Singh, "Effects of interleukin-1 receptor antagonist on tumor stroma in experimental uveal melanoma," *Investigative Ophthalmology and Visual Science*, vol. 52, no. 8, pp. 5529–5535, 2011.

[17] R. Rosen, T. Vagaggini, Y. Chen, and D.-N. Hu, "Zeaxanthin inhibits hypoxia-induced VEGF secretion by RPE cells through decreased protein levels of hypoxia-inducible factors-1α," *BioMed Research International*, vol. 2015, Article ID 687386, 11 pages, 2015.

[18] R. A. Kowluru, B. Menon, and D. L. Gierhart, "Beneficial effect of zeaxanthin on retinal metabolic abnormalities in diabetic rats," *Investigative Ophthalmology and Visual Science*, vol. 49, no. 4, pp. 1645–1651, 2008.

[19] H. L. Ramkumar, J. Tuo, F. de Shen et al., "Nutrient supplementation with n3 polyunsaturated fatty acids, lutein, and zeaxanthin decrease A2E accumulation and VEGF expression in the retinas of Ccl2/Cx3cr1-deficient mice on Crb1rd8 background," *Journal of Nutrition*, vol. 143, no. 7, pp. 1129–1135, 2013.

[20] P. Fernández-Robredo, S. Recalde, G. Arnáiz et al., "Effect of zeaxanthin and antioxidant supplementation on vascular endothelial growth factor (VEGF) expression in apolipoprotein-e deficient mice," *Current Eye Research*, vol. 34, no. 7, pp. 543–552, 2009.

[21] R. A. Kowluru, Q. Zhong, J. M. Santos, M. Thandampallayam, D. Putt, and D. L. Gierhart, "Beneficial effects of the nutritional supplements on the development of diabetic retinopathy," *Nutrition and Metabolism*, vol. 11, no. 1, article 8, 2014.

[22] S. Dithmar, D. M. Albert, and H. E. Grossniklaus, "Animal models of uveal melanoma," *Melanoma Research*, vol. 10, no. 3, pp. 195–211, 2000.

[23] J. Y. Niederkorn, J. Mellon, M. Pidherney, E. Mayhew, and R. Anand, "Effect of anti-ganglioside antibodies on the metastatic spread of intraocular melanomas in a nude mouse model of human uveal melanoma," *Current Eye Research*, vol. 12, no. 4, pp. 347–358, 1993.

[24] D. Ma, G. P. Luyten, T. M. Luider, and J. Y. Niederkorn, "Relationship between natural killer cell susceptibility and metastasis of human uveal melanoma cells in a murine model," *Investigative Ophthalmology and Visual Science*, vol. 36, no. 2, pp. 435–441, 1995.

[25] D. Ma, G. P. Luyten, T. M. Luider, M. J. Jager, and J. Y. Niederkorn, "Association between NM23-H1 gene expression and metastasis of human uveal melanoma in an animal model," *Investigative Ophthalmology and Visual Science*, vol. 37, no. 11, pp. 2293–2301, 1996.

[26] Z. Liang, W. Zhan, A. Zhu et al., "Development of a unique small molecule modulator of CXCR4," *PLoS ONE*, vol. 7, no. 4, Article ID e34038, 2012.

[27] H. Yang, M. J. Jager, and H. E. Grossniklaus, "Bevacizumab suppression of establishment of micrometastases in experimental ocular melanoma," *Investigative Ophthalmology and Visual Science*, vol. 51, no. 6, pp. 2835–2842, 2010.

[28] H. Li, H. Alizadeh, and J. Y. Niederkorn, "Differential expression of chemokine receptors on uveal melanoma cells and their metastases," *Investigative Ophthalmology and Visual Science*, vol. 49, no. 2, pp. 636–643, 2008.

[29] I. Notting, J. Buijs, R. Mintardjo et al., "Bone morphogenetic protein 7 inhibits tumor growth of human uveal melanoma in vivo," *Investigative Ophthalmology and Visual Science*, vol. 48, no. 11, pp. 4882–4889, 2007.

[30] R. S. Apte, J. Y. Niederkorn, E. Mayhew, and H. Alizadeh, "Angiostatin produced by certain primary uveal melanoma cell lines impedes the development of liver metastases," *Archives of Ophthalmology*, vol. 119, no. 12, pp. 1805–1809, 2001.

[31] D. Ma, R. D. Gerard, X.-Y. Li, H. Alizadeh, and J. Y. Niederkorn, "Inhibition of metastasis of intraocular melanomas by adenovirus-mediated gene transfer of plasminogen activator inhibitor type 1 (PAI-1) in an athymic mouse model," *Blood*, vol. 90, no. 7, pp. 2738–2746, 1997.

[32] S. Heegaard, M. Spang-Thomsen, and J. U. Prause, "Establishment and characterization of human uveal malignant melanoma xenografts in nude mice," *Melanoma Research*, vol. 13, no. 3, pp. 247–251, 2003.

[33] P. R. van Ginkel, S. R. Darjatmoko, D. Sareen et al., "Resveratrol inhibits uveal melanoma tumor growth via early mitochondrial dysfunction," *Investigative Ophthalmology and Visual Science*, vol. 49, no. 4, pp. 1299–1306, 2008.

[34] A. Béliveau, M. Bérubé, P. Carrier, C. Mercier, and S. L. Guérin, "Tumorigenicity of the mixed spindle-epithelioid SP6.5 and epithelioid TP17 uveal melanoma cell lines is differentially related to alpha5beta1 integrin expression," *Investigative Ophthalmology and Visual Science*, vol. 42, no. 12, pp. 3058–3065, 2001.

[35] J. F. Marshall, D. C. Rutherford, L. Happerfield et al., "Comparative analysis of integrins in vitro and in vivo in uveal and cutaneous melanomas," *British Journal of Cancer*, vol. 77, no. 4, pp. 522–529, 1998.

[36] E. Musi, G. Ambrosini, E. de Stanchina, and G. K. Schwartz, "The phosphoinositide 3-kinase α selective inhibitor BYL719 enhances the effect of the protein kinase C inhibitor AEB071 in GNAQ/GNA11-mutant uveal melanoma cells," *Molecular Cancer Therapeutics*, vol. 13, no. 5, pp. 1044–1053, 2014.

[37] S. Hu, Q. Luo, B. Cun et al., "The pharmacological NF-κB inhibitor BAY11-7082 induces cell apoptosis and inhibits the migration of human uveal melanoma cells," *International Journal of Molecular Sciences*, vol. 13, no. 12, pp. 15653–15667, 2012.

[38] A. K. Samadi, S. M. Cohen, R. Mukerji et al., "Natural withanolide with aferin A induces apoptosis in uveal melanoma cells by suppression of Akt and c-MET activation," *Tumour Biology*, vol. 33, no. 4, pp. 1179–1189, 2012.

[39] R. Folberg, L. Leach, K. Valyi-Nagy et al., "Modeling the behavior of uveal melanoma in the liver," *Investigative Ophthalmology and Visual Science*, vol. 48, no. 7, pp. 2967–2974, 2007.

[40] M. Tardif, J. Coulombe, D. Soulières, A. P. Rousseau, and G. Pelletier, "Gangliosides in human uveal melanoma metastatic process," *International Journal of Cancer*, vol. 68, no. 1, pp. 97–101, 1996.

[41] R. E. MacLaren, R. A. Pearson, A. MacNeil et al., "Retinal repair by transplantation of photoreceptor precursors," *Nature*, vol. 444, no. 7116, pp. 203–207, 2006.

[42] S. J. Kang, Q. Zhang, S. R. Patel et al., "In vivo high-frequency contrast-enhanced ultrasonography of choroidal melanoma in rabbits: imaging features and histopathologic correlations," *British Journal of Ophthalmology*, vol. 97, no. 7, pp. 929–933, 2013.

[43] P. Bonicel, J. Michelot, F. Bacin et al., "Establishment of IPC 227 cells as human xenografts in rabbits: a model of uveal melanoma," *Melanoma Research*, vol. 10, no. 5, pp. 445–450, 2000.

[44] P. E. Liggett, G. Lo, K. J. Pince, N. A. Rao, S. G. Pascal, and J. Kan-Mitchel, "Heterotransplantation of human uveal melanoma," *Graefe's Archive for Clinical and Experimental Ophthalmology*, vol. 231, no. 1, pp. 15–20, 1993.

[45] H. E. Grossniklaus, B. C. Barron, and M. W. Wilson, "Murine model of anterior and posterior ocular melanoma," *Current Eye Research*, vol. 14, no. 5, pp. 399–404, 1995.

[46] S. Dithmar, D. Rusciano, and H. E. Grossniklaus, "A new technique for implantation of tissue culture melanoma cells in a murine model of metastatic ocular melanoma," *Melanoma Research*, vol. 10, no. 1, pp. 2–8, 2000.

[47] M. Yanoff and B. S. Fine, *Ocular Pathology: A Text and Atlas*, J. B. Lippincott Company, Philadelphia, Pa, USA, 1989.

[48] J. Molnár, N. Gyémánt, I. Mucsi et al., "Modulation of multidrug resistance and apoptosis of cancer cells by selected carotenoids," *In Vivo*, vol. 18, no. 2, pp. 237–244, 2004.

[49] M. Maccarrone, M. Bari, V. Gasperi, and B. Demmig-Adams, "The photoreceptor protector zeaxanthin induces cell death in neuroblastoma cells," *Anticancer Research*, vol. 25, no. 6, pp. 3871–3876, 2005.

[50] M. D. Kars, O. D. Işeri, U. Gunduz, and J. Molnar, "Reversal of multidrug resistance by synthetic and natural compounds in drug-resistant MCF-7 cell lines," *Chemotherapy*, vol. 54, no. 3, pp. 194–200, 2008.

[51] Y. Kozuki, Y. Miura, and K. Yagasaki, "Inhibitory effects of carotenoids on the invasion of rat ascites hepatoma cells in culture," *Cancer Letters*, vol. 151, no. 1, pp. 111–115, 2000.

[52] P.-H. Baudelet, A.-L. Gagez, J.-B. Bérard et al., "Antiproliferative activity of *Cyanophora paradoxa* pigments in melanoma, breast and lung cancer cells," *Marine Drugs*, vol. 11, no. 11, pp. 4390–4406, 2013.

[53] A. P. Firdous, E. R. Sindhu, V. Ramnath, and R. Kuttan, "Anticarcinogenic activity of meso-zeaxanthin in rodents and its possible mechanism of action," *Nutrition and Cancer*, vol. 65, no. 6, pp. 850–856, 2013.

Childbearing May Increase the Risk of Nondiabetic Cataract in Chinese Women's Old Age

Manqiong Yuan,[1,2] Yaofeng Han,[1,2] Ya Fang,[1,2] and Cheng-I Chu[3]

[1]State Key Laboratory of Molecular Vaccinology and Molecular Diagnostics, School of Public Health, Xiamen University, Xiamen 361102, China
[2]Key Laboratory of Health Technology Assessment in Fujian Province University, School of Public Health, Xiamen University, Xiamen 361102, China
[3]Department of Public Health, Tzu Chi University, Hualien 97004, Taiwan

Correspondence should be addressed to Ya Fang; fangya@xmu.edu.cn

Academic Editor: Kathryn P. Burdon

Backgrounds. Ocular changes may arise during pregnancy and after childbirth, but very few studies have reported the association between childbearing and cataract among older adults. *Methods.* 14,292 individuals aged 60+ years were recruited in Xiamen, China, in 2013. Physician-diagnosed cataract and diabetes status were assessed by a self-reported questionnaire. Childbearing status was measured by number of children (NOC). Structural equation modeling (SEM) analysis was conducted to examine the relationships among NOC, diabetes, and cataract. Gender-specific logistic models regressing nondiabetic cataract on NOC were performed by adjusting some covariates. *Results.* 14,119 participants had complete data, of whom 5.01% suffered from cataract, with higher prevalence in women than men (6.41% versus 3.51%). Estimates of SEM models for women suggested that both NOC and diabetes were risk factors for cataract and that no correlation existed between NOC and diabetes. Women who had one or more children faced roughly 2–4 times higher risk of nondiabetic cataract than their childless counterparts (OR [95% CI] = 3.88 [1.24, 17.71], 3.21 [1.04, 14.52], 4.32 [1.42, 19.44], 4.41 [1.46, 19.74], and 3.98 [1.28, 18.10] for having 1, 2, 3, 4-5, and 6 or more children, resp.). *Conclusions.* Childbearing may increase the risk of nondiabetic cataract in Chinese women's older age.

1. Introduction

According to the two latest WHO assessments, cataract has consistently been the leading cause of world blindness, which was responsible for around 48% and 51% of blindness in 2002 [1] and 2010 [2], respectively. Biological ageing plays the most crucial role in the development of cataract [3–5]. China, the most populous country, has been experiencing an unprecedented ageing due to a lower birth rate [6] and longer life expectancy [7]. About 15.5% of the entire Chinese were aged 60+ years in 2014, a figure much higher than the threshold for ageing society (10%). Therefore as an age-related disease, cataract requires increased and urgent attention in China [8, 9].

Besides age, many other related factors, such as diabetes and gender, have also been well-addressed in previous studies [10–13]. It has been demonstrated that diabetics faced 2-5 times greater risk of developing cataracts than the nondiabetic counterparts [12]. Additionally, gender diversity in the prevalence of cataract has also been frequently reported and most studies showed greater prevalence among females than males [11]. Hormonal differences between men and women may mainly contribute to such gender diversity [10, 14], but the reasons were still not fully understood.

Ocular changes may arise during pregnancy due to the modifications of hormone, metabolism, and weight [15]. Although most of the changes are reversible, some are occasionally permanent which may in turn cumulatively affect women's vision at their older ages [16]. A study revealed that there was a significant association between parity and the risk of cataract among middle- and older age women [17]. However, the evidence is scant since very few studies have directly reported the link between childbearing and cataract, especially for women in their old ages. In this study, we aim to (1) test the relationship between childbearing and cataract among the older women and (2) examine whether diabetes is a mediator in this relationship.

2. Methods

2.1. Study Population. As previously described [18], we conducted a large scale cross-sectional survey among 14,292 older adults aged 60+ years in Xiamen, China, in 2013. The participants were enrolled by a multistage sampling procedure. In the first stage, all 38 subdistricts in Xiamen were selected. In stage 2, one-third of communities were randomly sampled from each subdistrict and a total of 173 communities were included in the end. The randomization of these communities was performed by computer-generated random numbers. In stage 3, participants were conveniently selected from each community by controlling for gender and age composition. The number of individuals to be sampled in each community was determined according to its proportion of eligible older adults. Participants' demographic characteristics, activities of daily living, physical health, psychological health, and social support were assessed by a structural questionnaire, which was finished by a face-to-face interview. Written informed consent was obtained by each participant and our study was approved by the ethical review committee of School of Public Health, Xiamen University.

2.2. Measurements. The primary outcomes in this study were whether the participants suffered from physician-diagnosed cataract and diabetes. They were assessed by the same item: "Do you suffer from the following physician-diagnosed chronic diseases? (check all that apply)." Cataract and diabetes were two of the fifteen listed chronic diseases. Only if the option was ticked, we assume the participant suffered from the corresponding chronic disease. In Xiamen, for medical screening purposes, people who were aged 60 years or older can participate in an annual physical examination for free in recent years, including blood pressure and blood glucose checks, and an ocular examination. Moreover, some self-reported chronic diseases were reported to be highly correlated with physician's records [19]. Therefore, the reliability of self-reported diabetes and cataract in the elderly should be potentially ensured (see Supplementary 1 for the reason in detail in Supplementary Material available online at http://dx.doi.org/10.1155/2015/385815). The nondiabetic cataracts in our study referred to the individuals who suffered from cataract but did not have diabetes. The exposure of interest was childbearing status which was measured by number of children (NOC). It was assessed by the item of "How many children have you had?" Numerical response was obtained and was classified into six levels: 0, 1, 2, 3, 4-5, and 6 or more. Additionally, some basic information (gender, age, residence, education, and marital status), life habits (dietary salt intake, smoking history, and alcohol drinking), and hypertension status were included as covariates (see Table 1 for the details of the classification of the variables). We considered the hypertension status as a covariate because it has also been frequently reported to have relationship to cataract [20].

2.3. Analytical Strategies. First, we summarized the characteristics of participants by cataract status using descriptive statistics (mean and standard deviation for age and counts and proportions for the other categorical characteristics). Chi-square tests were performed to assess the relationship between cataract and all the other covariates. Second, to identify the relationships among NOC, diabetes, and cataract in women, Stata v 13.0 was used to perform structural equation modeling (SEM). The reason we tested their relationships was due to the concern that diabetes may be a mediator in the relationship between NOC and cataract. The SEM for this mediation model for the ith participant ($1 \leq i \leq n$) is given by

$$\text{logit}\left[\text{Probability}\left(D_i\right)\right] = \beta_0 + \beta_1 \text{NOC}_i + \varepsilon_i,$$
$$\text{logit}\left[\text{Probability}\left(C_i\right)\right] \quad (1)$$
$$= \gamma_0 + \gamma_1 D_i + \gamma_2 \text{NOC}_i + \boldsymbol{\gamma_3}^{\text{T}}\text{Covariates} + \delta_i,$$

where the outcome D_i is diabetic status, C_i is cataract status, β_0, β_1, γ_0, γ_1, γ_2, and $\boldsymbol{\gamma_3}^{\text{T}}$ are the regression coefficients, *Covariates* are the nine covariates described above, and ε_i and δ_i are the random errors. We assume that the error terms (ε_i, δ_i) are uncorrelated. Third, we presented the prevalence of cataract by line chart under the six levels of NOC, stratified by gender and diabetes status. Fourth, logistic regressions were carried out to model the cataract status on the NOC among the participants without diabetes, stratified by gender and adjusted by the nine covariates mentioned above. $P < 0.05$ indicated that the associations were statistically significant in our study.

3. Results

Among the 14,292 participants, 14,119 had complete data on all variables mentioned above and were included in the following analyses. Descriptive statistics of characteristics stratified by gender and cataract status were presented in Table 1. Among 14,119 valid participants, the prevalence of cataract was 5.01%, with an obviously higher prevalence in women than men (6.41% versus 3.51%). The average age was significantly higher in cataract participants than in those without cataract for both men and women ($P < 0.001$). An increase trend of prevalence of cataract was presented as NOC grew for women and ranged from 3.10% for the childless to 9.09% for those who had six or more children. However, such trend disappeared in men. About ten percent of participants suffered from diabetes, of whom the prevalence values of cataract were 4.48% for men and 9.26% for women, which were both higher than their nondiabetic counterparts. Approximately thirty percent of participants reported to have hypertension and 6.85% of them reported to have cataract. Significantly higher prevalence of cataract was presented in hypertensive participants than nonhypertensive groups for both men and women. Female participants who had salt-heavy diet, were illiterate, were single or widowed, and had quit drinking had significantly higher prevalence of cataract ($P < 0.05$). However, for male participants, except for the

TABLE 1: Summary of gender stratified basic characteristics of 14,119 participants.

Characteristic	Male (N = 6,806)				Female (N = 7,313)			
	Noncataract	Cataract	[a]Prevalence (%)	[b]P	Noncataract	Cataract	[a]Prevalence (%)	[b]P
Total, N	6567	239	3.51		6844	469	6.41	
Age, mean (SD)/years	70.81 (7.73)	75.00 (7.42)		<0.001	71.75 (8.78)	75.75 (8.49)		<0.001
NOC, N (%)				0.141				<0.001
0	242 (3.69)	13 (5.44)	5.10		125 (1.83)	4 (0.85)	3.10	
1	1110 (16.90)	37 (15.48)	3.23		904 (13.21)	49 (10.45)	5.14	
2	1924 (29.30)	55 (23.01)	2.78		1662 (24.28)	83 (17.70)	4.76	
3	1706 (25.98)	69 (28.87)	3.89		1880 (27.47)	131 (27.93)	6.51	
4 or 5	1306 (19.89)	57 (23.85)	4.18		1753 (25.61)	150 (31.98)	7.88	
6 or more	279 (4.25)	8 (3.35)	2.79		520 (7.60)	52 (11.09)	9.09	
Diabetes status, N (%)				0.177				<0.001
Nondiabetic	5991 (91.23)	212 (88.70)	3.42		6148 (89.83)	398 (84.86)	6.08	
Diabetic	576 (8.77)	27 (11.30)	4.48		696 (10.17)	71 (15.14)	9.26	
Hypertension status, N (%)				0.012				<0.001
Nonhypertensive	4668 (71.08)	152 (63.60)	3.15		4785 (69.92)	265 (56.50)	5.25	
Hypertensive	1899 (28.92)	87 (36.40)	4.38		2059 (30.08)	204 (43.50)	9.01	
Dietary salt intake, N (%)				0.975				0.006
Salt-light (<6 g/day)	2618 (39.87)	97 (40.59)	3.57		3463 (50.6)	233 (49.68)	6.30	
Salt-medium (6–18 g/day)	3313 (50.45)	120 (50.21)	3.50		2975 (43.47)	191 (40.72)	6.03	
Salt-heavy (≥18 g/day)	636 (9.68)	22 (9.21)	3.34		406 (5.93)	45 (9.59)	9.98	
Residence, N (%)				0.159				0.532
City	3158 (48.09)	126 (52.72)	3.84		3371 (49.25)	238 (50.75)	6.59	
Rural	3409 (51.91)	113 (47.28)	3.21		3473 (50.75)	231 (49.25)	6.24	
Education, N (%)				0.146				<0.001
Illiterate	1103 (16.8)	42 (17.57)	3.67		3223 (47.09)	267 (56.93)	7.65	
Primary	2348 (35.75)	88 (36.82)	3.61		1824 (26.65)	119 (25.37)	6.12	
Junior high school	1634 (24.88)	45 (18.83)	2.68		952 (13.91)	35 (7.46)	3.55	
Senior high school and beyond	1482 (22.57)	64 (26.78)	4.14		845 (12.35)	48 (10.23)	5.38	
Occupation, N (%)				0.485				0.395
Employed	2059 (31.35)	86 (35.98)	4.01		1441 (21.05)	88 (18.76)	5.76	
Farmer	2905 (44.24)	101 (42.26)	3.36		2764 (40.39)	195 (41.58)	6.59	
Jobless	331 (5.04)	11 (4.60)	3.22		1337 (19.54)	103 (21.96)	7.15	
Others	1272 (19.37)	41 (17.15)	3.12		1302 (19.02)	83 (17.70)	5.99	
Marital status, N (%)				0.433				<0.001
Inmarriage	5575 (84.89)	200 (83.68)	3.46		3839 (56.09)	208 (44.35)	5.14	
Single	147 (2.24)	9 (3.77)	5.77		31 (0.45)	3 (0.64)	8.82	
Divorced	81 (1.23)	2 (0.84)	2.41		76 (1.11)	3 (0.64)	3.80	
Widowed	764 (11.63)	28 (11.72)	3.54		2898 (42.34)	255 (54.37)	8.09	
Smoking history, N (%)				<0.001				0.293
Never	2139 (32.57)	80 (33.47)	3.61		6340 (92.64)	437 (93.18)	6.45	
Sometimes	1558 (23.72)	48 (20.08)	2.99		300 (4.38)	15 (3.20)	4.76	
Often	2113 (32.18)	61 (25.52)	2.81		137 (2.00)	9 (1.92)	6.16	
Quit	757 (11.53)	50 (20.92)	6.20		67 (0.98)	8 (1.71)	10.67	

TABLE 1: Continued.

Characteristic	Male ($N = 6,806$)				Female ($N = 7,313$)			
	Noncataract	Cataract	[a]Prevalence (%)	[b]P	Noncataract	Cataract	[a]Prevalence (%)	[b]P
Alcohol Drinking, N (%)				0.235				0.025
Never	2873 (43.75)	106 (44.35)	3.56		6141 (89.73)	423 (90.19)	6.44	
Sometimes	2544 (38.74)	87 (36.40)	3.31		607 (8.87)	33 (7.04)	5.16	
Often	654 (9.96)	20 (8.37)	2.97		45 (0.66)	4 (0.85)	8.16	
Quit	496 (7.55)	26 (10.88)	4.98		51 (0.75)	9 (1.92)	15.00	

[a]Prevalence of cataract.
[b]P value of chi-square test to assess the relationship between cataract and the other variables.
NOC: number of children; BMI: body mass index.

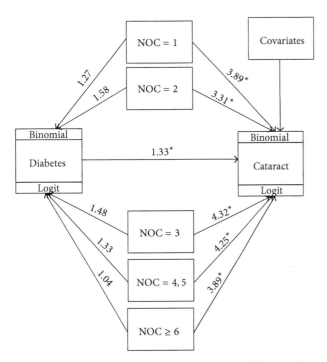

FIGURE 1: Path diagram of structural equation modeling to depict the relationships among number of children (NOC), diabetes, cataract, and the other nine covariates. The covariates included age, hypertension status, dietary salt intake, residence, education, occupation, marital status, smoking history, and alcohol drinking ($^*P < 0.05$).

hypertensive status, only smoking history was significantly associated with cataract status. Unexpectedly, men who had quit smoking presented highest prevalence, and those who smoked often showed lowest one.

As descriptive results shown above, both diabetes and having more children increase the risk of cataract for older women. To test whether diabetes is a mediator in the relationship between NOC and cataract, mediation analysis with SEM was performed. Figure 1 presented the path diagram with estimated odds ratios (OR), which represented the SEM models for female elderly (equation (1)). Diabetic women had a statistically higher risk (OR = 1.33) of cataract than their nondiabetic counterparts. Those who had one or more children faced roughly 2-4 times higher risk of cataract than the childless women. However, all the paths between NOC and diabetes were not significant, indicating that diabetes should not be a mediator in the relationship between NOC and cataract. The details of the estimates of the SEM models can be found in Supplementary 2.

The prevalence of cataract under the six levels of NOC stratified by gender and diabetic status was depicted by line chart in Figure 2. The left panel was the prevalence of cataract among the 12,749 nondiabetic participants. A notably increased prevalence (solid line) appeared as NOC grew for nondiabetic older women, but it disappeared among the nondiabetic older men (dotted line). Moreover, the nondiabetic females had higher prevalence of cataract than nondiabetic males at all levels of NOC except among the childless participants. The right panel was the prevalence of cataract among 1,370 diabetic participants. At all the levels of NOC, diabetic females had obvious higher prevalence of cataract than diabetic males. The increased trend of prevalence as having more children disappeared for diabetic female and male participants.

Table 2 presented the ORs with corresponding 95% confidence intervals (CIs) obtained from logistic regression models for nondiabetic participants stratified by gender. For both nondiabetic women and men, age was a crucial risk factor for developing cataract. The older women who had one or more children faced roughly 2-4 times higher risk of nondiabetic cataract than their childless counterparts (OR [95% CI] = 3.88 [1.24, 17.71], 3.21 [1.04, 14.52], 4.32 [1.42, 19.44], 4.41 [1.46, 19.74], and 3.98 [1.28, 18.10] for having 1, 2, 3, 4-5, and 6 or more children, resp.). However, among the nondiabetic older men, the ORs seemed to decrease as NOC grew, although they were not statistically significant. Hypertension, salt-heavy diet, and living in a city were risk factors for women but not for men. Unexpectedly, having quit smoking was a risk factor, and being widowed was a protect factor for men only.

4. Discussion

The findings in this study indicated that childbearing may increase the risk of nondiabetic cataract in women's old age. After controlling for the potential confounders, nondiabetic women who had one or more children faced roughly 2-4 times higher risk of cataract than the childless. Moreover, SEM analysis suggested that diabetes was not a mediator in

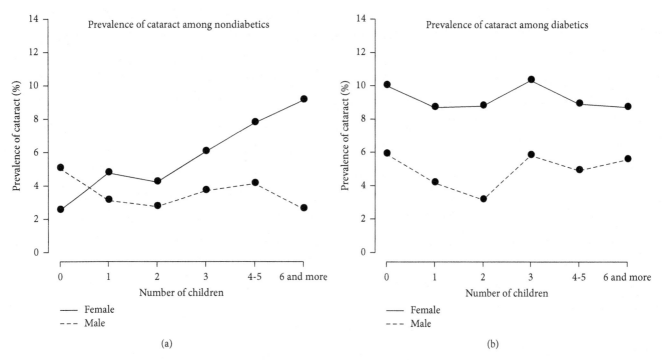

FIGURE 2: Line charts of the prevalence of cataract under the six levels of number of children, stratified by gender and diabetes status. The left panel was the prevalence of cataract among the 12,749 nondiabetic participants while the right one was among 1,370 diabetic participants.

the relationship between NOC and cataracts. These results may contribute to the existing body of literature on identifying the risk factor of cataract among the older individuals.

The pathomechanism underlying the association between childbearing and cataract remains unclear. However, some possible explanations for the childbearing effect in older women may be speculated; these include (1) pregnancy-induced estrogen changes [21]. Some investigators believed that estrogen played a protective role in controlling the development of cataract [10]. A previous study indicated that the risk of cortical cataract increased by about 5% for each one year increment in age at menarche and that the risk decreased by 11% for each five years of age older at menopause [22]. Therefore, we may postulate that the increased risk of cataract for women having more children is due to a reduction in lifetime exposure to circulating estrogens induced by each pregnancy and breastfeeding. (2) Postpartum obesity may be another important risk factor of cataract for women in their later life [23, 24]. A previous study presented that the average gestational weight gains for Chinese women (17.3 ± 4.9 kg, 17.4 ± 4.4 kg, and 15.7 ± 5.1 kg for women of low, moderate, and high prepregnancy body mass index, resp.) [25] were much higher than the recommended criteria [26] (13–16.7 kg, 11–16.4 kg, and 7.1–14.4 kg, resp.). (3) Various ocular changes occur during pregnancy, including decreased sensitivity of the cornea, enlarged blind spots, and bitemporal loss [27, 28]. The cumulative effect of those asymptomatic and subtle ocular changes may also contribute to the development of cataract for women in later life. (4) A complex of other risk factors, such as the stress for taking care of many children, may also increase the risk of cataract. However, in either case, more physiological studies were in great need to fully elucidate the mechanism.

In line with many previous studies [29–31], cataract was more common in women than men, with the prevalence of 6.41% versus 3.51% in the present study. Such difference is often addressed by the estrogen deficiency [10] or biomass cooking fuels [32]. However, this explanation could not fully elucidate our results. In the present study the prevalence of cataract among childless women was notably lower than that among childless men (3.1% versus 5.1%). This result may further indicate that childbearing was an important risk factor of cataract among older women. A study has directly stated that the risk of cataract in young women (35–45 years) increased by an estimated 20% for each additional birth [33]. Moreover, older women (45–86 years) were observed to have 11.3% higher risk of cataract for each additional live birth in a recent cohort study [17]. Among the nondiabetic women, the prevalence of cataract grew as they had more children, but such trend disappeared among the women with diabetes. In other words, the effect of childbearing on cataract among the female older adults may be mediated or covered by the effect of diabetes. Cataract was the second most ocular common complication of diabetes [34], and the effect of diabetes on cataract should be direct and obvious. However, the childbearing occurred at women's younger age and its effect on age-related cataract may be cumulative and subtle. Therefore the effect of childbearing on cataract is easy to be neglected or covered by other stronger risk factors.

Consistent with many previous studies [35–37], our findings identified hypertension, salt-heavy diet, living in a city, and having quit smoking as risk factors for development

TABLE 2: Odds ratio (OR) with 95% confidence intervals (CIs) of gender-specific logistic regressions for nondiabetic datasets.

Characteristic (reference)	Male ($N = 6{,}203$)		Female ($N = 6{,}546$)	
	OR	95% CI	OR	95% CI
Age	1.08***	1.06–1.11	1.04***	1.03–1.06
NOC (0)				
1	0.95	0.39–2.57	3.88*	1.24–17.71
2	0.69	0.29–1.83	3.21*	1.04–14.52
3	0.77	0.33–2.02	4.32*	1.42–19.44
4 or 5	0.67	0.28–1.77	4.41*	1.46–19.74
6 or more	0.30*	0.09–0.95	3.98*	1.28–18.10
Hypertension status (nonhypertensive)				
Hypertensive	1.24	0.92–1.67	1.68***	1.35–2.08
Dietary salt intake (salt-light (<6 g/day))				
Salt-medium (6–18 g/day)	1.15	0.85–1.56	1.07	0.86–1.33
Salt-heavy (≥18 g/day)	0.96	0.56–1.60	1.68**	1.12–2.46
Residence (city)				
Rural	0.91	0.55–1.49	0.73*	0.53–1.00
Education (illiterate)				
Primary	1.35	0.90–2.07	0.91	0.68–1.2
Junior high school	1.18	0.70–1.98	0.46**	0.27–0.75
Senior high school and beyond	1.50	0.86–2.64	0.69	0.42–1.11
Occupation (employed)				
Farmer	1.20	0.69–2.12	1.06	0.68–1.67
Jobless	1.10	0.50–2.25	1.02	0.68–1.54
Others	0.88	0.56–1.37	0.83	0.56–1.23
Marital status (inmarriage)				
Single	1.49	0.50–4.28	2.80	0.41–11.66
Divorced	0.75	0.12–2.53	0.88	0.21–2.46
Widowed	0.60*	0.37–0.94	0.97	0.75–1.24
Smoking history (never)				
Sometimes	0.85	0.55–1.30	0.56*	0.29–0.99
Often	1.07	0.71–1.62	0.64	0.26–1.34
Quit	1.92*	1.21–3.02	1.01	0.35–2.46
Alcohol drinking (never)				
Sometimes	1.11	0.79–1.56	1.05	0.68–1.55
Often	1.22	0.70–2.06	1.55	0.44–4.17
Quit	0.94	0.53–1.60	1.61	0.50–4.36

*P value < 0.05, **P value < 0.01, ***P value < 0.001.
NOC: number of children; BMI: body mass index.

of cataract. Salt-heavy diet has been well-addressed to be related to hypertension [38, 39], which may increase the risk of development of the posterior subcapsular cataracts [40, 41]. As for smoking, it had been consistently stated to be associated with both nuclear and posterior subcapsular cataract [35]. In this study, having quit smoking was a risk factor for older men which might be due to the smoking history in their younger age. Some investigators found that risk of cataract remains elevated for many years following smoking cessation [42]. Unexpectedly, we found men who smoked often had obviously lower prevalence of cataract than those who never smoked (2.81% versus 3.61%). Such paradoxical result has also been presented in other studies [43]. To find the reason, we further analyzed our data and found that individuals who smoked often were significantly younger than those who never smoked (69.45 years versus 71.78 years, $P < 0.01$), especially among men (69.12 years versus 71.77 years, $P < 0.01$). Therefore, age, the most critical risk factor of cataract, probably confounded the relationship between cataract and smoking history. This speculation was further validated in the following regression model for men where OR for smoking often was higher than never smoking (1.07 versus 1.00), after controlling for age and other impact factors. Another possible explanation is that some related chronic diseases can prompt smoking cessation for older adults, and the current smokers may have or believe they have relatively better physician conditions. However, this speculation cannot be validated in this study due to our cross-sectional survey and limited measurements. To fully uncover the relationship between smoking and cataract, variables such as smoking pack-years, age of smoking cessation, and the reason(s) for smoking cessation are in great need. Despite the fact that abovementioned risk factors of cataracts were well-demonstrated, limited studies have elucidated the gender-specified risk factors. Our results suggested that salt-heavy diet and hypertension were the risk factors for nondiabetic female only and on the contrary, having quit smoking was for nondiabetic male only. More precise study design and analyses were needed to explore such gender disparities.

The findings in the present study have uncovered the relationship between childbearing and cataract in older adults. They may open new research challenges to detect the risk factors of senile cataract. Nevertheless, some limitations should be acknowledged. First, the chronic conditions were obtained by a self-reported question. As a result, we may have underestimated the true prevalence of cataract and diabetes. However, substantial agreement was found in a study comparing subjects' self-reported diabetes with information from medical records [19]. Some studies demonstrated that self-reported diabetes was >92% reliable over time [44] and it was a reliable proxy for medical record review [45]. The difference between self-reporting and true prevalence of cataract has been evaluated in Supplementary 1, and the reliability of self-reported cataract in this study may also be potentially ensured. Second, to exclude the diabetes-induced cataracts, the data of the participants with diabetes were all removed from our regression models. However, some of participants may have cataract prior to diabetes or the cataracts were not diabetes-induced, and as a result, the complete exclusion may consequently result in some bias. Nevertheless, such bias was restricted, since only 71 (less than 1%) female participants had both cataract and diabetes. Third, there are three primary types of age-related cataracts (nuclear, cortical, and posterior subcapsular), and each may have its own somewhat varying causes [37, 41]. However, the types of cataracts were not asked in our survey and therefore we cannot specify which type(s) of cataract were accounted for in relation to childbearing.

5. Conclusions

This study has revealed a relationship between childbearing status and the risk of cataract among Chinese elderly, and diabetes was not a mediator in this relationship. As a result, we should pay more attention to the eyes care for the women during pregnancy and after childbirth.

Conflict of Interests

The authors declare no conflict of interests.

Authors' Contribution

Manqiong Yuan analyzed the data and wrote and revised the paper; Yaofeng Han and Cheng-I Chu reviewed and revised the paper; Ya Fang conceived and designed the study and critically revised the paper.

Acknowledgments

This work was supported by the Xiamen Committee on Ageing Fund (Grant no. XDHT2013357A) and National Natural Science Foundation of China (Grant no. 81402768).

References

[1] S. Resnikoff, D. Pascolini, D. Etya'ale et al., "Global data on visual impairment in the year 2002," *Bulletin of the World Health Organization*, vol. 82, no. 11, pp. 844–851, 2004.

[2] D. Pascolini and S. P. Mariotti, "Global estimates of visual impairment: 2010," *The British Journal of Ophthalmology*, vol. 96, no. 5, pp. 614–618, 2012.

[3] P. J. Foster, T. Y. Wong, D. Machin, G. J. Johnson, and S. K. L. Seah, "Risk factors for nuclear, cortical and posterior subcapsular cataracts in the Chinese population of Singapore: the Tanjong Pagar Survey," *The British Journal of Ophthalmology*, vol. 87, no. 9, pp. 1112–1120, 2003.

[4] B. Bergman, H. Nilsson-Ehle, and J. Sjöstrand, "Ocular changes, risk markers for eye disorders and effects of cataract surgery in elderly people: a study of an urban Swedish population followed from 70 to 97 years of age," *Acta Ophthalmologica Scandinavica*, vol. 82, no. 2, pp. 166–174, 2004.

[5] M. S. Nowak and J. Smigielski, "The prevalence of age-related eye diseases and cataract surgery among older adults in the city of Lodz, Poland," *Journal of Ophthalmology*, vol. 2015, Article ID 605814, 7 pages, 2015.

[6] Y. Cai, "China's below-replacement fertility: government policy or socioeconomic development?" *Population and Development Review*, vol. 36, no. 3, pp. 419–440, 2010.

[7] P. Liu, C. Li, Y. Wang et al., "The impact of the major causes of death on life expectancy in China: a 60-year longitudinal study," *BMC Public Health*, vol. 14, article 1193, 2014.

[8] H. Sasaki, Y. B. Shui, M. Kojima et al., "Characteristics of cataracts in the Chinese singaporean," *Journal of Epidemiology*, vol. 11, no. 1, pp. 16–23, 2001.

[9] M. Oles and P. Oles, "Coping style and quality of life in elderly patients with vision disturbances," *Journal of Ophthalmology*, vol. 2014, Article ID 584627, 6 pages, 2014.

[10] C. Younan, P. Mitchell, R. G. Cumming, J. Panchapakesan, E. Rochtchina, and A. M. Hales, "Hormone replacement therapy, reproductive factors, and the incidence of cataract and cataract surgery: the Blue Mountains Eye Study," *American Journal of Epidemiology*, vol. 155, no. 11, pp. 997–1006, 2002.

[11] S. Tsai, W. Hsu, C. Cheng, J. Liu, and P. Chou, "Epidemiologic study of age-related cataracts among an elderly chinese population in Shih-Pai, Taiwan," *Ophthalmology*, vol. 110, no. 6, pp. 1089–1095, 2003.

[12] M. A. Javadi and S. Zarei-Ghanavati, "Cataracts in diabetic patients: a review article," *Journal of Ophthalmic & Vision Research*, vol. 3, no. 1, pp. 52–65, 2008.

[13] A. Pollreisz and U. Schmidt-Erfurth, "Diabetic cataract—pathogenesis, epidemiology and treatment," *Journal of Ophthalmology*, vol. 2010, Article ID 608751, 8 pages, 2010.

[14] K. Lai, J. Cui, S. Ni et al., "The effects of postmenopausal hormone use on cataract: a meta-analysis," *PLoS ONE*, vol. 8, no. 10, Article ID e78647, 2013.

[15] M. Gotovac, S. Kaštelan, and A. Lukenda, "Eye and pregnancy," *Collegium Antropologicum*, vol. 37, supplement 1, pp. 189–193, 2013.

[16] P. Garg and P. Aggarwal, "Ocular changes in pregnancy," *Nepalese Journal of Ophthalmology*, vol. 4, no. 1, pp. 150–161, 2012.

[17] Y. Tian, J. Wu, G. Xu et al., "Parity and the risk of cataract: a cross-sectional analysis in the Dongfeng-Tongji cohort study," *The British Journal of Ophthalmology*, 2015.

[18] W. Chen, Y. Fang, F. Mao et al., "Assessment of disability among the elderly in Xiamen of China: a representative sample survey of 14,292 older adults," *PLoS ONE*, vol. 10, no. 6, Article ID e0131014, 2015.

[19] Y. Okura, L. H. Urban, D. W. Mahoney, S. J. Jacobsen, and R. J. Rodeheffer, "Agreement between self-report questionnaires and medical record data was substantial for diabetes, hypertension, myocardial infarction and stroke but not for heart failure," *Journal of Clinical Epidemiology*, vol. 57, no. 10, pp. 1096–1103, 2004.

[20] A. Paunksnis, F. Bojarskiene, A. Cimbalas, L. R. Cerniauskiene, D. I. Luksiene, and A. Tamosiunas, "Relation between cataract and metabolic syndrome and its components," *European Journal of Ophthalmology*, vol. 17, no. 4, pp. 605–614, 2007.

[21] F. Mu, H. Eliassen, S. Tworoger, S. Hankinson, and S. Missmer, "Reproductive history in relation to plasma sex steroid hormone, prolactin, and growth factor concentrations in premenopausal women," *Fertility and Sterility*, vol. 100, no. 3, supplement, p. S328, 2013.

[22] B. E. K. Klein, "Lens opacities in women in Beaver Dam, Wisconsin: is there evidence of an effect of sex hormones?" *Transactions of the American Ophthalmological Society*, vol. 91, pp. 517–544, 1993.

[23] E. P. Gunderson, M. Murtaugh, C. E. Lewis, C. P. Quesenberry, D. S. West, and S. Sidney, "Excess gains in weight and waist circumference associated with childbearing: the Coronary Artery Risk Development in Young Adults Study (CARDIA)," *International Journal of Obesity*, vol. 28, no. 4, pp. 525–535, 2004.

[24] E.-S. Tai, L. S. Lim, T. Aung et al., "Relation of age-related cataract with obesity and obesity genes in an Asian population," *The American Journal of Epidemiology*, vol. 169, no. 10, pp. 1267–1274, 2009.

[25] W. Wang, F. Chen, J. Mi et al., "Gestational weight gain and its relationship with birthweight of offspring," *Chinese Journal of Obstetrics and Gynecology*, vol. 48, no. 5, pp. 321–325, 2013.

[26] W. Wong, N. L. Tang, T. Lau, and T. Wong, "A new recommendation for maternal weight gain in Chinese women," *Journal of the American Dietetic Association*, vol. 100, no. 7, pp. 791–796, 2000.

[27] M. R. Razeghinejad, T. Y. Tania Tai, S. J. Fudemberg, and L. J. Katz, "Pregnancy and glaucoma," *Survey of Ophthalmology*, vol. 56, no. 4, pp. 324–335, 2011.

[28] R. B. Dinn, A. Harris, and P. S. Marcus, "Ocular Changes in Pregnancy," *Obstetrical & Gynecological Survey*, vol. 58, no. 2, pp. 137–144, 2003.

[29] R. Raman, S. S. Pal, J. S. K. Adams, P. K. Rani, K. Vaitheeswaran, and T. Sharma, "Prevalence and risk factors for cataract in diabetes: sankara nethralaya diabetic retinopathy epidemiology and molecular genetics study, report no. 17," *Investigative Ophthalmology & Visual Science*, vol. 51, no. 12, pp. 6253–6261, 2010.

[30] G. N. Rao, R. Khanna, and A. Payal, "The global burden of cataract," *Current Opinion in Ophthalmology*, vol. 22, no. 1, pp. 4–9, 2011.

[31] Y. H. Shih, H. Y. Chang, M. I. Lu, and B. S. Hurng, "Time trend of prevalence of self-reported cataract and its association with prolonged sitting in Taiwan from 2001 and 2013," *BMC Ophthalmology*, vol. 14, article 128, 2014.

[32] V. K. Shalini, M. Luthra, L. Srinivas et al., "Oxidative damage to the eye lens caused by cigarette smoke and fuel smoke condensates," *Indian Journal of Biochemistry & Biophysics*, vol. 31, no. 4, pp. 261–266, 1994.

[33] D. C. Minassian, V. Mehra, and A. Reidy, "Childbearing and risk of cataract in young women: an epidemiological study in central India," *The British Journal of Ophthalmology*, vol. 86, no. 5, pp. 548–550, 2002.

[34] D. Ivancić, Z. Mandić, J. Barać, and M. Kopić, "Cataract surgery and postoperative complications in diabetic patients," *Collegium Antropologicum*, vol. 29, supplement 1, pp. 55–58, 2005.

[35] S. S. DeBlack, "Cigarette smoking as a risk factor for cataract and age-related macular degeneration: a review of the literature," *Optometry*, vol. 74, no. 2, pp. 99–110, 2003.

[36] A. G. Abraham, N. G. Condon, and E. West Gower, "The new epidemiology of cataract," *Ophthalmology clinics of North America*, vol. 19, no. 4, pp. 415–425, 2006.

[37] T. H. Rim, M. H. Kim, W. C. Kim, T. I. Kim, and E. K. Kim, "Cataract subtype risk factors identified from the Korea National Health and Nutrition Examination survey 2008–2010," *BMC Ophthalmology*, vol. 14, article 4, 2014.

[38] F. J. Haddy and M. B. Pamnani, "Role of dietary salt in hypertension," *Journal of the American College of Nutrition*, vol. 14, no. 5, pp. 428–438, 1995.

[39] N. Dalai, H. Cui, M. Yan, G. Rile, S. Li, and X. Su, "Risk factors for the development of essential hypertension in a Mongolian population of China: a case-control study," *Genetics and Molecular Research*, vol. 13, no. 2, pp. 3283–3291, 2014.

[40] J. S. Tan, J. J. Wang, and P. Mitchell, "Influence of diabetes and cardiovascular disease on the long-term incidence of cataract: the Blue Mountains eye study," *Ophthalmic Epidemiology*, vol. 15, no. 5, pp. 317–327, 2008.

[41] G. M. Richter, M. Torres, F. Choudhury, S. P. Azen, and R. Varma, "Risk factors for cortical, nuclear, posterior subcapsular, and mixed lens opacities: the Los Angeles latino eye study," *Ophthalmology*, vol. 119, no. 3, pp. 547–554, 2012.

[42] D. E. Flaye, K. N. Sullivan, T. R. Cullinan, J. H. Silver, and R. A. F. Whitelocke, "Cataracts and cigarette smoking. The City Eye Study," *Eye*, vol. 3, no. 4, pp. 379–384, 1989.

[43] A. E. Yawson, E. M. Ackuaku-Dogbe, N. A. H. Seneadza et al., "Self-reported cataracts in older adults in Ghana: sociodemographic and health related factors," *BMC Public Health*, vol. 14, no. 1, article 949, 2014.

[44] A. L. Schneider, J. S. Pankow, G. Heiss, and E. Selvin, "Validity and reliability of self-reported diabetes in the atherosclerosis risk in communities study," *American Journal of Epidemiology*, vol. 176, no. 8, pp. 738–743, 2012.

[45] N. Goldman, I.-F. Lin, M. Weinstein, and Y.-H. Lin, "Evaluating the quality of self-reports of hypertension and diabetes," *Journal of Clinical Epidemiology*, vol. 56, no. 2, pp. 148–154, 2003.

High Levels of 17β-Estradiol Are Associated with Increased Matrix Metalloproteinase-2 and Metalloproteinase-9 Activity in Tears of Postmenopausal Women with Dry Eye

Guanglin Shen and Xiaoping Ma

Department of Ophthalmology, Zhongshan Hospital, Fudan University, 180 Fenglin Road, Shanghai 200032, China

Correspondence should be addressed to Xiaoping Ma; xiaopingma@126.com

Academic Editor: Chuanqing Ding

Purpose. To determine the serum levels of sex steroids and tear matrix metalloproteinases (MMP) 2 and 9 concentrations in postmenopausal women with dry eye. *Methods.* Forty-four postmenopausal women with dry eye and 22 asymptomatic controls were enrolled. Blood was drawn and analyzed for serum levels of sex steroids and lipids. Then, the following tests were performed: tear collection, Ocular Surface Disease Index (OSDI) questionnaire, fluorescein tear film break-up time (TBUT), corneal fluorescein staining, Schirmer test, and conjunctival impression cytology. The conjunctival mRNA expression and tear concentrations of MMP-2 and MMP-9 were measured. *Results.* Serum 17β-estradiol levels were significantly higher in the dry eye subjects than in the controls ($P = 0.03$), whereas there were no significant differences in levels of testosterone, dehydroepiandrosterone sulfate (DHEA-S), and progesterone. Tear MMP-2 and MMP-9 concentrations ($P < 0.001$), as well as the MMP-9 mRNA expression in conjunctival samples ($P = 0.02$), were significantly higher in dry eye subjects than in controls. Serum 17β-estradiol levels were positively correlated with tear MMP-2 and MMP-9 concentrations and negatively correlated with Schirmer test values. *Conclusions.* High levels of 17β-estradiol are associated with increased matrix metalloproteinase-2 and metalloproteinase-9 activity in tears of postmenopausal women with dry eye.

1. Introduction

Epidemiological data have shown that dry eye becomes more frequent with age in both sexes and that women are at a higher risk of dry eye than men [1–3]. The higher prevalence of dry eye in women has been partly attributed to hormonal changes that occur with menstruation, pregnancy, lactation, menopause [4–7], and use of medications such as contraceptives and hormone replacement therapy (HRT) [8]. Sex hormones have been suggested to play a key role in maintaining ocular surface homeostasis.

Ocular surface tissues have been found to be specific targets for sex hormones. Androgen, estrogen, and progesterone receptors have been identified in human lacrimal glands [9], meibomian glands [9, 10], and cornea and conjunctiva [11, 12]. Androgens influence the structure and function of the lacrimal and meibomian glands and exert a significant anti-inflammatory effect on the ocular surface [13, 14]. In contrast, despite the large number of studies, the impact of estrogen and progesterone on the ocular surface tissues is still controversial [15, 16]. Dry eye in postmenopausal women is characterized by both high and low serum estrogen levels and conflicting results [8, 17, 18] have been reported concerning the effect of HRT on the signs and symptoms of dry eye in women. Whether dry eye in females is caused by estrogen excess or deficiency, androgen deficiency or estrogen/androgen relative imbalance remains to be determined.

Matrix metalloproteinases (MMPs) are a family of proteolytic enzymes that function to maintain and remodel tissue architecture. In addition to their normal roles in tissue remodeling, MMP-2 and MMP-9 are known to be critical extracellular matrix remodeling enzymes in wound healing and diseases of the ocular surface [19]. There are many factors regulating MMP expression, including sex steroids, cytokines, growth factors, and cellular interactions and transformation. Sex steroids such as estrogen and testosterone have been shown to regulate MMP-2 and MMP-9 expression. Previous studies have shown that estrogen administration increases the expression of MMP-2 and MMP-9 in immortalized human corneal epithelial cells and the lacrimal glands of ovariectomized rabbits or rats [20–22]. It has also been confirmed that MMP activity is upregulated by estrogen in other tissues. For example, estrogen stimulates MMP-2 expression in human granulosa-lutein cells and vascular smooth cells [23] as well as MMP-9 expression in human mesangial cells [24]. Testosterone administration, on the other hand, has been shown to decrease MMP-2 activity in the lacrimal glands of ovariectomized rats [22]. Hence, further studies are required to determine the relationship between sex steroid levels and MMPs in humans.

The aim of this study was to determine the serum sex steroid levels, including 17β-estradiol, testosterone, dehydroepiandrosterone sulfate (DHEA-S), and progesterone, in postmenopausal women with dry eye. Furthermore, we investigated the relationship between sex steroid levels and MMP-2 and MMP-9 activity in tears.

2. Materials and Methods

2.1. Subjects. Between January 2015 and July 2015, dry eye subjects were consecutively recruited from the outpatient clinic and normal control subjects were recruited from a health checkup population at Zhongshan Hospital of Fudan University. This case-control study was approved by the local Ethical Committee and conducted in accordance with the Declaration of Helsinki. Written informed consent was obtained from each participant before starting the study procedures.

Postmenopausal women aged over 50 years were recruited and later categorized into two groups: the dry eye group and the control group. "Postmenopausal" was defined as no menses for at least 1 year. During a preliminary visit, medical history was assessed, and a comprehensive ophthalmic examination was performed on all participants to ensure eligibility. Dry eye was diagnosed if the subject fulfilled at least two of the following criteria: Ocular Surface Disease Index (OSDI) [25] score > 20, fluorescein tear film break-up time (TBUT) ≤ 5 seconds, and corneal fluorescein staining score > 3 according to the National Eye Institute (NEI) grading scale [26]. The age-matched asymptomatic control subjects exhibited normal results on all of the above measures.

Exclusion criteria for both groups included (1) ceased menses due to autoimmune disorders, smoking, or hysterectomy; (2) a history of Sjogren's syndrome (SS), diabetes, or other systemic disorders known to affect the ocular surface; (3) a history of HRT, contact lens use, or ocular surgery; (4) the use of any topical ocular medication or systemic medication known to exacerbate dry eye; and (5) the presence of anterior segment abnormality or active eye disease other than dry eye.

2.2. Study Protocol. Blood was drawn from each participant by phlebotomists at the Department of Clinical Laboratory, Zhongshan Hospital. Then, tears were collected from the participants, the OSDI questionnaire was administered to the participants, and a series of dry eye tests were performed in the following order: fluorescein TBUT, corneal fluorescein staining, Schirmer test, and conjunctival impression cytology. There was at least a 5-minute gap between each test. Dry eye tests were performed by the same researcher to maintain consistency. Application of artificial tears or other ocular lubricants was discontinued 3 days before each participant's study visit. The temperature and humidity of the examination room were controlled at a range from 20°C to 24°C and from 40% to 50%, respectively. For each subject, the right eye was used for analysis.

2.3. Laboratory Blood Analysis. Blood samples were drawn from all participants at 8:00 a.m. following an overnight fast. Serum levels of sex steroids (17β-estradiol, total testosterone, DHEA-S, and progesterone) were measured using a chemiluminescence method. The limit of detection for the steroids was as follows: 17β-estradiol 5.0 pg/mL (18.35 pmol/L), testosterone 0.087 nmol/L, DHEA-S 0.003 μmol/L, and progesterone 0.095 nmol/L. A serum lipid profile, including total cholesterol, triglycerides, high-density lipoprotein- (HDL-) cholesterol, and low-density lipoprotein- (LDL-) cholesterol, was also obtained as it may influence sex steroid levels [27].

2.4. Tear Sample Collection. Tear samples were collected using disposable 5 μL microcapillary tubes (Microcaps; Drummond Scientific Co., Broomall, PA) without anesthesia. Approximately 5 μL of tear fluids was gathered from the inferior temporal tear meniscus from each eye. Care was taken to ensure that the lid margin, cornea, or conjunctiva was not touched, to avoid as much as possible reflex tears. The tear flow rate was controlled during the process, and only samples with a flow rate of 1–5 μL/min were used for further tests. Tears from both eyes were pooled together and transferred into a 1.5 mL Eppendorf tube and then immediately stored at −80°C until further examination.

2.5. Quantification of MMP-2 and MMP-9 in Tear Samples. Total MMP-2 and MMP-9 (pro- and active forms) concentrations in extracted tear samples were each determined using commercially available quantitative sandwich ELISA kits (Quantikine; R&D Systems, Inc., Minneapolis, MN). Sample preparation and analysis were performed according to the manufacturer's instructions. Tear fluid of precise volume from each sample was transferred and diluted 1 : 20. The final results were corrected according to the dilution factor.

2.6. Assessments of Dry Eye. Dry eye symptoms were assessed using the OSDI questionnaire, which has previously been validated as a reliable method for measuring the severity of dry eye [25]. The OSDI consists of 12 questions about symptoms experienced within the previous week and yields scores ranging from 0 (least severe) to 100 (most severe).

Fluorescein TBUT was measured by instilling 5 μL of 2% sodium fluorescein solution and calculating the time between the last complete blink and the appearance of the first dry spot in the stained tear film. Three consecutive measurements were conducted, and the average value was taken.

TABLE 1: Demographics and clinical characteristics in patients with dry eye and normal controls.

Characteristics	Dry eye group ($n = 44$)	Control group ($n = 22$)	P value
Age (years)	63.2 ± 7.4	60.7 ± 5.3	0.18
Duration of menopause (years)	11.2 ± 8.0	10.3 ± 5.9	0.81
BMI	22.9 ± 2.2	22.6 ± 2.1	0.70
Lipid profile			
Total cholesterol (mmol/L)	4.5 ± 0.8	4.7 ± 1.0	0.47
Triglycerides (mmol/L)	1.5 ± 0.6	1.6 ± 0.5	0.33
HDL-cholesterol (mmol/L)	1.1 ± 0.3	1.1 ± 0.2	0.36
LDL-cholesterol (mmol/L)	2.8 ± 0.8	3.0 ± 0.9	0.28
OSDI (points)	39.5 ± 24.4	14.0 ± 8.4	<0.001
Fluorescein TBUT (s)	2.5 ± 1.1	9.8 ± 3.9	<0.001
Corneal fluorescein staining (points)	3.1 ± 2.5	0.3 ± 0.4	<0.001
Schirmer test (mm/5 min)	7.1 ± 5.6	12.6 ± 6.2	<0.001

BMI = body mass index, HDL = high-density lipoprotein, LDL = low-density lipoprotein, OSDI = Ocular Surface Disease Index, and TBUT = tear film break-up time.

Corneal fluorescein staining was evaluated under cobalt blue illumination following fluorescein instillation. Corneal staining was assessed using the NEI scale, where grades of 0–3 were assigned for five regions of the corneal surface, up to a total of 15 points.

Then, Schirmer test (without anesthesia) was performed with sterile strips inserted at the border of the medial to the lateral third of the lower lid margin with the lids closed. The moistened length was measured after 5 minutes.

2.7. Conjunctival Impression Cytology. Conjunctival epithelial cells were collected via impression cytology as previously described [28]. Briefly, after administration of topical anesthetic (0.5% proparacaine hydrochloride; Alcon), two sterile membrane filters (6 × 6 mm, Millipore) were gently placed onto the inferotemporal and superotemporal bulbar conjunctiva. Gentle pressure was applied to the filters for 10 seconds using blunt smooth edged forceps. The membranes were then gently removed from the eye and transferred into an Eppendorf tube containing TRIzol reagent (Invitrogen; Carlsbad, CA). The samples were then stored at −80°C until processing.

2.8. Real-Time PCR. Total RNA in conjunctival cell samples was isolated using TRIzol Reagent (Invitrogen) and then reverse-transcribed with Prime-Script RT Master mix (Takara, Otsu, Japan). Gene expression was detected by quantitative real-time PCR using primers for MMP-2, MMP-9, and glyceraldehyde 3-phosphate dehydrogenase (GADPH). The primer sequences used were as follows: MMP-2 (sense: 5′-AGCGAG-TGGATGCCGCCTTTAA-3′; antisense: 5′-CATTCCAGG-CATCTGCGATGAG-3′); MMP-9 (sense: 5′-GCCACTACT-GTGCCTTTGAGTC-3′; antisense: 5′-CCCTCAGAGAAT-CGCCAGTACT-3′); and GADPH (sense: 5′-GTCTCCTCT-GACTTCAACAGCG-3′; antisense: 5′-ACCACCCTGTTG-CTGTAGCCAA-3′). Reactions were performed using the Roche LightCycler 480 System (Roche, Indianapolis, IN) in combination with a SYBR Premix Ex Taq Kit (Takara) according to the manufacturer's instructions. The relative gene expression was calculated using the Comparative C_T Method and standardizing levels to GADPH mRNA.

2.9. Data Analysis. Statistical analysis was performed using SPSS version 20.0 (SPSS Inc., Chicago, IL). Descriptive statistics were presented as the mean ± standard deviation (SD). The sample size (at least 15 eyes at each group) was determined to detect 20% difference in sex steroid levels, with $\alpha = 0.05$ and $\beta = 0.20$. Some values of 17β-estradiol levels were below the limit of assay quantitation (5 pg/mL). Thus, we categorized subjects by 17β-estradiol levels less than 5 pg/mL and by 17β-estradiol levels of 5 pg/mL or greater for analysis. Differences in demographics and measurements between the 2 groups were assessed using Mann-Whitney test for continuous measures and Pearson's chi-squared test for categorical factors. Spearman's rank correlation coefficients between parameters were calculated. $P < 0.05$ was considered statistically significant.

3. Results

3.1. Characteristics of Subjects. A total of 66 postmenopausal women (66 eyes, mean age 62.4 ± 6.8 years) were enrolled in this study. Among the 66 subjects, 44 subjects were identified as having dry eye based on the diagnostic criteria, and 22 normal control subjects were included for comparison. Baseline demographics and clinical characteristics in patients with dry eye and normal controls are presented in Table 1. No significant differences were noted between the 2 study groups in terms of age, duration of menopause, body mass index (BMI), or lipid profile (total cholesterol, triglycerides, HDL-cholesterol, and LDL-cholesterol). All 66 women had normal weight (BMI range: 18.5–25) and cholesterol levels. The results of OSDI, fluorescein TBUT, corneal fluorescein staining, and Schirmer test differed significantly between the dry eye group and the control group ($P < 0.001$).

3.2. Serum Levels of Sex Steroids. The serum levels of sex steroids in the dry eye group and the control group are

TABLE 2: Comparison of serum levels of sex steroids between the dry eye group and the normal control group.

Laboratory test	Dry eye group ($n = 44$)	Control group ($n = 22$)	P value
17β-Estradiol (pg/mL)			0.03*
<5	29	20	
≥5	15	2	
Testosterone (nmol/L)	0.60 ± 0.41	0.40 ± 0.24	0.08
DHEA-S (μmol/L)	3.53 ± 1.93	3.15 ± 1.30	0.57
Progesterone (nmol/L)	0.79 ± 0.53	0.63 ± 0.39	0.34

*Pearson's chi-squared test.

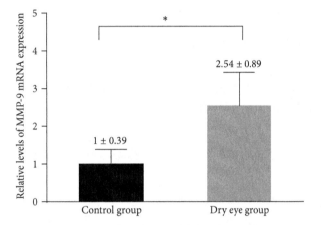

FIGURE 1: Real-time PCR results of relative levels of MMP-9 mRNA expression in conjunctival cytology samples obtained from patients with dry eye and normal controls. Values were presented as mean ± SD. *Significant difference with $P < 0.05$.

presented in Table 2. This study showed detectable levels of 17β-estradiol (≥5 pg/mL) in 15 dry eye subjects (34% of subjects) and 2 normal controls (9% of subjects). 17β-Estradiol levels were significantly higher in the dry eye subjects than in the controls ($\chi^2 = 4.79$, $P = 0.03$). Levels of testosterone, DHEA-S, and progesterone were higher in the dry eye group, but differences did not reach a level of significance ($P = 0.08$, $P = 0.57$, and $P = 0.34$, resp.).

3.3. MMP-2 and MMP-9 Gene Expression.
The results of MMP mRNA expression in conjunctival epithelia were obtained by impression cytology from dry eye subjects and normal controls. Significantly higher levels of MMP-9 mRNA were observed in dry eye subjects than in normal controls ($P = 0.02$, Figure 1). MMP-2 transcripts were undetectable in the samples obtained from normal subjects and those obtained from dry eye subjects.

3.4. MMP-2 and MMP-9 Concentrations in Tears.
The concentrations of MMP-2 and MMP-9 in the tears of all subjects are shown in Figure 2. The two MMPs tested were detected in all of the samples. The tear concentrations of MMP-2 and MMP-9 in the dry eye group were significantly greater than those in the control group ($P < 0.001$).

3.5. Correlation of Sex Steroid Levels with MMP-2 and MMP-9 Tear Concentrations and Clinical Tests.
Table 3 shows the correlation of sex steroids levels with MMP-2 and MMP-9 tear concentrations and clinical tests in the dry eye group. Specifically, the results of the correlation between 17β-estradiol and other test parameters were calculated from the data gathered from 15 dry eye subjects who had detectable levels of 17β-estradiol. The analysis of the other three sex steroids was conducted in all 44 dry eye subjects. The levels of 17β-estradiol positively correlated with tear concentrations of MMP-2 and MMP-9. The results of Schirmer test showed a significant negative correlation with 17β-estradiol (Figure 3). The levels of testosterone showed a weak negative correlation with TBUT results but no correlation with the results of other tests. The levels of DHEA-S and progesterone showed no correlations with the results of the other tests.

4. Discussion

The prevalence of dry eye is higher in females, especially in postmenopausal women [1]. This fact indicates that sex steroid imbalance is related to the onset and development of dry eye. However, the role of sex steroids in dry eye is complex and remains to be fully understood. Our results demonstrate that the serum levels of 17β-estradiol were significantly higher in postmenopausal women with dry eye than in controls, whereas the levels of testosterone, DHEA-S, and progesterone between the two groups were not significantly different.

Only a few studies have investigated the levels of sex steroids in postmenopausal women with dry eye. Tamer et al. [29] evaluated androgen levels in dry eye patients both with meibomian gland dysfunction (MGD) and without MGD and compared these levels with those of normal control subjects. Total testosterone levels were not significantly different among the three groups, which is consistent with our results. The study also reported lower levels of bioavailable testosterone, DHEA, and DHEA-S in MGD patients than in controls, whereas there was no significant difference between non-MGD dry eye patients and controls. Another small-sample study [30] also found no significant difference in total testosterone levels between postmenopausal women with dry eye and controls. Inconsistent with our findings, a recent study [31] reported that the serum levels of 17β-estradiol and total testosterone were significantly lower in evaporative dry eye patients than in controls. In patients with SS, the disease is not associated with significant alterations in serum levels of testosterone, estrone, or estradiol, whereas DHEA and DHEA-S levels were significantly reduced [32]. However, another study showed no significant difference in DHEA and DHEA-S levels in patients with SS [32, 33].

In our study, we did not subdivide dry eye patients into MGD or non-MGD categories. This could partially explain the differences in sex steroids levels between the current study and previous studies. It would be worth looking at aqueous deficient and evaporative dry eye separately. Other possible factors for the conflicting results among these studies are limited number of subjects, racial differences, and variations in the duration of menopause. In addition, serum sex steroids could not reflect the total estrogen and androgen pool in

TABLE 3: Spearman correlation of sex steroid levels with tear MMP concentrations and clinical tests.

Parameters	MMP-2		MMP-9		OSDI		TBUT		Corneal staining		Schirmer test	
	ρ	P	ρ	P	ρ	P	ρ	P	ρ	P	ρ	P
17β-Estradiol	0.67	0.006*	0.58	0.03*	−0.07	0.80	−0.38	0.17	−0.09	0.74	−0.58	0.02*
Testosterone	0.28	0.12	0.21	0.24	0.14	0.41	−0.32	0.04*	0.17	0.28	0.02	0.91
DHEA-S	0.004	0.98	0.16	0.38	0.31	0.06	−0.09	0.58	−0.16	0.32	−0.05	0.75
Progesterone	0.07	0.72	0.06	0.77	0.24	0.16	−0.15	0.34	−0.10	0.56	0.02	0.90

DHEA-S = dehydroepiandrosterone sulfate, MMP = matrix metalloproteinase, OSDI = Ocular Surface Disease Index, and TBUT = tear film break-up time.
*Significant difference with $P < 0.05$
ρ: Spearman's correlation coefficient.

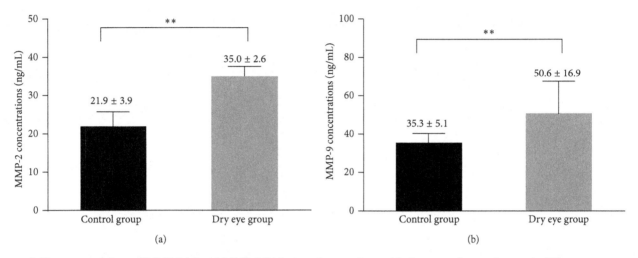

FIGURE 2: The concentrations of MMP-2 (a) and MMP-9 (b) in tears from patients with dry eye and normal controls. Values were presented as mean ± SD. **Significant difference with $P < 0.001$.

postmenopausal women [34]. It should be noted that humans are unique in possessing adrenal glands that secrete large amounts of DHEA and DHEA-S, which are then converted into androgens and estrogens by steroidogenic enzymes in peripheral tissues and thereby permit target tissues to adjust the amount of active sex hormones according to local requirements [34]. The human ocular surface has been shown to contain mRNAs for steroidogenic enzymes, which are necessary for the local synthesis and metabolism of androgens and estrogens [11]. Therefore, the human ocular surface may be among the many peripheral tissues and be a source of sex steroids.

Versura et al. [6] reported that ocular surface function impairment is greatest when estrogen levels are highest as this impairment occurs during the follicular phase in the menstrual cycle. We found that the levels of estrogen in dry eye patients were still higher than those of age-matched controls after menopause. In another study, 11 out of 20 asymptomatic postmenopausal women developed dry eye symptoms after three months of HRT (estrogen/progesterone) use, whereas symptomatic women were not relieved of dry eye by HRT [35]. A large population-based study of 25,665 postmenopausal women found an increased risk of dry eye in women using HRT, particularly among those using estrogen alone [8]. These data support the hypothesis that estrogen has detrimental effects on the ocular surface.

Inflammation is a common factor that underlies many causes of dry eye. This study assessed the ocular surface expression of MMP-2 and MMP-9, molecules strictly related to the inflammatory process [21]. MMP-9 activity has also been considered to be a better biomarker of dry eye disease severity than traditional clinical signs and is associated with disruption of corneal epithelial barrier function [36, 37].

In this study, quantitative real-time PCR showed that the conjunctival expression of MMP-9 was significantly higher in dry eye patients than in controls, similar to the results of Chotikavanich et al. [36], which found an increasing trend in MMP-9 expression in dry eye subjects stratified by severity level. However, we were unable to detect MMP-2 expression in the conjunctival epithelium in our present study, which is possibly explained by the lower MMP-2 production in the conjunctiva than in other ocular surface tissues [38]. In addition, a lower amount of total RNA was obtained by impression cytology, which may have decreased sensitivity.

Increased MMP-2 and MMP-9 production has been observed in the tear fluid collected from patients with systemic dry eye and from those with nonsystemic dry eye [37, 39]. Consistent with previous findings, we also found that the tear concentrations of MMP-2 and MMP-9 in dry eye subjects were significantly higher than those in controls.

We also observed that the levels of 17β-estradiol were correlated positively with tear concentrations of MMP-2 and

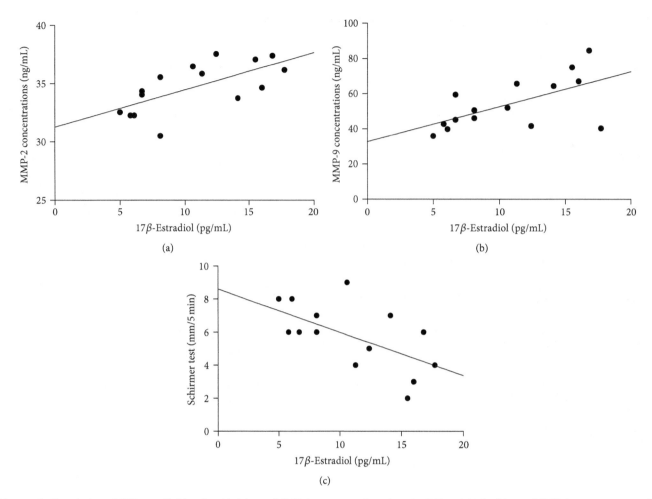

FIGURE 3: Correlation of 17β-estradiol levels with (a) tear MMP-2 concentrations ($\rho = 0.67$, $P = 0.006$); (b) tear MMP-9 concentrations ($\rho = 0.58$, $P = 0.03$); and (c) Schirmer test results ($\rho = -0.58$, $P = 0.02$). Spearman's rank correlation coefficients were calculated in 15 dry eye subjects who had detectable levels of 17β-estradiol.

MMP-9. This finding indicates that 17β-estradiol stimulates the activity of MMP-2 and MMP-9 in tears of patients with dry eye. The source of tear-derived MMP-2 and MMP-9 has not been established. Corneal epithelial cells [19] and lacrimal glands [21] have been found to synthesize both MMP-2 and MMP-9 in the ocular surface system. A recent study has shown that the major sources of tear-derived MMP-2 and MMP-9 following corneal wounding are the lacrimal gland and conjunctival-associated lymphoid tissue, whereas the corneal epithelium, stromal keratocytes, and conjunctival epithelium including goblet cells contribute little to tear-derived MMP-2 and MMP-9, and the meibomian glands do not appear to contribute at all [38]. Therefore, we postulate that 17β-estradiol may have effects on the promotion of inflammation in the lacrimal gland and conjunctival epithelium and may increase the activity of MMP-2 and MMP-9 in tears of patients with dry eye.

The rationale for our postulation is supported by previous studies on 17β-estradiol effects in ocular surface tissues. Suzuki and Sullivan have reported that 17β-estradiol upregulated the gene expression of proinflammatory cytokines and MMP-2, MMP-7, and MMP-9 in SV40 immortalized human corneal epithelial cells (HCEs) after 6 and/or 24 hours of hormone treatment [20]. However, 17β-estradiol effects on gene expression are not translated into changes in MMP-2 and MMP-9 activity in the culture of either SV40 HCEs or primary corneal epithelial cell cultures [40]. On the other hand, an animal study showed that estrogen treatment of ovariectomized rabbits significantly upregulates the expression and activity of MMP-2 and MMP-9 in the lacrimal gland [21]. A more recent study also demonstrated that systemic estradiol administration increases MMP-2 expression in lacrimal glands of ovariectomized rats [22]. Moreover, in the present study, 17β-estradiol was found to have a negative correlation with Schirmer test results but no correlation with the results of OSDI or corneal staining. Consistent with our result, Mathers et al. also reported a negative correlation between serum estradiol levels and tear production in postmenopausal women [4]. These results indicate that 17β-estradiol leads to regressive, inflammatory changes of the lacrimal gland, and, thus, tear production is reduced.

A limitation of our study is the fact that the method used to assess serum 17β-estradiol levels was not sensitive enough because many values were below the limit of detection. Further studies with larger subject numbers and with more sensitive analytical techniques are needed.

5. Conclusions

In conclusion, this study demonstrated that serum levels of 17β-estradiol were higher in postmenopausal women with dry eye than in controls. Levels of 17β-estradiol positively correlated with tear MMP-2 and MMP-9 concentrations and negatively correlated with Schirmer test results. We postulate that 17β-estradiol upregulates MMP-2 and MMP-9 production in the lacrimal gland and MMP-9 production in the conjunctival epithelium and thus increases the activity of MMP-2 and MMP-9 in tears of dry eye subjects. Our results support the findings from animal studies that showed upregulation of MMP levels following estradiol treatment.

Disclosure

Guanglin Shen is the first author.

Conflict of Interests

The authors declare that there is no conflict of interests regarding the publication of this paper.

Acknowledgment

This work is supported by the research grant from the Shanghai Municipal Commission of Health and Family Planning (Grant no. 2011Z-11/3).

References

[1] J. A. Smith, J. Albenz, C. Begley et al., "The epidemiology of dry eye disease: report of the Epidemiology Subcommittee of the International Dry Eye WorkShop (2007)," *Ocular Surface*, vol. 5, no. 2, pp. 93–107, 2007.

[2] C. A. McCarty, A. K. Bansal, P. M. Livingston, Y. L. Stanislavsky, and H. R. Taylor, "The epidemiology of dry eye in Melbourne, Australia," *Ophthalmology*, vol. 105, no. 6, pp. 1114–1119, 1998.

[3] E.-M. Chia, P. Mitchell, E. Rochtchina, A. J. Lee, R. Maroun, and J. J. Wang, "Prevalence and associations of dry eye syndrome in an older population: the Blue Mountains Eye study," *Clinical and Experimental Ophthalmology*, vol. 31, no. 3, pp. 229–232, 2003.

[4] W. D. Mathers, D. Stovall, J. A. Lane, M. B. Zimmerman, and S. Johnson, "Menopause and tear function: the influence of prolactin and sex hormones on human tear production," *Cornea*, vol. 17, no. 4, pp. 353–358, 1998.

[5] P. Versura and E. C. Campos, "Menopause and dry eye. A possible relationship," *Gynecological Endocrinology*, vol. 20, no. 5, pp. 289–298, 2005.

[6] P. Versura, M. Fresina, and E. C. Campos, "Ocular surface changes over the menstrual cycle in women with and without dry eye," *Gynecological Endocrinology*, vol. 23, no. 7, pp. 385–390, 2007.

[7] P. Kramer, V. Lubkin, W. Potter, M. Jacobs, G. Labay, and P. Silverman, "Cyclic changes in conjunctival smears from menstruating females," *Ophthalmology*, vol. 97, no. 3, pp. 303–307, 1990.

[8] D. A. Schaumberg, J. E. Buring, D. A. Sullivan, and M. Reza Dana, "Hormone replacement therapy and dry eye syndrome," *The Journal of the American Medical Association*, vol. 286, no. 17, pp. 2114–2119, 2001.

[9] E. M. Rocha, L. A. Wickham, L. A. Da Silveira et al., "Identification of androgen receptor protein and 5α-reductase mRNA in human ocular tissues," *British Journal of Ophthalmology*, vol. 84, no. 1, pp. 76–84, 2000.

[10] B. Esmaeli, J. T. Harvey, and B. Hewlett, "Immunohistochemical evidence for estrogen receptors in meibomian glands," *Ophthalmology*, vol. 107, no. 1, pp. 180–184, 2000.

[11] F. Schirra, T. Suzuki, D. P. Dickinson, D. J. Townsend, I. K. Gipson, and D. A. Sullivan, "Identification of steroidogenic enzyme mRNAs in the human lacrimal gland, meibomian gland, cornea, and conjunctiva," *Cornea*, vol. 25, no. 4, pp. 438–442, 2006.

[12] L. A. Wickham, J. Gao, I. Toda, E. M. Rocha, M. Ono, and D. A. Sullivan, "Identification of androgen, estrogen and progesterone receptor mRNAs in the eye," *Acta Ophthalmologica Scandinavica*, vol. 78, no. 2, pp. 146–153, 2000.

[13] D. A. Sullivan, B. D. Sullivan, M. D. Ullman et al., "Androgen influence on the meibomian gland," *Investigative Ophthalmology & Visual Science*, vol. 41, no. 12, pp. 3732–3742, 2000.

[14] D. A. Sullivan, L. Block, and J. D. O. Pena, "Influence of androgens and pituitary hormones on the structural profile and secretory activity of the lacrimal gland," *Acta Ophthalmologica Scandinavica*, vol. 74, no. 5, pp. 421–435, 1996.

[15] S. Truong, N. Cole, F. Stapleton, and B. Golebiowski, "Sex hormones and the dry eye," *Clinical and Experimental Optometry*, vol. 97, no. 4, pp. 324–336, 2014.

[16] P. Versura, G. Giannaccare, and E. C. Campos, "Sex-steroid imbalance in females and dry eye," *Current Eye Research*, vol. 40, no. 2, pp. 162–175, 2015.

[17] K.-S. Na, D. H. Jee, K. Han, Y.-G. Park, M. S. Kim, and E. C. Kim, "The ocular benefits of estrogen replacement therapy: a population-based study in postmenopausal Korean women," *PLoS ONE*, vol. 9, no. 9, Article ID e106473, 2014.

[18] A. A. Jensen, E. J. Higginbotham, G. M. Guzinski, I. L. Davis, and N. J. Ellish, "A survey of ocular complaints in postmenopausal women," *Journal of the Association for Academic Minority Physicians*, vol. 11, no. 2-3, pp. 44–49, 2000.

[19] D.-Q. Li, B. L. Lokeshwar, A. Solomon, D. Monroy, Z. Ji, and S. C. Pflugfelder, "Regulation of MMP-9 production by human corneal epithelial cells," *Experimental Eye Research*, vol. 73, no. 4, pp. 449–459, 2001.

[20] T. Suzuki and D. A. Sullivan, "Estrogen stimulation of proinflammatory cytokine and matrix metalloproteinase gene expression in human corneal epithelial cells," *Cornea*, vol. 24, no. 8, pp. 1004–1009, 2005.

[21] C. Zylberberg, V. Seamon, O. Ponomareva, K. Vellala, M. Deighan, and A. M. Azzarolo, "Estrogen up-regulation of metalloproteinase-2 and -9 expression in rabbit lacrimal glands," *Experimental Eye Research*, vol. 84, no. 5, pp. 960–972, 2007.

[22] X. Song, P. Zhao, G. Wang, and X. Zhao, "The effects of estrogen and androgen on tear secretion and matrix metalloproteinase-2 expression in lacrimal glands of ovariectomized rats," *Investigative Ophthalmology and Visual Science*, vol. 55, no. 2, pp. 745–751, 2014.

[23] C. S. Wingrove, E. Garr, I. F. Godsland, and J. C. Stevenson, "17β-Oestradiol enhances release of matrix metalloproteinase-2 from human vascular smooth muscle cells," *Biochimica et*

Biophysica Acta (BBA)—Molecular Basis of Disease, vol. 1406, no. 2, pp. 169–174, 1998.

[24] M. Potier, S. J. Elliot, I. Tack et al., "Expression and regulation of estrogen receptors in mesangial cells: influence on matrix metalloproteinase-9," *Journal of the American Society of Nephrology*, vol. 12, no. 2, pp. 241–251, 2001.

[25] R. M. Schiffman, M. D. Christianson, G. Jacobsen, J. D. Hirsch, and B. L. Reis, "Reliability and validity of the ocular surface disease index," *Archives of Ophthalmology*, vol. 118, no. 5, pp. 615–621, 2000.

[26] M. A. Lemp, "Report of the National Eye Institute/Industry workshop on clinical trials in dry eyes," *The CLAO Journal*, vol. 21, no. 4, pp. 221–232, 1995.

[27] W. L. Miller and R. J. Auchus, "The molecular biology, biochemistry, and physiology of human steroidogenesis and its disorders," *Endocrine Reviews*, vol. 32, no. 1, pp. 81–151, 2011.

[28] R. Singh, A. Joseph, T. Umapathy, N. L. Tint, and H. S. Dua, "Impression cytology of the ocular surface," *British Journal of Ophthalmology*, vol. 89, no. 12, pp. 1655–1659, 2005.

[29] C. Tamer, H. Oksuz, and S. Sogut, "Androgen status of the nonautoimmune dry eye subtypes," *Ophthalmic Research*, vol. 38, no. 5, pp. 280–286, 2006.

[30] M. C. B. Duarte, N. T. Pinto, H. Moreira, A. T. R. Moreira, and D. Wasilewski, "Total testosterone level in postmenopausal women with dry eye," *Arquivos Brasileiros De Oftalmologia*, vol. 70, no. 3, pp. 465–469, 2007.

[31] C. Gagliano, S. Caruso, G. Napolitano et al., "Low levels of 17-β-oestradiol, oestrone and testosterone correlate with severe evaporative dysfunctional tear syndrome in postmenopausal women: a case-control study," *British Journal of Ophthalmology*, vol. 98, no. 3, pp. 371–376, 2014.

[32] D. A. Sullivan, A. Bélanger, J. M. Cermak et al., "Are women with Sjögren's syndrome androgen-deficient?" *Journal of Rheumatology*, vol. 30, no. 11, pp. 2413–2419, 2003.

[33] M. T. Brennan, V. Sankar, R. A. Leakan et al., "Sex steroid hormones in primary Sjögren's syndrome," *The Journal of Rheumatology*, vol. 30, no. 6, pp. 1267–1271, 2003.

[34] F. Labrie, A. Bélanger, V. Luu-The et al., "DHEA and the intracrine formation of androgens and estrogens in peripheral target tissues: its role during aging," *Steroids*, vol. 63, no. 5-6, pp. 322–328, 1998.

[35] U. Erdem, O. Ozdegirmenci, E. Sobaci, G. Sobaci, U. Göktolga, and S. Dagli, "Dry eye in post-menopausal women using hormone replacement therapy," *Maturitas*, vol. 56, no. 3, pp. 257–262, 2007.

[36] S. Chotikavanich, C. S. de Paiva, de Quan Li et al., "Production and activity of matrix metalloproteinase-9 on the ocular surface increase in dysfunctional tear syndrome," *Investigative Ophthalmology & Visual Science*, vol. 50, no. 7, pp. 3203–3209, 2009.

[37] K. R. Vandermeid, S. P. Su, K. W. Ward, and J.-Z. Zhang, "Correlation of tear inflammatory cytokines and matrix metalloproteinases with four dry eye diagnostic tests," *Investigative Ophthalmology and Visual Science*, vol. 53, no. 3, pp. 1512–1518, 2012.

[38] A. Petznick, M. C. Madigan, Q. Garrett, D. F. Sweeney, and M. D. M. Evans, "Contributions of ocular surface components to matrix-metalloproteinases (MMP)-2 and MMP-9 in feline tears following corneal epithelial wounding," *PLoS ONE*, vol. 8, no. 8, Article ID e71948, 2013.

[39] A. Solomon, D. Dursun, Z. Liu, Y. Xie, A. Macri, and S. C. Pflugfelder, "Pro- and anti-inflammatory forms of interleukin-1 in the tear fluid and conjunctiva of patients with dry-eye disease," *Investigative Ophthalmology and Visual Science*, vol. 42, no. 10, pp. 2283–2292, 2001.

[40] T. Suzuki and D. A. Sullivan, "Comparative effects of estrogen on matrix metalloproteinases and cytokines in immortalized and primary human corneal epithelial cell cultures," *Cornea*, vol. 25, no. 4, pp. 454–459, 2006.

Safety and Efficacy of Adding Fixed-Combination Brinzolamide/Timolol Maleate to Prostaglandin Therapy for Treatment of Ocular Hypertension or Glaucoma

Anton Hommer,[1] Douglas A. Hubatsch,[2] and Juan Cano-Parra[3]

[1]*Private Office, Vienna, Austria*
[2]*Alcon Laboratories, Inc., Fort Worth, TX 76134, USA*
[3]*Hospital Municipal de Badalona, 08911 Barcelona, Spain*

Correspondence should be addressed to Anton Hommer; a.hommer@aon.at

Academic Editor: Gianluca Manni

Purpose. To evaluate the safety and efficacy of adding brinzolamide 1%/timolol maleate 0.5% fixed combination (BTFC) to a prostaglandin analog (PGA). *Methods.* This was a 12-week, open-label, single-arm study of patients with open-angle glaucoma or ocular hypertension with intraocular pressure (IOP) not sufficiently controlled after ≥4 weeks of PGA monotherapy. The primary outcome was mean IOP change from baseline at week 12. Other outcomes included IOP change from baseline at week 4, percentage of patients achieving IOP ≤18 mmHg at week 12, and patient experience survey responses at week 12. *Results.* Forty-seven patients were enrolled and received treatment. The most commonly used PGAs were latanoprost (47%) and travoprost (32%). Mean ± SD IOP was decreased at week 12 (17.2 ± 4.1 mmHg) compared with baseline (23.1 ± 3.0 mmHg; $P < 0.001$, paired t-test); IOP at week 4 was 17.2 ± 3.3 mmHg. At week 12, 70% of patients achieved IOP ≤18 mmHg. Patient-reported symptoms (e.g., pain and redness) were mostly unchanged from baseline. Twenty-eight adverse events (AEs) were reported; the most frequently reported AE was headache (3 events in 2 patients). *Conclusion.* Adjunctive BTFC + PGA therapy was effective and well tolerated. IOP decreased by 6 mmHg at weeks 4 and 12.

1. Introduction

Elevated intraocular pressure (IOP) is the major risk factor for development of primary open-angle glaucoma (POAG), and higher IOP levels are associated with increased risk of glaucoma-related blindness [1, 2]. Lowering IOP with pharmacologic therapy reduces the rate of disease progression (e.g., optic neuropathy) and visual field loss and reduces the risk of conversion from ocular hypertension (OH) to glaucoma [2–4]. Pharmacotherapy is usually initiated with a single ocular hypotensive agent [2], and prostaglandin analogs (PGAs) or β-blockers are frequently prescribed as initial monotherapy because of their IOP-lowering efficacy and safety profiles [5].

However, many patients require multiple IOP-lowering agents to achieve or maintain sufficient IOP reduction [4]. Combining glaucoma medications with complementary mechanisms of action may further reduce IOP. PGAs (e.g., latanoprost, travoprost, and bimatoprost) reduce IOP by increasing uveoscleral and, to a lesser extent, trabecular aqueous humor outflow, whereas β-blockers (e.g., timolol) and carbonic anhydrase inhibitors (brinzolamide, dorzolamide) decrease aqueous humor production [2]. Increasing the number of individual medications that patients must self-administer increases treatment complexity and may reduce adherence to glaucoma medication regimens [6, 7]. For patients with IOP insufficiently controlled with a single medication, adding a fixed-combination adjunctive therapy to their monotherapy provides additive IOP-lowering efficacy with only 2 medication bottles (versus 3 with individual agents). Glaucoma treatment guidelines typically suggest stepwise addition of 1 ocular hypotensive medication at a time for patients who require additional IOP reduction [8–10]; however, adding a fixed-combination glaucoma medication to monotherapy has been reported to be well tolerated and effective [11].

Brinzolamide 1%/timolol maleate 0.5% fixed-combination ophthalmic suspension (BTFC; AZARGA, Alcon Laboratories, Inc., Fort Worth, TX) has been demonstrated to effectively lower IOP in patients with POAG or OH, including those transitioned because of insufficient reduction in IOP with previous therapy [12].

The purpose of this study was to evaluate the efficacy and safety of adding BTFC to PGA monotherapy in patients with POAG or OH who were responsive to but inadequately controlled by their PGA monotherapy.

2. Methods

2.1. Study Design and Treatment. This was a 12-week, prospective, interventional, single-arm, open-label study conducted at 5 sites in Austria and Spain from March 2011 to April 2013 (registration identifiers: ClinicalTrials.gov, NCT01263444; EudraCT, 2010-022948-21). The study consisted of 3 visits: a screening/baseline visit and follow-up visits conducted after 4 weeks (±3 days) and 12 weeks (±3 days) of treatment. Follow-up visits were scheduled for approximately the same time of day as the baseline visit (±1 hour). At the conclusion of the baseline visit, patients were instructed to continue their PGA therapy and to self-administer 1 drop of BTFC (10 mg/mL [1.0%] brinzolamide/5 mg/mL [0.5%] timolol) into the study eye(s) twice daily at 8 AM and 8 PM for 12 weeks. The 8 PM dose was instilled at a 5-minute interval from the once-daily PGA dose. For eyes not qualifying for inclusion in the study, IOP was required to be controlled either with no pharmacologic intervention or with prostaglandin monotherapy. Patients using contact lenses during the study were instructed to remove lenses for instillation of study medication and to wait ≥15 minutes after instillation before reinsertion.

This study was approved by the Ethikkommission der Stadt Wien (Austria) and CEIC Fundación Oftalmológica del Mediterráneo (Spain) and was performed in compliance with the ethical principles of the Declaration of Helsinki and Good Clinical Practice. Before screening, patients provided written informed consent using an ethics board-approved consent form.

2.2. Patients. Eligible patients were aged ≥18 years with an existing clinical diagnosis of OH, POAG, or pigment dispersion glaucoma in both eyes. Additional inclusion criteria were IOP responsive to but insufficiently controlled by PGA monotherapy after ≥4 weeks of treatment before screening; baseline IOP (on PGA therapy) ≥20 mmHg in at least 1 eye (the study eye) and ≤35 mmHg in both eyes; and best-corrected visual acuity (BCVA) of 6/60 Snellen (1.0 log MAR) or better in each eye.

Key exclusion criteria were medical history of allergy, hypersensitivity, or poor tolerance to any components of the study medications; any primary or secondary glaucoma other than POAG, OH, or pigment dispersion glaucoma; narrow angle with complete or partial closure in either eye; progressive retinal or optic nerve disease other than glaucoma; corneal dystrophies or concurrent conjunctivitis, keratitis, or uveitis in either eye; history or risk of uveitis or cystoid macular edema; history of herpes simplex; any abnormality in the study eye preventing reliable applanation tonometry or fundus/anterior chamber examination; intraocular conventional or laser surgery <3 months before screening; any cardiac or pulmonary condition that precluded safe administration of a topical β-blocker; any use of corticosteroids ≤30 days before the study or during the study; use of any carbonic anhydrase inhibitor; severely impaired renal function; hyperchloremic acidosis; myasthenia gravis; and participation in any other investigational study ≤30 days before baseline. Women who were pregnant, lactating, or of childbearing potential and not using a reliable method of birth control were also excluded. For patients using systemic medications that may affect IOP (e.g., oral β-blockers, α-agonists and blockers, angiotensin-converting enzyme inhibitors, and calcium channel blockers), a stable course was required for ≥7 days before baseline and throughout the study.

2.3. Efficacy Outcomes and Assessments. The primary efficacy outcome was the mean change in IOP from baseline, when patients were receiving PGA monotherapy, to week 12, when patients were receiving BTFC plus PGA. Other assessments included the mean change in IOP from baseline to week 4, percentage of patients reaching the target IOP of ≤18 mmHg at week 12, and mean change in patient experience survey responses from baseline to week 12. IOP measurements were performed at baseline, week 4, and week 12 by Goldmann applanation tonometry; tonometers were calibrated before patient screening was initiated, and IOP measurements for individual patients were performed by the same operator using the same tonometer at all visits. The patient experience survey was administered at the baseline visit and at week 12. Symptom severity was defined as minimal (symptom present but barely noticeable), mild (symptom definitely present but does not limit activity), moderate (symptom present and severe enough to partially limit activity), or severe (symptom present and is incapacitating).

2.4. Safety Outcomes and Assessments. Safety was assessed by monitoring adverse event (AE) reports. Ocular signs and BCVA at weeks 4 and 12 were also assessed. Ocular signs were assessed in both eyes at each study visit by slit-lamp biomicroscopy of the eyelids, conjunctiva, cornea, iris, anterior chamber, and lens. Findings were graded as 0.5 (trace), 1 (mild), 2 (moderate), or 3 (severe). BCVA was measured using a Snellen visual acuity chart at each study visit; if >1 error occurred on a given line, values were rounded up.

2.5. Statistical Analyses. Efficacy outcomes were analyzed in the intent-to-treat (ITT) population (i.e., all patients who received study medication and had at least 1 on-therapy study visit) and in the per-protocol (PP) population (i.e., all patients who received study medication, completed all study visits, and had no major protocol deviations) using data from the study eye. Safety outcomes were analyzed using data for all patients who received study medication.

Mean IOP change from baseline measured at week 12 was analyzed by 2-sided paired t-tests; results at week 4 were considered supportive data. Changes in patient experience survey responses were evaluated by 1-way analysis of variance. Demographic information, percentages of patients with IOP ≤18 mmHg versus >18 mmHg, and safety data were summarized descriptively. Statistical analyses were performed using SAS (SAS Institute, Cary, NC, USA) by an independent biostatistician; $P < 0.05$ was considered statistically significant.

A power calculation determined that completion of the study by ≥40 patients was sufficient to detect a difference in mean IOP ≥1.5 mmHg (week 12 versus baseline; SD = 2.8 mmHg) with 90% power. To ensure that ≥40 patients completed the study, the target enrollment was 50 patients.

3. Results

3.1. Patients. Forty-seven patients were enrolled and included in the safety and ITT data sets; 38 patients completed the study. Most patients were aged ≥66 years (72.3%, $n = 34/47$), and approximately half were female (51.1%, $n = 24/47$). Patient diagnoses at enrollment were OH, 66.0% ($n = 31$); POAG, 55.3% ($n = 26$); and pigment dispersion glaucoma, 2.1% ($n = 1$). Two diagnoses were reported for some patients, causing total diagnoses to exceed 100%. Latanoprost was the most frequently used PGA therapy (46.8%, $n = 22/47$), followed by travoprost (31.9%, $n = 15/47$), bimatoprost (17.0%, $n = 8/47$), and tafluprost (4.3%, $n = 2/47$). Nine patients discontinued from the study; 8 discontinuations were because of AEs, and 1 patient withdrew consent. One patient was excluded from the PP data set ($n = 37$) because of a protocol deviation (i.e., exclusion criteria: corneal dystrophy).

3.2. Efficacy Outcomes. Efficacy data were similar in the ITT and PP data sets; results for the ITT population are presented. IOP (mean ± SD) was 23.1 ± 3.0 mmHg at baseline ($n = 47$; range, 20.0–32.0 mmHg), 17.2 ± 3.3 mmHg at week 4 (range, 10.0–25.0 mmHg), and 17.2 ± 4.1 mmHg at week 12 ($n = 40$; range, 10.0–28.0 mmHg). The overall mean ± SD IOP reduction from baseline was 6.0±3.2 mmHg at week 12 ($P < 0.001$); similar results were observed at week 4 (Figure 1). Analysis by PGA type for travoprost and latanoprost verified that the decrease from baseline at week 12 was significant for both (5.1 ± 3.4 mmHg and 7.1 ± 2.9 mmHg, resp.; $P < 0.001$ for both). At week 12, 70% of patients achieved the target IOP of ≤18 mmHg. At baseline, no patients had IOP ≤18 mmHg (Figure 2).

There were no significant differences between baseline and week 12 in the number of patients who reported experiencing a symptom or event on the patient experience survey (Table 1). At week 12, there was a nonsignificant decrease from baseline in pain severity in or around the eyes when exposed to light ($P = 0.072$). Among patients who reported stinging or burning (baseline, $n = 14/47$; week 12, $n = 12/39$), there was a difference in symptom severity between baseline and week 12 ($P = 0.035$). At baseline, 21.4% of patients reported severity of this symptom as "minimal," 64.3% as "mild," and 14.3% as "moderate." At week 12, 53.9%, 15.4% and 30.8% of patients reported minimal, mild, and moderate severity, respectively.

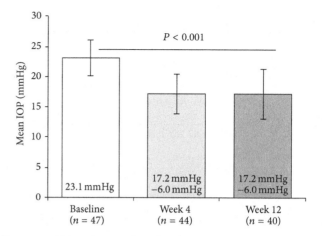

FIGURE 1: IOP reduction from baseline at weeks 4 and 12. Bars represent mean IOP ± SD; mean IOP reduction from baseline is indicated inside bars. IOP = intraocular pressure. Baseline versus week 12, $P < 0.001$; 1-way analysis of variance with a post hoc, 2-sided paired t-test.

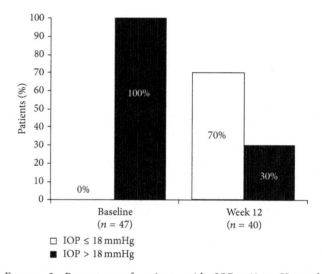

FIGURE 2: Percentage of patients with IOP ≤18 mmHg and >18 mmHg at baseline and week 12. Patient percentages are indicated inside bars. IOP = intraocular pressure.

3.3. Safety Outcomes. A total of 28 AEs were reported by 21 patients (Table 2); 16 AEs (57.1%) were determined to be related or possibly related to the study medication. One serious AE (moderate pseudostenocardia related to study medication) occurred and led to study discontinuation. Seven additional patients discontinued because of AEs (allergic conjunctivitis; tiredness and insomnia; rhinitis sicca; headache, metallic taste, ocular foreign body sensation, blurred vision, and 1 unspecified AE; stomachache; headache; and eye pain). Nearly all AEs were mild or moderate in severity (96.4%, $n = 27/28$), and 96.4% of AEs resolved by

TABLE 1: Patient experience survey data.

	Incidence and severity	Patients, n (%)[*]		P value
		Baseline $n = 47$	Week 12 $n = 39$	
Do you experience or have you noticed		At this moment	Immediately following instillation of study medication	
Pain in or around your eyes when exposed to light?	Yes	5 (10.6)	5 (12.8)	0.753[†]
	Minimal	0	1 (20.0)	0.072[‡]
	Mild	0	1 (20.0)	
	Moderate	1 (20.0)	3 (60.0)	
	Severe	4 (80.0)	0	
Blurred or dim vision?	Yes	9 (19.2)	14 (35.9)	0.081[†]
	Minimal	5 (55.6)	6 (42.9)	0.733[‡]
	Mild	2 (22.2)	3 (21.4)	
	Moderate	2 (22.2)	5 (35.7)	
	Severe	0	0	
Stinging or burning?	Yes	14 (29.8)	12 (30.8)	0.921[†]
	Minimal	3 (21.4)	7 (53.9)	0.035[‡]
	Mild	9 (64.3)	2 (15.4)	
	Moderate	2 (14.3)	4 (30.8)	
	Severe	0	0	
A feeling that something is in your eyes or under your lids?	Yes	11 (23.4)	11 (28.2)	0.611[†]
	Minimal	2 (18.2)	4 (40.0)	0.385[‡]
	Mild	4 (36.4)	4 (40.0)	
	Moderate	5 (45.5)	2 (20.0)	
	Severe	0	0	
Deep pain in or around your eyes?	Yes	3 (6.4)	3 (7.7)	0.812[†]
	Minimal	0	1 (33.3)	0.368[‡]
	Mild	1 (33.3)	0	
	Moderate	2 (66.7)	2 (66.7)	
	Severe	0	0	
Redness in your eyes[§]?	Yes	13 (27.7)	11 (28.2)	0.955[†]
	Minimal	5 (38.5)	3 (27.3)	0.366[‡]
	Mild	4 (30.8)	7 (63.6)	
	Moderate	3 (23.1)	1 (9.1)	
	Severe	1 (7.7)	0	

[*] For each question, the percentage of "yes" responses was calculated based on the group size, and severity data were calculated as the percentage of patients who responded "yes."
[†] Numbers of "yes" responses at week 12 versus baseline were analyzed by 1-way analysis of variance.
[‡] Symptom severity responses at week 12 versus baseline were analyzed by 1-way analysis of variance.
[§] Causes of redness were not specified.

the end of the study. The most frequently reported AE was headache (3 events reported for 2 patients).

Slit-lamp observations were similar among visits. At baseline, observations for eyelids, conjunctiva, cornea, iris, anterior chamber, and fundus were normal for most patients (57.4% to 100.0%); abnormalities were reported as "trace" or "mild" for most eyes. Examination of the lens at baseline was abnormal for most patients (72.3%); however, most abnormalities were reported as "trace" or "mild." BCVA was unchanged from baseline to week 4 or week 12.

4. Discussion

Reducing IOP to minimize disease progression is the standard of care for glaucoma and OH. Several studies have demonstrated that maintaining sufficiently low IOP may slow or prevent progression of visual field defects. For many patients, long-term monotherapy does not maintain target IOP, and many patients benefit from a combination of 3 ocular hypotensive agents [4, 12]. The goal of this study was to evaluate the safety and efficacy of adding adjunctive

TABLE 2: Adverse events (safety population).

	Episodes, n (%) n = 28
Patients experiencing ≥1 adverse event, n (%)*	21 (44.7)
Adverse event severity	
Mild	23 (82.1)
Moderate	4 (14.3)
Severe	1 (3.6)
Adverse event	
Headache	3 (10.7)
Allergic conjunctivitis	1 (3.6)
Allergic rhinitis	1 (3.6)
Ankle pain	1 (3.6)
Burning/eyelid swelling	1 (3.6)
Blurred vision	1 (3.6)
Conjunctival discomfort	1 (3.6)
Corneal superficial keratitis	1 (3.6)
Crusting of lashes	1 (3.6)
Dry eye	1 (3.6)
Eye pain	1 (3.6)
Lid erythema	1 (3.6)
Metallic taste	1 (3.6)
Ocular foreign body sensation	1 (3.6)
Pseudostenocardia†	1 (3.6)
Punctate keratopathy	1 (3.6)
Rhinitis sicca	1 (3.6)
Scheduled knee total endoprosthesis due to gonarthrosis	1 (3.6)
Stomachache	1 (3.6)
Subjective poorer vision	1 (3.6)
Tinnitus	1 (3.6)
Tiredness and insomnia	1 (3.6)
Trace keratitis	1 (3.6)
Upper respiratory infection	1 (3.6)
Worsening of dorsal pain	1 (3.6)
Unknown‡	1 (3.6)

*Calculated as the percentage of patients in the safety population (n = 47).
†Serious adverse event.
‡A description was not available for 1 event in 1 patient.

BTFC in patients with open-angle glaucoma or OH who had insufficient IOP reduction with PGA monotherapy alone.

At baseline, when patients were receiving only PGA monotherapy, mean IOP was 23.1 mmHg. After 12 weeks of adjunctive BTFC therapy, mean IOP decreased by 6.0 mmHg to 17.2 mmHg. This reduction was observed at week 4 and was maintained through study completion. IOP was >18 mmHg in all patients at baseline, but at week 12, 70% of patients achieved the target IOP of ≤18 mmHg. The most common AE was headache, which was reported by 2 patients, and nearly all AEs were mild or moderate in severity. BCVA and slit-lamp biomicroscopy observations were unchanged from baseline throughout the study.

Maintaining IOP levels ≤18 mmHg may decrease the risk of glaucoma progression. A meta-analysis of 5 retrospective studies of patients with POAG or exfoliative glaucoma with ≥5 years of follow-up demonstrated that glaucoma progressed in 51% of patients with IOP >18 mmHg, whereas 78% of patients with mean IOP of 18 mmHg did not progress [3]. In general, as mean IOP increased above 18 mmHg, the percentage of patients who remained stable decreased; likewise, at mean IOP levels below 18 mmHg, the percentage of patients who remained stable increased [3]. In the current study, only 30% of patients failed to achieve IOP ≤18 mmHg after 12 weeks of BTFC adjunctive to a PGA, which was a marked improvement from baseline. Rates of visual field decline have been shown to decrease with even small reductions in IOP [13, 14]. The Early Manifest Glaucoma Trial demonstrated that for every 1 mmHg decrease in IOP, the progression risk decreases by as much as 10% [14]. These studies suggest that the additive IOP-lowering efficacy of BTFC adjunctive to PGA therapy described in the current study may decrease risk of glaucoma progression by reducing IOP in patients not sufficiently controlled with PGA therapy alone.

Our findings are in agreement with previous reports describing increased IOP-lowering efficacy of 3-medication combinations that included a PGA, a carbonic anhydrase inhibitor, and a β-blocker [15–17]. In the current study, most patients were receiving latanoprost or travoprost at enrollment; adding adjunctive BTFC reduced mean IOP by an additional 6 mmHg from levels achieved with the PGA monotherapy. Previously, the stepwise IOP-lowering efficacy of travoprost monotherapy, fixed-combination travoprost/timolol, and fixed-combination travoprost/timolol plus brinzolamide was assessed in a single-arm, open-label study of patients with POAG or OH [16]. After a washout period, travoprost monotherapy decreased mean diurnal IOP by 6.2 mmHg; fixed-combination travoprost/timolol reduced IOP by an additional 3.1 mmHg, and adding brinzolamide to the fixed combination further reduced IOP by 1.9 mmHg [16]. Mean diurnal IOP with travoprost/timolol plus adjunctive brinzolamide was 5.0 mmHg lower than levels achieved with travoprost monotherapy [16]. An observer-masked, placebo-controlled crossover comparison of patients with open-angle glaucoma responsive to but insufficiently controlled with latanoprost monotherapy demonstrated that fixed-combination dorzolamide/timolol adjunctive to latanoprost reduced 24-hour mean IOP by 5.6 mmHg from levels that were maintained with latanoprost alone [17]. Similar 3-medication combinations have also shown increased IOP-lowering efficacy compared with fixed combinations of 2 ocular hypotensive agents; mean IOP reductions with travoprost/timolol plus adjunctive brinzolamide or dorzolamide/timolol plus adjunctive latanoprost ranged from 1.9 mmHg to 5.2 mmHg compared with the fixed combinations alone [15, 18].

The AEs observed in this study were consistent with the known side effects of BTFC and topical PGAs [19, 20]. Nearly all AEs were mild in severity, and the most frequently reported AE was headache. Most ocular symptoms and events reported by patients were similar at baseline and week 12;

there was a nonsignificant improvement in pain severity in or around eyes during light exposure at week 12. No changes from baseline in slit-lamp observations or BCVA were observed.

Potential limitations of this study include the single-arm, open-label design and 12-week study duration. Patients' baseline IOP may have been influenced by noncompliance with the prior medication, and adherence to study medication may have been increased because of participation in a clinical trial. Future studies with multiarm or crossover designs and longer follow-up durations would be valuable.

The use of different PGAs in this study was intentional, as it was meant to reflect clinical practice where a variety of PGAs are used based on the patient's profile and the physician's preference. Although not powered to show differences between groups, analysis by PGA type (travoprost and latanoprost) verified that IOP decreased significantly for both treatment groups when BTFC was added. However, if a specific PGA and brinzolamide/timolol combination were not to lower IOP, the effect would be masked because the mean change in IOP was calculated across all PGA types.

In conclusion, BTFC adjunctive therapy reduced IOP when added to a PGA in patients with OH or POAG whose IOP was poorly controlled with PGA monotherapy alone. IOP reductions were evident after 4 weeks of combined BTFC plus PGA therapy and were maintained through 12 weeks. BTFC was well tolerated, and the ocular AEs reported were consistent with the current BTFC safety profile. Adding adjunctive BTFC therapy may provide a safe and effective option for patients requiring additional IOP reduction beyond that provided by a PGA.

Conflict of Interests

Anton Hommer has received research support from Alcon, Allergan, and Santen; has received honoraria or consultation fees from Alcon, Allergan, Bausch & Lomb, Heidelberg, Merck, and Santen; and has participated in speakers bureaus sponsored by Alcon, Allergan, Merck, and Santen. Douglas A. Hubatsch is an employee of Alcon. Juan Cano-Parra has received research support from Alcon. This study was sponsored by Alcon Research, Ltd., Fort Worth, TX, USA. Medical writing support was provided by Heather D. Starkey, Ph.D., of Complete Healthcare Communications, Inc. (Chadds Ford, PA), and was funded by Alcon.

References

[1] D. Peters, B. Bengtsson, and A. Heijl, "Factors associated with lifetime risk of open-angle glaucoma blindness," *Acta Ophthalmologica*, vol. 92, no. 5, pp. 421–425, 2014.

[2] C. A. B. Webers, H. J. M. Beckers, R. M. M. A. Nuijts, and J. S. A. G. Schouten, "Pharmacological management of primary open-angle glaucoma: second-line options and beyond," *Drugs and Aging*, vol. 25, no. 9, pp. 729–759, 2008.

[3] W. C. Stewart, A. E. Kolker, E. D. Sharpe et al., "Long-term progression at individual mean intraocular pressure levels in primary open-angle and exfoliative glaucoma," *European Journal of Ophthalmology*, vol. 18, no. 5, pp. 765–770, 2008.

[4] M. A. Kass, D. K. Heuer, E. J. Higginbotham et al., "The Ocular Hypertension Treatment Study: a randomized trial determines that topical ocular hypotensive medication delays or prevents the onset of primary open-angle glaucoma," *Archives of Ophthalmology*, vol. 120, no. 6, pp. 701–713, 2002.

[5] P. N. Schacknow and J. R. Samples, "Medications used to treat glaucoma," in *The Glaucoma Book*, P. N. Schacknow and J. R. Samples, Eds., vol. 4, pp. 583–628, Springer, New York, NY, USA, 2010.

[6] F. Djafari, M. R. Lesk, P. J. Harasymowycz, D. Desjardins, and J. Lachaine, "Determinants of adherence to glaucoma medical therapy in a long-term patient population," *Journal of Glaucoma*, vol. 18, no. 3, pp. 238–243, 2009.

[7] A. L. Robin, G. D. Novack, D. W. Covert, R. S. Crockett, and T. S. Marcic, "Adherence in glaucoma: objective measurements of once-daily and adjunctive medication use," *American Journal of Ophthalmology*, vol. 144, no. 4, pp. 533–540, 2007.

[8] European Glaucoma Society, *Terminology and Guidelines for Glaucoma*, European Glaucoma Society, 2014, http://www.eugs.org/eng/EGS_guidelines.asp.

[9] National Institute of Clinical Excellence, *Glaucoma: Diagnosis and Management of Chronic Open Angle Glaucoma and Ocular Hypertension*, 2014, http://guidance.nice.org.uk/CG85/Guidance/pdf/English.

[10] American Academy of Ophthalmology Glaucoma Panel, *Preferred Practice Pattern Guidelines. Primary Open-Angle Glaucoma*, American Academy of Ophthalmology, San Francisco, Calif, USA, 2010.

[11] A. G. P. Konstas, G. Holló, A.-B. Haidich et al., "Comparison of 24-hour intraocular pressure reduction obtained with brinzolamide/timolol or brimonidine/timolol fixed-combination adjunctive to travoprost therapy," *Journal of Ocular Pharmacology and Therapeutics*, vol. 29, no. 7, pp. 652–657, 2013.

[12] I. Lanzl and T. Raber, "Efficacy and tolerability of the fixed combination of brinzolamide 1% and timolol 0.5% in daily practice," *Clinical Ophthalmology*, vol. 5, no. 1, pp. 291–298, 2011.

[13] B. C. Chauhan, F. S. Mikelberg, P. H. Artes et al., "Canadian Glaucoma Study: 3. Impact of risk factors and intraocular pressure reduction on the rates of visual field change," *Archives of Ophthalmology*, vol. 128, no. 10, pp. 1249–1255, 2010.

[14] M. C. Leske, A. Heijl, M. Hussein, B. Bengtsson, L. Hyman, and E. Komaroff, "Factors for glaucoma progression and the effect of treatment: the Early Manifest Glaucoma Trial," *Archives of Ophthalmology*, vol. 121, no. 1, pp. 48–56, 2003.

[15] I. Goldberg, J. G. Crowston, M. C. Jasek, J. A. Stewart, and W. C. Stewart, "Intraocular pressure-lowering efficacy of brinzolamide when added to travoprost/timolol fixed combination as adjunctive therapy," *Journal of Glaucoma*, vol. 21, no. 1, pp. 55–59, 2012.

[16] G. Holló and P. Kóthy, "Intraocular pressure reduction with travoprost/timolol fixed combination, with and without adjunctive brinzolamide, in glaucoma," *Current Medical Research and Opinion*, vol. 24, no. 6, pp. 1755–1761, 2008.

[17] A. G. P. Konstas, D. Mikropoulos, A. T. Dimopoulos, G. Moumtzis, L. A. Nelson, and W. C. Stewart, "Second-line therapy with dorzolamide/timolol or latanoprost/timolol fixed combination versus adding dorzolamide/timolol fixed combination to latanoprost monotherapy," *British Journal of Ophthalmology*, vol. 92, no. 11, pp. 1498–1502, 2008.

[18] A. Akman, A. Cetinkaya, Y. A. Akova, and A. Ertan, "Comparison of additional intraocular pressure-lowering effects of

latanoprost vs brimonidine in primary open-angle glaucoma patients with intraocular pressure uncontrolled by timolol-dorzolamide combination," *Eye*, vol. 19, no. 2, pp. 145–151, 2005.

[19] AZARGA, *(Brinzolamide 1%/Timolol 0.5% Fixed Combination). Full Prescribing Information*, Alcon Laboratories, Surrey, UK, 2013.

[20] C. L. Alexander, S. J. Miller, and S. R. Abel, "Prostaglandin analog treatment of glaucoma and ocular hypertension," *Annals of Pharmacotherapy*, vol. 36, no. 3, pp. 504–511, 2002.

Risk Factors in Normal-Tension Glaucoma and High-Tension Glaucoma in relation to Polymorphisms of Endothelin-1 Gene and Endothelin-1 Receptor Type A Gene

Dominika Wróbel-Dudzińska,[1] Ewa Kosior-Jarecka,[1] Urszula Łukasik,[1] Janusz Kocki,[2] Agnieszka Witczak,[3] Jerzy Mosiewicz,[3] and Tomasz Żarnowski[1]

[1]*Department of Diagnostics and Microsurgery of Glaucoma, Medical University, Chmielna 1, 20-079 Lublin, Poland*
[2]*Department of Clinical Genetics, Medical University, Radziwiłłowska 11, 20-080 Lublin, Poland*
[3]*Department of Internal Diseases, Medical University, Staszica 16, 20-081 Lublin, Poland*

Correspondence should be addressed to Dominika Wróbel-Dudzińska; ddudzinska@interia.pl

Academic Editor: Gianluca Scuderi

The aim of the research is to analyse the influence of polymorphisms of endothelin-1 gene and endothelin-1 receptor type A gene on the clinical condition of patients with primary open angle glaucoma. *Methods.* 285 Polish patients took part in the research (160 normal-tension glaucoma and 125 high-tension glaucoma). DNA was isolated by standard methods and genotype distributions of four polymorphisms in genes encoding endothelin-1 (K198N) and endothelin-1 receptor type A polymorphisms (C1222T, C70G, and G231A) were determined. Genotype distributions were compared between NTG and HTG groups. The clinical condition of participants was examined for association with polymorphisms. *Results.* A similar frequency of occurrence of the polymorphic varieties of the studied genes was observed in patients with NTG and HTG. There is no relation between NTG risk factors and examined polymorphisms. NTG patients with TT genotype of K198N polymorphism presented with the lowest intraocular pressure in comparison to GG + GT genotype ($p = 0.03$). In NTG patients with CC genotype of C1222T polymorphism ($p = 0.028$) and GG of C70G polymorphism ($p = 0.03$) the lowest values of mean blood pressure were observed. *Conclusions.* The studied polymorphic varieties (K198N, C1222T) do have an influence on intraocular pressure as well as arterial blood pressure in NTG patients.

1. Introduction

The term "glaucoma" describes a group of diseases that result in progressive and irreparable optic nerve damage characterised by typical advancing changes in the optic disc and ensuing visual field defects. Normal-tension glaucoma (NTG) is a particular kind of glaucoma with a characteristic glaucomatous cupping of the optic disc, visual field defects, open anterior chamber angle, and intraocular pressure classified as normal.

Elevated intraocular pressure is one of the most important risk factors in glaucoma development. However, its reduction in patients with normal-tension glaucoma does not entirely prevent the disease from advancing. Research done by the Collaborative Normal-Tension Glaucoma Study Group (CNTGSG) suggests other factors that play a role in the pathogenesis of glaucomatous optic neuropathy. Special attention is paid to primary vascular dysregulation since its symptoms, such as low arterial blood pressure, cold extremities, Raynaud's syndrome, and migraines, often are present in persons with normal-tension glaucoma [1].

So far, scientific research has resulted in a few theories explaining the pathomechanism of glaucomatous optic neuropathy.

Mechanical theory assumes that elevated intraocular pressure (IOP), the main risk factor in glaucomatous optic neuropathy, plays an important role in the optic nerve damage. In 1957 Von Graefe noticed that there exists a relation between elevated intraocular pressure and deformation of the lamina cribrosa [2]. Numerous studies have proven that high intraocular pressure causes cribriform plate abnormalities, which cause pressure and subsequent damage of the axons of retinal ganglion cells which pass through the plate [3].

According to the vascular theory, glaucomatous optic neuropathy is triggered by a variety of systemic and local vascular factors leading to low ophthalmic perfusion and ischemia. Among systemic factors we can list the following: hypertension and hypotension, cardiovascular diseases, diabetes, and cerebral circulation disorders [4]. Topical factors causing ischemia are as follows: low blood perfusion pressure and anatomical abnormalities of vessels supplying the eyeball [5]. Examination of the fundus of the eye reveals changes resulting from ischemia: sphincter optic disk haemorrhages, notching, focal areas of choroidal atrophy, and slower retinal flow shown by an angiogram.

Excitotoxicity theory posits that there are many processes which contribute to the development of glaucomatous optic neuropathy, for example, the toxic influence of cell mediators, neurotrophin deficiency, ischemia, or apoptosis. Ischemia, caused by autoregulation mechanism disorders and endothelium dysfunction, stimulates the release of ET-1, norepinephrine, and nitric oxide (NO), which in turn influence the blood flow in the optic disc. Subsequent reperfusion results in a considerable rise in free oxygen radicals and nitrogen compound concentration. NMDA receptor is then activated which fuels NO synthesis and radicals production. Toxic peroxynitrates, produced in the process, lead to retinal ganglion cell apoptosis.

Endothelin-1 (ET-1), discovered by Yanagisawa et al. in 1988 [6], the strongest vasoconstrictive agent in the human body, takes part in regulating ocular blood flow, the outflow of aqueous humour from the anterior chamber, and, as a result, intraocular pressure. It also assists in retinal ganglion cell apoptosis [7, 8]. Endothelin influences 2 kinds of receptors (related to protein G): ET_AR and ET_BR, which have the opposite effect. Numerous *in vitro* research has demonstrated that ET-1 can be found in the corneal epithelium, endothelium cells, pigmented part of ciliary body, iris, trabecular meshwork, lens, choroid, retinal pigment epithelium, retinal ganglion cells, and astrocytes [9, 10]. ET_A receptors have been identified in the retinal and choroidal vessels as well as in the iris, whereas ET_B receptors have been found in the retinal neurons, glia, and ciliary body. Both kinds of receptors can be found in the lamina cribrosa, which suggests that ET-1 plays an important role in local extracellular matrix remodelling and vascular wall stress regulation [11]. Therefore, ET-1 level and gene polymorphism might be crucial in the pathogenesis of glaucoma. The aim of this study is to find a relation between polymorphisms of ET-1 gene and ET-1 receptor type A and their influence on clinical condition of patients with normal-tension glaucoma and high-tension glaucoma (HTG).

2. Material and Methods

285 Polish Caucasian patients treated at the Department of Diagnostics and Microsurgery of Glaucoma in Lublin (Poland) between 2009 and 2013 took part in the study. To demonstrate the differences between the two types of primary open-angle glaucoma patients were divided into two groups: those diagnosed with normal-tension glaucoma (160 patients, including 110 women and 50 men) and those presenting with high-tension glaucoma (HTG) and intraocular pressure above 21 mmHg (125 patients, including 87 women and 38 men). Patients were accepted for the study only if they had been previously informed about the aim and scope of the research, expressed their consent for participating in the study, and met the following criteria. The investigation was conducted in compliance with the tenets of the Declaration of Helsinki.

Criteria for diagnosing high-tension glaucoma (with high intraocular pressure) are as follows: diagnosed glaucomatous optic neuropathy based on changes in the optic disc and visual field defects, open anterior chamber angle in gonioscopy, and intraocular pressure above 21 mmHg at the time of diagnosis evaluated on the basis of a 24-hour intraocular pressure monitoring. In the case of NTG intraocular pressure at the time of diagnosis was below 21 mmHg.

A comprehensive ophthalmic examination was performed in both groups. Visual acuity was tested using Snellen charts. Intraocular pressure was measured by means of an applanation tonometer. An ultrasound pachymeter was used to measure the thickness of cornea. All patients were also given a biomicroscopic examination with a slit lamp. To assess anterior chamber angle a gonioscopy was performed using a Zeiss gonioscope. Schaffer classification was applied in evaluating the width of the angle. Examination of the fundus of the eye made it possible to assess the optic disc structure, presence of peripapillary atrophy, notching of the neuroretinal rim, and optic disc haemorrhages. Moreover, patients with best corrected visual acuity equal to or better than 0.1 had their visual field analysed using Humphrey perimeter and 30-2 SITA-Fast strategy. Results were considered credible if the sum of falsely positive and falsely negative answers was lower than 15%. When assessing the results of visual field analysis, the mean deviation (MD) at the time of diagnosis (expressed in decibels, dB) was taken into account. Prior to clinical examination patients were asked whether they had been diagnosed with hypertension, hypotension, diabetes mellitus, or any cardiovascular disorders (migraine, cold extremities).

DNA was isolated from peripheral blood leukocytes by means of QIAamp DNA Blood Midi Kit (QIAGEN Inc., Germany). DNA concentration was measured using NanoDrop 2000/2000c Spectrophotometer V1.0 (Thermo Fisher Scientific). TaqMan SNP probe (Applied Biosystems) and CFX96 Real-Time PCR Detection System thermal cycler (Bio-Rad) were used to assay 4 polymorphisms of the single nucleotide of the endothelin-1 gene (K198N) and endothelin-1 receptor type A (C1222T, C70G, and G231A). DNA amplification was obtained by means of a Real-Time Polymerase Chain Reaction (details in Tables 1 and 2). Real-Time PCR Thermal Cycler is equipped with optical system which makes it possible to track PCR process in real time. To this end, fluorochrome-labelled molecular TaqMan probes (oligonucleotides of about 20–30 bp length) complementary to replicated DNA sequences and to PCR product were used. At the end of $5'$ probe there is a fluorescent dye and at

TABLE 1: Standard amplification report.

	AmpliTaq Gold Enzyme Activation	PCR 40 cycles	
	HOLD	Denaturation	Annealing/extending
Time	10 minutes	15 seconds	1 minute
Temperature	95°C	92°C	60°C

TABLE 2: Reaction mixture composition.

Ingredient	Volume in μL/well
TaqMan Universal PCR Master Mix	12.5
Stock of SNP	1.25
Isolated patient's DNA (10 ng)	11.25
Total	25
Buffer: 10 mM Tris-HCl, 1 mM EDTA, pH 8.0, DNase-free water	

TABLE 3: Demographic and clinical characteristics data.

	NTG	HTG	p value
Gender (females : men)	110 : 50	87 : 38	$p > 0.05$
Age (years)	72.01 ± 11,61	75.85	$p = 0.02$
BCVA	0.65	0.5	$p < 0.05$
IOP (mmHg)	17.29 ± 2.93	24.65 ± 7.78	$p < 0.005$
c/d ratio	0.79	0.8	$p = 0.53$
Haemorrhage	16%	4.3%	$p = 0.02$
Notches	50.7%	16.3%	$p < 0.0001$
PPA	21.7%	13.4%	$p > 0.05$
MD (dB)	−8.56 ± 6,26	−13.83 ± 7.01	$p < 0.005$
Cold extremities	75.6%	28.6%	$p = 0.018$
Low blood pressure	69.7%	16.7%	$p = 0.039$
Migraine	38.6%	0%	$p = 0.036$

the end of $3'$ a quencher. The dyes that were used in the study were FAM (6-carboxyfluorescein) and VIC (ABI company trademark, USA) and the quencher was TAMRA (6-carboxytetramethylrhodamine). The composition of the reaction mixture and its parameters are shown in Table 2.

K198N polymorphism of the endothelin-1 gene (rs 5370) leads to transversion of purine guanine (G) into pyrimidine thymine (T) in nucleotide 5665 in exon 5 (Lys/Asn change in codon 198). C1222T polymorphism of the endothelin-1 receptor type A gene (rs 5343), involving transition of pyrimidine cytosine (C) into thymine (T), concerns nucleotide 1363 in exon 8 in $3'$ untranslated region ($3'$UTR). C70G polymorphism of the endothelin-1 receptor type A gene (rs 5335) is a transversion of pyrimidine cytosine (C) into purine guanine (G) and is located in $3'$ untranslated region ($3'$UTR). This polymorphism concerns nucleotide 211 in exon 8. Point mutation changes the chemical structure of DNA; however, its function still remains unknown. Polymorphism of the EDN R_A G231A gene, which involves transition of purine guanine into adenine, is located in exon 1 in $5'$ untranslated region ($5'$UTR).

In order to assess patients' arterial blood pressure rhythm a 24-hour ambulatory blood pressure monitoring was conducted using an ABPM device.

Statistical analysis of the obtained results was conducted by means of the IBM SPSS Statistica 19 and Statistica 10 software. The value of $p < 0,05$ was considered statistically significant.

3. Results

Differences in age and sex in both study groups were not demonstrated. More demographics data are presented in Table 3.

Table 4 shows the frequency of occurrence of particular polymorphic variations in the studied genes. The distributions in NTG and HTG groups were consistent with the Hardy-Weinberg equilibrium. Homozygous wild type GG genotype of K198N polymorphism of the endothelin-1 gene was observed in 198 patients (69.7%), homozygous mutant TT genotype in 11 patients (3.9%), and heterozygous GT genotype in 75 patients (26.4%). In male patients homozygous GG genotype was more frequent in patients with HTG rather than in patients with NTG (65.8% vs. 54%). A statistically significant difference was demonstrated in the frequency of occurrence of GG genotype in men from the study groups (χ^2 test, $p < 0.05$). GT genotype was more frequent in men with NTG rather than with HTG (40% versus 28.9%). The difference was statistically significant (χ^2 test, $p < 0.05$).

When analysing C1222T polymorphism it was observed that in both groups homozygous wild type CC genotype appeared in 100 patients (35.2%), homozygous mutant TT genotype in 41 patients (14.4%), and heterozygous CT genotype in 143 patients (50.4%). TT genotype was more frequent in men with NTG rather than with HTG (22% versus 13.2%).

There was no statistically significant difference in the frequency of occurrence of particular genotypes of C70G and G231A polymorphisms in both study groups (χ^2 test, $p > 0.05$).

When comparing both groups in terms of the frequency of occurrence of C70G and G231A polymorphisms with relation to patients' gender, no statistically significant differences were found (χ^2 test, $p > 0.05$) (Tables 5 and 6).

When comparing both groups in terms of the frequency of occurrence of particular genotypes of the researched polymorphisms, no statistically significant differences were found (χ^2 test, $p > 0.05$).

3.1. Influence of the Studied Polymorphisms on Clinical Condition

(i) Intraocular Pressure. Intraocular pressure differed statistically significantly between the two groups (Student's t-test, $p < 0.05$). When analysing K198N polymorphism the lowest intraocular pressure, 13.7 mmHg, was observed in the group of patients with NTG with TT genotype and the highest pressure, 17.6 mmHg, in patients with GG genotype (ANOVA test, $p = 0.03$). There were no statistically significant differences between intraocular pressure and the

TABLE 4: Frequency of allelic variants of polymorphisms of ET and EDN RA gene in NTG and HTG patients.

Patients (%)	K198N GG	K198N TT	K198N GT	C1222T CC	C1222T TT	C1222T CT	C70G CC	C70G GG	C70G CG	G231A GG	G231A AA	G231A GA
NTG	107 (66.9%)	7 (4.4%)	46 (28.7%)	56 (35%)	25 (15.6%)	79 (49.4%)	27 (16.9%)	44 (27.5%)	89 (55.6%)	83 (51.9%)	6 (3.8%)	71 (44.4%)
HTG	91 (73.4%)	4 (3.2%)	29 (23.3%)	44 (35.5%)	16 (12.9%)	64 (51.6%)	21 (16.9%)	36 (29%)	67 (54%)	65 (52.4%)	5 (4%)	54 (43.5%)

TABLE 5: Frequency of allelic variants of polymorphisms of ET and EDN RA gene in female and male NTG patients.

NTG Patients (%)	K198N GG	K198N TT	K198N GT	C1222T CC	C1222T TT	C1222T CT	C70G CC	C70G GG	C70G CG	G231A GG	G231A AA	G231A GA
F	80 (72.7%)	4 (3.6%)	26 (23.6%)	40 (36.4%)	14 (12.7%)	56 (50.9%)	18 (16.4%)	32 (29.1%)	60 (54.5%)	55 (50%)	4 (3.6%)	51 (46.4%)
M	27 (54%)	3 (6%)	20 (40%)	16 (32%)	11 (22%)	23 (46%)	9 (18%)	12 (24%)	29 (58%)	28 (56%)	2 (4%)	20 (40%)

TABLE 6: Frequency of allelic variants of polymorphisms of ET and EDN RA gene in female and male HTG patients.

HTG Patients (%)	K198N			C1222T			C70G			G231A	
	GG	TT	GT	CC	TT	CT	CC	GG	CG	GG	AA	GA
F	66 (76.6%)	2 (2.3%)	18 (20.9%)	31 (36%)	11 (12.8%)	44 (51.2%)	12 (14%)	27 (31.4%)	47 (54.7%)	3 (50%)	4 (4.7%)	39 (45.3%)
M	25 (65.8%)	2 (5.3%)	11 (28.9%)	13 (34.2%)	5 (13.2%)	20 (52.6%)	9 (23.7%)	9 (23.7%)	20 (52.6%)	22 (57.9%)	1 (2.6%)	15 (39.5%)

TABLE 7: Maximum intraocular pressure (IOP) according to the allelic variants of studied polymorphisms.

IOP (mmHg)	K198N			C1222T			C70G			G231A		
	GG	TT	GT	CC	TT	CT	CC	GG	CG	GG	AA	GA
NTG	17.6	13.7	17	16.6	16.4	16.4	17.4	16.4	17.6	16.9	14.8	16
HTG	19.5	24.5	25.8	26.6	21.5	25.5	27.7	21.9	25.6	25.1	33	22.7

TABLE 8: Mean deviation at the moment of diagnosis (dB).

	NTG		HTG		Student's t-test	
	M	SD	M	SD	t	p
Mean deviation (dB)	−8.58	6.26	−13.83	7.01	5.708	0.000

occurrence of particular genotypes of C1222T, C70G, and G231A polymorphisms in the study groups (ANOVA test, $p > 0.05$). Interestingly, the highest intraocular pressure was observed in patients with HTG with AA genotype of G231A polymorphism, whereas in patients with NTG and with the same genotype intraocular pressure was one of the lowest (14.8 mmHg), however, without statistical significance (Student's t-test, $p > 0.05$) (Table 7).

(ii) Visual Field. Average value of the mean deviation (MD) at the time of diagnosis was −8.58 dB in the group of patients with normal-tension glaucoma and −13.83 dB in the group of patients with high-tension glaucoma. Average value of MD at the time of glaucoma diagnosis was statistically significant in both study groups (Student's t-test, $p < 0.005$). There was no relation between the stage of glaucoma and the occurrence of particular genotypes of the studied polymorphisms (Table 8).

(iii) Influence of Gene Polymorphisms on Vascular Risk Factors (Tables 3 and 9). Optic disk *haemorrhages* were present in 27 patients (18.7%) from the NTG group and 4 patients (4.3%) from the HTG group (χ^2 test with Yates's correction for continuity, $p = 0.02$).

Notching of the neuroretinal rim was observed in 50.7% of patients (70 persons) with normal-tension glaucoma and 16.3% of patients (14 persons) with high-tension glaucoma (χ^2 test, $p < 0.0001$). Moreover, in the group of patients with NTG, notching was statistically significantly more frequent in women than in men (75% versus 25%, χ^2 test, $p = 0.016$).

Peripapillary atrophy was present in 21.7% of patients with normal-tension glaucoma and 13.4% of patients with high-tension glaucoma. No statistically significant changes were demonstrated in peripapillary atrophy occurrence in both study groups (χ^2 test, $p > 0.05$).

In the group of patients with NTG there was no relation between the occurrence of polymorphic variations of the studied genes and the occurrence of risk factors such as optic disc haemorrhages, notching, or peripapillary atrophy (χ^2, $p > 0.05$).

Cold extremities are statistically significantly more frequent in patients with NTG (75.6%) than with HTG (28.6%), (χ^2 test with Yates's correction for continuity, $p = 0.018$). What is more, in both study groups these symptoms were more common in women (women with NTG, 79.4%, women with HTG, 40.0%; χ^2 test, $p = 0.059$) rather than in men (men with NTG, 50%, men with HTG, 0%; χ^2 test, $p = 0.19$).

Low arterial blood pressure presented much more often in the group of patients with NTG (69.7%) than in the group of patients with HTG (16.7%). The frequency of occurrence of low blood pressure in both study groups was statistically significantly different (χ^2 test with Yates's correction for continuity, $p = 0.039$). Additionally, in the group of patients with NTG low blood pressure was much more common in women (77.8%) than in men (33.3%), χ^2 test with Yates's correction for continuity, $p = 0.02$.

In both study groups only NTG patients complained of *migraines*, and they were predominantly women (χ^2 test with Yates's correction for continuity, $p = 0.036$).

No statistically significant relation was observed between symptoms such as cold extremities, low blood pressure and migraines, and the occurrence of particular genotypes of the studied polymorphisms in both groups (χ^2 test, $p > 0.05$).

3.2. Analysis of the Relation between the Occurrence of Endothelin-1 Gene K198N Polymorphism and Ambulatory Blood Pressure Monitoring Results (Table 10). Observed differences between the occurrence of GG and GT genotypes and maximum systolic pressure during the day as well as average systolic pressure during the day were close to being statistically significant. Maximum systolic pressure during the day for GG genotype was 159.4 ± 18.2 mmHg and for GT genotype 176.9 ± 42.8 mmHg, ANOVA test, $p = 0.065$. Average systolic pressure during the day for GG genotype was 127.4 ± 11.8 mmHg and for GT genotype 137.1 ± 21.6, ANOVA test, $p = 0.064$.

3.3. Analysis of the Relation between C1222T Polymorphism Genotypes of the Endothelin-1 Receptor Type A Gene and Ambulatory Blood Pressure Monitoring Results (Table 10). Maximum systolic pressure during the day was observed in patients with CT genotype (176.8 ± 33.1 mmHg) and the lowest in patients with homozygous CC genotype (152.3 ± 21.2 mmHg). The difference is statistically significant, ANOVA test, $p = 0.041$. Average systolic pressure during the day was highest in patients with heterozygous CT genotype (137.4 ± 16.6 mmHg) and lowest in persons with homozygous wild type CC genotype (123 ± 14.7 mmHg). The difference was statistically significant, ANOVA test, $p = 0.028$. An interesting observation is that average diastolic pressure at night was highest in patients with homozygous mutant TT genotype (72.4 ± 15.2 mmHg) and the lowest in patients with homozygous wild type CC genotype (61.3 ± 6 mmHg).

TABLE 9: Relation between glaucoma risk factors and polymorphic variants in NTG patients.

Patients (%)	NTG											
		K198N			C1222T			C70G			G231A	
	GG	TT	GT	CC	TT	CT	CC	GG	CG	GG	AA	GA
Haemorrhages	21.2% (21)	16.7% (1)	15% (6)	18% (9)	9.1% (2)	22.3% (16)	15.4% (4)	20.5% (8)	30% (15)	23% (17)	0% (0)	15.6% (10)
Notches	20% (1)	49.5% (48)	64.1% (25)	49% (24)	54.5% (12)	54.2% (38)	48% (12)	51.3% (19)	54.4% (43)	52.1% (38)	50% (3)	53.3% (33)
Low blood pressure	59.1% (13)	100% (1)	90% (9)	58.3% (7)	60% (3)	81.3% (13)	57.4% (4)	58.3% (7)	85.7% (12)	68.8% (11)	0% (0)	75% (12)
Cold extremities	67.9% (19)	100% (1)	83.3% (10)	62.5% (10)	71.4% (5)	83.3% (15)	66.7% (6)	62.5% (10)	87.5% (14)	71.4% (15)	0% (0)	78.9% (15)
Migraine	32.6% (14)	100% (1)	53.8% (7)	33.3% (7)	44.4% (4)	40.7% (11)	50% (6)	29.4% (5)	39.3% (11)	32.3% (10)	50% (1)	45.8% (11)

TABLE 10: Relation between mean blood pressure (BP) (mmHg) and polymorphic variants in NTG patients.

NTG	K198N			C1222T			C70G			G231A		
	GG	TT	GT	CC	TT	CT	CC	GG	CG	GG	AA	GA
Maximum systolic BP day	159.4	—	176.9	152.3	157.5	176.8	157	155.5	173.3	160.6	167	172.2
Mean systolic BP day	127.4	—	137.1	123	126.3	137.4	125.85	124	135.8	128.14	136.16	113.46
Mean diastolic BP day	75.3	—	80.2	76.83	77.85	77.02	76.55	75.65	78.14	76.54	80.5	77.5
Mean systolic BP night	111.98	—	112.96	105.4	115.05	115.05	111.7	103.8	116.45	113.6	114.83	109.7
Mean diastolic BP night	65.3	—	67.07	61.3	72.4	65.4	69.2	60.5	66.89	66.2	65.16	65.6

The difference was close to being statistically significant, ANOVA test, $p = 0.055$.

3.4. Analysis of the Relation between C70G Polymorphism Genotypes of the Endothelin-1 Receptor Type A Gene and Ambulatory Blood Pressure Monitoring Results (Table 10). The highest average systolic pressure during the day was observed in persons with heterozygous CG genotype (135.8 ± 10.36 mmHg) and the lowest in patients with homozygous mutant GG genotype (124 ± 25.73 mmHg), ANOVA test, $p = 0.088$. The lowest average systolic pressure at night was observed in patients with homozygous GG genotype (103.8 ± 9.91 mmHg) and the highest in patients with heterozygous CG genotype (116.45 ± 15.62 mmHg), ANOVA test, $p = 0.081$.

When comparing G231A polymorphism genotypes of the endothelin-1 receptor type A gene and ambulatory blood pressure monitoring results, no statistically significant differences were shown.

4. Discussion

Polymorphisms of the endothelin-1 gene are in the centre of attention of many scientists from different fields of medicine. Unfortunately, among all studies available in international literature there are only few concerning their relation to the development and occurrence of glaucoma.

Many reports confirm that endothelin-1 has its part in the pathogenesis of glaucoma by influencing local blood flow in the eyeball, as well as regulating intraocular pressure and retinal ganglion cell apoptosis. Hence, it seems justified to search for a relation between ET-1 gene and ET-1 receptor type A polymorphisms and the development and occurrence of glaucomatous optic neuropathy, especially normal-tension glaucoma, whose risk factors are related to vasoconstriction.

In our research, when comparing the frequency of occurrence of particular genotypes of K198N polymorphism of the endothelin-1 gene, C1222T, C70G, and G231A of endothelin-1 gene receptor type A, no statistically significant differences were demonstrated between the study groups (normal-tension glaucoma and high-tension glaucoma), also taking into account the patients' gender. So far, not many publications referring to the above-mentioned issue have been released.

Ishikawa et al. compared the frequency of occurrence of the polymorphisms of the endothelin-1 gene and its receptors among Japanese population. 426 patients with open-angle glaucoma (including 176 persons with primary open-angle glaucoma and 250 patients with normal-tension glaucoma) and 225 healthy persons participated in the research. They were able to show statistically significant differences in the frequency of occurrence of KK genotype of K198N polymorphism in the study groups (KK genotype was more common in patients with open-angle glaucoma than in healthy patients (53.2% versus 43.8%, $p = 0.022$)) [12]. Interestingly, in our research we observed that the frequency of occurrence of homozygous wild type GG genotype (69.7%) was much higher than occurrence of mutant TT genotype (3.9%) of K198N polymorphism (107 patients with NTG and 91 with POAG) ($p < 0.05$). In addition, homozygous wild type genotype was more common in women (76.7% in POAG versus 72.7% in NTG) rather than in men (66% POAG versus 54% NTG) ($p > 0.05$). The above results might suggest a possible relation between K198N polymorphism of the endothelin-1 gene and glaucoma occurrence. Further research including healthy patients should be conducted to confirm this hypothesis.

Furthermore, Ishikawa et al. demonstrated that CC genotype of C1222T polymorphism of the endothelin-1 receptor type A gene was much more common among healthy patients (healthy patients 61.2% versus patients with glaucoma 52.6%, $p = 0.036$) [12]. In our research we observed the occurrence of homozygous CC genotype in 35.2% of patients (56 persons with NTG and 44 persons with POAG). Differences in the frequency of occurrence of the above-mentioned genotypes between our study group and Ishikawa's study group might be a result of a racial difference.

When analysing the frequency of occurrence of particular polymorphisms the researchers were not able to show their relation to gender, as was also the case in our research [12].

Genetic background of glaucoma development was the subject of a research by Kim et al., who studied polymorphisms of the endothelin-1 gene and its receptors in Korean population. Their study group were 67 patients with normal-tension glaucoma and 100 healthy persons (not treated for glaucoma). The following pattern of C1222T polymorphism genotypes was obtained: CC genotype was observed in 46.3% of patients with NTG (31 persons) and 49% from the control group (49 persons), CT genotype was present in 38.8% of patients with NTG (26 persons) and in 46% of healthy persons (46 persons), and mutant TT genotype was observed in 14.9% of patients with NTG (10 persons) and in 5% from the control group (5 persons) ($p = 0.028$). In our research we obtained a similar pattern of genotypes: CC genotype was present in 35% of patients with NTG (56 persons), CT genotype in 49.4% (79 persons), and TT genotype in 15.6% (25 persons). Later, the researchers compared the frequency of occurrence of C70G and G231A polymorphisms. They were unable to obtain statistically significant results. To sum up, on the basis of the findings the authors of the study were able to confirm a relation between C1222T polymorphism of the endothelin-1 receptor type A and the development of NTG in Korean population [14].

When comparing study groups with regard to the intraocular pressure at the time of diagnosis, a statistically significant difference was observed. In the group with normal-tension glaucoma average intraocular pressure at the time of diagnosis was 17.9 mmHg and in the group with primary open-angle glaucoma 24.65 mmHg, $p < 0.005$. The observed relation confirms an accurate choice of patients for the study groups. Similar report came from Häntzschel et al., who observed intraocular pressure of 18.8 ± 2.04 mmHg for NTG and 29.6 ± 7.9 mmHg for POAG, $p = 0.001$ [15].

Our research showed a lack of statistically significant differences between the occurrence of particular genotypes of C1222T, C70G, and G231A polymorphisms of the endothelin-1 receptor type A and the intraocular pressure at the time of diagnosis.

However, the lowest intraocular pressure at the time of diagnosis was observed in patients with normal-tension glaucoma and homozygous mutant TT genotype of K198N polymorphism (13.7 ± 2.6 mmHg) in comparison to other genotypes (GG genotype 16.8 ± 3.7 mmHg and GT genotype 16.1 ± 3.8 mmHg) ($p = 0.03$).

When analysing the relation between polymorphisms of the endothelin-1 gene and its receptors, Kim et al. noticed a statistically significant difference in the level of the intraocular pressure at the time of diagnosis of NTG between persons with AA genotype of G231A polymorphism (14.0 ± 2.8 mmHg) and GG + GA genotypes (16.2 ± 2.3 mmHg) ($p = 0.047$) [14]. We observed similar levels of intraocular pressure depending on G231A polymorphism genotypes of the endothelin-1 receptor type A gene. The lowest intraocular pressure at the time of diagnosis was in patients with normal-tension glaucoma and AA genotype (14.8 ± 4.80 mmHg) as compared to GG genotype (16.9 ± 3.4 mmHg) or GA genotype (16.0 ± 4.0 mmHg). Nevertheless, the relation was not statistically significant ($p = 0.241$). According to above data the presence of homozygous mutant AA genotype of G231A polymorphism might be a good prognostic factor for patient with NTG. The function of this polymorphism is still unknown; then further research is needed to explain it.

When comparing the occurrence of C70G polymorphism genotypes in patients with normal-tension glaucoma, Ishikawa et al. did not notice any differences in intraocular pressure between particular genotypes (GG genotype 16.5 mmHg, CC + CG genotypes 17.0 mmHg) [12]. Similar results were obtained in our research. Intraocular pressure in patients with normal-tension glaucoma presents as follows: in patients with GG genotype intraocular pressure was 16.4 mmHg, in patients with CC genotype was 17.4 mmHg, and in patients with heterozygous CG genotype was 17.6 mmHg ($p = 0.28$).

In our study glaucoma, at the time of diagnosis, was less advanced according to MD in the group of patients with normal-tension glaucoma (-8.58 ± 6.26 dB) than in patients with high-tension glaucoma (-13.83 ± 7.01 dB) ($p < 0.0001$). Häntzschel et al., while analysing visual field defects and loss of retinal nerve fibres, observed smaller visual field defect in patients with normal-tension glaucoma than in patients with primary open-angle glaucoma (NTG MD -3.69 dB versus POAG MD -9.77 dB, $p = 0.0001$) [15]. Our research seems to confirm the above observation (NTG MD -4.18 dB versus POAG MD -7.18 dB, $p = 0.015$).

The pathogenesis of optic disc haemorrhages is not yet known. It is not clear which vessels they originate from: arterioles, venules, or capillaries. One of theories claims that sudden changes of pressure in stiff scleral vessels lead to their mechanical tear. Others point to the role of primary vascular dysregulation. Elevated level of ET-1 and MMP-9 might spread from the choroid to the optic disk causing vasoconstriction, ischemia, and blood-brain barrier disruption. Such sequence of events might explain optic disk haemorrhages in patients with normal-tension glaucoma [16]. What is more, persistent vasospasms cause microinfarctions which in turn lead to visual field defects [17]. We found no statistically significant differences in the frequency of optic disc haemorrhages depending on the studied K198N polymorphisms of the endothelin-1 gene and C1222T, C70G, and G231A of the endothelin-1 receptor type A gene. Nevertheless, optic disc haemorrhages tended to occur more often in patients with wild type GG genotype of G231A polymorphism in both study groups and mutant GG genotype of C70G polymorphism in patients with high-tension glaucoma. It is worth noticing that optic disc haemorrhages do not occur in patients with mutant AA genotype of G231A polymorphism in both study groups. This might suggest that the presence of mutant AA genotype protects patients with normal-tension glaucoma against vasoconstricting factors. This is the first study about a relation between K198N polymorphisms of the endothelin-1 gene and C1222T, C70G, and G231A of the endothelin-1 receptor type A gene and the occurrence of optic disc haemorrhages.

For many years the influence of blood pressure on the development of glaucomatous optic neuropathy, especially normal-tension glaucoma, has been extensively studied. It has been pointed out in many works that hemodynamic parameters such as reduced ocular blood flow and fluctuations in ocular perfusion pressure, nocturnal fall of blood pressure, autoregulation dysfunctions, and migraines, might be the reason for ischemia and optic nerve damage [18]. Ambulatory blood pressure monitoring of patients with glaucoma makes it possible to observe the modifiable disease risk factors.

Ocular perfusion pressure, understood as a difference between average arterial blood pressure and intraocular pressure, is a crucial parameter for supplying optic nerve in necessary elements. A research conducted by Ramli et al. showed that patients with normal-tension glaucoma had much lower parameters of nocturnal blood pressure and ocular perfusion pressure than healthy persons, which only supports the great importance of ischemia theory in the pathogenesis of normal-tension glaucoma [19, 20].

On the basis of a research by Barbados Eye Study and Framingham Eye Study, diastolic perfusion pressure was acknowledged to be the most permanent vascular risk factor in the development of glaucomatous optic neuropathy [21], whereas the researchers of the Early Manifest Glaucoma Trial deemed low systolic pressure to be a factor predisposing to glaucoma progression [22].

Following Flammer, who found that nocturnal blood pressure dips are the only risk factor in patients with rapidly developing optic nerve damage in NTG, we investigate systemic blood pressure abnormalities in this group. On the basis of the interview obtained from patients and their medical history we noticed that low blood pressure was presented much more often in NTG group (69.7%) than in HTG group (16.7%) ($p = 0.039$). Taking into account the low pressure as a risk factor for normal-tension glaucoma pathogenesis, it seemed advisable to determine the relationship between systemic blood pressure values and presence of studied polymorphisms only in NTG group. We analysed the relation between the occurrence of particular genotypes of the studied K198N polymorphisms of the endothelin-1 gene, C1222T, C70G, and G231A of the endothelin-1 receptor type A, and ambulatory blood pressure monitoring results. In the case of K198N polymorphism a much higher maximum systolic blood pressure and average systolic blood pressure during the day were observed in patients with heterozygous GT genotype rather than those with homozygous wild type genotype. The difference was close to being statistically significant ($p = 0.06$). In order to confirm the preliminary observations, the study group should be larger.

In the case of C1222T polymorphism a statistically significantly higher maximum systolic blood pressure during the day and average systolic blood pressure during the day were observed in the group of patients with heterozygous CT genotype (176.8 ± 33.1 mmHg and 137.4 ± 16.6 mmHg) in comparison to homozygous CC genotype (152.3 ± 21.2 mmHg and 123 ± 14.7 mmHg) ($p = 0.041$ and $p = 0.028$). Interestingly, the highest average nocturnal diastolic pressure was observed in patients with homozygous mutant TT genotype (72.4 ± 15.2 mmHg) and the lowest with homozygous wild type CC genotype (61.3 ± 6 mmHg). The difference was close to statistical significance ($p = 0.055$).

Undoubtedly, polymorphisms of the studied genes do have an influence on the level of arterial blood pressure and its regulation. The above observations might point at the existence of autoregulation mechanisms dysfunction, vascular dysregulation, or even the dysfunction of vascular endothelium responsible for endothelin release. The mechanisms by which those polymorphisms affect function remain to be examined and clarified since functional studies are not yet available.

5. Conclusion

In patients with NTG and HTG a similar frequency of occurrence of polymorphic variants of the studied genes was observed. The is no relation between NTG risk factors and K198N, C1222T, C70G, and G231A polymorphisms. The studied polymorphic variants have an influence on the level of intraocular pressure and arterial blood pressure in patients with NTG. Endothelin might play an important role in glaucoma pathogenesis. Giving a better knowledge of risk factors of NTG will give us more effective tools for preventing its development or even minimizing the glaucomatous damage.

Conflict of Interests

None of the authors have any commercial interests in the subject of the paper nor in entities discussed in the paper.

Acknowledgments

The paper was supported by Grant no. 179 from the Medical University of Lublin and used equipment was purchased as part of the following project: The Equipment of Innovative Laboratories Doing Research on New Medicines Used in the Therapy of Civilization and Neoplastic Diseases within the Operational Program Development of Eastern Poland 2007–2013, Priority Axis I Modern Economy, Operations I.3 Innovation Promotion.

References

[1] Collaborative Normal-Tension Glaucoma Study Group, "Comparison of glaucomatous progression between untreated patients with normal-tension glaucoma and patients with therapeutically reduced intraocular pressures," *American Journal of Ophthalmology*, vol. 126, no. 4, pp. 487–497, 1998.

[2] A. Von Graefe, "Über die Iridectomie bei Glaucom und über den glaucomatosen Prozess," *Graefe's Archive for Clinical and Experimental Ophthalmology*, vol. 3, no. 2, pp. 456–465, 1857.

[3] R. C. Zeimer and Y. Ogura, "The relation between glaucomatous damage and optic nerve head mechanical compliance," *Archives of Ophthalmology*, vol. 107, no. 8, pp. 1232–1234, 1989.

[4] J. Czajkowski and M. Pilas-Pomykalska, "Występowanie naczyniowych czynników ryzyka w populacji chorych na jaskrę-badanie epidemiologiczne z lat 2002-2003," in *Wyniki Badań Ankietowych 18 645 Chorych*, wydanie specjalne, Okulistyka, 2005.

[5] J. Caprioli and A. L. Coleman, "Blood flow in glaucoma discussion.: blood pressure, perfusion pressure, and glaucoma," *American Journal of Ophthalmology*, vol. 149, no. 5, pp. 704–712, 2010.

[6] M. Yanagisawa, H. Kurihara, S. Kimura et al., "A novel potent vasoconstrictor peptide produced by vascular endothelial cells," *Nature*, vol. 332, no. 6163, pp. 411–415, 1988.

[7] T. J. Good and M. Y. Kahook, "The role of endothelin in the pathophysiology of glaucoma," *Expert Opinion on Therapeutic Targets*, vol. 14, no. 6, pp. 647–654, 2010.

[8] I. O. Haefliger, E. Dettmann, R. Liu et al., "Potential role of nitric oxide and endothelin in the pathogenesis of glaucoma," *Survey of Ophthalmology*, vol. 43, no. 6, pp. 51–58, 1999.

[9] B. C. Chauhan, "Endothelin and its potential role in glaucoma," *Canadian Journal of Ophthalmology*, vol. 43, no. 3, pp. 356–360, 2008.

[10] Y. Z. Shoshani, A. Harris, M. M. Shoja et al., "Endothelin and its suspected role in the pathogenesis and possible treatment of glaucoma," *Current Eye Research*, vol. 37, no. 1, pp. 1–11, 2012.

[11] H.-Y. Chen, Y.-C. Chang, W.-C. Chen, and H.-Y. Lane, "Association between plasma endothelin-1 and severity of different types of glaucoma," *Journal of Glaucoma*, vol. 22, no. 2, pp. 117–122, 2013.

[12] K. Ishikawa, T. Funayama, Y. Ohtake et al., "Association between glaucoma and gene polymorphism of endothelin type A receptor," *Molecular Vision*, vol. 11, pp. 431–437, 2005.

[13] L. W. Herndon, J. S. Weizer, and S. S. Stinnett, "Central corneal thickness as a risk factor for advanced glaucoma damage," *Archives of Ophthalmology*, vol. 122, no. 1, pp. 17–21, 2004.

[14] S. H. Kim, J. Y. Kim, D. M. Kim et al., "Investigations on the association between normal tension glaucoma and single nucleotide polymorphisms of the endothelin-1 and endothelin receptor genes," *Molecular Vision*, vol. 12, pp. 1016–1021, 2006.

[15] J. Häntzschel, N. Terai, F. Sorgenfrei, M. Haustein, K. Pillunat, and L. E. Pillunat, "Morphological and functional differences between normal-tension and high-tension glaucoma," *Acta Ophthalmologica*, vol. 91, no. 5, pp. 386–391, 2013.

[16] D. Gherghel, S. Orgül, K. Gugleta, and J. Flammer, "Retrobulbar blood flow in glaucoma patients with nocturnal over-dipping in systemic blood pressure," *American Journal of Ophthalmology*, vol. 132, no. 5, pp. 641–647, 2001.

[17] Y. Delaney, T. E. Walshe, and C. O'Brien, "Vasospasm in glaucoma: clinical and laboratory aspects," *Optometry and Vision Science*, vol. 83, no. 7, pp. 406–414, 2006.

[18] N. Plange, M. Kaup, L. Daneljan, H. G. Predel, A. Remky, and O. Arend, "24-h blood pressure monitoring in normal tension glaucoma: night-time blood pressure variability," *Journal of Human Hypertension*, vol. 20, no. 2, pp. 137–142, 2006.

[19] S. Mroczkowska, A. Benavente-Perez, A. Negi, V. Sung, S. R. Patel, and D. Gherghel, "Primary open-angle glaucoma vs normal-tension glaucoma: the vascular perspective," *JAMA Ophthalmology*, vol. 131, no. 1, pp. 36–43, 2013.

[20] N. Ramli, B. S. Nurull, N. N. Hairi, and Z. Mimiwati, "Low nocturnal ocular perfusion pressure as a risk factor for normal tension glaucoma," *Preventive Medicine*, vol. 57, pp. S47–S49, 2013.

[21] M. C. Leske, "Incidence of open angle glaucoma: the Barbados Eye Studies. The Barbados Eye Group," *Archives of Ophthalmology*, vol. 119, pp. 89–98, 2001.

[22] M. C. Leske, A. Heijl, L. Hyman, B. Bengtsson, L. Dong, and Z. Yang, "Predictors of long-term progression in the early manifest glaucoma trial," *Ophthalmology*, vol. 114, no. 11, pp. 1965–1972, 2007.

Scheimpflug Imaging Parameters Associated with Tear Mediators and Bronchial Asthma in Keratoconus

Dorottya Pásztor,[1] Bence Lajos Kolozsvári,[1] Adrienne Csutak,[1] András Berta,[1] Ziad Hassan,[2] Beáta Andrea Kettesy,[1] Péter Gogolák,[3] and Mariann Fodor[1]

[1]Department of Ophthalmology, University of Debrecen, Debrecen 4012, Hungary
[2]Orbident Refractive Surgery and Medical Center, Debrecen 4012, Hungary
[3]Department of Immunology, University of Debrecen, Debrecen 4012, Hungary

Correspondence should be addressed to Mariann Fodor; mfodor@med.unideb.hu

Academic Editor: Vito Romano

Purpose. To determine associations between mediators in tears in the whole spectrum of keratoconus (KC); to explore connections between mediators and Scheimpflug parameters; to examine correlations between Scheimpflug parameters and bronchial asthma. *Methods.* Tear samples were collected from 69 patients and 19 controls. Concentrations of mediators—IL-6, -10; CXCL8, CCL5; MMP-9, -13; TIMP-1; t-PA, PAI-1—were measured by Cytometric Bead Array. Measured Pentacam parameters include keratometry values (K_1, K_2, K_{max}), corneal thickness (Pachy Pupil, Apex, Min), and elevations and indices (including Belin-Ambrósio deviation (BAD-D)). *Results.* A number of significant positive associations were observed between pairs of mediator concentrations. Significant positive correlations were found between BAD-D and CXCL8/MMP-9 and K_2 and MMP-9. Significant negative associations were explored between Pachy Min and CXCL8/t-PA. Significant associations were found between pairs of mediators (IL-6 and CXCL8; CCL5 and CXCL8/MMP-9; TIMP-1 and MMP-9/-13/t-PA; t-PA and CXCL8/CCL5/PAI-1) and the severity of KC. Significant positive correlation between asthma and the severity of KC was explored. *Conclusion.* Cooperation of different mediators in tears all taking part in the complex pathomechanism of keratoconus was revealed. Our research verifies that inflammation plays a crucial role in the pathogenesis of KC. Additionally this study confirms the effect of bronchial asthma on keratoconus.

1. Introduction

Keratoconus (KC) is usually a bilateral, progressive ectatic corneal disorder, usually appearing in puberty [1–3]. The corneal stroma becomes thinner and protrudes, causing the typical conical shape that leads to irregular astigmatism, myopia, and the decrease of visual acuity [1–3]. The apex of the protrusion can most commonly be found in inferotemporal orientation from the center of the cornea [1, 2]. The incidence of KC is around 1 : 2,000 in the general population [2]. The etiology of the disease is not yet known in detail [1–4].

Classically, KC is considered to be a noninflammatory disease [1]. However, recent studies have suggested that inflammatory factors play a key role in the pathomechanism of the disorder [4]. Elevated levels of interleukin- (IL-) 1b, IL-4, IL-5, IL-6, IL-8, and IL-17; tumor necrosis factor (TNF)-α, -β; interferon- (IFN-) γ; matrix metalloproteinase- (MMP-) 1, MMP-3, MMP-7, MMP-9, and MMP-13; Cathepsin B; and Lipocalin-1 have been found in the tears of patients with keratoconus [4–11]. Decreased levels of IL-4, IL-10, IL-12, and IL-13; TNF-α; IFN-γ; Chemokine (C-C motif) ligand 5 (CCL5/RANTES, regulated on activation, normal T cell expressed and secreted); lipophilin C; lipophilin A; lactoferrin; α-fibrinogen; zinc-α2-glycoprotein (ZAG); immunoglobulin A (IgA); immunoglobulin κ-chain (IGKC); polymeric immunoglobuline receptor (PIGR); phospholipase A2; cystatin S; cystatin SN and cystatin SA have also been found in the tear fluid [4, 8, 10–14]. Kenney et al. have found a decreased level of tissue inhibitor of metalloproteinase-1 (TIMP-1) in KC corneas, compared to normal corneas [15].

In addition, an association between KC and bronchial asthma has been identified almost 50 years earlier [16]. Several studies have demonstrated a strong association between KC, asthma, and other immune disorders, pointing to the crucial role of the immune system in the pathogenesis of keratoconus [17, 18].

In the past few decades, slit-imaging technologies provided further improvement in corneal imaging. Nowadays, we can measure not only the front but also the back surface of the cornea with pachymetric mapping and can typify corneal architecture in three dimensions. Furthermore, Ambrósio et al. established numerous indices to improve the screening of the ectasia [19, 20].

There are only a few preliminary studies examining the association between mediators (mainly cytokines) in the tear fluid and the severity of keratoconus. Lema and Durán analyzed 28 eyes [5], Jun et al. checked 18 patients [13], and Kolozsvári et al. studied only 14 keratoconic eyes [21]. In a recent study, Shetty et al. [22] examined the association between MMP-9, IL-6, TNF-α, and different stages of KC. The crucial limitations of these studies [5, 13, 21, 22] are the small number of patients, or the few examined mediators, or the lack of subclinical cases.

In the present study, our goals were to determine associations between the different types of mediators in tear fluid—IL-6, IL-10, chemokine (C-X-C motif) ligand 8 (CXCL8)/IL-8, CCL5/RANTES, MMP-9, MMP-13, TIMP-1, tissue plasminogen activator (t-PA), and plasminogen activator inhibitor (PAI-1)—in the whole spectrum of keratoconic eyes (suspect, subclinical, and manifest cases of keratoconus) and normal eyes. An additional goal was to explore associations between these mediators and the Scheimpflug parameters which characterize the severity of keratoconus. Our aim was also to examine the relationship between the Scheimpflug imaging parameters and bronchial asthma in keratoconus.

2. Patients and Methods

2.1. Subjects and Clinical Examinations. In this prospective study, patients with keratoconus and normal subjects were recruited from the Outpatient Unit, Department of Ophthalmology, Faculty of Medicine, University of Debrecen, Hungary.

We examined patients with keratoconus at all stages (severe, moderate, and mild KC, subclinical KC or forme fruste KC) and normal, control patients. We have categorized the participants based on the clinical stage of keratoconus, but group allocation was not a factor in the analysis. An eye was diagnosed as having keratoconus where it had one or a combination of the following clinical signs: central or paracentral stromal thinning of the cornea, conical protrusion, Fleischer's ring, Vogt's striae by slit-lamp examination, and topographic changes [23]. The stages of KC were divided between mild, if the steepest keratometric reading (K_2) was <45 diopters (D); moderate, when K_2 was between 45 and 52 D; and severe if K_2 was >52 D [13, 24]. At present, there are no specific or universally accepted criteria categorizing an eye as having subclinical KC or forme fruste KC (FFKC). The criteria for diagnosing subclinical KC or FFKC were defined as one or a combination of the following clinical signs: if it was the fellow eye of a patient with keratoconus and had a normal cornea on slit-lamp examination (in several cases, keratoplasty or corneal cross-linking was performed on the keratoconic eye), or using a Pentacam, the BAD-D (Belin-Ambrósio deviation index) [20], ART Max (Maximum Ambrósio's Relational Thickness) [19], and PPI Ave (Average Pachymetric Progression Index) [19]; or where the back elevation values at the thinnest location (B.Ele.Th.) were not in the normal range of the Pentacam; or where the criteria of KC did not apply but the maximum keratometric reading of the front surface (K_{max} Front) was more than 47 D.

We included a randomly selected eye from each participant, although both eyes were examined. Eye selection was based on generating random values using Microsoft Excel set to produce numeric indicators with equal probabilities for either eye. Altogether, 69 patients (mean (SD) age 30.7 (10.3), range 13–68 years) with the following diagnoses—severe KC: 25, moderate KC: 21, mild KC: 5 and subclinical KC: 18—and 19 normal controls (mean (SD) age 31.7 (11.5), range 18–67 years) were enrolled in the study. The 69 eyes of the patients represented the whole spectrum of the abnormal, ectatic, and keratoconic corneas, although no such group allocation was made.

The exclusion criteria included the existence of active inflammatory or infective systemic or ocular disease, eye rubbing, and current treatment with systemic or local anti-inflammatory drugs. Those eyes that were affected by previous ocular surgery or trauma, as well as those patients who were pregnant or lactating during the course of the study, were also excluded. Written informed consent from each participant, as well as permission from the University of Debrecen Institutional Ethics Committee, was obtained prior to enrollment. The tenets of the Declaration of Helsinki were followed in all procedures during the study.

Both eyes of each participant underwent ophthalmological evaluation, including clinical history (especially bronchial asthma and contact lens usage), automated kerato-refractometry (KR-8900; Topcon Co, Tokyo, Japan), uncorrected and corrected distance visual acuity determinations, slit-lamp biomicroscopy (under low illumination to avoid reflex tearing), Rotating Scheimpflug tomography (Pentacam HR, Oculus Optikgeräte GmbH, Wetzlar, Germany), and nonstimulated tear sample collection with glass capillaries.

2.2. Pentacam Measurements. All eyes were examined with a Pentacam HR (software version 1.16r26 and 1.17r139) without the application of any eye drops. Three sequential scans were taken in each eye by the same trained examiner. In short, the patients were asked to keep both eyes open and fixate on the target, in the center of the blue fixation beam. The examiner with the joystick then focuses and obtains a correct alignment with the corneal apex and a perfect focus, and the instrument automatically takes 25 Scheimpflug images within two seconds. The quality of images was checked under the quality specification (QS) window and only the correct measurements ("QS" reads "OK") were accepted; if the comments were marked yellow or red, the examination was repeated [25, 26].

The following parameters were exported to Microsoft Excel (Microsoft Corp, Redmond, Washington): Holladay equivalent keratometry values in the flat (K_1) and steep (K_2) meridian; maximal keratometry of the front surface (K_{max} Front); corneal astigmatism (Astig); corneal thickness at the pupil's center (Pachy Pupil), at the apex (Pachy Apex) and at the thinnest point of the cornea (Pachy Min); Index of Surface Variation (ISV); Index of Vertical Asymmetry (IVA); Keratoconus Index (KI); Central Keratoconus Index (CKI); Index of Height Asymmetry (IHA); Index of Height Decentration (IHD); front and back elevation at the thinnest location (F.Ele.Th. and B.Ele.Th.); minimal, maximal, and average pachymetric progression indices (PPI Min, PPI Max, and PPI Ave); Ambrósio's Relational Thickness (ART); and Belin-Ambrósio deviation index (BAD-D).

2.3. Tear Collection and Analysis. Nontraumatic tear collection was carried out using sterile thin glass microcapillary tubes from the inferior meniscus, without anesthetic drops or stimulation. Tears were collected for two minutes and then promptly transferred to Eppendorf tubes and frozen at $-80°C$ without centrifugation, within 15 minutes of collection. The samples were stored until they were analyzed. In all cases, the total volume of collected tear samples was registered. We calculated tear volumes from the length of the tear column in the tube.

In tear samples, the concentrations of IL-6, IL-10, CXCL8/IL-8, CCL5/RANTES, MMP-9, MMP-13, TIMP-1, t-PA, and PAI-1 were measured using the Cytometric Bead Array method. Combined FlowCytomix Simplex Kits were used with the suitable FlowCytomix Basic Kit, with minor modifications to the manufacturer's orders (eBioscience, Bender Med Systems GmbH, Vienna, Austria) [27]. Briefly stated, 12.5 μL of tear samples (diluted samples, if necessary) or serial dilutions of mixed standard cytokines were added to a 12.5 μL suspension of fluorescent cytokine capture beads in multiwell filter microplates. Added to the wells were 12.5 microliters of biotin-conjugated anti-cytokine antibodies, after which the plates were incubated for two hours on a microplate shaker. The wells were emptied and washed with a vacuum filtration manifold. Phycoerythrin-conjugated streptavidin was added to the plate wells, followed by an additional incubation period of one hour and washed as described before. A 150 μL assay buffer was applied to the wells, after which multiparametric data acquisition was executed using a FACS Array cytometer (BD Biosciences Immunocytometry Systems, San Jose, CA). The data were analyzed with the FlowCytomix Pro 2.3 software (eBioscience). Additional serial dilutions of the standard were applied to achieve better sensitivity and modified standard curves were thus generated in the analysis. The subsequent detection limits were as follows: IL-6: 1.2 pg/mL; IL-10: 1.9 pg/mL; CXCL8 (IL-8): 0.5 pg/mL; CCL5 (RANTES): 25 pg/mL; MMP-9: 95 pg/mL; MMP-13: 50 pg/mL; TIMP-1: 28 pg/mL; t-PA: 4.8 pg/mL; and PAI-1: 13.5 pg/mL.

2.4. Statistical Analysis. We categorized the participants for descriptive purposes based on clinical severity (group allocation was not used as a variable in the analysis). Mediator concentration variables were inspected for the distribution shape and natural log transformed (for t-PA and PAI-1, square root transformed) to improve normality. Similarly, Pentacam parameters were subjected to one of these transformations if that improves distributional symmetry.

Pentacam parameters were unified in a composite index referred to as the Standardized Pentacam Score. This was calculated by centering, standardizing, and direction correcting the source variables (so that the higher values invariably represent more severe pathologies), running a principal component analysis and deriving the first principal component.

Associations between all possible pairs of mediator levels, as well as those between mediators in the tear fluid and Scheimpflug parameters, were evaluated using simple linear regression, including a quadratic term by a curvature in the relationship, if required. Associations between pairs of mediators and the Standardized Pentacam Score were assessed using multiple linear regressions adjusted for age, the presence of asthma, and contact lens usage. Mediator variables were used in linear and quadratic forms, and interactions between those terms were also included in order to accommodate the model to curvatures in the outcome space. Relationships were expressed as the overall significance of the mediator pair effect and also as additive differences in the Standardized Pentacam Score at sample-covered locations, defined by mediator pair concentrations versus an arbitrary reference point.

3. Results

3.1. Associations between Mediator Levels in the Tear Fluid. A number of significant positive associations were observed between pairs of mediator concentrations in tear fluid collected from KC patients and subjects with normal eyes, as shown in Table 1.

3.2. Associations between Mediators in the Tear Fluid and Scheimpflug Parameters. Significant positive associations were found between BAD-D and CXCL8, BAD-D and MMP-9, and K_2 and MMP-9. Significant negative associations were found between Pachy Min and CXCL8 and Pachy Min and t-PA (Table 2).

3.3. Associations between Pairs of Mediators and the Standardized Pentacam Score (A Composite Parameter Calculated from Pentacam Readings). A significant association was found between the TIMP-1 concentration, the MMP-9 concentration, and the Standardized Pentacam Score: the combination of high TIMP-1 and low MMP-13 levels was characterized by a low score, while high levels of both mediators—as well as low TIMP-1 concentrations coupled with moderate MMP-9 levels—were associated with an elevated score (Table 3).

Significant associations were also found between the concentrations of a number of other pairs of mediators and the Standardized Pentacam Score as shown in Table 4.

TABLE 1: Significant positive associations between the concentrations of the different tear mediators.

	IL-6 (pg/mL)	IL-10 (pg/mL)	CXCL8 (pg/mL)	CCL5 (pg/mL)	MMP-9 (ng/mL)	MMP-13 (ng/mL)	TIMP-1 (ng/mL)	t-PA (pg/mL)	PAI-1 (ng/mL)
IL-6 (pg/mL)		$p < 0.0001$	$p < 0.0001^*$	$p < 0.0001$	$p = 0.0203$	$p < 0.0001^*$	$p < 0.0001^*$	$p < 0.0001^*$	$p < 0.0001$
IL-10 (pg/mL)			$p < 0.0001$	$p < 0.0001$		$p < 0.0001$		$p < 0.0001$	$p < 0.0001^*$
CXCL8 (pg/mL)				$p < 0.0001$	$p < 0.0001$	$p < 0.0001$	$p < 0.0001$	$p < 0.0001^*$	$p < 0.0001$
CCL5 (pg/mL)					$p < 0.0001$			$p < 0.0001^*$	$p < 0.0001$
MMP-9 (ng/mL)						$p < 0.0001$	$p < 0.0001$		
MMP-13 (ng/mL)							$p = 0.0001^*$	$p < 0.0001$	$p < 0.0001^*$
TIMP-1 (ng/mL)								$p < 0.0001^*$	$p < 0.0001^*$
t-PA (pg/mL)									$p < 0.0001^*$
PAI-1 (ng/mL)									

IL: interleukin; CXCL8: chemokine (C-X-C motif) ligand 8 = IL-8; CCL5: chemokine (C-C motif) ligand 5 = RANTES: regulated on activation, normal T cell expressed and secreted; MMP: matrix metalloproteinase; TIMP-1: tissue inhibitor of metalloproteinase-1; t-PA: tissue plasminogen activator; PAI-1: plasminogen activator inhibitor (shape of relationship: linear, *quadratic**).

TABLE 2: Significant associations between tear mediators and Pentacam indices.

	CXCL8 (pg/mL)	MMP-9 (ng/mL)	t-PA (pg/mL)
BAD-D	$p = 0.020$	$p = 0.005$	
K_2 F		$p = 0.031$	
Pachy Min	**$p = 0.027$**		**$p = 0.023$**

BAD-D: Belin-Ambrósio deviation index; KI: keratoconus Index; K_2 F: Holladay equivalent keratometry value in the steep meridian on the front surface; Pachy Min: corneal thickness at the thinnest point of the cornea; CXCL8: chemokine (C-X-C motif) ligand 8 = IL-8: interleukin-8; MMP-9: matrix metalloproteinase-9; t-PA: tissue plasminogen activator (bold values represent negative correlations).

3.4. The Effect of Bronchial Asthma on Standardized Pentacam Score.

There was a history of asthma in five patients (7.25%) and one of contact lens usage in 15 patients (21.74%). A strong, significant positive association between asthma and the Standardized Pentacam Score was found by linear regression adjusted for age and contact lens usage. Asthmatic patients' scores were, on average, an estimated 5.7 units (95% CI: 2.0 to 9.4, $p = 0.003$)—or 1.32 standard deviations—higher than those of subjects without the condition.

4. Discussion

To the best of our knowledge, this is the first study that aimed to reveal associations between pairs of mediators and the severity of keratoconus, evaluated using a Pentacam. Despite the intensive clinical and biochemical investigations, the pathogenesis of keratoconus is not yet known in detail. Classically, keratoconus was considered a noninflammatory disease [1]; however, recently published articles have suggested that inflammation is involved in the pathogenesis of KC [4, 7–14]. In the tear fluid of keratoconic patients, elevated levels of IL-6, TNF-α, and MMP-9 were detected, and IL-6 and TNF-α levels were also elevated in subclinical cases [5, 6]. Jun et al. found high level of IL-6 and low levels of IL-12, TNF-α, IFN-γ, IL-4, IL-13, and CCL5 in the tear fluid of KC patients [13]. Partly in line with these results, increased tear levels of MMP-1, MMP-3, MMP-7, MMP-9, and MMP-13; IL-4, IL-5, IL-6, and IL-8, and TNF-α, -β were found in keratoconus [9]. In keratoconic corneas, a decrease in TIMP-1 mRNA was reported [15]. Only few studies investigated the associations between a range of cytokines in the tear fluid and the severity of keratoconus. The limitations of these reports are the small number of patients, or the few examined mediators, or the lack of subclinical cases [5, 13, 21, 22].

In the current study, we have determined the associations between nine mediators (IL-6, IL-10, CXCL8/IL-8, CCL5/RANTES, MMP-9, MMP-13, TIMP-1, t-PA, and PAI-1) in the tear fluid of keratoconic patients covering the whole spectrum of the disease (from subclinical to manifest keratoconus). In accordance with earlier studies, we proved that different mediators—including cytokines, chemokines, enzymes, and inhibitors—in the tear fluid cooperate and take part in a complex immunological network [4, 5, 7–14, 21]. Significant associations were explored between the concentrations of different mediators (between IL-6 and CXCL8; between CCL5, CXCL8, and MMP-9; between TIMP-1, MMP-9, MMP-13, and t-PA; and between t-PA, CXCL8, CCL5, and PAI-1) and the Standardized Pentacam Score, which is a composite index statistically unifying all Pentacam parameters. As far as we know, there are no studies evaluating the association between different tear mediators and Pachy Min and also BAD-D, which was designed to present comprehensive data based on anterior and posterior corneal elevation and a pachymetric evaluation. Our results support the linkage between the complex network of the various mediators and the comprehensive Pentacam indices. Based on our results, inflammation not only seems to be involved in the pathogenesis of keratoconus, but also plays a crucial role in the pathological corneal processes from the initial stage to the final one. We have found only a few significant associations between the single mediators and Pentacam indices, highlighting the fact that mediators, including cytokines, take part in a complex cascade. The examined mediators overlap, neutralize and enhance the effects of one another. It is in line with evidence showing that various multitargeted mediators in the serum collaborate

TABLE 3: Additive differences in the Standardized Pentacam Score at various locations defined by TIMP-1 concentration (ng/mL) and MMP-13 concentration (ng/mL) versus the indicated reference point, as estimated by linear regression adjusted for age, the presence of asthma, and contact lens usage.

		TIMP-1 (ng/mL)					
		12.18	20.09	33.12	54.60	90.02	148.41
MMP-13 (ng/mL)	33.12	$p > 0.05$	$p > 0.05$	$p > 0.05$	$p > 0.05$	$p > 0.05$	Reference point
	54.60	4.96 [0.27; 9.64] $p = 0.038$	$p > 0.05$	$p > 0.05$	$p > 0.05$	$p > 0.05$	$p > 0.05$
	90.02	4.30 [0.021; 8.59] $p = 0.049$	$p > 0.05$	$p > 0.05$	$p > 0.05$	$p > 0.05$	$p > 0.05$
	148.41	N/A	N/A	$p > 0.05$	$p > 0.05$	$p > 0.05$	$p > 0.05$
	244.69	N/A	N/A	$p > 0.05$	3.93 [0.084; 7.79] $p = 0.045$	4.60 [0.69; 8.51] $p = 0.022$	4.43 [0.29; 8.58] $p = 0.037$

Square brackets indicate 95% confidence intervals; N/A indicates insufficient sample coverage for estimation.

TABLE 4: Significant associations between pairs of mediators and the Standardized Pentacam Score.

	IL-6 (pg/mL)	CCL5 (pg/mL)	TIMP-1 (ng/mL)	t-PA (pg/mL)
CXCL8 (pg/mL)	$p = 0.014$	$p = 0.028$		$p = 0.024$
CCL5 (pg/mL)				$p = 0.026$
MMP-9 (ng/mL)		$p = 0.04$	$p = 0.001$	
MMP-13 (ng/mL)			$p = 0.043$	
t-PA (pg/mL)			$p = 0.014$	
PAI-1 (ng/mL)				$p = 0.02$

IL: interleukin; CXCL8: chemokine (C-X-C motif) ligand 8 = IL-8; CCL5: chemokine (C-C motif) ligand 5 = RANTES: regulated on activation, normal T cell expressed and secreted; MMP: matrix metalloproteinase; TIMP-1: tissue inhibitor of metalloproteinase-1; t-PA: tissue plasminogen activator; PAI-1: plasminogen activator inhibitor.

in different diseases, suggesting that examination of only one or a few mediators is not enough to explore complex immunopathological processes [13, 28, 29].

MMPs are zinc-dependent endopeptidases, which participate in degrading and remodeling the extracellular matrix, thereby maintaining its integrity during normal conditions. Nevertheless, under pathological conditions, MMPs can support tissue destruction and other inflammatory reactions. TIMP-1 is the inhibitor of MMPs, which prevents pro-MMP activation and, furthermore, presents antiapoptotic properties [15, 30, 31]. MMP-13 was categorically reported in keratoconus, suggesting that it plays a role in intra- and extracellular pathological collagen destruction [32]. Additionally, proMMP-13 activation is partially inhibited by TIMP-1 [33]. In line with these studies, we have found significant associations between TIMP-1 concentration, MMP-13 concentration, and the Standardized Pentacam Score. The combination of high TIMP-1 and low MMP-13 levels was characterized by a low score, while high levels of both mediators—as well as low TIMP-1 concentrations coupled with moderate MMP-9 levels—were associated with elevated scores. Additionally, significant positive associations were found between MMP-9 and BAD-D, and also with K_2.

Based on our study and others, the collagenolytic milieu of the human cornea seems to be more complex than expected. Further studies are required to understand the exact mechanisms of collagenases and inhibitors.

An active form of t-PA converts plasminogen to plasmin and can also degrade several components of the extracellular matrix, triggering the activation of the MMP pathway. Numerous interactions have been observed between the fibrinolytic and MMP systems taking part in proteolytic activation. Plasminogen activators are partially regulated by PAIs, inhibiting this cascade system and, therefore, influencing KC progression [34]. Different growth factors and cytokines induce the PAI-1 gene and inhibit the activity of the t-PA enzyme. In addition, PAs could affect the proteolytic inactivation of growth factors [35]. Significant associations between the severity of keratoconus and pairs of t-PA/TIMP-1 and t-PA/PAI were detected in our study. In addition to this observation, significant negative associations were found between the corneal thickness at the thinnest point of the cornea and t-PA.

Apart from the elements of the proteolytic and fibrinolytic systems, we have examined different cytokines, such as the proinflammatory IL-6 and chemokine CXCL8/IL-8 and the anti-inflammatory Th2 cytokine IL-10 [13]; we found that all of these cytokines cooperate with each other and play a crucial role in the pathogenesis of KC. The significant positive association between BAD-D and CXCL8 and the significant negative correlation between Pachy Min and CXCL8 highlight the roles of the chemokines.

Bronchial asthma is a chronic airway inflammatory disease. The infiltration of eosinophils, mastocytes, and T lymphocytes and the release of several inflammatory mediators play an important role in asthma's pathogenesis [36, 37]. Different proteins are altered in the serum of these patients, such as IgE; IL-1, IL-4, IL-6, IL-8, and IL-13; CCL5; TNF-α; MMP-9; TIMP-1; t-PA; and serum Angiopoietin-1 [36, 38–43]. Due to an increase in the number of known mediators, additional anti-inflammatory options are becoming available in the therapy of asthma. The connection between asthma and other atopic diseases with keratoconus was first published almost 50 years ago and has been confirmed several times since then [16–18]. We found a strong significant positive association between asthma and the severity of keratoconus, meaning that asthmatic patients have 5.7 higher score than nonasthmatic subjects. Based on our study, bronchial asthma has an impact on the severity of keratoconus. This result albeit was a secondary outcome of our study and confirms the previous hypothesis related to the connection between KC and asthma. Further larger randomized studies are required to verify this strong correlation.

The strengths of our study are the large number of participants (88 subjects) and the consideration of a wide range of tear mediators that could be associated with Pentacam parameters. Our study has limitations, such as the lack of examination of enzyme activities, as well as the fact that we did not examine the progression of keratoconus and the effect of asthma medication. In addition, this study does not exclude the role of other inflammatory molecules in the pathophysiology of KC. It would be interesting to measure more and different types of mediators, but this remains to be determined in subsequent studies. However, several new correlations can be revealed from our results that can be the basis for further study of this topic.

5. Conclusion

Keratoconus has a complex pathomechanism, in which many different cytokines, chemokines, enzymes, and inhibitors are involved. This study reveals the cooperation of the different mediators in tear fluid all taking part in this complex immunological network. As far as we know, this is the first study to reveal associations between tear mediators and BAD-D or Pachy Min. Our study confirms that inflammation is involved in the pathogenesis of keratoconus. As a next step, the precise role of these mediators needs to be defined, as well as examination of the progression of KC and exploration of other mediators' functions. These studies might then serve as a platform for finding targets for local inhibition of pathological corneal thinning, or eventual treatment. In addition, our study confirms the effect of bronchial asthma on keratoconus. Further prospective studies are required to examine the effect of the systemic treatment of asthma on the pathomechanism of keratoconus.

Conflict of Interests

The authors declare that there is no conflict of interests regarding the publication of this paper.

References

[1] J. H. Krachmer, R. S. Feder, and M. W. Belin, "Keratoconus and related non-inflammatory corneal thinning disorders," *Survey of Ophthalmology*, vol. 28, no. 4, pp. 293–322, 1984.

[2] Y. S. Rabinowitz, "Keratoconus," *Survey of Ophthalmology*, vol. 42, no. 4, pp. 297–319, 1998.

[3] A. E. Davidson, S. Hayes, A. J. Hardcastle, and S. J. Tuft, "The pathogenesis of keratoconus," *Eye*, vol. 28, no. 2, pp. 189–195, 2014.

[4] V. Galvis, T. Sherwin, A. Tello, J. Merayo, R. Barrera, and A. Acera, "Keratoconus: an inflammatory disorder?" *Eye*, vol. 29, no. 7, pp. 843–859, 2015.

[5] I. Lema and J. A. Durán, "Inflammatory molecules in the tears of patients with keratoconus," *Ophthalmology*, vol. 112, no. 4, pp. 654–659, 2005.

[6] I. Lema, T. Sobrino, J. A. Durán, D. Brea, and E. Díez-Feijoo, "Subclinical keratoconus and inflammatory molecules from tears," *British Journal of Ophthalmology*, vol. 93, no. 6, pp. 820–824, 2009.

[7] C. Pannebaker, H. L. Chandler, and J. J. Nichols, "Tear proteomics in keratoconus," *Molecular Vision*, vol. 16, pp. 1949–1957, 2010.

[8] A. Acera, E. Vecino, I. Rodríguez-Agirretxe et al., "Changes in tear protein profile in keratoconus disease," *Eye*, vol. 25, no. 9, pp. 1225–1233, 2011.

[9] S. A. Balasubramanian, S. Mohan, D. C. Pye, and M. D. P. Willcox, "Proteases, proteolysis and inflammatory molecules in the tears of people with keratoconus," *Acta Ophthalmologica*, vol. 90, no. 4, pp. e303–e309, 2012.

[10] S. A. Balasubramanian, V. C. Wasinger, D. C. Pye, and M. D. Willcox, "Preliminary identification of differentially expressed tear proteins in keratoconus," *Molecular Vision*, vol. 19, pp. 2124–2134, 2013.

[11] R. Sorkhabi, A. Ghorbanihaghjo, N. Taheri, and M. H. Ahoor, "Tear film inflammatory mediators in patients with keratoconus," *International Ophthalmology*, vol. 35, no. 4, pp. 467–472, 2015.

[12] I. Lema, D. Brea, R. Rodríguez-González, E. Díez-Feijoo, and T. Sobrino, "Proteomic analysis of the tear film in patients with keratoconus," *Molecular Vision*, vol. 16, pp. 2055–2061, 2010.

[13] A. S. Jun, L. Cope, C. Speck et al., "Subnormal cytokine profile in the tear fluid of keratoconus patients," *PLoS ONE*, vol. 6, no. 1, Article ID e16437, 2011.

[14] S. A. Balasubramanian, D. C. Pye, and M. D. P. Willcox, "Levels of lactoferrin, secretory IgA and serum albumin in the tear film of people with keratoconus," *Experimental Eye Research*, vol. 96, no. 1, pp. 132–137, 2012.

[15] M. C. Kenney, M. Chwa, S. R. Atilano et al., "Increased levels of catalase and cathepsin V/l2 but decreased TIMP-1 in keratoconus corneas: evidence that oxidative stress plays a role in this disorder," *Investigative Ophthalmology and Visual Science*, vol. 46, no. 3, pp. 823–832, 2005.

[16] D. W. Sabiston, "The association of keratoconus, dermatitis and asthma," *Transactions of the Ophthalmological Society of New Zealand*, vol. 18, pp. 66–71, 1966.

[17] A. Y. Nemet, S. Vinker, I. Bahar, and I. Kaiserman, "The association of keratoconus with immune disorders," *Cornea*, vol. 29, no. 11, pp. 1261–1264, 2010.

[18] I. Merdler, A. Hassidim, N. Sorkin, S. Shapira, Y. Gronovich, and Z. Korach, "Keratoconus and allergic diseases among Israeli adolescents between 2005 and 2013," *Cornea*, vol. 34, no. 5, pp. 525–529, 2015.

[19] R. Ambrósio Jr., A. L. C. Caiado, F. P. Guerra et al., "Novel pachymetric parameters based on corneal tomography for diagnosing keratoconus," *Journal of Refractive Surgery*, vol. 27, no. 10, pp. 753–758, 2011.

[20] R. Ambrósio Jr., I. Ramos, B. Lopes et al., "Assessing ectasia susceptibility prior to LASIK: the role of age and residual stromal bed (RSB) in conjunction to Belin-Ambrósio deviation index (BAD-D)," *Revista Brasileira de Oftalmologia*, vol. 73, no. 2, pp. 75–80, 2014.

[21] B. L. Kolozsvári, G. Petrovski, P. Gogolák et al., "Association between mediators in the tear fluid and the severity of keratoconus," *Ophthalmic Research*, vol. 51, no. 1, pp. 46–51, 2014.

[22] R. Shetty, A. Ghosh, R. R. Lim et al., "Elevated expression of matrix metalloproteinase-9 and inflammatory cytokines in keratoconus patients is inhibited by cyclosporine A," *Investigative Ophthalmology & Visual Science*, vol. 56, no. 2, pp. 738–750, 2015.

[23] Y. S. Rabinowitz, "Videokeratographic indices to aid in screening for keratoconus," *Journal of Refractive Surgery*, vol. 11, no. 5, pp. 371–379, 1995.

[24] I. Lema, J. A. Durán, C. Ruiz, E. Díez-Feijoo, A. Acera, and J. Merayo, "Inflammatory response to contact lenses in patients with keratoconus compared with myopic subjects," *Cornea*, vol. 27, no. 7, pp. 758–763, 2008.

[25] K. Miháltz, I. Kovács, Á. Takács, and Z. Z. Nagy, "Evaluation of keratometric, pachymetric, and elevation parameters of keratoconic corneas with pentacam," *Cornea*, vol. 28, no. 9, pp. 976–980, 2009.

[26] Ö. Ö. Uçakhan, V. Çetinkor, M. Özkan, and A. Kanpolat, "Evaluation of Scheimpflug imaging parameters in subclinical keratoconus, keratoconus, and normal eyes," *Journal of Cataract and Refractive Surgery*, vol. 37, no. 6, pp. 1116–1124, 2011.

[27] M. Fodor, B. L. Kolozsvári, G. Petrovski et al., "Effect of contact lens wear on the release of tear mediators in keratoconus," *Eye and Contact Lens*, vol. 39, no. 2, pp. 147–152, 2013.

[28] K. E. Clark, H. Lopez, B. A. Abdi et al., "Multiplex cytokine analysis of dermal interstitial blister fluid defines local disease mechanisms in systemic sclerosis," *Arthritis Research and Therapy*, vol. 17, article 73, 2015.

[29] B. Mickiewicz, P. Tam, C. N. Jenne et al., "Integration of metabolic and inflammatory mediator profiles as a potential prognostic approach for septic shock in the intensive care unit," *Critical Care*, vol. 19, no. 1, article 11, 2015.

[30] F. J. Matthews, S. D. Cook, M. A. Majid, A. D. Dick, and V. A. Smith, "Changes in the balance of the tissue inhibitor of matrix metalloproteinases (TIMPs)-1 and -3 may promote keratocyte apoptosis in keratoconus," *Experimental Eye Research*, vol. 84, no. 6, pp. 1125–1134, 2007.

[31] T. Sakimoto and M. Sawa, "Metalloproteinases in corneal diseases: degradation and processing," *Cornea*, vol. 31, no. 11, pp. S50–S56, 2012.

[32] Z. Mackiewicz, M. Määttä, M. Stenman, L. Konttinen, T. Tervo, and Y. T. Konttinen, "Collagenolytic proteinases in keratoconus," *Cornea*, vol. 25, no. 5, pp. 603–610, 2006.

[33] V. Knäuper, L. Bailey, J. R. Worley, P. Soloway, M. L. Patterson, and G. Murphy, "Cellular activation of proMMP-13 by MT1-MMP depends on the C-terminal domain of MMP-13," *FEBS Letters*, vol. 532, no. 1-2, pp. 127–130, 2002.

[34] H. R. Lijnen, "Elements of the fibrinolytic system," *Annals of the New York Academy of Sciences*, vol. 936, pp. 226–236, 2001.

[35] J.-D. Vassalli, A.-P. Sappino, and D. Belin, "The plasminogen activator/plasmin system," *The Journal of Clinical Investigation*, vol. 88, no. 4, pp. 1067–1072, 1991.

[36] W. Stankiewicz, M. P. Dabrowski, A. Chcialowski, and T. Plusa, "Cellular and cytokine immunoregulation in patients with chronic obstructive pulmonary disease and bronchial asthma," *Mediators of Inflammation*, vol. 11, no. 5, pp. 307–312, 2002.

[37] N. A. Hanania, "Targeting airway inflammation in asthma: current and future therapies," *Chest*, vol. 133, no. 4, pp. 989–998, 2008.

[38] E. Banach-Wawrzeńczyk, A. Dziedziczko, and D. Rość, "Fibrinolysis system in patients with bronchial asthma," *Medical Science Monitor*, vol. 6, no. 1, pp. 103–107, 2000.

[39] Y. Higashimoto, Y. Yamagata, S. Taya et al., "Systemic inflammation in COPD and asthma: similarities and differences," *The Journal of the Japanese Respiratory Society*, vol. 46, no. 6, pp. 443–447, 2008.

[40] S. Saad-El-Din Bessa, G. H. Abo El-Magd, and M. M. Mabrouk, "Serum chemokines RANTES and monocyte chemoattractant protein-1 in Egyptian patients with atopic asthma: relationship to disease severity," *Archives of Medical Research*, vol. 43, no. 1, pp. 36–41, 2012.

[41] P. Hodsman, C. Ashman, A. Cahn et al., "A phase 1, randomized, placebo-controlled, dose-escalation study of an anti-IL-13 monoclonal antibody in healthy subjects and mild asthmatics," *British Journal of Clinical Pharmacology*, vol. 75, no. 1, pp. 118–128, 2013.

[42] K.-Y. Moon, P.-H. Lee, S.-W. Park, C.-S. Park, and A.-S. Jang, "Serum angiopoietin is associated with lung function in patients with asthma: a retrospective cohort study," *BMC Pulmonary Medicine*, vol. 14, no. 1, article 143, 2014.

[43] K. Grzela, W. Zagorska, A. Krejner et al., "Prolonged treatment with inhaled corticosteroids does not normalize high activity of Matrix Metalloproteinase-9 in exhaled breath condensates of children with asthma," *Archivum Immunologiae et Therapiae Experimentalis*, vol. 63, no. 3, pp. 231–237, 2015.

Usefulness of Surgical Media Center as a Cataract Surgery Educational Tool

Tomoichiro Ogawa, Takuya Shiba, and Hiroshi Tsuneoka

Department of Ophthalmology, The Jikei University School of Medicine, 3-25-8 Nishishinbashi, Minato-ku, Tokyo 105-0003, Japan

Correspondence should be addressed to Tomoichiro Ogawa; tomo-to@seagreen.ocn.ne.jp

Academic Editor: Lisa Toto

Purpose. This study retrospectively analyzed cataract surgeries to examine the usefulness of Surgical Media Center (SMC) (Abbott Medical Optics Inc.), a new cataract surgery recording device, for training of cataract surgery. *Methods.* We studied five hundred cataract surgeries conducted with a phacoemulsification system connected to the SMC. After surgery, the surgical procedures were reviewed, with changes in aspiration rate, vacuum level, and phaco power displayed as graphs superimposed on the surgical video. We examined whether use of SMC is able to demonstrate the differences in technique between experienced and trainee operators, to identify inappropriate phacoemulsification techniques from analyzing the graphs, and to elucidate the cause of intraoperative complications. *Results.* Significant differences in the time taken to reach maximum vacuum and the speed of increase in vacuum during irrigation and aspiration were observed between experienced and trainee operators. Analysis of the graphs displayed by SMC detected inappropriate phacoemulsification techniques mostly in cases operated by trainee operators. *Conclusions.* Using SMC, it was possible to capture details of cataract surgery objectively. This recording device allows surgeons to review cataract surgery techniques and identify the cause of intraoperative complication and is a useful education tool for cataract surgery.

1. Introduction

With technological advances in phacoemulsification instruments, emulsification and aspiration of the crystalline lens through even smaller incisions are now possible [1–6]. These instruments play very important roles in cataract surgeries. During surgery, information such as the amount of ultrasound generated by the instrument and the vacuum level achieved can be presented on the intraoperative video image using video overlay. However, the conventional overlay displays ultrasound power, vacuum pressure, and aspiration rate at one instant only, and it is difficult to capture how phaco power and vacuum change over time. To address this issue, a new generation cataract surgery recording device, the Surgical Media Center (SMC) (Abbott Medical Optics Inc.), was developed. The SMC is a cataract surgical data management tool designed for use with phaco systems such as Sovereign, Sovereign Compact, and Signature (Abbott Medical Optics Inc.). The SMC consists of a computer installed with dedicated software that records the intraoperative images from the surgical microscope together with phaco power, vacuum level, and aspiration rate over time during the surgery and displays the data as graphs synchronized with the surgical video (Figure 1). Since the graphs are recorded simultaneously with the surgical video, review of the video after surgery provides clear information of how the changes in phaco power, aspiration rate, and vacuum level over time affect the process of phacoemulsification. In addition, the state of foot pedal depression is also displayed, allowing surgeons to assess the surgical manipulations objectively (Figure 2). Recently, High-Definition Surgical Media Center (HD-SMC) (Abbott Medical Optics Inc.) with improved image quality has been launched, allowing detailed observation of cataract surgery procedures in high-definition images.

Surgical recording devices with the above-mentioned features should be widely used as an educational tool for learners of cataract surgery. However, there are few reports on detailed analysis of these devices and their educational usefulness in training cataract surgeons. In this study, we examined the practical advantages of the new cataract surgery

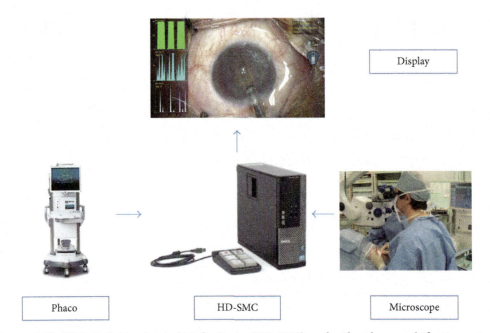

Figure 1: The High-Definition Surgical Media Center (HD-SMC) used with a phacoemulsification system.

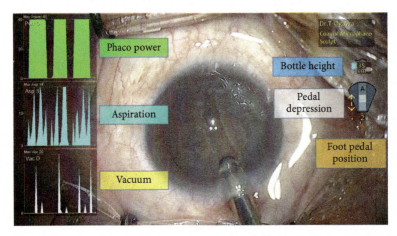

Figure 2: An example of display by the High-Definition Surgical Media Center (HD-SMC).

recording devices, SMC and HD-SMC, and verified that these devices are useful educational tools for cataract surgery.

2. Patients and Methods

2.1. Patients. Three hundred and sixty-eight patients (500 eyes) who underwent cataract surgery using Sovereign, Sovereign Compact, or Signature at the Jikei Medical University School of Medicine between April 2008 and July 2014 were analyzed. Surgeries were conducted by three experienced cataract surgeons and three surgeons who were learning the surgical techniques (trainee operators).

2.2. Methods. Phacoemulsification was conducted using a phacoemulsification system (Sovereign, Sovereign Compact, or Signature) connected to a surgical microscope and a surgical data recording device (SMC or HD-SMC). After surgery, the changes in phaco power, vacuum level, and aspiration rate over time recorded by the SMC or HD-SMC were displayed in graphs synchronized with the surgical video.

An experienced operator was defined as a surgeon who had conducted cataract surgeries in over 300 eyes per year and in a total of over 2000 eyes. A trainee operator was defined as a surgeon who had conducted cataract surgeries in a total of less than 200 eyes. Six surgeons conducted cataract surgeries during the study period: three were experienced and three were trainees.

This study aimed to examine whether SMC or HD-SMC is able to demonstrate the difference in techniques between experienced and trainee operators, to identify inappropriate phacoemulsification techniques from analyzing the graphs, and to elucidate the cause of intraoperative complications such as posterior capsule rupture.

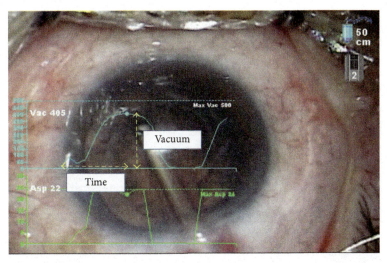

Figure 3: Changes in vacuum level over time during irrigation and aspiration (IA).

To compare the performance of experienced and trainee operators, 20 cases of cataract with grade 2 nucleus hardness (Emery-Little classification) performed by each of the 6 surgeons were selected. During irrigation and aspiration (IA), the time taken for vacuum to increase from 0 to a plateau and the peak vacuum level were measured three times. The speed of increase in vacuum was calculated by dividing maximum vacuum level by the time to each maximum vacuum (Figure 3). For Trainee Operator 1, maximum vacuum, time to maximum vacuum, and speed of increase in vacuum were determined for the subsequent 40 cataract surgeries. Statistical analysis was performed using Kruskal-Wallis test. A p value less than 0.05 was considered significant. The data were measured by a staff member not related to the operators or to the study.

In addition, the three experienced operators analyzed the relationship between the surgical video and surgical parameter data displayed in the overlays in cases, where phacoemulsification of nucleus or aspiration of cortex was difficult, and in cases with intraoperative complications.

3. Results

3.1. Comparison between Experienced and Trainee Operators. The speed of increase in vacuum level is shown in Table 1. The mean time to reach maximum vacuum during I/A was 1.49 ± 0.45 sec in experienced operators and 2.80 ± 0.98 sec in trainee operators, with a significant difference between two groups ($p < 0.001$). The mean maximum vacuum was 314 ± 70 mmHg in experienced operators and 300 ± 65 mmHg in trainee operators, with no significant difference between two groups ($p = 0.226$). The mean speed of vacuum increase was 225 ± 76 mmHg/sec in experienced operators and 115 ± 35 mmHg/sec in trainee operators and was significantly higher in experienced operators ($p < 0.001$).

Intragroup comparison was also conducted for the group of experienced operators and the group of trainee operators. In the group of experienced operators, time to reach maximum vacuum and speed of vacuum increase were not significantly different between operators, but maximum vacuum was significantly lower in Operator 2 compared to Operators 1 and 3 (both $p < 0.001$). In the group of trainee operators, there were no significant differences in time to reach maximum vacuum, maximum vacuum, and speed of vacuum increase between operators.

For Trainee Operator 1, the time to reach maximum vacuum and speed of increase were 1.54 ± 0.39 sec and

Table 1: Time to maximum vacuum (time), maximum vacuum level (vacuum), and speed of increase in vacuum level (speed).

(a)

	Time (sec)	Vacuum (mmHg)	Speed (mmHg/sec)
Experienced	$1.49 \pm 0.45^{*a}$	314 ± 70	$225 \pm 76^{*d}$
Operator 1	1.54 ± 0.38	$367 \pm 41^{*b}$	257 ± 90
Operator 2	1.32 ± 0.47	$242 \pm 50^{*bc}$	199 ± 62
Operator 3	1.62 ± 0.45	$334 \pm 47^{*c}$	222 ± 63
Trainee	$2.80 \pm 0.98^{*a}$	300 ± 65	$115 \pm 35^{*d}$
Operator 1	2.64 ± 0.68	321 ± 52	126 ± 28
Operator 2	3.42 ± 1.18	311 ± 57	99 ± 30
Operator 3	2.15 ± 1.00	268 ± 74	120 ± 40

$^{*}p < 0.001$, Kruskal-Wallis test. $n = 20$ for each operator. The same superscripted letters indicate that they are compared to each other.

(b)

	Time (sec)	Vacuum (mmHg)	Speed (mmHg/sec)
Trainee Operator 1			
1–20 (operations)	$2.64 \pm 0.68^{*ef}$	321 ± 52	$126 \pm 28^{*gh}$
21–40 (operations)	$1.54 \pm 0.39^{*e}$	306 ± 29	$208 \pm 44^{*g}$
41–60 (operations)	$1.50 \pm 0.26^{*f}$	297 ± 32	$202 \pm 36^{*h}$

$^{*}p < 0.001$, Kruskal-Wallis test. The same superscripted letters indicate that they are compared to each other.

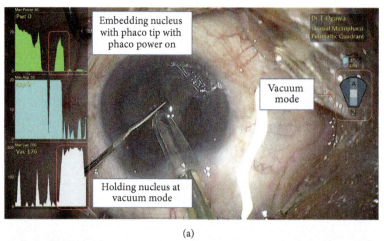

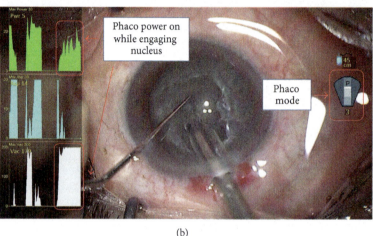

Figure 4: Nucleus fragmentation technique. (a) Correct nucleus fragmentation technique. (b) Case 1, inappropriate nucleus fragmentation technique.

306 ± 29 mmHg/sec, respectively, for the 21st to 40th cataract surgeries (intermediate group) and were 1.50 ± 0.26 sec and 297 ± 32 mmHg/sec for the 41st to 60th cataract surgeries (latter group). The time was significantly reduced and the speed was significantly increased in these subsequent operations compared to the first 20 operations.

3.2. Analysis of SMC Graphs and Inappropriate Phacoemulsification Techniques. Analysis of the graphs recorded by SMC revealed inappropriate phacoemulsification techniques. The relationship between SMC parameter data and surgical video is demonstrated in representative examples below.

3.2.1. Inappropriate Nucleus Fragmentation Procedure. The correct method to fracture the nucleus is first to embed the phaco tip into the nucleus with a short blast of phaco, then stop phaco power, and engage the nucleus under vacuum mode (Figure 4(a)). In a case of inappropriate technique (Case 1, Figure 4(b)), the SMC overlay showed that phaco power remained elevated while the nucleus was being engaged. Hence, SMC revealed that the operator was generating ultrasound while engaging the nucleus.

3.2.2. Inappropriate Cortex Aspiration. When cortex aspiration is executed smoothly, vacuum increases steeply reaching a high level within a short time (Figure 5(a)). In Case 2 (Figure 5(b)) in which there was difficulty with cortex aspiration due to insufficient occlusion of the phaco tip and inadequate depression of the foot pedal, the vacuum curve (arrow 1) increased sluggishly reaching a low maximum level.

3.2.3. Inappropriate Trenching. In trenching, nonoccluded aspiration is usually conducted so that the phaco tip does not penetrate the nucleus; hence the vacuum level does not increase. In Case 3 (Figure 6), the vacuum level was elevated (arrow) during trenching, indicating nonoccluded aspiration as not being achieved.

3.3. Intraoperative Complication. The causes of intraoperative complications including posterior capsule rupture were examined by analyzing SMC data.

Posterior Capsule Rupture during Bimanual IA. In Case 4 (Figure 7), the surgical video depicted only the occurrence of posterior capsule rupture during IA but provided no

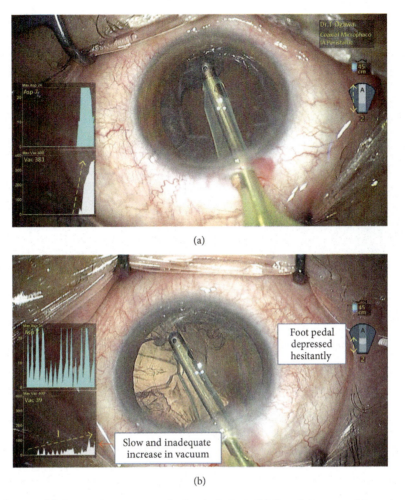

Figure 5: Aspiration of cortex. (a) Appropriate cortex aspiration technique. (b) Case 2, inappropriate cortex aspiration technique.

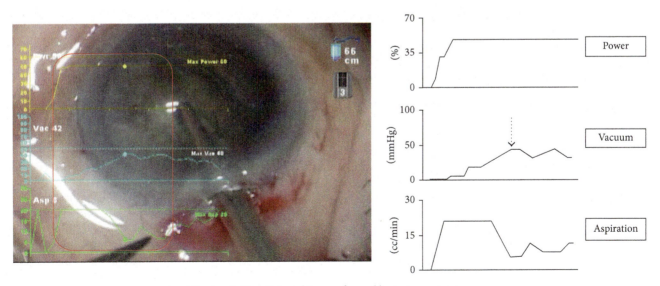

Figure 6: Case 3, trenching performed by trainee operator.

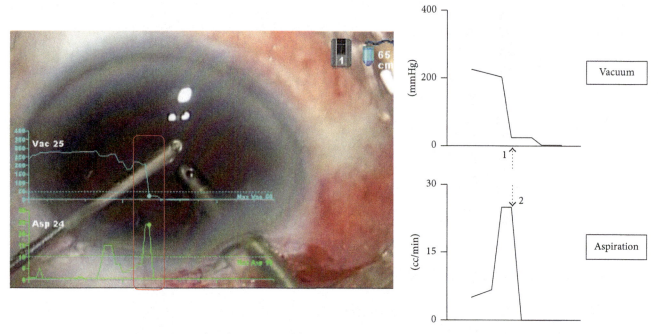

FIGURE 7: Accidental aspiration of the posterior capsule during aspiration of cortex.

more information. The SMC overlay, however, showed that while the cortex was aspirated and occlusion at the IA tip was released, the vacuum level dropped (arrow 1) while the aspiration rate increased abruptly (arrow 2). These findings indicated that a surge occurred, which aspirated the posterior capsule accidentally, resulting in posterior capsule rupture.

4. Discussion

In SMC and HD-SMC, users can choose any method to display the system data such as phaco power, vacuum level, and aspiration rate. In other words, it is possible to display only those data that are necessary. The format of presentation can be selected either as line graphs (Figure 2) or as bar graphs. The point on the line graph is synchronized with the video image displayed at the same time. Since the data before and after that time point are also displayed, the changes in each parameter over time are clearly depicted. The present study aimed at capturing the techniques and the changes in different parameters during cataract surgery. Therefore we chose to display the data in line graphs that are efficient in demonstrating temporal changes. The x- and y-axes of these line graphs can also be set at will, and the maximum value for the y-axes as well as the speed of progression of the point on the graph can also be selected freely. In other words, when one wishes to inspect the surgical video closely, the graphs can be reduced in size and moved to a location of the screen not overlapping with the video image. When one wishes to examine the changes in the curves in detail, the graph size can be increased and the progression of the graph can be delayed. Depending on what information one desires to obtain from SMC or HD-SMC, the method of display can be selected freely.

Conventional video overlay systems can only display phaco power, vacuum, and aspiration rate of an instant. Therefore the greatest merit of SMC and HD-SMC is the visualization of changes in various parameters over time. When the latest SMC is connected to Signature, the state of foot pedal control can also be visualized, which allows better understanding of the condition of the phacoemulsification device and the operator's manipulations.

Previous reports on cataract surgery education described surgical training using simulations or the necessity of feedback in cataract surgical education [7–16]. There is no report on cataract surgery training using actual intraoperative findings as teaching material. In the present study, we examined the usefulness of SMC and HD-SMC that are capable of displaying detailed and objective surgical parameters in training cataract surgery.

First, we examined whether the surgical recording devices are capable of showing the differences of technical competence between experienced and trainee operators, focusing on the changes in vacuum level during IA. Experienced operators and trainee operators differed significantly in the time taken to reach maximum vacuum and the speed of increase in vacuum level. This difference is also illustrated in Case 2. Because of the lack of experience in cataract surgery, trainee operators are not skillful in operating the foot pedal and hence are unable to control the increase in vacuum by depressing the foot pedal. The SMC recordings showed that trainee operators did not depress the foot pedal sufficiently at the beginning and increased the depressing slowly thereafter. Moreover, surgical videos showed that experienced operators ensured that the IA tip was occluded. Therefore, use of SMC revealed that, in addition to foot pedal control, whether the IA tip is properly occluded also contributes to the difference in speed of vacuum increase.

For Trainee Operator 1, after the first 20 operations, she underwent technical retraining using the SMC aiming to perform IA more effectively. Thereafter, the mean time to reach maximum vacuum, maximum vacuum, and speed of vacuum increase were determined for every 20 consecutive operations. The results showed that as the number of operations increased, the time to reach maximum vacuum was shortened and the speed of increase was improved. These findings imply that, through instructions using the SMC, the operator achieved appropriate pedal control and proper occlusion of the IA tip.

Therefore, the time to reach maximum vacuum and the speed of increase in vacuum may be regarded as indicators for evaluation of the skillfulness of handling the operation device. Educating trainees on the status of pedal control and occlusion of the IA tip based on the values of the above parameters is useful in training surgical techniques.

Using SMC or HD-SMC, inappropriate phacoemulsification techniques were detected; most of the cases were performed by trainee operators.

In Case 1, during nucleus fragmentation, the operator generated ultrasound while trying to engage the nucleus. With the phaco power turned on, the nucleus continued to be fragmented, and it was difficult to stabilize the nucleus with the phaco tip. After the surgery, we reviewed the SMC records with the operator. We found that the operator did not have a good understanding of the principle of nucleus fragmentation, and, during routine surgeries, he was not able to stabilize the nucleus properly and had trouble with nucleus fragmentation. After reviewing the surgical technique using the SMC overlays, he generated ultrasound while embedding the phaco tip into the nucleus; once inside the nucleus, he engaged the nucleus on vacuum mode only. Using this method, he succeeded to conduct nucleus fragmentation reliably.

Case 2 was a case in which cortex aspiration was not smooth. The vacuum curve (arrow 1) increased slowly and reached a low maximum level. The reason was that the operator had not acquired the skills to control the foot pedal and to predict the vacuum response to pedal depression. Worried about accidentally aspirating the capsule, he depressed the foot pedal hesitantly.

Moreover, to increase the vacuum effectively, the IA tip opening has to be occluded properly. The video revealed that the IA tip opening was not occluded sufficiently, which resulted in inadequate increase in vacuum. After viewing the SMC recording, the operator was able to depress the foot pedal stronger than before and ensure that the tip opening was well occluded, achieving more efficient vacuum increase.

In Case 3, a trainee operator performed trenching. Even during trenching, vacuum continued to increase (arrow). Under this condition, nonoccluded aspiration cannot be obtained. In order to perform surgery safety, the operator must ensure complete open aspiration. In addition, decreasing the vacuum setting reduces the risk when occluded aspiration occurs. This case illustrates the usefulness of SMC in reviewing surgical technique and set values for the machine.

By viewing surgical videos, it is possible to have general idea about basic techniques such as manipulation of the hand piece or the hook. However, detailed operations such as the pressure applied to the foot pedal, the intensity of ultrasound generated, and their timing cannot be learnt from conventional surgical videos.

When an operator has problem with performing cataract surgery but does not know the reason, use of the SMC allows the operator to visualize his/her own surgical technique and to compare his/her techniques with the correct techniques. It is easy to comprehend which surgical techniques require improvement. The SMC is thus useful in training surgical techniques and further upgrading of surgical skills.

Moreover, various complications including posterior capsule rupture tend to occur during training. Case 4 illustrates the occurrence of posterior capsule rupture during surgery performed by a trainee operator. The SMC recording clearly showed that posterior capsule rupture was caused by a surge. Using conventional recording devices, one can visualize the occurrence of posterior capsule rupture but cannot understand why it happened. Therefore, there is a possibility that the same complication may occur again in future surgeries. However, reviewing the SMC recording with the operator revealed that the operator lacked knowledge on surge. Taking this opportunity, the operator understood the importance of foot pedal control for surge prevention and was able to put it in practice thereafter. Thus, this case demonstrates that SMC is useful for analyzing the cause of intraoperative complication of posterior capsule rupture and for improving surgical technique.

The present study had a limitation. We used the time taken to reach maximum vacuum and the speed of increase in vacuum as parameters to indicate the technical competence of operators. We hypothesized that skillful control of the foot pedal and timely occlusion of the phaco tip are reflected by a shorter time to reach maximum vacuum and higher speed of vacuum increase. However, further studies are required to investigate the validity of these parameters.

5. Conclusion

In the present study, use of SMC or HD-SMC that shows the time courses of phaco power, vacuum, and aspiration rate as well as the state of foot pedal depression superimposed on surgical video allowed more detailed and objective assessments of surgical techniques compared to conventional video overlays. The SMC was able to demonstrate the differences in techniques between experienced and trainee operators, detect inappropriate phacoemulsification techniques by analyzing the graphs, and elucidate the cause of intraoperative complication. Since this recording device allows the review of cataract surgery techniques and identification of the causes of intraoperative complications, it is a valuable tool for educating trainee surgeons on cataract surgery.

Conflict of Interests

The authors declare that there is no conflict of interests regarding the publication of this paper.

References

[1] M. Wilczynski, I. Drobniewski, A. Synder, and W. Omulecki, "Evaluation of early corneal endothelial cell loss in bimanual microincision cataract surgery (MICS) in comparison with standard phacoemulsification," *European Journal of Ophthalmology*, vol. 16, no. 6, pp. 798–803, 2006.

[2] J. Wang, E.-K. Zhang, W.-Y. Fan, J.-X. Ma, and P.-F. Zhao, "The effect of micro-incision and small-incision coaxial phacoemulsification on corneal astigmatism," *Clinical and Experimental Ophthalmology*, vol. 37, no. 7, pp. 664–669, 2009.

[3] S. Masket, L. Wang, and S. Belani, "Induced astigmatism with 2.2- and 3.0-mm coaxial phacoemulsification incisions," *Journal of Refractive Surgery*, vol. 25, no. 1, pp. 21–24, 2009.

[4] H. Tsuneoka, T. Shiba, and Y. Takahashi, "Feasibility of ultrasound cataract surgery with a 1.4 mm incision," *Journal of Cataract and Refractive Surgery*, vol. 27, no. 6, pp. 934–940, 2001.

[5] H. Tsuneoka, T. Shiba, and Y. Takahashi, "Ultrasonic phacoemulsification using a 1.4 mm incision: clinical results," *Journal of Cataract and Refractive Surgery*, vol. 28, no. 1, pp. 81–86, 2002.

[6] M. Wilczynski, E. Supady, L. Piotr, A. Synder, D. Palenga-Pydyn, and W. Omulecki, "Comparison of surgically induced astigmatism after coaxial phacoemulsification through 1.8 mm microincision and bimanual phacoemulsification through 1.7 mm microincision," *Journal of Cataract and Refractive Surgery*, vol. 35, no. 9, pp. 1563–1569, 2009.

[7] J. Bergqvist, A. Person, A. Vestergaard, and J. Grauslund, "Establishment of a validated training programme on the Eyesi cataract simulator. A prospective randomized study," *Acta Ophthalmologica*, vol. 92, no. 7, pp. 629–634, 2014.

[8] S. L. Cremers, J. B. Ciolino, Z. K. Ferrufino-Ponce, and B. A. Henderson, "Objective Assessment of Skills in Intraocular Surgery (OASIS)," *Ophthalmology*, vol. 112, no. 7, pp. 1236–1241, 2005.

[9] K. C. Golnik, A. Haripriya, H. Beaver et al., "Cataract surgery skill assessment," *Ophthalmology*, vol. 118, no. 10, pp. 2094–2094.e2, 2011.

[10] A. Naseri and D. F. Chang, "Assessing the value of simulator training on residency performance," *Journal of Cataract and Refractive Surgery*, vol. 38, no. 1, pp. 188–189, 2012.

[11] R. Pokroy, E. Du, A. Alzaga et al., "Impact of simulator training on resident cataract surgery," *Graefe's Archive for Clinical and Experimental Ophthalmology*, vol. 251, no. 3, pp. 777–781, 2013.

[12] S. Puri and S. Sikder, "Cataract surgical skill assessment tools," *Journal of Cataract and Refractive Surgery*, vol. 40, no. 4, pp. 657–665, 2014.

[13] H. Saedon, "An analysis of ophthalmology trainees' perceptions of feedback for cataract surgery training," *Clinical Ophthalmology*, vol. 8, pp. 43–47, 2013.

[14] S. Sikder, K. Tuwairqi, E. Al-Kahtani, W. G. Myers, and P. Banerjee, "Surgical simulators in cataract surgery training," *British Journal of Ophthalmology*, vol. 98, no. 2, pp. 154–158, 2014.

[15] A. Spiteri, R. Aggarwal, T. Kersey, L. Benjamin, A. Darzi, and P. Bloom, "Phacoemulsification skills training and assessment," *British Journal of Ophthalmology*, vol. 94, no. 5, pp. 536–541, 2010.

[16] L. Steeples, K. Mercieca, and K. Smyth, "Consent for cataract surgery training: a national trainers' survey," *Eye*, vol. 26, no. 5, pp. 666–670, 2012.

Visual and Refractive Outcomes of a Toric Presbyopia-Correcting Intraocular Lens

Alice T. Epitropoulos[1,2]

[1] The Eye Center of Columbus, 262 Neil Avenue, Columbus, OH 43215, USA
[2] The Ohio State University, Columbus, OH, USA

Correspondence should be addressed to Alice T. Epitropoulos; aepitrop@columbus.rr.com

Academic Editor: Santiago Garcia-Lazaro

Purpose. To evaluate outcomes in astigmatic patients implanted with the Trulign (Bausch + Lomb) toric presbyopia-correcting intraocular lens (IOL) during cataract surgery in a clinical practice setting. *Methods.* Retrospective study in 40 eyes (31 patients) that underwent cataract extraction and IOL implantation in a procedure using intraoperative wavefront aberrometry guidance (ORA system). Endpoints included uncorrected visual acuity (VA), reduction in refractive cylinder, accuracy to target, axis orientation, and safety. *Results.* At postoperative month 1, refractive cylinder was ≤0.50 D in 97.5% of eyes (≤1.00 D in 100%), uncorrected distance VA was 20/25 or better in 95%, uncorrected intermediate VA was 20/25 or better in 95%, and uncorrected near VA was 20/40 (J3 equivalent) or better in 92.5%. Manifest refraction spherical equivalent was within 1.00 D of target in 95% of eyes and within 0.50 D in 82.5%. Lens rotation was <5° and best-corrected VA was 20/25 or better in all eyes. *Conclusion.* The IOL effectively reduced refractive cylinder and provided excellent uncorrected distance and intermediate vision and functional near vision. Refractive predictability and rotational stability were exceptional. Implantation of this toric presbyopia-correcting IOL using ORA intraoperative aberrometry provides excellent refractive and visual outcomes in a standard of care setting.

1. Introduction

Corneal astigmatism affects a significant proportion of patients undergoing cataract surgery; studies have estimated that 22% to 25% of cataract patients have more than 1.50 D of corneal astigmatism [1, 2]. Because residual postoperative refractive astigmatism compromises visual outcomes, concurrent reduction of astigmatism is vital to achieving patient satisfaction following cataract surgery. Techniques to assist with reduction of astigmatism include limbal relaxing incisions (LRIs), astigmatic keratotomy, excimer or femtosecond laser refractive surgery, and toric intraocular lenses (IOLs) [3].

Toric IOLs are generally a predictable treatment for astigmatism [3] and their use prevents the development of irregular astigmatism that may result from corneal manipulation, as well as potential complications associated with incisions, such as exacerbation of dry eye, variable wound healing, and infection. Toric IOLs also have the advantage of potential reversibility. Several monofocal toric IOLs are available. These IOLs effectively reduce astigmatism [4, 5], but if corrected for distance VA, patients typically still rely on glasses for computer work and reading.

Premium lenses, either accommodative or multifocal, address presbyopia and provide a broader range of vision. The Trulign toric IOL (Bausch + Lomb, Bridgewater, NJ, USA) is a toric modification of the Crystalens accommodative IOL (Bausch + Lomb) with a toric optic on the posterior surface. The IOL was designed to reduce postoperative refractive cylinder and provide improved distance, intermediate, and near vision. The aspheric optic of the parent IOL provides excellent image sharpness [6] and depth of focus [7]. On the basis of favorable refractive and visual outcomes in a FDA registration trial [8], in 2013, the Trulign toric IOL became the first premium presbyopia-correcting toric IOL available for use in the United States.

The objective of this study was to evaluate the efficacy and safety of the Trulign toric IOL in astigmatic cataract patients implanted with the IOL in a standard of care, clinical practice setting.

2. Materials and Methods

2.1. Patients. This retrospective, noncomparative study involved patients who underwent phacoemulsification and implantation of the Trulign toric IOL in one or both eyes at The Eye Center of Columbus (Columbus, OH, USA) between August 2013 and October 2014. The study was approved by the Mount Carmel Institutional Review Board and was conducted in accordance with the tenets of the Declaration of Helsinki. All patients provided informed consent before undergoing surgery.

The inclusion criteria included patients who underwent phacoemulsification and implantation of the Trulign toric IOL; use of the intraoperative wavefront aberrometer (ORA System; WaveTec Vision, Alcon, Aliso Viejo, CA, USA) was required. Eyes that underwent procedures concomitant with the phacoemulsification and lens implantation were excluded.

2.2. Intraocular Lens. The Trulign toric IOL (model BL1UT, Bausch + Lomb) is a silicone multipiece IOL that is a toric modification of the Crystalens accommodative IOL; the only differences are that the posterior surface of the optic is toric, and the anterior surface of the optic has two marks that indicate the flat meridian of the lens and aid in alignment. The plate haptics are hinged adjacent to the optic and have small polyimide loop haptics. The overall diameter of the IOL is 11.5 mm and the optic diameter is 5.0 mm. The toric presbyopia-correcting IOL is available in spherical equivalent (SE) powers ranging from +10.00 to +33.00 D in 0.50 D increments, with cylindrical powers of 1.25 D, 2.00 D, and 2.75 D at the lens plane (estimated cylindrical powers of 0.83 D, 1.33 D, and 1.83 D, resp., at the corneal plane). The recommended starting A-constant is 119.1.

2.3. Preoperative Assessment. A comprehensive eye examination conducted preoperatively included a detailed history, slit-lamp biomicroscopy, and ophthalmoscopy. Patients were administered the validated Standard Patient Evaluation of Eye Dryness (SPEED) questionnaire [9] to screen for the presence of ocular surface disease, and patients with ocular surface disease began treatment tailored to the type and severity of dry eye. Dry eye treatments used most commonly were fish oil (reesterified omega-3 fatty acids), thermal pulsation, topical corticosteroid, topical cyclosporine, and punctal occlusion. Treatment was continued until the ocular surface was healthy enough to generate accurate measurements (on average, 4–6 weeks).

Keratometry, topography, axial length, and anterior chamber depth measurements were taken to determine the power of IOL to be implanted. If topography and keratometry measurements were not consistent, the surgery was delayed. The Trulign calculator [10] estimated the toric IOL cylinder power and lens axis orientation needed to best correct for the predicted corneal cylinder, based on keratometry, the incision location, and a predicted magnitude of surgically induced astigmatism (SIA) of 0.30 diopters.

2.4. Surgical Technique. All surgeries were performed by one surgeon (Alice T. Epitropoulos) under topical anesthesia using standard phacoemulsification technique. Cardinal reference marks to help with axis of lens placement were made preoperatively on the limbus at 12, 3, 6, and 9 o'clock meridians of the cornea. A Mastel marker (Mastel Precision Surgical Instruments, Inc., Rapid City, SD) was used to mark the steep axis of astigmatism as determined by preoperative testing. A 2.8 mm clear corneal, three-plane incision was created temporally at 10° in left eyes and 190° in right eyes. A cohesive ophthalmic viscoelastic device (OVD) (ProVisc; Alcon, Fort Worth, TX, USA) was injected into the anterior chamber, and a round anterior continuous curvilinear capsulorhexis of 5.2–5.5 mm was created manually around the visual axis with Utrata forceps. Coaxial phacoemulsification and extraction of the cataract was performed using an Alcon Infiniti phacoemulsification unit (Alcon, Fort Worth, TX, USA). Meticulous cortical cleanup was followed by polishing of the anterior and posterior capsule using the Whitman/Shephard Capsule Polisher (Bausch + Lomb). Intraoperative wavefront aberrometry was used in all surgeries to corroborate the preoperative assessments of sphere and cylinder in the aphakic eye, and also to confirm correct alignment of the axis of the IOL. When the recommendation of ORA differed from that of preoperative measurements and the Trulign calculator, we decided which recommendation to follow on a case-by-case basis. Most often when there was a discrepancy, we used a compromise halfway between the differing recommendations.

The presbyopia-correcting toric IOL was placed in the capsular bag, spun to ensure that the haptics were at the equator, and then rotated to obtain correct alignment relative to the markings on the cornea and the steep axis of astigmatism. A posttoric measurement was taken using the intraoperative aberrometer to evaluate and aid in the final placement of the toric IOL. After the toric lens placement was confirmed and finalized, all OVD was removed from the eye including behind the IOL. We confirmed that the Trulign IOL was vaulted posteriorly in the capsule, and the toric alignment was once again verified. The wound was tested for integrity and if not watertight, the incision was closed with either a suture or sealant (ReSure; Ocular Therapeutix, Inc., Bedford, MA).

2.5. Postoperative Assessment. All patients were followed for a minimum of 1 month after surgery. Preoperative and postoperative month 1 data were collected from patient charts for analysis. When available, data also were collected from follow-up at 3–13 months after surgery.

The main outcome measures included corneal and manifest refractive cylinder, refractive predictability, uncorrected distance visual acuity (UDVA), uncorrected intermediate visual acuity (UIVA) measured at 70–80 cm, uncorrected near visual acuity (UNVA) measured at 40 cm, IOL rotational stability, and safety parameters (adverse events, surgical complications, and best-corrected visual acuity (BCVA)). As part of the safety evaluation, patients were evaluated for visual disturbances, and all patients were asked specifically if they had any problems with night vision.

Rotational stability of the lens was evaluated at a slit-lamp (Haag-Streit, Mason, OH) that has degree marks labeled on the beam, which allows measurement of the toric IOL axis when the slit beam is aligned with the toric IOL axis markings in a dilated eye [11].

3. Results

This case series included 40 eyes in 31 patients. The mean (± standard deviation, SD) age of the patients was 71.2 ± 5.2 years (range: 57–80). Thirteen patients (41.9%) were male and 18 (58.1%) female. Five eyes were post-LASIK, 2 eyes had a history of epiretinal membrane, 2 eyes had mild irregular astigmatism that was not felt to be associated with substantial visual disturbance, and 1 eye had a history of macular pucker and trans-pars plana vitrectomy. The surgeon considered all eyes to have potential for 20/32 or better BCVA. Mean preoperative K cylinder was 1.77 D (range from 0.63 to 2.77 D). Mean preoperative manifest refraction spherical equivalent (MRSE) was −1.01 D (range from −6.25 to 3.13 D). Mean axial length was 24.4 mm (range from 22 to 27 mm). All eyes were implanted with the toric presbyopia-correcting IOL during routine cataract surgery.

The mean target MRSE for operated eyes was −0.30 D (range, plano to −0.64 D). The target MRSE was between plano and −0.30 in 55% of eyes and between plano and −0.50 D in 87.5% of eyes. Intraoperative aberrometry results affected the selection of the spherical or cylindrical power of IOL used, or the alignment of the lens, in approximately half of the eyes. There were no intraoperative surgical complications.

3.1. Refractive Outcomes.
At postoperative month 1, mean MRSE was −0.12 D. Mean (± SD) corneal cylinder was 1.52 ± 0.60 D, and mean refractive cylinder was 0.17 ± 0.23 D. At each lens cylinder power (1.25, 2.00, and 2.75 D), the toric lens effectively neutralized the effects of corneal cylinder on postoperative refraction (Figure 1). Refractive cylinder at postoperative month 1 was ≤0.5 D in 97.5% (39/40) of eyes and ≤1.00 D in all 40 eyes (Figure 2).

The IOL demonstrated good refractive predictability (Figure 3). At postoperative month 1, MRSE was within 0.50 D of the target MRSE in 82.5% (33/40) of eyes and within 1.00 D of the target MRSE in 95% (38/40) of eyes. In the 15 eyes with longer-term follow-up, MRSE was within 0.50 D of the target MRSE in 80% (12/15) of eyes and within 1.00 D of the target MRSE in 86.7% (13/15) of eyes at 3–13 months after surgery.

3.2. Visual Outcomes.
At postoperative month 1, UDVA was 20/20 or better in 75% (30/40) of eyes and 20/25 or better in 95% (38/40) of eyes (Figure 4). UDVA in the remaining 2 eyes was worse than 20/40. One of these eyes had a MRSE of −1.50 D, and UDVA was 20/70; however, the patient

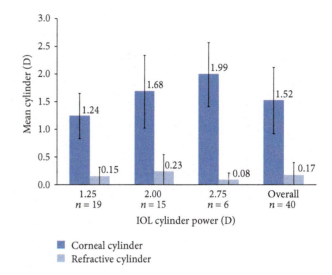

Figure 1: Mean corneal and refractive cylinder at postoperative month 1.

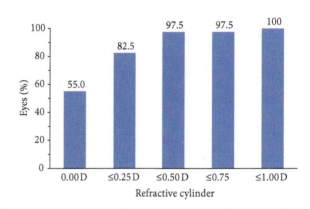

Figure 2: Frequency distribution of residual refractive cylinder at postoperative month 1.

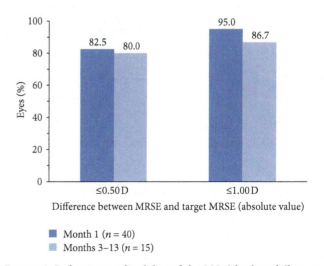

Figure 3: Refractive predictability of the IOL (absolute difference between MRSE and target MRSE). IOL: intraocular lens; MRSE: manifest refraction spherical equivalent.

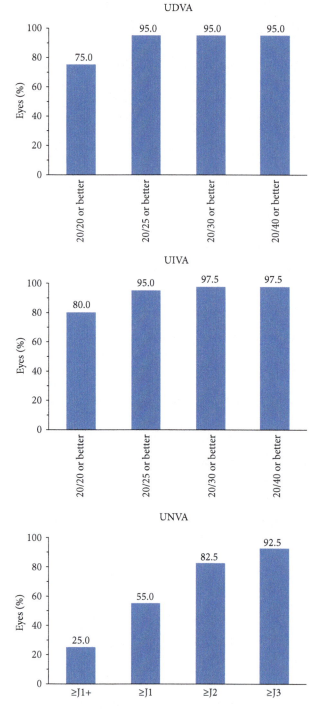

FIGURE 4: Uncorrected distance, intermediate, and near visual acuity (UDVA, UIVA, and UNVA) at postoperative month 1.

enjoyed her excellent uncorrected reading vision. Her UIVA was 20/16, and UNVA was 20/20. The other patient had unexpected hyperopia (MRSE was +1.38 D). Both patients were offered an IOL exchange but were satisfied with using glasses and declined the lens exchange.

Intermediate visual acuity results were exceptional. At postoperative month 1, UIVA was 20/20 or better in 80% (32/40) of eyes, 20/25 or better in 95% (38/40) of eyes, and 20/40 or better in 97.5% (39/40) of eyes (Figure 4). Near visual acuity results were also favorable. Overall, 92.5% (37/40) of all eyes had UNVA of J3 or better at postoperative month 1 (Figure 4), and UNVA in the remaining 3 eyes was J5.

Quality of vision was excellent in all eyes. There were no complaints of glare, halos, problems with night vision, or other visual disturbances.

3.3. Rotational Stability. At the postoperative month 1 evaluation, lens rotation was <5° in all eyes.

3.4. Safety. There were no unexpected adverse events related to the procedure or lens. One eye with a history of epiretinal membrane developed early capsular fibrosis that required Nd:YAG laser capsulotomy. Another eye with a history of irregular astigmatism had residual refractive cylinder noted at postoperative day 7. The lens was in the original position where we placed it (it had not rotated). Using the Berdahl & Hardten Toric IOL Calculator [12], we determined that the lens needed to be rotated from 95 to 120 degrees to better neutralize the cylinder. We performed a secondary surgical intervention rotating the lens 25°. MRSE was plano and UDVA was 20/20 in the eye at postoperative month 1.

BCVA was 20/20 or better in 92.5% (37/40) of eyes and 20/25 or better in all 40 eyes at postoperative month 1.

4. Discussion

The presbyopia-correcting, toric IOL demonstrated excellent refractive predictability in this study. The IOL effectively neutralized the postoperative corneal cylinder, with mean postoperative refractive cylinder reduced to near zero. Visual outcomes were favorable. The targeted MRSE of plano to −0.64 D helped to achieve acceptable near vision without compromising distance vision. Uncorrected distance and intermediate visual acuity and quality of vision were excellent.

The results of this study are consistent with the favorable safety and efficacy outcomes demonstrated in the FDA registration trial of the lens [8]. The inclusion and exclusion criteria for this study were chosen to have a study population somewhat similar to the study population in the FDA trial yet still reflect real-world clinical practice. The mean age of patients in this study was similar to that in the registration trial, but the ophthalmic histories of patients in this study were more complicated, reflecting real-world clinical practice. Altogether, 25% of eyes in this study would have been excluded from the registration trial because of irregular corneal astigmatism (the toric IOL is recommended for use in patients with regular astigmatism only), previous refractive surgery, macular pathology, and previous vitrectomy. Although eyes with these characteristics are generally not considered to be candidates for a premium lens, in our experience, the toric lens can be used successfully in such eyes when patients are appropriately counseled and have realistic expectations.

Despite the inclusion of eyes that would not have been eligible for a multifocal lens, the refractive and visual outcomes in this study were outstanding. The mean residual refractive cylinder at postoperative month 1 was 0.17 D in this series, compared with a postoperative month 4–6 mean residual cylinder value of 0.43 D (all toric IOL powers) in the registration trial [13]. The residual refractive cylinder was ≤0.50 D for 97.5% of eyes in this study, and 55% of eyes had complete resolution of astigmatism, compared with 70.9% of eyes with residual refractive cylinder ≤0.50 D and 34.3% of eyes with complete resolution of astigmatism in the registration trial [8]. The refractive predictability of the lens was outstanding in both studies. Postoperative MRSE was within 0.50 D of the target in 82.5% of eyes in this study and 73.7% of eyes in the FDA registration trial [13].

In this case series, 95% of eyes achieved 20/25 or better UDVA and 95% achieved 20/25 or better UIVA, compared with 72.4% and 86.6%, respectively, in the registration trial [8]. Quality outcomes were particularly evident in assessments of near vision. In this case series, 55% of eyes achieved UNVA of ≥J1 (20/25 Snellen equivalent) and 92.5% achieved UNVA of ≥J3 (20/40 Snellen equivalent). In the registration trial, 17.9% of eyes achieved UNVA of 20/25 (J1) or better, and 70.1% achieved UNVA of 20/40 (J3) or better [8].

Outcomes in this case series met or surpassed those in the registration trial in all categories, and UNVA was improved without compromising distance vision. To some degree, this is expected because of the greater variability of target MRSE used. The outstanding UDVA, UIVA, and UNVA outcomes in this case series might also be explained in part by the emphasis we placed on obtaining reliable biometry and topography measurements. Ocular surface disease was treated preoperatively to maximize the accuracy of the preoperative measurements, and, in a few patients, surgery was delayed due to inconsistent measurements. Also, intraoperative wavefront aberrometry was used in all surgeries for corroboration of preoperative measurements. When there was a discrepancy between preoperative and ORA calculations, the surgeon determined which calculations to use, and use of the ORA calculations did not necessarily always result in better outcomes. Nonetheless, use of intraoperative wavefront aberrometry influenced the choice of lens power or axis placement in approximately half of the cases and may have improved our outcomes overall.

Lens positioning and rotational stability is crucial because even small errors in positioning or rotation have the potential to affect the uncorrected visual acuity. The rotational stability of the toric lens was excellent in this case series, as well as in the registration trial. The FDA trial utilized photographs to evaluate for rotational stability. In the FDA registration trial, 96.1% of the implants rotated less than 5 degrees from implantation to 4–6 months postoperatively [8]. The polyimide loop haptics allow for excellent rotational stability with this IOL platform. Meticulous cortical cleanup is critical in preventing capsular fibrosis. Rigorous polishing of the anterior and posterior capsule removes the stimulus for the anterior capsule to fibrose and contract, minimizing the potential for the lens to move or tilt. We recommend early Nd:YAG laser capsulotomy for capsular fibrosis that develops, because asymmetric fibrosis can shift the lens in an asymmetric manner.

The toric IOL, built on the accommodative Crystalens IOL platform, provided excellent visual quality in this case series. The aspheric optics of the parent lens have been associated with excellent quality of vision, including better contrast sensitivity and fewer problems with glare and halos, compared with multifocal lenses [14]. Because multifocal IOLs are often associated with loss of contrast sensitivity [15], they may not perform as well at night and should not be implanted in patients with macular pathology [3]. Unfortunately, it is difficult to predict whether a patient will develop macular pathology. An accommodative IOL can be used for patients with macular pathology, and the toric IOL can be used in patients with preoperative corneal astigmatism who desire an excellent range of vision. It is also an ideal lens for cataract patients with preoperative corneal astigmatism and a monofocal lens in the contralateral eye, who desire a broader range of vision.

A limitation of this study is the lack of a control group, which is a common limitation in a retrospective case series study design. Multifocal toric IOLs are not yet available for use in the United States, but future prospective studies should evaluate the Trulign toric IOL compared with a multifocal toric IOL in patients with preoperative corneal astigmatism who desire a range in vision and would accept either the Trulign toric or a multifocal toric IOL.

5. Conclusions

The availability of a premium presbyopia-correcting IOL that offers toric correction is an important advancement in patient care. In this case series, the novel toric IOL provided excellent UDVA and UIVA and functional UNVA. The lens effectively and predictably reduced refractive astigmatism and demonstrated excellent rotational stability, and no patient had visual disturbances. Use of this presbyopia-correcting toric IOL can provide excellent refractive and visual outcomes in a standard of care, clinical practice setting. This toric IOL is an excellent option for astigmatic patients undergoing cataract surgery who desire a wide range of vision along with quality night vision.

Disclosure

Alice T. Epitropoulos is a consultant to Bausch + Lomb and has received research support from Bausch + Lomb. This research was presented in part at the American Society of Cataract & Refractive Surgery (ASCRS) Annual Meeting, April 17–21, 2015, San Diego, CA, USA.

Conflict of Interests

The author declares no financial or proprietary interest in any material or method mentioned.

Acknowledgment

This research was supported by an investigator-initiated grant from Bausch + Lomb.

References

[1] T. Ferrer-Blasco, R. Montés-Micó, S. C. Peixoto-de-Matos, J. M. González-Méijome, and A. Cerviño, "Prevalence of corneal astigmatism before cataract surgery," *Journal of Cataract and Refractive Surgery*, vol. 35, no. 1, pp. 70–75, 2009.

[2] X. Yuan, H. Song, G. Peng, X. Hua, and X. Tang, "Prevalence of corneal astigmatism in patients before cataract surgery in Northern China," *Journal of Ophthalmology*, vol. 2014, Article ID 536412, 7 pages, 2014.

[3] B. V. Ventura, L. Wang, M. P. Weikert, S. B. Robinson, and D. D. Koch, "Surgical management of astigmatism with toric intraocular lenses," *Arquivos Brasileiros de Oftalmologia*, vol. 77, no. 2, pp. 125–131, 2014.

[4] N. Garzón, F. Poyales, B. O. de Zárate, J. L. Ruiz-García, and J. A. Quiroga, "Evaluation of rotation and visual outcomes after implantation of monofocal and multifocal toric intraocular lenses," *Journal of Refractive Surgery*, vol. 31, no. 2, pp. 90–97, 2015.

[5] D. K. Lam, V. W. Chow, C. Ye, P. K.-F. Ng, Z. Wang, and V. Jhanji, "Comparative evaluation of aspheric toric intraocular lens implantation and limbal relaxing incisions in eyes with cataracts and ≤3 dioptres of astigmatism," *British Journal of Ophthalmology*, 2015.

[6] J. S. Pepose, D. Wang, and G. E. Altmann, "Comparison of through-focus image quality across five presbyopia-correcting intraocular lenses (an American Ophthalmological Society thesis," *Transactions of the American Ophthalmological Society*, vol. 109, pp. 221–231, 2011.

[7] M. J. Kim, L. Zheleznyak, S. MacRae, H. Tchah, and G. Yoon, "Objective evaluation of through-focus optical performance of presbyopia-correcting intraocular lenses using an optical bench system," *Journal of Cataract and Refractive Surgery*, vol. 37, no. 7, pp. 1305–1312, 2011.

[8] J. S. Pepose, J. Hayashida, J. Hovanesian et al., "Safety and effectiveness of a new toric presbyopia-correcting posterior chamber silicone intraocular lens," *Journal of Cataract and Refractive Surgery*, vol. 41, no. 2, pp. 295–305, 2015.

[9] W. Ngo, P. Situ, N. Keir, D. Korb, C. Blackie, and T. Simpson, "Psychometric properties and validation of the standard patient evaluation of eye dryness questionnaire," *Cornea*, vol. 32, no. 9, pp. 1204–1210, 2013.

[10] Toric calculator, July 2015, http://trulign.com/professionals/en-us/toriccalculator.aspx.

[11] V. E. George and D. S. George, "Axis measurement strip for Haag-Streit BM900 series slitlamp," *Journal of Cataract and Refractive Surgery*, vol. 40, no. 10, pp. 1584–1587, 2014.

[12] "Toric Results Analyzer," http://astigmatismfix.com.

[13] J. Hayashida, "Effectiveness Endpoints. Trulign Toric Accommodating Intraocular Lens. US FDA Ophthalmic Devices Advisory Committee Meeting Sponsor Presentation. 08 April 2013," http://www.fda.gov/AdvisoryCommittees/ucm340995.htm.

[14] R. Ang, G. Martinez, E. Cruz, A. Tiongson, and A. Dela Cruz, "Prospective evaluation of visual outcomes with three presbyopia-correcting intraocular lenses following cataract surgery," *Clinical Ophthalmology*, vol. 7, pp. 1811–1823, 2013.

[15] D. Calladine, J. R. Evans, S. Shah, and M. Leyland, "Multifocal versus monofocal intraocular lenses after cataract extraction," *Cochrane Database of Systematic Reviews*, vol. 9, Article ID CD003169, 2012.

A Head-Mounted Spectacle Frame for the Study of Mouse Lens-Induced Myopia

Yangshun Gu,[1] Baisheng Xu,[1] Chunfei Feng,[2] Yang Ni,[3] Qin Wu,[1] Chixin Du,[1] Nan Hong,[1] Peng Li,[3] Zhihua Ding,[3] and Bo Jiang[1]

[1]Department of Ophthalmology, First Affiliated Hospital, College of Medicine, Zhejiang University, Hangzhou, Zhejiang 310003, China
[2]Department of Operation Room, First Affiliated Hospital, College of Medicine, Zhejiang University, Hangzhou, Zhejiang 310003, China
[3]State Key Lab of Modern Optical Instrumentation, Department of Optical Engineering, Zhejiang University, Hangzhou, Zhejiang 310027, China

Correspondence should be addressed to Bo Jiang; drjiangbo@hotmail.com

Academic Editor: Terri L. Young

The mouse model has been widely employed to explore the mysteries of myopia. For now, existing techniques for induction of experimental myopia in mice can be classified into three types: (1) devices directly glued to the fur; (2) devices attached using a combination of glue and sutures; (3) devices attached using a skull-mounted apparatus. These techniques each have its advantages, disadvantages when considering the devices stability, safety, complexity, effectiveness, and so forth. Thus, techniques for myopia induction in mice have yet to be further refined to popularize the applications. In this pilot study, we introduce a new head fixation device named the head-mounted spectacle frame apparatus for the study of mouse lens-induced myopia. Surgical procedures for device attachment were relatively simple and easy to learn in our study. Effective myopia induction was validated by retinoscopy refraction and axial length measurement using optical coherence tomography. In addition, it showed improved compliance and reliable safety when compared to the published methods. The head-mounted spectacle frame apparatus provides a new choice for the study of lens-induced myopia in mouse. It also allows for the use of form deprivation, making it attractive for future experimental mouse myopia trials.

1. Introduction

For the past half century, myopia has emerged as an extremely important health issue and the related literature has increased exponentially [1, 2]. And epidemiological data suggested that the prevalence and incidence of myopia were increasingly high, causing serious social and economic burdens [3]. So both scientists and ophthalmologists showed great interest and applied significant effort to elucidate the mechanism of myopia development.

As an important component in the field of myopia research, animal model has greatly expanded our knowledge on the visual regulation of refractive development [4, 5]. These animal models such as monkeys, chicks, tree shrews, fish, and guinea pigs each have its advantages and disadvantages [6–8]. However, presently consensus has not been established yet regarding which model is ideal. Recently, the establishment of mouse model of myopia has contributed to a recent surge in interest and revealed several essential findings [9–11]. The mouse model offers a highly efficient model in which to study the genetic and environmental basis of the growth of the eye, as well as gene-environment interactions [12–14]. Nevertheless, available techniques for device attachment in mice are limited. In methods using sutures, glue, or a combination of techniques, the goggle or defocusing lens may be easily scratched off and lead to poor ocular health [11, 15, 16]. Other researchers introduced an Elizabethan collar to avoid troublesome scratches, but

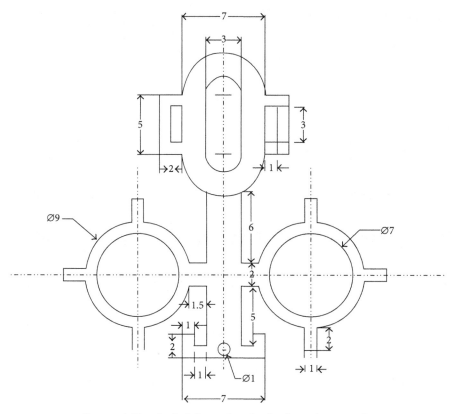

FIGURE 1: The physical dimensions for the frame (unit: mm).

the collar may seriously impact the animal's activity and systemic health [11, 17]. The head-mounted goggle apparatus was reported to be highly stable and efficient. However, the components of goggle apparatus were not convenient fabrication and the surgical procedures were complicated [18].

Then, the purpose of this study is to introduce a simple head fixation device for myopia induction in mice that (1) can be attached with simplified procedures, (2) should keep stable for a certain period of time, (3) effectively induce experimental myopia, and (4) is reliably secured to the eye and whole health.

2. Materials and Methods

2.1. Design of the Head Fixation Device. The head fixation device is composed of two parts, the nylon connector and the metal spectacle frame. The nylon connector, including M3 × 8 nylon screws, gaskets, and caps, was designed and produced (Shanghai Zhisheng Plastic Co., Ltd.). The spectacle frames were first designed using Rhinoceros software (Version 5.0, Robert McNeel & Associates; Figure 1) and then were made of 304 stainless steel by laser cutting (Versolsolar Hangzhou Co., Ltd.). A single spectacle frame has four functional components including the (1) kidney-shaped slotted hole for position control, (2) rounded lens clip for experimental lens fixation, (3) nose pad for strengthening fixation, and (4) connecting rod for integration. The spectacle frames underwent manual shaping to be attached to the mouse head; the physical dimensions and a computer representation of the 3D shape for the frame are shown in Figures 1 and 2.

2.2. Surgical Procedures

(1) The mice were anesthetized by intraperitoneal injection of 4% chloral hydrate (10 mg/kg, Figure 3(a)).

(2) The dorsal cranial fur was shaven; the surgical area was cleaned with Betadine (Figure 3(b)).

(3) A middle line incision (8–10 mm) was made to expose the dorsal cranial surface of the skull.

(4) The exposed fascia and periosteum were removed from the coronal suture to the sagittal suture, and the surface was cleaned and dried (Figure 3(c)).

(5) The screw was sutured to the bilateral temporal muscle, cervical trapezius muscle, and frontal skin with 6-0 nylon sutures (Figure 3(d)).

(6) The incision was sutured with 6-0 nylon suture, and antibiotic ointments were applied (Figure 3(e)).

(7) The gasket and screw were fixed to supply a platform supporting the spectacle frame (Figure 3(f)).

(8) The spectacle frame was placed on the head, and the cap was screwed in and adjusted to position the lens clip (Figure 3(g)).

(9) The fixation was strengthened by suturing the nose pad to the skin, and the experimental lenses were fixed (Figure 3(h)).

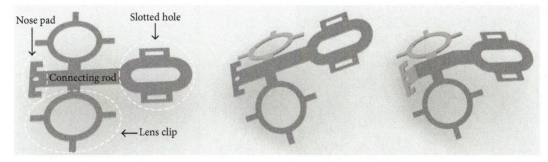

Figure 2: A schematic of the spectacle frame showing the functional components including the slotted hole, lens clip, nose pad, and connecting rod. And a brief visualization of the 3D shape is present.

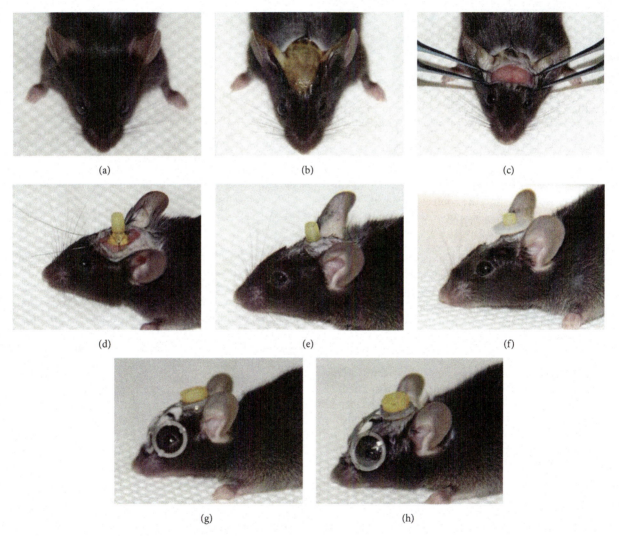

Figure 3: Simplified operation procedures of the head-mounted spectacle frame apparatus: (a) general anesthesia; (b) incision preparation; (c) exposure of the skull and muscle; (d) suturing the screw; (e) suturing the incision; (f) fixing the gasket; (g) fixing the spectacle frame; and (h) fixing the experimental lenses.

2.3. Experimental Design. Male C57BL6J mice aged postnatal 28 days (P28) underwent baseline retinoscopy refraction and axial length measurement using a custom-built optical coherence tomography (OCT), which has been detailed in [19, 20] (Figure 4). Two groups were set in the current study. In the experimental group ($n = 25$), myopia was monocularly induced with the head-mounted spectacle frame over the right eye using a −15.0 diopter (D) lens (Hangzhou Boston Optics Co., Ltd.); no defocusing lens or plano lens was fixed to the left lens clip. In the control group ($n = 10$), no

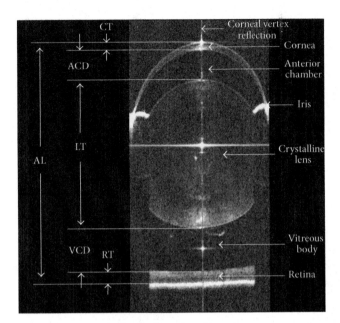

Figure 4: The schematic diagram of axial length measurement from the anterior corneal surface to the retinal pigment epithelium along the corneal vertex reflection.

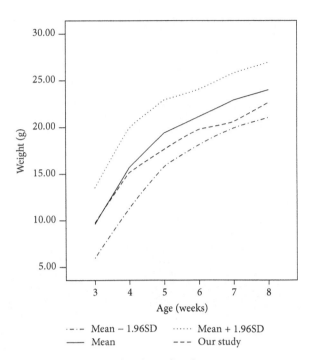

Figure 5: A body weight chart for the mice in experimental group. Reference values (mean, mean ± 1.96SD) were obtained from the JAX LAB (http://jaxmice.jax.org/support/weight/000664.html). The mean weight of mice in experimental group falls between the reference mean and mean − 1.96SD.

spectacle frame or lens was fixed. The experimental mice were housed in isolation, and the control mice were housed in groups of five. The body weight was measured weekly in experimental group from the time of purchase (P21) to the sacrifice date (P56). All mice were exposed to a 12 h light : 12 h dark cycle and checked daily for 28 days to assess the defocusing lens position stability. Then mice aged P56 were refracted and measured again to assess the effectiveness of myopia induction. In addition, a coronal segment of the tissue corresponding to the locations of the underlying screws was serially sectioned and H&E stained.

2.4. Ethics Statement. This study was approved by the Institutional Animal Care and Use Committee (IACUC) at Zhejiang University (Permit number: Zju201306-1-01-066). All experimental procedures were conducted in accordance with the Guidelines for the Care and Use of Laboratory Animals of Zhejiang University. All mice were sacrificed by an anesthetic overdose, and all efforts were made to minimize suffering.

3. Results

There were no intraoperative complications, and none of the animals experienced postoperative incision infection. The mice wearing head-mounted spectacle frames appeared to have normal activity and were well groomed and freely feeding (see video in Supplementary Material available online at http://dx.doi.org/10.1155/2016/8497278). Mice weights were monitored weekly, and weight gain of mice in experimental group was appropriate when compared with the reference values from the JAX LAB (Figure 5).

There were two situations to be noted in the assessment of device stability, a spectacle frame "lost" and an entire apparatus "lost." In these cases, the defocusing lens could flip away from the eye and allowed for some normal visual input, which required timely intervention. The "lost" of spectacle frame was always the result of a loosened screw cap or nose pad and could be retightened in minutes. An entire "lost" apparatus was usually caused by frequent scratching, tissue reaction, or accidental clamping with the cage, and the nylon connector and spectacle frame should be refixated under general anesthesia. In this study (Table 1), 2 cases of spectacle frame loss but no entire apparatus loss were found in the first week (P29–P35), 8 cases of spectacle frame loss and 2 cases of entire apparatus loss occurred in the second week (P36–P42), 12 cases of spectacle frame loss and 3 cases of entire apparatus loss occurred in the third week (P43–P49), and 13 cases of spectacle frame loss and 3 cases of entire apparatus loss occurred in the fourth week (P50–P56). With this technique, 9/30 mice lost the spectacle frame or entire apparatus once, 14/30 mice lost the spectacle frame or entire apparatus twice, and 2/30 lost the spectacle frame or entire apparatus three times during the 28 days induction period. In the first two weeks, no mice lost the spectacle frame or entire apparatus three or more times. Our apparatus stability was relatively superior to the way that directly glued to the fur and was essentially the same as the head-mounted goggling apparatus reported by Faulkner et al. [18] (Table 2).

Refractive error data in Table 3 demonstrated no significant difference between the right and left eyes in the experimental group at P28 (0.08 ± 1.26 D; paired t-test $p = 0.75$) or in the controls (0.70 ± 1.34 D; paired t-test $p = 0.13$).

TABLE 1: Stability assessment of the head-mounted spectacle frame apparatus.

Experimental duration	# times spectacle frame was lost	# times entire apparatus was lost	# times defocusing lens was lost[a]
First week	2	0	2
Second week	8	2	10
Third week	12	3	15
Fourth week	13	3	16
Total	35	8	43

[a]Times defocusing lens was lost indicate the total of times spectacle frame was lost and times entire apparatus was lost.

TABLE 2: A comparison of the reported apparatus stability and the head-mounted spectacle frame.

Compliance (# times defocusing lens was lost)	≤2	≥3
Our apparatus	30/30	0/30
Head-mounted goggling apparatus [18]	24/28	4/28
Glued to the fur [18]	13/30	17/30

Our apparatus versus the head-mounted goggling apparatus, Fisher's Exact Test, $p = 0.0482$.
Our apparatus versus the glued to the fur technique, Fisher's Exact Test, $p < 0.001$.

28 days later, the right eye of mice in experimental group showed a significant myopic shift compared to the left eye (-4.90 ± 2.17 D; paired t-test $p = 1.69 \times 10^{-9}$), but not found in the control group (-0.90 ± 1.37 D; paired t-test $p = 0.07$). The axial length measurements using OCT (Table 3) showed no significant difference between the right and left eyes in both experimental (0.004 ± 0.034 mm; paired t-test $p = 0.58$) and control group (0.004 ± 0.016 mm; paired t-test $p = 0.48$) at P28. After the induction period, the right eyes of mice in experimental group were significantly longer than the contralateral eyes (0.025 ± 0.037 mm; paired t-test $p = 0.002$), while no significant difference was found in the controls (-0.013 ± 0.031 mm; paired t-test $p = 0.22$).

Postmortem evaluation showed general reactive hyperplasia of the skin and no obvious alteration of the skull underlying the screws. Histological examination revealed chronic inflammation of the hypoderm due to the foreign body reaction in the H&E stained sections when compared with the normal controls, and the skull at the screw locations appeared healthy with no bony destruction (Figure 6).

4. Discussion

It is generally known that form deprivation and lens defocusing are the two classical methods for myopia induction in animal, and they were also reported to be used in the study of mouse myopia [9, 21]. No matter which method is chosen, existing techniques for device attachment can be shared. In this study, we used the lens-induced myopia model for the reason of renewed interest that myopia progression in humans and animals can be altered through optical intervention [5, 22].

A literature survey showed that Tejedor and de la Villa made the first attempts by lid-suturing to induce deprivation myopia in mouse; however, it was not suitable for defocusing lens attachment [15]. Later, Schaeffel et al. introduced the method that goggles directly glued to the fur around the eye, and it was improved by Barathi et al. to be used in lens-induced myopia [16, 17]. The method using glue was technically simple, but the device stability was not reliable enough and may lead to poor ocular health. Thus, Tkatchenko et al. reported a further refined technique, using a combination of glue and sutures [11]. Although the application of this method may not be restrained by mouse age and the effectiveness of myopia induction was reported to be good, no compliance data was shown. And our informal observations revealed that the stability has yet to be improved. Then some researchers used plastic collar to improve stability; however, it would inevitably affect the physical activity and whole health [11, 17]. Faulkner et al. developed a noncontact head-mounted goggle apparatus for the study of murine myopia [18]. It was reported to have satisfactory position stability and effective induction. However, the surgical procedures for the delicate device were quite complicated and time consuming and may lead to skull or brain injury. In addition, it was not suitable to be used in younger mouse with fragile skull, which may also make restriction on its popularity. Thus, it is still necessary to invent an easily operated, safe, and effective device for the myopia induction in mice.

Thus we developed the head-mounted spectacle frame and introduced a relatively easy-to-learn fixation method. Firstly, this device is lightweight (the nylon connector, spectacle frame, and defocusing lens amount to 0.50–0.60 grams) and could enhance the compliance of spectacle frame wearing. Comparing with the head-mounted goggle apparatus, our research results demonstrated at least evenly matched position stability. In our study, there were still situations that indicated that the defocusing lens was not permanently fixed, and the ability to maintain device stability tended to decrease with extended induction time. Therefore, it was of great importance to tighten the screws when operating and to check the fitting situation carefully during the experimental period. Secondly, our device showed satisfactory safety. The body weight gradually increased during the experimental period, with no obvious difference with the reference values. With sutures fixation but not skull implantation, there were only chronic subdermal inflammations found at the screw locations, but no pathological change in the skull or adjacent brain. Thirdly, and perhaps most importantly, our device and method induced myopic shift and axial elongation in the experimental eyes. Literatures have shown that a -10 D lens fitted over the mouse eye could induce a refractive shift of -13.03 D in 46 days (P10–P56) under a 12 : 12 h light : dark cycle [16], and a -25 lens induced a 14.6 D myopic shift in 21 days (P24–P45) under constant light [11]. In this study, the myopic shift of 4.90 D in 28 days (P29–P56) is relatively small and is approximately equal to that reported by Faulkner et al. using a head-mounted goggling apparatus (5.66 D myopic shift in 14 days of form deprivation) [18]. Many

Table 3: Results of retinoscopy refraction and axial length measurements.

	Age	Relative refraction (diopters)		Axial length (mm)	
		OD-OS	p value*	OD-OS	p value*
Experimental group	P28	0.08 ± 1.26	0.753	0.004 ± 0.034	0.577
	P56	−4.90 ± 2.17	1.69×10^{-9}	0.025 ± 0.037	0.002
Control group	P28	0.70 ± 1.34	0.132	0.004 ± 0.016	0.482
	P56	−0.90 ± 1.37	0.068	−0.013 ± 0.031	0.220

Experimental group: $n = 25$; control group: $n = 10$.
OD-OS: values indicated the difference between the right and left eyes.
*Student's paired t-test.

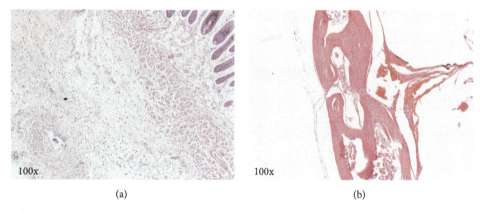

Figure 6: H&E stained sections of the skin (a) and the skull (b) at the screw sites. Note the reactive hyperplasia of the subcutaneous tissue, and the absence of a glaucomatous reaction or destructive changes to the skull.

explanations may contribute to the reduced effectiveness, such as species variability of the mice, a later induction initiation, or others. In any case, the head-mounted spectacle frame apparatus is reliable and practicable. In addition, our device is economical and the surgical procedures are easy to learn, for only requiring commonly used microscopic suture materials but not professional equipment. This is also a beneficial aspect of our device and method in consideration of the popularization.

Some limitations should be considered in the current study. First, the physical dimensions of the one-piece frame were fixed in this study, which may not be compatible with mouse younger than P28. Thus frames with optimized physical dimensions adapting to younger mice during the susceptible period for myopia induction could substantially increase a future use of this device. Second, the introduced method is a rather invasive procedure, which requires recovery and infection and pain management. Thus design of inflammation and pain management may be necessary in further study. Third, although other reported methods and procedures were not easy to duplicate, it was still of significance to make comparison between these methods and our method at the same time, including effectiveness, security. And experiments along these lines are currently in progress in our laboratory.

In summary, we described a novel apparatus named the head-mounted spectacle frame apparatus and represented a simplification of the currently employed head fixation techniques for study of myopia in mouse. Our results demonstrated several advantages, including the improved compliance, effective myopia induction, and reliable security. The new method also has the potential to test form deprivation myopia. All of these features would likely prove useful in small animal models among investigators studying experimental myopia trials.

Conflict of Interests

The authors declare that there is no conflict of interests regarding the publication of this paper.

Authors' Contribution

Yangshun Gu, Baisheng Xu, and Bo Jiang conceived and designed the experiments. Yangshun Gu, Baisheng Xu, Chunfei Feng, Qin Wu, Yang Ni, and Bo Jiang performed the experiments. Yangshun Gu, Baisheng Xu, Chunfei Feng, Nan Hong, and Bo Jiang analyzed the data. Qin Wu, Yang Ni, Chixin Du, Peng Li, and Zhihua Ding contributed reagents/materials/analysis tools. Yangshun Gu, Baisheng Xu, and Bo Jiang wrote the paper. Yang Ni, Chixin Du, Peng Li, and Zhihua Ding designed the software used in OCT imaging analysis.

Acknowledgments

This work was supported by the National Natural Science Foundation of China (Grant nos. 81200717, 61475143, and

61335003); the Specialized Research Fund for the Doctoral Program of Higher Education (Grant no. 20120101120027); Zhejiang Provincial Natural Science Foundation of China (LY14F050007). The authors are grateful to Jianxin Wang (Versolsolar Hangzhou Co., Ltd.) for advice and technical assistance on the design of head-mounted spectacle frame apparatus.

References

[1] I. G. Morgan, K. Ohno-Matsui, and S.-M. Saw, "Myopia," *The Lancet*, vol. 379, no. 9827, pp. 1739–1748, 2012.

[2] C.-T. Xu, S.-Q. Li, Y.-G. Lü, and B.-R. Pan, "Development of biomedical publications on ametropia research in PubMed from 1845 to 2010: a bibliometric analysis," *International Journal of Ophthalmology*, vol. 4, no. 1, pp. 1–7, 2011.

[3] T. R. Fricke, B. A. Holden, D. A. Wilson et al., "Global cost of correcting vision impairment from uncorrected refractive error," *Bulletin of the World Health Organization*, vol. 90, no. 10, pp. 728–738, 2012.

[4] W. N. Charman, "Myopia revisited, 2010–2015," *Ophthalmic and Physiological Optics*, vol. 35, no. 6, pp. 637–642, 2015.

[5] E. L. Smith III, L.-F. Hung, and B. Arumugam, "Visual regulation of refractive development: insights from animal studies," *Eye*, vol. 28, no. 2, pp. 180–188, 2014.

[6] M. H. Edwards, "Animal models of myopia. A review," *Acta Ophthalmologica Scandinavica*, vol. 74, no. 3, pp. 213–219, 1996.

[7] X. T. Zhou and J. Qu, "Selection of animal model in myopia research," *Zhonghua Yan Ke Za Zhi*, vol. 41, no. 6, pp. 486–487, 2005.

[8] W. Shen, M. Vijayan, and J. G. Sivak, "Inducing form-deprivation myopia in fish," *Investigative Ophthalmology and Visual Science*, vol. 46, no. 5, pp. 1797–1803, 2005.

[9] M. T. Pardue, R. A. Stone, and P. M. Iuvone, "Investigating mechanisms of myopia in mice," *Experimental Eye Research*, vol. 114, pp. 96–105, 2013.

[10] X. T. Zhou, J. Qu, and F. Lu, "Dose the mice is ideal animal myopia model?" *Zhonghua Yan Ke Za Zhi*, vol. 44, no. 7, pp. 584–586, 2008.

[11] T. V. Tkatchenko, Y. Shen, and A. V. Tkatchenko, "Mouse experimental myopia has features of primate myopia," *Investigative Ophthalmology and Visual Science*, vol. 51, no. 3, pp. 1297–1303, 2010.

[12] H. Park, C. C. Tan, A. Faulkner et al., "Retinal degeneration increases susceptibility to myopia in mice," *Molecular Vision*, vol. 19, pp. 2068–2079, 2013.

[13] R. Chakraborty, H. n. Park, A. M. Hanif, C. S. Sidhu, P. M. Iuvone, and M. T. Pardue, "ON pathway mutations increase susceptibility to form-deprivation myopia," *Experimental Eye Research*, vol. 137, pp. 79–83, 2015.

[14] M. T. Pardue, A. E. Faulkner, A. Fernandes et al., "High susceptibility to experimental myopia in a mouse model with a retinal on pathway defect," *Investigative Ophthalmology and Visual Science*, vol. 49, no. 2, pp. 706–712, 2008.

[15] J. Tejedor and P. de la Villa, "Refractive changes induced by form deprivation in the mouse eye," *Investigative Ophthalmology and Visual Science*, vol. 44, no. 1, pp. 32–36, 2003.

[16] V. A. Barathi, V. G. Boopathi, E. P. H. Yap, and R. W. Beuerman, "Two models of experimental myopia in the mouse," *Vision Research*, vol. 48, no. 7, pp. 904–916, 2008.

[17] F. Schaeffel, E. Burkhardt, H. C. Howland, and R. W. Williams, "Measurement of refractive state and deprivation myopia in two strains of mice," *Optometry and Vision Science*, vol. 81, no. 2, pp. 99–110, 2004.

[18] A. E. Faulkner, M. K. Kim, P. M. Iuvone, and M. T. Pardue, "Head-mounted goggles for murine form deprivation myopia," *Journal of Neuroscience Methods*, vol. 161, no. 1, pp. 96–100, 2007.

[19] Y. Ni, B. Xu, L. Wu et al., "Assessment of full-eye response to osmotic stress in mouse model in vivo using optical coherence tomography," *Journal of Ophthalmology*, vol. 2015, Article ID 568509, 8 pages, 2015.

[20] P. Li, Z. Ding, Y. Ni et al., "Visualization of the ocular pulse in the anterior chamber of the mouse eye *in vivo* using phase-sensitive optical coherence tomography," *Journal of Biomedical Optics*, vol. 19, no. 9, Article ID 090502, 2014.

[21] I. G. Morgan, R. S. Ashby, and D. L. Nickla, "Form deprivation and lens-induced myopia: are they different?" *Ophthalmic and Physiological Optics*, vol. 33, no. 3, pp. 355–361, 2013.

[22] P. R. Sankaridurg and B. A. Holden, "Practical applications to modify and control the development of ametropia," *Eye*, vol. 28, no. 2, pp. 134–141, 2014.

Apelin Protects Primary Rat Retinal Pericytes from Chemical Hypoxia-Induced Apoptosis

Li Chen,[1,2] Yong Tao,[1,2] Jing Feng,[1,2] and Yan Rong Jiang[1,2]

[1]Department of Ophthalmology, People's Hospital, Peking University, 11 Xizhimen South Street, Xicheng District, Beijing 100044, China
[2]Key Laboratory of Vision Loss and Restoration, Beijing Key Laboratory of Diagnosis and Therapy of Retinal and Choroid Diseases, Ministry of Education, 11 Xizhimen South Street, Xicheng District, Beijing 100044, China

Correspondence should be addressed to Yan Rong Jiang; drjyr@gmail.com

Academic Editor: Juliana L. Dreyfuss

Pericytes are a population of cells that participate in normal vessel architecture and regulate permeability. Apelin, as the endogenous ligand of G protein-coupled receptor APJ, participates in a number of physiological and pathological processes. To date, the effect of apelin on pericyte is not clear. Our study aimed to investigate the potential protection mechanisms of apelin, with regard to primary rat retinal pericytes under hypoxia. Immunofluorescence staining revealed that pericytes colocalized with APJ in the fibrovascular membranes dissected from proliferative diabetic retinopathy patients. In the *in vitro* studies, we first demonstrated that the expression of apelin/APJ was upregulated in pericytes under hypoxia, and apelin increased pericytes proliferation and migration. Moreover, knockdown of apelin in pericyte was achieved via lentivirus-mediated RNA interference. After the inhibition of apelin, pericytes proliferation was inhibited significantly in hypoxia culture condition. Furthermore, exogenous recombinant apelin effectively prevented hypoxia-induced apoptosis through downregulating active-caspase 3 expression and increasing the ratio of B cell lymphoma-2 (Bcl-2)/Bcl-2 associated X protein (Bax) in pericytes. These results suggest that apelin suppressed hypoxia-induced pericytes injury, which indicated that apelin could be a potential therapeutic target for retinal angiogenic diseases.

1. Introduction

Pericytes are a population of contractile cells that surround the endothelial cells of microvessel [1]. Genetic studies have shown that pericytes exert multiple effects on the vasculature: they participate in vascular development, maturation, and remodeling, and they also contribute to normal architecture and regulate permeability [1–3]. Retina, a light sensitive layer lining at the back of the eye, has the highest pericyte density around the body [4]. Recently, pericytes have received considerable attention as an active player in the pathological mechanisms of retinal angiogenic diseases, such as diabetic retinopathy (DR) and retinopathy of prematurity (ROP) [5, 6]. DR is one of the most common and important chronic microvascular complications in individuals with diabetes mellitus, which will give rise to blindness in uncontrolled conditions. Numerous studies have shown that the primary morphological change in the diabetic retina is the dysfunction and loss of pericytes [7]. The absence of pericytes destabilizes retinal vessels, making them more susceptible to hypoxia-induced sprouting [7, 8]. Others showed that pericytes are also involved in pathological retinal angiogenesis in a murine model of ROP [9]. Therefore, pericytes are currently under consideration as therapeutic targets for the treatment of retinal angiogenic diseases.

Apelin, a natural ligand for an orphan G protein-coupled receptor APJ, is widely expressed in various tissues, including brain, heart, lung, kidney, uterus, and ovary [10, 11], and is reported to be involved in the regulation of multiple physiological functions [12]. The studies of apelin-deficient mice and Xenopus laevis embryos indicate that apelin is involved in the regulation of vasculogenesis and angiogenesis [13, 14]. Hara et al. showed that the size of choroidal neovascular membrane lesions was decreased in apelin gene knockout mice [15], and *in vitro* studies have shown that apelin induced proliferation and migration of vascular smooth muscle cells (VSMCs) and suppresses VSMCs apoptosis induced by serum deprivation via APJ/PI3-K/Akt signaling pathways [16, 17]. In endothelial cells apelin also significantly enhanced migration, proliferation, and capillary-like tube formation [18]. Besides, our previous studies showed that apelin significantly enhanced the viability, migration, and proliferation of Müller cells and retinal pigment epithelium (RPE) cells through the pathway of MAPK/Erk and PI3-K/Akt [19–21].

Hypoxia has been widely used as a typical apoptosis insult to a variety of cell types [22]. Hypoxia has been shown to induce rat pancreatic β-cell apoptosis through Bcl-2/Bax pathway [23]. Previous studies demonstrated that apelin suppressed apoptosis in osteoblastic cell, human osteoblasts, and bone marrow mesenchymal cells through regulation of Bcl-2/Bax via PI3-K pathway [24–26]. Moreover, apelin reduced cytochrome c release from mitochondria to cytoplasm and activation of caspase 3. These results explained apelin protected cells via various mechanisms.

However, whether apelin has protective effects on rat primary pericytes has not been explored. We propose a putative role for apelin in the viability and apoptosis of pericytes and conducted this study to investigate whether apelin could exert protective effects on primary rat retinal pericytes under hypoxia.

2. Materials and Methods

2.1. Reagents. Exogenous recombinant apelin-13 peptide was purchased from Sigma (St. Louis, MO). The makers of pericytes were PDGFR-B (ab69506, Abcam, US), NG2 (SC-20162, Santa Cruz, CA), and Desmin (ab6322, Abcam, US). Anti-apelin and anti-APJ were purchased from Abcam company (ab59469, ab125213, and ab84296, Abcam, US), respectively. CellTiter 96 AQueous One Solution was used in cell Proliferation Assay (Promega, US). Lentiviral vector knockout of apelin was constructed and purchased from GeneChem Co., Ltd. (Shanghai, China). Bcl-2 and Bax antibody were obtained from Cell Signaling Technology (#2870; #2772, CST, US).

2.2. Primary Rat Pericyte Cells Isolation, Culture, and Treatment. All experiments were performed in accordance with the Research Ethics Committees of the People's Hospital, Peking University, China. We isolated primary rat retinal pericyte cells from the retinal microvessel of Sprague-Dawley (SD) rats, using a modified method of previously published articles [27–29]. Briefly, eyes from SD rats (4–6 weeks, 150–200 g) were incubated with cold Dulbecco's phosphate-buffered saline (PBS) containing penicillin-streptomycin antibiotic (500 U/mL) for 10 min. The retinas were removed and cut into 1×1 mm small pieces and then incubated with collagenase I (Roche Applied Science, Mannheim, Germany) for 30–45 min at 37°C. The digested retina were filtered through 70 μm and 40 μm nylon mesh (Falcon, BD, US) and then centrifuged. Rat retinal pericytes were purified with Dynabeads Pan Mouse IgG (Invitrogen Dynal AS, Norway) according to the instructions. Before use, we washed the Dynabeads (25 μL) in Dulbecco's Modified Eagle's Media (DMEM) (Hyclone, US), and we added 1 μL mouse anti-desmin monoclonal antibody (ab6322, abcam, US) and then incubated them overnight at 4°C. The cell pellets were suspended in DMEM containing 10% fetal bovine serum (Gibco, US) and incubated with Dynabeads conjugated mouse anti-desmin monoclonal antibody for 30 min at 37°C, with gentle rotation. After washing, the bead-bound pericytes in pericyte medium (Sciencell Inc., US) were suspended at 37°C in a humidified atmosphere of a 5% CO_2 incubator. Pericytes between passages three and five were used throughout the study.

In chemical hypoxia-induced pericytes injury models, 150 μmol $CoCl_2$ was used according to the previous report [21]. In the viability assay, we treated pericytes with different concentrations of apelin (10, 100, and 1000 ng/mL) and knockdown of apelin was performed via lentivirus vector. We incubated control group cells in pericyte medium.

2.3. Immunofluorescent Staining. Immunofluorescent staining of membranes tissue was described in our previous published study [20, 30]. Briefly, 12 fibrovascular membranes with proliferative diabetic retinopathy were surgically obtained during vitrectomy. In a similar manner, 10 macular preretinal membranes were obtained and served as control. Immunofluorescence staining was performed on the frozen sections of the fibrovascular membranes and of the control membranes by staining with rabbit anti-apelin (ab59469, 1:100, Abcam, US) or rabbit anti-APJ (ab84296, 1:200, Abcam, US). The human patients study protocol was approved by the Ethical Committee and Institutional Review Board of Peking University People's Hospital (Beijing, China) and was conducted in accordance with the Declaration of Helsinki. Written informed consent was obtained from each study subject.

Pericytes which were cultured on cover slides (Fisher, US) were fixed with 4% paraformaldehyde and incubated in 0.3% H_2O_2 and 0.1% triton X-100 to quench endogenous peroxidase activity and penetrate the cytomembrane. Then, the cells were incubated in 3% blocking goat serum for 1 h and then incubated with anti-PDGFR-β (ab69506, 1:100, Abcam, US), NG2 (SC-20162, 1:100, Santa Cruz, CA), desmin (ab6322, 1:200, Abcam, US), apelin (1:100, Abcam, US), and APJ (1:200, Abcam, US) overnight at 4°C. The following day, pericytes were incubated with the relevant fluorescence-conjugated secondary antibody (1:200, Invitrogen, US) for 2 h at room temperature. Images were obtained with Nikon 50i fluorescent microscope (Nikon, Tokyo, Japan) under 200x magnifications.

2.4. Lentivirus-Mediated shRNA Knockdown of Apelin Expression and Transfection. The knockdown of Apelin (Rattus, NM_031612.2, GI:52345441) was induced by a lentivirus-mediated RNA interference vector (GeneChem Co., Ltd., Shanghai, China). The small interfering RNA (siRNA) target sequences were selected: #1, 5′-GAGGAGAGATAG-AAACAGA-3′; #2, 5′-GGAGGATGTTGGCTGAGAA-3′; #3, 5′-GTTTGCCTTTCTTGACAAA-3′; and #4, 5′-CAG-ATGAGTTCTCTTCTCT-3′. The lentivirus-GFP (LV-GFP) which included the GFP gene and did not include the apelin interference sequence served as negative control. For lentivirus transduction, pericytes were cultured at 5×10^4 cells/well into 6-well culture plates. After being grown to 70% confluence, cells were transduced with shRNA lentivirus at a multiplicity of infection (MOI) of 100. Cells were harvested at 24 hours after infection, and transfection efficiency was evaluated by immunofluorescence staining. The knockdown efficiency of apelin was evaluated by RT-PCR and western blot analysis.

2.5. Cell Viability/Cell Proliferation. Pericyte viability was measured by MTS assay, according to the manufacturer's instructions (CellTiter 96 AQueous One Solution Assay; Promega, Madison, WI, US). 5000 cells/well were seeded into a 96-well plate and incubated with different concentrations of apelin (1, 100, and 1000 ng/mL) for 24 h. At the end of the incubation, 10 μL MTS solution was added into each well and incubated for 1 h. The absorbance wavelength was evaluated with microculture plate reader (Model 550; Bio-Rad, Tokyo, Japan) at 490 nm (OD_{490}). Each experiment was performed in five wells and repeated at least three times.

2.6. Edu Assay. Pericytes proliferation was assessed using a Cell-Light EdU Apollo 643 *in vitro* Imaging Kit (RuiBo. Inc., Guangzhou, China). Briefly, 1×10^4 cells/well, which was pretreated with apelin, was plated in 96-well plates for 24 h. Following the incubation interval, 10 μmol 5-ethynyl-2′-deoxyuridine (Edu) medium was added to each well and incubated for 2 h. After washing twice with PBS, pericytes were fixed with 4% paraformaldehyde for 30 min and washed with 2 mg/mL glycine solution for 5 min in order to neutralize paraformaldehyde and assure a good staining system. The cells were incubated in 100 μL 1x Apollo staining solution for 30 min and the nuclei were dyed with Hoechst 33342. The images were obtained under 10x magnification, using a Nikon 50i fluorescent microscope. Each experiment was performed in five wells and repeated at least three times.

2.7. Cell Migration/Transwell Assay. Transwell assay was used for evaluating cell migration assays. Briefly, 100 μL of pericyte suspension (1×10^5 cells/mL) was added to the upper chamber and 600 μL medium containing apelin, hypoxia medium, or DMEM (control) to the lower chamber, respectively. The chambers were incubated for 6 h at 37°C. The filters were fixed with 4% paraformaldehyde for 15 min and we subjected the nuclei to DAPI staining for 10 min. The remaining cells on the upper surface of the filter were removed by wiping with a cotton swab. The number of migrated cells were quantified by counting in five random fields (10x magnification), using a Nikon 50i fluorescence microscope. The data are shown as the mean ± standard deviation (SD). Each experiment was repeated at least three times.

2.8. TUNEL Assay. Pericyte apoptosis after hypoxia was evaluated by terminal deoxynucleotidyl transferase-mediated dUTP nick end-labeling (TUNEL) assay. TUNEL staining was performed on cell coverslips using a commercial kit (In Situ Cell Death Detection Kit; Roche Applied Science, USA), according to the manufacturer's recommended instructions. TUNEL-positive cell nuclei were visualized as green fluorescence and images performed under 10x magnification. Finally, the percentage of TUNEL-positive cells was calculated in five microscopic fields of each slide.

2.9. Quantitative Real-Time PCR. Total RNA was isolated from cultured pericytes using Trizol reagent (Invitrogen, CA, US), and we determined the concentration and integrity of total RNA with UV spectrophotometry (NANODROP 2000C, Thermo, US). We used the Fermentas reverse transcription system (Fermentas, St. Leon-Rot, Germany) to reverse RNA (1 μg) into first strand cDNA, using a real-time PCR system (PikoReal 96 PCR system, Thermo Scientific). The PCR solution system contained 1 μL of cDNA (1 : 20 diluted), specific primers 1 μL (10 pmol), 3 μL DEPC-water, and 5 μL of SYBR Select Master Mix (Invitrogen), with a final volume of 10 μL. Each sample was measured in triplicate wells. Primers used were as follows: β-actin Forward: 5′-TGGCTCTATCCTGGCCTCACT-3′, β-actin Reverse: 5′-GCTCAGTAACAGTCCGCCTAGAA-3′; rat apelin Forward: 5′-GATGGAGAAAGGCGAAGAAAG-3′, rat apelin Reverse: 5′-GGTGAGAGATGAGACCACTTGT-3′. The standard PCR conditions included 2 min at 50°C and 10 min at 95°C, followed by 35 cycles of extension at 95°C for 15 s, 60°C for 30 s, and 72°C for 30 s. The mRNA expression was normalized to the expression level of ACTB. We calculated the changes in mRNA expression according to the $2^{-\Delta\Delta CT}$ method, with $\Delta CT = C_{Target\ gene} - CT_{ACTB}$ and $\Delta\Delta CT = \Delta C_{Treatment} - \Delta CT_{Control}$. Each experiment was repeated at least three times.

2.10. Western Blot Analysis. Pericytes were harvested and lysed in RIPA buffer (1% Nonidet P-40, 0.5% sodium deoxycholate, 0.1% SDS in PBS) and centrifuged at 15,000 rpm for 15 min at 4°C. The membranes were blocked with 5% nonfat milk for 1 h and then incubated overnight at 4°C with primary antibody: rabbit anti-Bcl-2, (#2870; 1 : 1000, CST); rabbit anti-Bax, (#2772; 1 : 1000; CST); rabbit anti-Apelin (ab125213; 1 : 500; abcam); and rabbit anti-APJ (ab84296; 1 : 1000, abcam). The membranes were incubated with goat anti-rabbit horse-radish peroxidase- (HRP-) conjugated secondary antibody (1 : 3000, DAKO, Japan) for 1 h at room temperature. The density of each band was analyzed with Image J software. Each experiment was repeated at least three times.

2.11. Statistical Analysis. The results were expressed as mean ± SD. Difference between two groups was compared with an independent sample *t*-test (SPSS17.0 software, Chicago, IL). Two-tailed $P < 0.05$ was considered to indicate statistical significance. Differences among groups were assessed using one-way analysis of variance (ANOVA), followed by Dunnett's test. A value of $P < 0.05$ was considered as significantly different. We repeated all experiments at least three times, and representative experiments are shown.

3. Results

3.1. Immunohistochemical Expression of APJ in Fibrovascular Membranes. Expression of APJ was detected in the specimens of all fibrovascular membranes of the proliferative diabetic retinopathy (PDR) group with strong staining for APJ (Figure 1). Colocalization of pericyte markers desmin and APJ were observed in all specimens of the PDR group

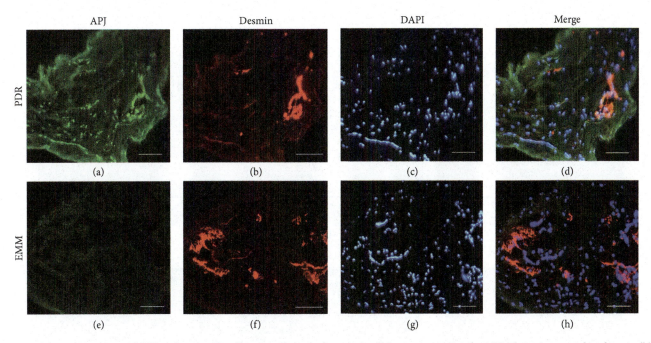

Figure 1: Immunostaining of APJ and pericyte in fibrovascular membranes. (a–d) Immunostaining for APJ (a), pericyte marker desmin (b), and DAPI (c) in fibrovascular membranes from eyes with proliferative diabetic retinopathy. Staining intensities of APJ were strong and were colocalized with pericyte, as identified by desmin. (e–h) Staining of APJ (e), desmin (f), and DAPI (g) in epiretinal macular membranes (EMM) of control patients without diabetic retinopathy. None of APJ (e) and staining of desmin (f) were observed. Scale bar = 100 μm.

($n = 12$) (Figures 1(a)–1(d)). None of the membranes removed from the eyes of the epithelial macular membrane (EMM) group showed specific staining of APJ ($n = 10$) (Figures 1(e)–1(h)). Our previous study also demonstrated that vitreous concentrations of apelin were significantly higher in the PDR group than in the EMM group [30].

3.2. Cultivation and Identification of Primary Rat Retinal Pericytes.
Primary rat retinal pericytes were isolated by Magnetic Dynabeads and formed cell clusters floating in cell medium (Figure 2(A)). At day 7, the primary pericytes got adherence, and the colony formed and grew (Figure 2(B)). Generally, primary pericytes confluenced at about day 14. When pericytes were passaged, the growth and adherence became rapid obviously, which got adherence about 4-6 hours and passaged about 4-5 days. Primary rat retinal pericytes showed irregular triangular cell bodies, with thick filaments in the cytoplasm and a plump nucleus (Figure 2(C)). As specific markers for pericyte, desmin, PDGFR-β, and NG2 were used to confirm the purity of cultured primary rat pericyte cells, which was approximately 95% (Figure 3(b)).

3.3. Expression of Apelin and APJ Receptor in Pericytes.
Prior to exploring the effects of apelin in rat retinal pericytes, we carried out immunofluorescence staining to detect the expression of apelin/APJ in pericytes. We observed low apelin immunoreactivity in normal pericyte culture, which showed weak and diffuse expression in the cytoplasm (Figure 3(a)-(A), (B)). In similar way, the APJ staining was moderate, which was expressed in cytoplasm membrane (Figure 3(b)-(A), (B)). However, after exposure under hypoxia for 12 h, the expression of apelin represented obvious stronger cytoplasm staining (Figure 3(a)-(C), (D)), accompanied by expanding stronger APJ immunoreactivities in cytoplasm and cytoplasm membrane (Figure 3(b)-(C), (D)). In addition, the results of western blot about apelin and APJ under hypoxia support the change of immunofluorescence staining (Figures 3(c) and 3(d)). The expression of apelin and APJ under hypoxia was upregulated 2.5-fold and 1.9-fold, respectively ($P < 0.05$).

3.4. Detection of Interference Efficacy of Lentivirus-Apelin.
Quantitative Real-Time PCR in NRK-52E and IEC6 cells demonstrated that LV-Apelin (#4) was the most efficient shRNA, in which the RNA level of apelin was decreased by more than 70% (data was not shown). Then, we tested the knockdown efficiencies of LV-Apelin in pericytes. When MOI is 100, the result of immunofluorescence staining showed that interference efficacy achieved 90% (Figure 4(a)). After that, the qRT-PCR in pericyte revealed the apelin level was decreased by 75% in LV-apelin group compared to LV-GFP control group ($P < 0.01$) (Figure 4(b)). In a similar way, western blot demonstrated that the apelin level was downregulated by 64% ($P < 0.05$) (Figures 4(c) and 4(d)).

3.5. Apelin-Stimulated Cell Proliferation and Migration in Normoxia.
Experiments were performed to evaluate whether apelin had any effect on pericytes proliferation and migration in normoxia. Pericytes were incubated with apelin at different concentrations (1, 10, 100, and 1000 ng/mL) for 24 h. Among the various concentrations, MTS assay results show that 100 ng/mL group significantly increased pericytes viability, compared with the control groups (Figure 5(B)) (100 ng/mL

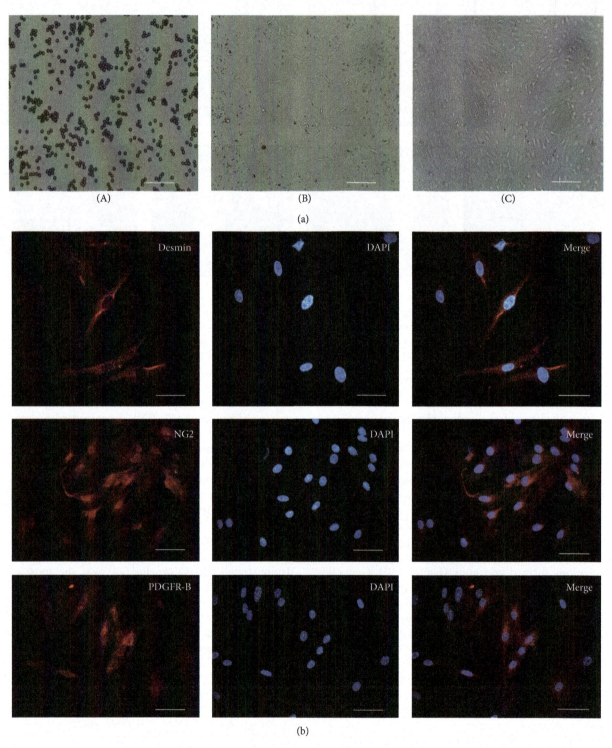

FIGURE 2: Morphology and immunofluorescent staining were identified in primary rat retinal pericytes. (a) Microscopic image of retinal pericytes, showing cell mass isolated by Dynabeads (A), at 7 days, pericytes got adherence and formed cells cluster (B), at passage 1 non-contact-inhibited growth of pericyte and irregular triangular cell bodies, with thick filaments in the cytoplasm and a plump nucleus (C). Scale bar = 200 μm. (b) Immunofluorescence staining with anti-desmin, NG2, and PDGFR-B antibody for primary rat retinal pericytes, respectively. Scale bar = 100 μm.

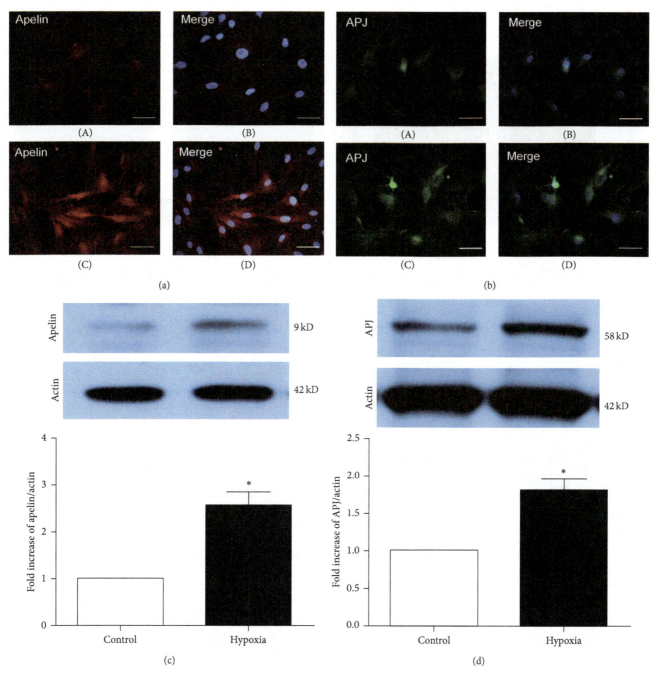

FIGURE 3: The cellular localization of apelin/APJ. (a) Apelin immunoreactivity was found weak and diffused in the cytoplasm of normal (A) but showed more intense cytoplasmic staining in hypoxic pericyte (C). Scale bar = 100 μm. Similarly, (b) compared with restricted cytomembrane expression in normal (A) and hypoxia (C) pericyte, APJ localization expanded and brightened in the cytoplasm and cytoplasm membrane (apelin in red, APJ in green, and DAPI in blue). Scale bar = 100 μm. (c) and (d) Western blot analysis shows that the expression of apelin and APJ under hypoxia was upregulated 2.5-fold and 1.9-fold, respectively ($P < 0.05$).

versus control, $^{**}P < 0.01$; 1000 ng/mL versus control, $^{*}P < 0.05$).

Edu experiment was used to detect pericyte proliferation at different concentrations of apelin (10 ng/mL and 100 ng/mL). The number of proliferative cells was significantly higher in the apelin-treated group, compared with the control group (Figure 5(A)).

In the cell migration assay, cells were measured in a modified Boyden Chamber in which pericytes migrated through a porous membrane. The mean number of migrated pericytes incubated with apelin (1–100 ng/mL) was significantly higher than the mean number of the control group ($P < 0.05$) (Figures 5(C) and 5(D)).

3.6. The Effects of Apelin and Lentivirus Knockdown Apelin for Cell Proliferation and Migration in Hypoxia.
Furthermore, we carried out experiment to study the effect of apelin for pericyte under hypoxia. We found that the viability of

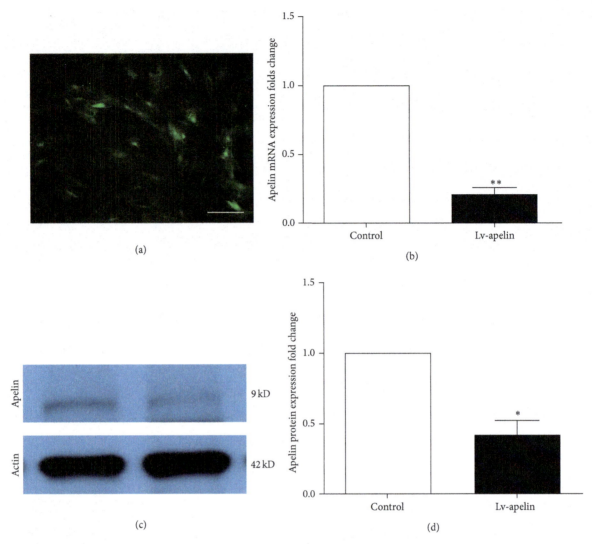

FIGURE 4: Pericytes transducted with Lentivirus-Apelin. (a) Immunofluorescence staining of LV-apelin infection in pericyte. Interference efficacy arrived about 90%, MOI = 100. Scale bar = 100 μm. (b) The mRNA expression of LV-Apelin was decreased by 75% after blocking by siRNA sequence ($P < 0.01$). (c and d). The western blot analysis shows that protein of expression of LV-Apelin decreased by 64% ($P < 0.05$).

pericytes incubated with $CoCl_2$ was decreased obviously time dependently. The viability of pericytes was reduced by 27% at 6 h and by 40% at 12 h after stimulation by 150 μmol/L $CoCl_2$, respectively. However, the viability of pericytes stimulated by apelin was significantly enhanced, compared with the $CoCl_2$ group (8 h versus control $^*P < 0.05$; 12 h versus control $^{**}P < 0.01$) (Figure 6(A)).

Our study showed that under hypoxia the viability of cells treated with apelin was significantly increased. Meanwhile, the viability of cells in the LV-apelin knockout group was significantly reduced ($CoCl_2$ versus apelin, $P < 0.05$; LV-GFP versus LV-apelin, $P < 0.05$; $CoCl_2$ versus LV-apelin, $P < 0.01$), which suggests that apelin can stimulate pericyte viability (Figure 6(B)). We also detected migration of pericytes under hypoxia. Compared with the control group, the mean number of migrated pericytes under hypoxia and combination with LV-apelin knockdown decreased significantly. However, in the group treated with apelin, the mean number of migrated pericytes was increased under hypoxia (Figures 6(C) and 6(D)).

3.7. Apelin Protected Pericytes against Apoptosis Induced by Hypoxia via Bcl-2/Bax Restoration and Caspase 3 Pathway. In the cell viability experiment, hypoxia resulted in a 27% decrease in pericyte viability. However, cell viability increased significantly in pericytes pretreated with 100 ng/mL of apelin for 12 h. To further evaluate the effects of apelin on cell death, we used TUNEL staining to detect DNA fragmentation and cell death in hypoxia-treated pericytes with and without apelin treatment. We pretreated pericytes with apelin for 12 h and then exposed these pericytes to hypoxia for 12 h. In the percentage of apoptotic cells showing green, approximately 30% of cell death was blocked by the apelin treatment (Figure 7).

Active-caspase 3 protein is one of the key executioners of apoptosis. As shown in Figure 8, active-caspase 3 protein

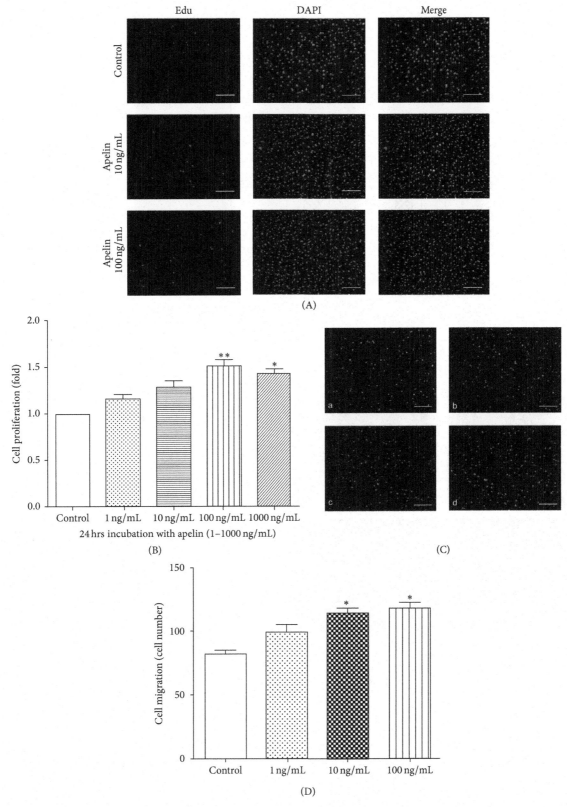

FIGURE 5: Effect of apelin on cell viability and migration under normoxia. (A) The Edu proliferation assay. Apollo staining (red) represents proliferating cells, and DAPI (blue) staining nuclei. Compared with the control group, the number of proliferating cells treated with apelin (10 or 100 ng/mL) increased significantly. Scale bar = 200 μm. (B) The folds of apelin-treated cell viability compared with the control group ($^*P < 0.05$, $^{**}P < 0.01$ versus untreated control); (C) and (D) pericyte migration in response to apelin treatment was measured using the transwell assay (a: control; b: 1 ng/mL; c: 10 ng/mL; d: 100 ng/mL, $^*P < 0.05$ versus untreated control). The data are expressed as means ± standard deviation (SD). Scale bar = 200 μm.

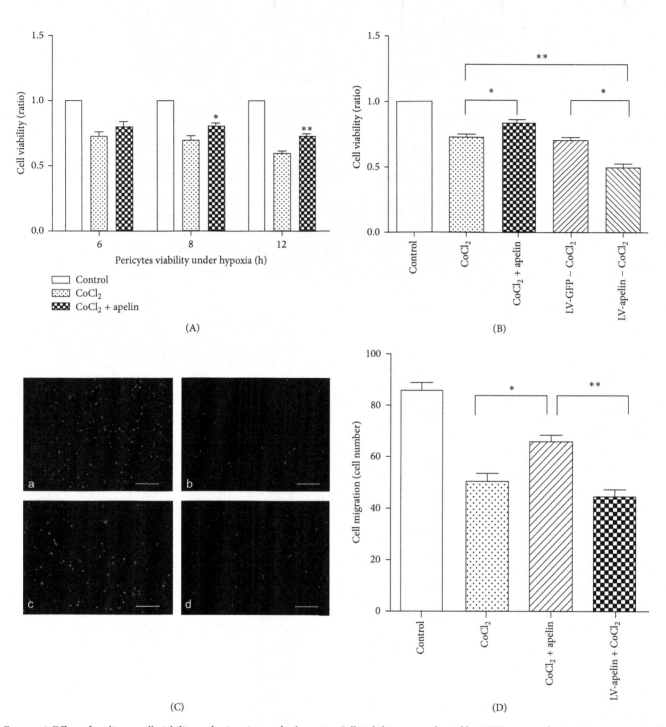

FIGURE 6: Effect of apelin on cell viability and migration under hypoxia. Cell viability was evaluated by MTS assay and migration was assessed with a transwell cell chamber. (A) In hypoxic pericytes, the viability of cells stimulated by apelin was significantly enhanced during 12 h (8 h versus $CoCl_2$ *$P < 0.05$; 12 h versus $CoCl_2$ **$P < 0.01$). (B) Viability of pericytes treated with apelin and LV-apelin knockout under hypoxia. Compared with the $CoCl_2$ group, viability was significantly increased in the apelin group ($P < 0.05$). Moreover, cell viability was significantly reduced in the LV-apelin knockout group (LV-GFP versus LV-apelin, $P < 0.05$; $CoCl_2$ versus LV-apelin, $P < 0.05$). (C) and (D) Pericyte migration induced by apelin under hypoxia (a: control; b: $CoCl_2$ 150 μmol; and c: $CoCl_2$ 150 μmol + apelin 100 ng/mL). The number of migrated cells per HPF is shown. Apelin versus $CoCl_2$ *$P < 0.05$. Scale bar = 200 μm.

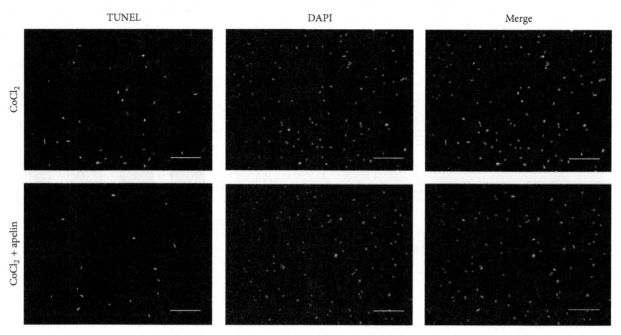

FIGURE 7: TUNEL staining was used to evaluate hypoxia-induced cell death. Cells were exposed to 100 ng/mL apelin for 12 h and then exposed to hypoxia for 12 h. Apoptotic nuclei were visualized by TdT-mediated dUTP nick end-labeling (TUNEL). Scale bar = 200 μm.

level significantly increased 12 h after hypoxia injury ($P < 0.001$, compared with the control group). Administration of apelin significantly decreased its levels after hypoxia injury ($P < 0.01$, compared with hypoxia group). The expression of active-caspase 3 in hypoxia combination with LV-Apelin knockdown was similar to hypoxia group and its levels significantly increased ($P < 0.01$, compared with control group) (Figures 8(a) and 8(b)).

Likewise, we also detect bcl-2 and Bax expression in pericyte. Western blot analysis showed that apelin dose-dependently induced Bcl-2 protein expression and down-regulated Bax protein expression in pericytes (Figures 8(c) and 8(d)). The antiapoptotic effect of apelin was through increased expression of Bcl-2 and reduced expression of Bax. In hypoxia group, the ratio of Bcl-2/Bax decreased 36% and LV-apelin group has a similar ratio ($P < 0.001$, compared with con. group). However, the ratio of Bcl-2/Bax in treatment with apelin group was significantly increased ($P < 0.001$, compared with hypoxia group) (Figures 8(e) and 8(f)).

4. Discussion

Apelin interacts with its specific receptor APJ, has multiple biological activities, and had been characterized in various tissues [31]. Previously, we proved that vitreous concentrations of apelin were significantly higher in the proliferative diabetic retinopathy (PDR) group. Likewise, apelin and APJ also colocalized with endothelial cells maker CD 31 in PDR [30]. In the present study, we further demonstrated that APJ was strong expressed in fibrovascular membranes of the PDR and was colocalized with pericytes. Therefore, apelin/APJ system was possibly involved in the pathological progression of PDR. However, the effect of apelin on apoptosis of primary retinal pericytes remains unknown. In order to study the effects of apelin in pericyte, primary rat pericytes were used here. Based on the current results, we proved the expression of apelin and APJ in pericytes and demonstrated that apelin and APJ are upregulated in hypoxia cultured condition. Knockdown of apelin inhibits proliferation and migration of pericytes. Moreover, exogenous recombinant apelin effectively prevented hypoxia-induced apoptosis through down-regulating the expression of active-caspase 3 and increased the ratio of Bcl-2/Bax in pericyte. These results establish the foundation for further study of diseases associated with ischemia and hypoxia.

As we all know, rodent is similar to human in genetic background. In previous published studies, primary cultured pericytes were mostly originated from bovine retina, which restricted further in vivo studies [32]. In the present study, we established a rodent- (rat-) based primary pericyte in vitro model. By using a magnetic beads isolation method, we obtained primary rat retinal pericytes successfully in the purity of 90%. As for marker of pericytes, alpha smooth muscle actin (α-SMA), tropomyosin desmin, nestin, sulfatide or nerve/glial antigen-2 (NG2) proteoglycan, platelet-derived growth factor receptor-B (PDGFR-B), aminopeptidase N (CD13), and the regulator of G-signaling 5 (RG5) are common pericyte markers [4, 33]. However, no single entirely pericyte-specific marker is known to date, and all markers currently used are dynamic in their expression and may be up- or downregulated in conjunction with developmental states, pathological reactions, and in vitro culturing conditions [4]. For example, pericytes on normal capillaries typically express desmin, but not SMA, whereas smooth muscle cells on arterioles and pericytes on venues are immunoreactive for both [34]. Therefore, we select three markers that sufficiently

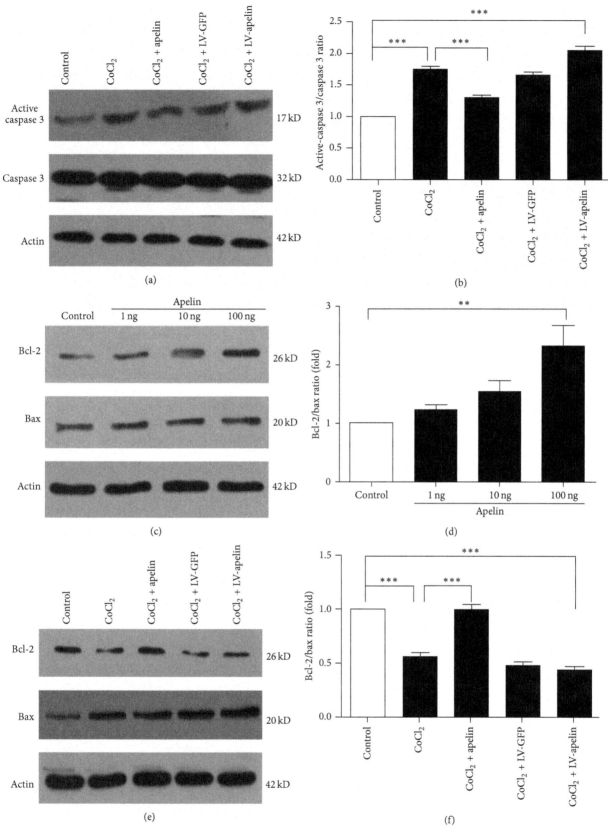

FIGURE 8: Effect of apelin on hypoxia-induced apoptosis in rat retinal pericytes. (a) Active-caspase 3 protein level significantly increased 12 h after hypoxia injury ($P < 0.001$). Apelin significantly decreased its levels after hypoxia injury ($P < 0.01$). (c and e) Effects of apelin on Bcl-2 and Bax protein expression in rat retinal pericytes. Cells were incubated with apelin and LV-apelin knockout under hypoxia. Western blot analysis was quantitated by densitometry of autoradiographs, and the relative mean ratio of Bcl-2/Bax was increased in apelin group ($P < 0.001$ versus con.) and reduced in Lv-apelin knockdown group ($P < 0.001$ versus con.).

identify pericytes in order to obtain highly pure rat retinal pericytes. In present study, pericytes uniformly expressed the cellular markers PDGFR-β, NG2 and desmin. Our results are consistent with Liu's study, who also proved these markers expressed in pericytes isolated from rats by mechanical morcellation and collagenase digestion [29].

Apelin/APJ is localized in a wide variety of tissues, including the endothelial cells of the primary blood vessels, neurons, and oligodendrocytes [18]. The lines of evidence show that apelin exerts its biological functions through its interaction with APJ. Knockout of apelin or APJ leads to the inhibition of both hypoxia-induced endothelial cell proliferation *in vitro* and hypoxia-induced vessel regeneration in the caudal fin regeneration of Fli-1 transgenic zebrafish [35]. Therefore, location of APJ in cells or tissues is very important with regard to apelin exerting its diverse functions. In the present study, through immunofluorescence staining, we first confirmed the expression of APJ in pericytes and hypoxia-induced upregulation of apelin and APJ. The results of this study showed that the expression of APJ was positive in pericytes, which is essential for apelin/APJ system and plays a role in pathological and physiological condition. This suggested that apelin might be involved in pericyte physiology and pathology.

Apelin was shown to have angiogenic activity in retinal endothelial cells, both *in vitro* and *in vivo* [18]. In our previous studies, we showed that apelin can enhance proliferation and migration of Müller cells and RPE cells [19, 21]. Eyries identified apelin as a hypoxia-inducible factor-1 (HIF-1) target gene and demonstrated that, under hypoxia, HIF-1 binds to the first intron of apelin, leading to upregulation of apelin expression [35]. In the present study, we observed that the viability and migration of pericytes incubated with various concentrations of apelin were enhanced. Under hypoxia exposure, pericytes viability decreased significantly with time-dependent manner and apelin can protect pericytes viability. Furthermore, knockdown of apelin led to a significant decrease in pericyte viability. These results further support the hypothesis that apelin is sensitive to hypoxia, playing a key role in hypoxia-induced pericyte proliferation and migration.

Many *in vitro* and *in vivo* insults, such as hypoxia and ischemia, trigger mixed cell death composed of both necrosis and apoptosis [31, 36]. Hypoxia-induced Bax upregulation, Bcl-2 downregulation, and caspase 3 activation in variety of cells were reversed by HIF-1 overexpression and lead to the acquisition of antiapoptotic properties [37–39]. The ratio of antiapoptotic to proapoptotic proteins, especially the Bcl-2/Bax ratio, determines susceptibility to apoptosis [40]. We therefore investigated whether these pathways were involved in the antiapoptotic effects of apelin in pericytes. Our result was consistent with previous studies, which indicated that Bcl-2/Bax apoptotic signaling pathways mediate the protective effects of the apelin/APJ system in vascular smooth muscle cells and osteoblasts [17, 24]. Caspases, cysteine proteases with aspartate specificity, are important mediators of apoptosis. Caspase 3 is effector caspase that is responsible for cleaving nucleases in addition to cellular substrates. We also revealed that apelin reduced caspase 3 activity, which suggests that apelin inhibits pericyte apoptosis through regulation of activity of caspase 3 and Bcl-2/Bax expression. Therefore, there is a growing consensus that apelin may be a promising therapeutic target against hypoxia/ischemia in the future.

In conclusion, this study demonstrated that apelin/APJ was expressed in PDR patient's membranes and in rat retinal pericytes. Apelin can protect pericytes against hypoxia-induced apoptosis through regulation of activation of caspase 3 and Bcl-2/Bax expression. These results indicated that apelin could be a potential therapeutic target for retinal angiogenic diseases.

5. Conclusion

Pericytes are a population of cells that are involved in normal vessel architecture and contraction and regulated blood flow. Hypoxia causes decreasing of pericytes viability in a time-dependent manner and induced pericytes apoptosis. However, apelin regulated function of pericytes under hypoxia inversely in a concentration-dependent manner and effectively prevented hypoxia-induced apoptosis through downregulating active-caspase 3 expression and increasing the ratio of Bcl-2/Bax.

Conflict of Interests

The authors declare that there is no conflict of interests regarding the publication of this paper.

Acknowledgments

This work has been supported by the National Natural Science Foundation of China (no. 81271027), EFSD/CDS/Lilly Grant (nos. 90561 and 94410), the Program for New Century Excellent Talents in University (no. NCET-12-0010), and Fok Ying Tong Education Foundation (Hong Kong).

References

[1] M. Hellström, H. Gerhardt, M. Kalén et al., "Lack of pericytes leads to endothelial hyperplasia and abnormal vascular morphogenesis," *The Journal of Cell Biology*, vol. 153, no. 3, pp. 543–554, 2001.

[2] P. Lindahl, B. R. Johansson, P. Levéen, and C. Betsholtz, "Pericyte loss and microaneurysm formation in PDGF-B-deficient mice," *Science*, vol. 277, no. 5323, pp. 242–245, 1997.

[3] P. Levéen, M. Pekny, S. Gebre-Medhin, B. Swolin, E. Larsson, and C. Betsholtz, "Mice deficient for PDGF B show renal, cardiovascular, and hematological abnormalities," *Genes & Development*, vol. 8, no. 16, pp. 1875–1887, 1994.

[4] A. Armulik, G. Genové, and C. Betsholtz, "Pericytes: developmental, physiological, and pathological perspectives, problems, and promises," *Developmental Cell*, vol. 21, no. 2, pp. 193–215, 2011.

[5] D. von Tell, A. Armulik, and C. Betsholtz, "Pericytes and vascular stability," *Experimental Cell Research*, vol. 312, no. 5, pp. 623–629, 2006.

[6] A. P. Hall, "Review of the pericyte during angiogenesis and its role in cancer and diabetic retinopathy," *Toxicologic Pathology*, vol. 34, no. 6, pp. 763–775, 2006.

[7] H.-P. Hammes, J. Lin, O. Renner et al., "Pericytes and the pathogenesis of diabetic retinopathy," *Diabetes*, vol. 51, no. 10, pp. 3107–3112, 2002.

[8] Y. Feng, F. vom Hagen, F. Pfister et al., "Impaired pericyte recruitment and abnormal retinal angiogenesis as a result of angiopoietin-2 overexpression," *Thrombosis and Haemostasis*, vol. 97, no. 1, pp. 99–108, 2007.

[9] S. Hughes, T. Gardiner, L. Baxter, and T. Chan-Ling, "Changes in pericytes and smooth muscle cells in the kitten model of retinopathy of prematurity: Implications for plus disease," *Investigative Ophthalmology and Visual Science*, vol. 48, no. 3, pp. 1368–1379, 2007.

[10] Y. Kawamata, Y. Habata, S. Fukusumi et al., "Molecular properties of apelin: tissue distribution and receptor binding," *Biochimica et Biophysica Acta—Molecular Cell Research*, vol. 1538, no. 2-3, pp. 162–171, 2001.

[11] M. de Falco, L. de Luca, N. Onori et al., "Apelin expression in normal human tissues," *In Vivo*, vol. 16, no. 5, pp. 333–336, 2002.

[12] A. Reaux, K. Gallatz, M. Palkovits, and C. Llorens-Cortes, "Distribution of apelin-synthesizing neurons in the adult rat brain," *Neuroscience*, vol. 113, no. 3, pp. 653–662, 2002.

[13] H. Kidoya, M. Ueno, Y. Yamada et al., "Spatial and temporal role of the apelin/APJ system in the caliber size regulation of blood vessels during angiogenesis," *The EMBO Journal*, vol. 27, no. 3, pp. 522–534, 2008.

[14] C. M. Cox, S. L. D'Agostino, M. K. Miller, R. L. Heimark, and P. A. Krieg, "Apelin, the ligand for the endothelial G-protein-coupled receptor, APJ, is a potent angiogenic factor required for normal vascular development of the frog embryo," *Developmental Biology*, vol. 296, no. 1, pp. 177–189, 2006.

[15] C. Hara, A. Kasai, F. Gomi et al., "Laser-induced choroidal neovascularization in mice attenuated by deficiency in the apelin-APJ system," *Investigative Ophthalmology and Visual Science*, vol. 54, no. 6, pp. 4321–4329, 2013.

[16] Q.-F. Liu, H.-W. Yu, L. You, M.-X. Liu, K.-Y. Li, and G.-Z. Tao, "Apelin-13-induced proliferation and migration induced of rat vascular smooth muscle cells is mediated by the upregulation of Egr-1," *Biochemical and Biophysical Research Communications*, vol. 439, no. 2, pp. 235–240, 2013.

[17] R.-R. Cui, D.-A. Mao, L. Yi et al., "Apelin suppresses apoptosis of human vascular smooth muscle cells via APJ/PI3-K/Akt signaling pathways," *Amino Acids*, vol. 39, no. 5, pp. 1193–1200, 2010.

[18] A. Kasai, N. Shintani, M. Oda et al., "Apelin is a novel angiogenic factor in retinal endothelial cells," *Biochemical and Biophysical Research Communications*, vol. 325, no. 2, pp. 395–400, 2004.

[19] D. Qin, X.-X. Zheng, and Y.-R. Jiang, "Apelin-13 induces proliferation, migration, and collagen I mRNA expression in human RPE cells via PI3K/Akt and MEK/Erk signaling pathways," *Molecular Vision*, vol. 19, pp. 2227–2236, 2013.

[20] Q. Lu, Y.-R. Jiang, J. Qian, and Y. Tao, "Apelin-13 regulates proliferation, migration and survival of retinal Müller cells under hypoxia," *Diabetes Research and Clinical Practice*, vol. 99, no. 2, pp. 158–167, 2013.

[21] X.-L. Wang, Y. Tao, Q. Lu, and Y.-R. Jiang, "Apelin supports primary rat retinal Müller cells under chemical hypoxia and glucose deprivation," *Peptides*, vol. 33, no. 2, pp. 298–306, 2012.

[22] A. Sendoel and M. O. Hengartner, "Apoptotic cell death under hypoxia," *Physiology*, vol. 29, no. 3, pp. 168–176, 2014.

[23] Y. Fang, Q. Zhang, J. Tan, L. Li, X. An, and P. Lei, "Intermittent hypoxia-induced rat pancreatic beta-cell apoptosis and protective effects of antioxidant intervention," *Nutrition & Diabetes*, vol. 4, no. 9, article e131, 2014.

[24] H. Xie, L.-Q. Yuan, X.-H. Luo et al., "Apelin suppresses apoptosis of human osteoblasts," *Apoptosis*, vol. 12, no. 1, pp. 247–254, 2007.

[25] S.-Y. Tang, H. Xie, L.-Q. Yuan et al., "Apelin stimulates proliferation and suppresses apoptosis of mouse osteoblastic cell line MC3T3-E1 via JNK and PI3-K/Akt signaling pathways," *Peptides*, vol. 28, no. 3, pp. 708–718, 2007.

[26] X. Zeng, S. P. Yu, T. Taylor, M. Ogle, and L. Wei, "Protective effect of apelin on cultured rat bone marrow mesenchymal stem cells against apoptosis," *Stem Cell Research*, vol. 8, no. 3, pp. 357–367, 2012.

[27] O. S. Kim, J. Kim, C.-S. Kim, N. H. Kim, and J. S. Kim, "KIOM-79 prevents methyglyoxal-induced retinal pericyte apoptosis in vitro and in vivo," *Journal of Ethnopharmacology*, vol. 129, no. 3, pp. 285–292, 2010.

[28] J. Cai, O. Kehoe, G. M. Smith, P. Hykin, and M. E. Boulton, "The angiopoietin/Tie-2 system regulates pericyte survival and recruitment in diabetic retinopathy," *Investigative Ophthalmology and Visual Science*, vol. 49, no. 5, pp. 2163–2171, 2008.

[29] G. Liu, C. Meng, M. Pan et al., "Isolation, purification, and cultivation of primary retinal microvascular pericytes: a novel model using rats," *Microcirculation*, vol. 21, no. 6, pp. 478–489, 2014.

[30] Y. Tao, Q. Lu, Y.-R. Jiang et al., "Apelin in plasma and vitreous and in fibrovascular retinal membranes of patients with proliferative diabetic retinopathy," *Investigative Ophthalmology & Visual Science*, vol. 51, no. 8, pp. 4237–4242, 2010.

[31] A. Y. Xiao, L. Wei, S. Xia, S. Rothman, and S. P. Yu, "Ionic mechanism of ouabain-induced concurrent apoptosis and necrosis in individual cultured cortical neurons," *The Journal of Neuroscience*, vol. 22, no. 4, pp. 1350–1362, 2002.

[32] E. Beltramo, E. Berrone, S. Giunti, G. Gruden, P. C. Perin, and M. Porta, "Effects of mechanical stress and high glucose on pericyte proliferation, apoptosis and contractile phenotype," *Experimental Eye Research*, vol. 83, no. 4, pp. 989–994, 2006.

[33] M. Krueger and I. Bechmann, "CNS pericytes: concepts, misconceptions, and a way out," *Glia*, vol. 58, no. 1, pp. 1–10, 2010.

[34] S. Morikawa, P. Baluk, T. Kaidoh, A. Haskell, R. K. Jain, and D. M. McDonald, "Abnormalities in pericytes on blood vessels and endothelial sprouts in tumors," *The American Journal of Pathology*, vol. 160, no. 3, pp. 985–1000, 2002.

[35] M. Eyries, G. Siegfried, M. Ciumas et al., "Hypoxia-induced apelin expression regulates endothelial cell proliferation and regenerative angiogenesis," *Circulation Research*, vol. 103, no. 4, pp. 432–440, 2008.

[36] L. Wei, D. J. Ying, L. Cui, J. Langsdorf, and S. Ping Yu, "Necrosis, apoptosis and hybrid death in the cortex and thalamus after barrel cortex ischemia in rats," *Brain Research*, vol. 1022, no. 1-2, pp. 54–61, 2004.

[37] B. Yang, K. He, F. Zheng et al., "Over-expression of hypoxia-inducible factor-1 alpha in vitro protects the cardiac fibroblasts from hypoxia-induced apoptosis," *Journal of Cardiovascular Medicine*, vol. 15, no. 7, pp. 579–586, 2014.

[38] B.-F. Wang, X.-J. Wang, H.-F. Kang et al., "Saikosaponin-D enhances radiosensitivity of hepatoma cells under hypoxic conditions by inhibiting hypoxia-inducible factor-1alpha," *Cellular Physiology and Biochemistry*, vol. 33, no. 1, pp. 37–51, 2014.

[39] A. Nishimoto, N. Kugimiya, T. Hosoyama, T. Enoki, T.-S. Li, and K. Hamano, "HIF-1α activation under glucose deprivation plays a central role in the acquisition of anti-apoptosis in human colon cancer cells," *International Journal of Oncology*, vol. 45, no. 6, pp. 2077–2084, 2014.

[40] Z. N. Oltvai, C. L. Milliman, and S. J. Korsmeyer, "Bcl-2 heterodimerizes in vivo with a conserved homolog, Bax, that accelerates programed cell death," *Cell*, vol. 74, no. 4, pp. 609–619, 1993.

Novice Reviewers Retain High Sensitivity and Specificity of Posterior Segment Disease Identification with iWellnessExam™

Samantha Slotnick,[1,2,3] Catherine Awad,[4,5] Sanjeev Nath,[6] and Jerome Sherman[2,3,6]

[1]*Private Practice, Scarsdale, NY 10583, USA*
[2]*SUNY State College of Optometry, New York, NY 10036, USA*
[3]*SUNY Eye Institute, Syracuse, NY 13202, USA*
[4]*Nova Southeastern University College of Optometry, Fort Lauderdale, FL 33314, USA*
[5]*University of Incarnate Word Rosenberg School of Optometry, San Antonio, TX 78229, USA*
[6]*Eye Institute & Laser Center, New York, NY 10065, USA*

Correspondence should be addressed to Samantha Slotnick; drslotnick@drslotnick.com

Academic Editor: Ireneusz Grulkowski

Introduction. Four novices to Spectral Domain Optical Coherence Tomography (SD-OCT) image review were provided a brief lecture on the interpretation of iVue iWellnessExam™ findings (available on iVue® SD-OCT, Optovue, Inc., Fremont, CA). For a cohort of 126 (Confirmed) Normal, 101 (Confirmed) Disease subjects, iWellnessExam™ OD, OS, and OU reports were provided. Each novice independently reviewed and sorted the subjects into one of four categories: normal, retinal disease, optic nerve (ON) disease, and retinal + ON disease. Their accuracy is compared between the novices and with an expert reviewer. *Results.* Posterior segment disease was properly detected by novices with sensitivities of 90.6%, any disease; 84.3%, retinal disease; 88.0%, ON disease; expert sensitivity: 96.0%, 95.5%, and 90.0%, respectively; specificity: 84.3%, novices; 99.2%, expert. Novice accuracy correlates best with clinical exposure and amount of time spent reviewing each image set. The novices' negative predictive value was 92.0% (i.e., very few false negatives). *Conclusions.* Novices can be trained to screen for posterior segment disease efficiently and effectively using iWellnessExam™ data, with high sensitivity, while maintaining high specificity. Novice reviewer accuracy covaries with both clinical exposure and time spent per image set. These findings support exploration of training nonophthalmic technicians in a primary medical care setting.

1. Introduction

A recently published article [1] on the specificity and sensitivity of disease identification utilizing the iVue iWellnessExam™ test revealed that the data provided were sufficient for a well-trained eye clinician to review and accurately detect disease in a very high percent of subjects with either retinal and/or optic nerve (ON) disease and to accurately confirm health in an extremely high percent of healthy controls. This SD-OCT scan obtains a substantial amount of data for the assessment of both central retina and optic nerve integrity simultaneously [2–7]. (review previous study for details) [1]. A follow-up pilot study was undertaken with the same set of data to determine whether novice review of the same SD-OCT data is an effective way to identify retinal and/or optic nerve disease and to confirm health in normal subjects.

The previous study was designed to measure the specificity and sensitivity of a well-trained optometric clinician, utilizing only data obtained on the iWellnessExam™ test, in the identification of retinal and optic nerve disease in a cohort of Confirmed Normal (CN) and Confirmed Disease (CD) subjects. Specificity data were obtained by evaluating patients within the Primary Care clinic at the University Eye Center (UEC) at SUNY State College of Optometry who were determined to be both without retinal and without ON disorder (CN subjects). Sensitivity data were obtained by evaluating patients within the Ocular Disease and Special Testing Service at the UEC with known central retinal

Table 1: Sensitivity and specificity of disease identification using only iWellnessExam™ data, by educational experience.

		Sensitivity		Specificity
	Any posterior seg. disease	Retinal disease	ON disease	Normal
Nonoptometric technician	81.2%	74.6%	88.0%	84.1%
Pre-1st yr, technician	93.1%	88.1%	96.0%	91.3%
1st yr student	94.1%	88.1%	76.0%	78.6%
3rd yr student	94.1%	86.6%	92.0%	83.3%
Expert	96.0%	95.5%	90.0%	99.2%
Average of novices	90.6 ± 6.3%	84.3 ± 6.5%	88.0 ± 8.6%	84.3 ± 5.2%

and/or optic nerve disorders (CD subjects). All glaucoma suspects were excluded from evaluation. SUNY IRB approval was obtained prior to the initiation of the study, and all subjects signed a SUNY IRB approved informed consent document.

2. Materials and Methods

Two groups of patients were examined: a "Confirmed Normal" (CN) cohort for the specificity aspect of the study (126 subjects) and a "Confirmed Disease" (CD) cohort for the sensitivity aspect of the study (101 subjects). Of the CD patients, 67 had retinal pathology; 50 had ON pathology. (Sixteen (16) fell into both categories, with both retinal and ON pathology.) No "glaucoma suspects" were included for evaluation, as their status as a normal or as an ON pathology subject could not be clearly established.

Data were obtained in the previous study, utilizing the iVue SD-OCT. It scans at 26,000 A-scans/second, with an axial resolution of 5 microns [8]. All analyses were made utilizing the iWellnessExam™, a one-step SD-OCT scan, which images a 7 mm × 7 mm area of the posterior pole centered on the fovea. The iWellnessExam™ report provides eight high-resolution cross-sectional retinal images, along with its data analysis results: a full retinal thickness map, a ganglion cell complex (GCC) map, and a report on Superior/Inferior (S/I) symmetry within the eye, and symmetry between eyes. Note that these scans were obtained and reviewed before the release of the normative database for the iVue system.

Four individuals who were novices at reviewing SD-OCT images were enlisted to participate in the clinical review of this data set. The novices were each of a different level of clinical and educational experience in the ophthalmic field.

(A) Nonoptometric Technician. This individual has served as a technician in studies involving retinal imaging technologies. He has no interest in pursuing a career in clinical optometry or ophthalmic research.

(B) Pre-1st-Year Student/Technician. This individual has been accepted into the professional program at the SUNY State College of Optometry. She has had 4 years of experience working in optometric and ophthalmological practices, including 18 months in an ophthalmological practice with 6 months as a technician, operating retinal scanning devices.

(C) 1st-Year Student. This individual was in the middle of his first year of the professional program at the SUNY State College of Optometry. Prior to entering optometry school, he spent one full year in an internship/research program, involved with the publication of unusual cases evaluated with cutting-edge ophthalmic technology.

(D) 3rd-Year Student. This individual was in the middle of her third year of the professional program at the SUNY State College of Optometry. She had previous experience in detecting PIL abnormalities on SD-OCT, based upon an unrelated independent study project.

These four novices were provided with a single, 1.5-hour lecture with author JS on the nature of the data obtained on iVue iWellnessExam™, and on both numerical and pictorial data interpretation. Prior to this lecture, none of the novices had any exposure to the iVue system.

Subject data sets were given a randomized code number, which served as the only identifier for each subject. Reviewers did not have access to any supplementary patient history, demographic, or clinical data. The novice reviewers were instructed to classify each subject into one of four categories: (1) normal, (2) retinal disease, (3) ON disease, and (4) retinal + ON disease. They were also requested to record the amount of time spent in review sessions so that an estimate of the amount of time spent per image could be made.

3. Results

Demographics and pathologies are listed in previous article [1].

Novice reviewers accurately identified disease (sensitivity) in 90.6 ± 6.3% of CD subjects and accurately identified health (specificity) in 84.3 ± 5.2% of CN subjects, utilizing only the iWellnessExam™ data. See Table 1 and Figures 1 and 2 for a detailed display of reviewer sensitivity and specificity data. Overall sensitivity for ocular disease improved with academic experience level.

Data were also evaluated for predictive value. These are measures of the reliability of a positive or a negative result on a test. Positive predictive value (PPV) is the percent of time that a positive test result will indicate disease. PPV is calculated as the number of true positives relative to the number of subjects who were *identified* as "positive" for the condition in question. Negative predictive value (NPV) is the percent of time that

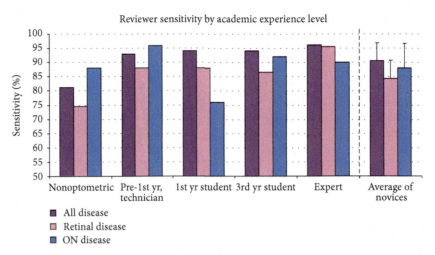

FIGURE 1: Sensitivity of reviewers for posterior segment disease identification, based on data provided with iWellnessExam™. Rightmost column set is an average of the performance of the four novices.

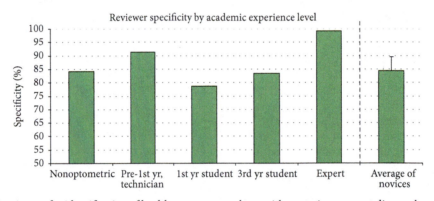

FIGURE 2: Specificity of reviewers for identification of healthy eyes among those with posterior segment disease, based on data provided with iWellnessExam™. Rightmost column is an average of the performance of the four novices.

a negative test result will indicate health. NPV is calculated as the number of true negatives relative to the number of subjects who were *identified* as "negative" for any condition. (Thus, a reviewer with high sensitivity for a disease, but who tends to over-refer, will identify more subjects as positive for a test than are truly positive. This will adversely impact the PPV.)

All novice reviewers demonstrated a greater PPV for the general category of disease than for either subcategory and a greater PPV for retinal disease than for ON disease (see Figure 3). This implies that overreferrals for disease primarily occurred in subjects who had only retinal disease (category 2) but were classified as category 4 (retinal + ON disease). The novices on the whole perform well on the most important factor: appropriate referral of patients who have any disease (82.4 ± 5.0%, with a range of 78–89%). Retinal disease overreferrals in patients with ON disease appear to abate with optometric education (3rd year more successful than 1st year at correctly identifying retinal disease). ON disease overreferral remains somewhat elevated in patients who have retinal disease. By contrast, all reviewers performed with a high NPV, ranging from 85% to 98% (see Figure 4; Table 2). If the novices identified a patient as normal, there was a 92.0 ± 4.8% chance that disease was not present.

With a small sample of novice reviewers, and with variations in their educational backgrounds, it is not easy to rank their relative exposures to ophthalmic conditions and expected disease identification ability. Plots of their performance were translated to Receiver Operator Characteristics (ROC) space. This evaluates each subject's false positive rate (1 − specificity) relative to their true positive rate (sensitivity). See Figure 5. Best overall performance is defined by minimizing the false positives while maximizing sensitivity, with the most desirable performance being plotted at the top left corner of the ROC space. ROC plots were used to compare (1) expert performance for overall disease and for the two subcategories of retinal and optic nerve disease (Figure 5(a)) and (2) the novices with the expert and with each other (Figure 5(b), all disease; Figure 5(c), retinal disease; Figure 5(d), optic nerve disease). For ease of comparison, the two-dimensional ROC findings are also presented as an accuracy rating. Accuracy is calculated as the sum of the true positives and true negatives divided by the sum of the total number of positives and negatives. Figure 6 compares the novices' accuracy, arranged by relative amount

TABLE 2: Statistics and positive and negative predictive value (PPV and NPV).

		Any disease	Retinal disease	Optic nerve disease
PPV	Nonoptometric	80.4%	71.4%	68.8%
PPV	Pre-1st yr, technician	89.5%	84.3%	81.4%
PPV	1st yr student	77.9%	68.6%	58.5%
PPV	3rd yr student	81.9%	73.4%	68.7%
PPV	*Expert*	*99.0%*	*98.5%*	*97.8%*
PPV	**Average of novices**	**82.4 ± 5.02%**	**74.4 ± 6.86%**	**69.3 ± 9.37%**
NPV	Nonoptometric	84.8%	86.2%	94.6%
NPV	Pre-1st yr, technician	94.3%	93.5%	98.3%
NPV	1st yr student	94.3%	92.5%	89.2%
NPV	3rd yr student	94.6%	92.1%	96.3%
NPV	*Expert*	*96.9%*	*97.7%*	*96.2%*
NPV	**Average of novices**	**92.0 ± 4.79%**	**91.1 ± 3.32%**	**94.6 ± 3.91%**

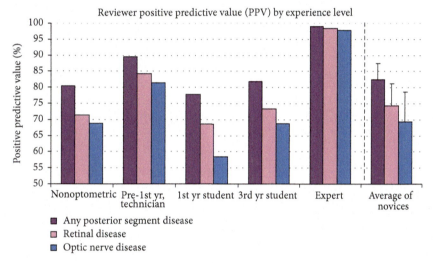

FIGURE 3: Reviewers' positive predictive value (PPV), based on data provided with iWellnessExam™. On average, novice reviewers were able to correctly predict whether a subject had disease 82 ± 5% of the time. There was a greater tendency for the novices to overrefer for optic nerve disease than for retinal disease, in all cases.

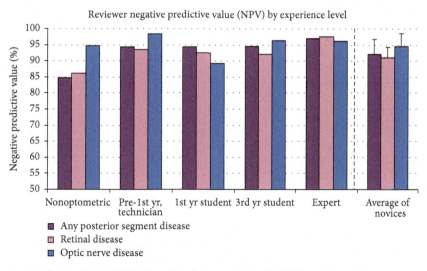

FIGURE 4: Reviewers' Negative Predictive Value (NPV), based on data provided with iWellnessExam™. On average, novice reviewers were able to correctly predict whether a subject was normal >90% of the time, with comparable performance to expert reviewer.

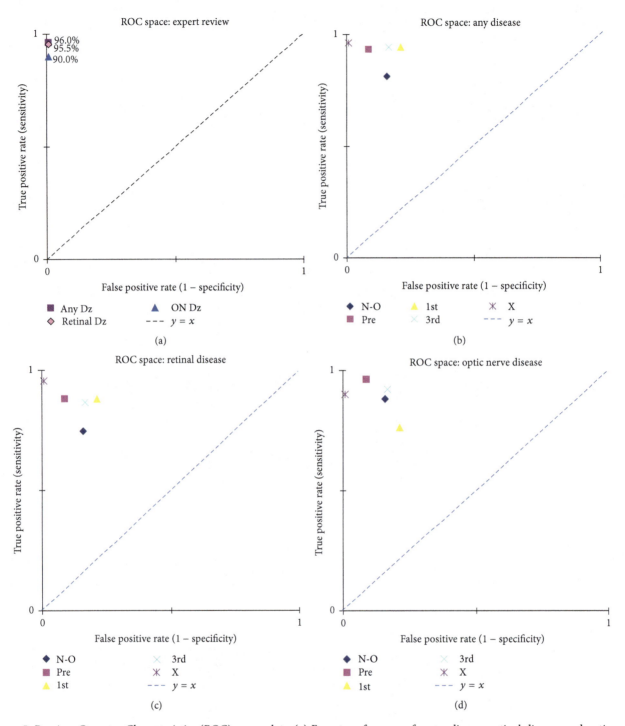

FIGURE 5: Receiver Operator Characteristics (ROC) space plots. (a) Expert performance for any disease, retinal disease, and optic nerve disease. (b–d) Comparison of all reviewers, including the expert, for (b) any disease, (c) retinal disease, and (d) ON disease. Key: N-O = nonoptometric technician; pre = pre-1st-year student/technician; 1st = 1st-year student; 3rd = 3rd-year student; X = expert. $y = x$: chance performance.

of time spent in optometric education. Figure 7 also compares their accuracy, rearranged to reflect their relative amount of clinical exposure time.

3.1. Time Spent per Image. Novice reviewers were asked to record the time they spent performing image review. The novices conducted image review over an average of 4 sittings (ranging from 2 to 6 sittings) and spent an average of 59 ± 13 sec per image set (range 49 to 77 sec per image set). See Table 3. There does seem to be a correlation between the amount of time spent per image set and the accuracy of the subject categorization among novices (see Figure 8).

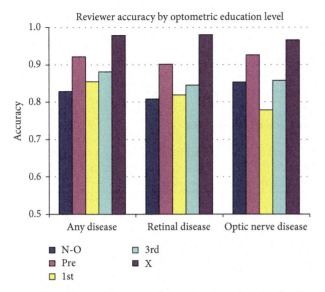

FIGURE 6: Reviewer accuracy by optometric education level.

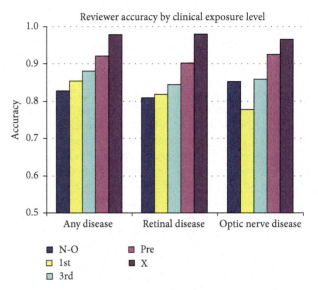

FIGURE 7: Reviewer accuracy by clinical exposure level.

TABLE 3: Time spent in data review, per subject (time not recorded when expert reviewed data).

	# of sittings	Time per subject (s)
Nonoptometric	6	50.1
Pre-1st yr, technician	3	76.8
1st yr student	6	48.9
3rd yr student	2	60.0
Average of novices	4.25	59.0 ± 12.9

4. Discussion

4.1. Effective Screening. Above all, a screening protocol needs to be capable of disease detection. The data obtained on iWellnessExam™ may complement the clinical data obtained in the course of a routine exam [1, 9–12]. Once disease is detected or suspected, appropriate referrals can be made for follow-up testing and clinical evaluation. The results here show that individuals who are novices at reviewing SD-OCT images can be trained in a short amount of time to achieve an impressive rate of detection of the presence of posterior segment disease, while maintaining high specificity for the affirmation of health in control subjects, using only the data provided on iWellnessExam™. Another study evaluating the learning curve of a novice relative to an expert in imaging interpretation showed a similar learning effect with good accuracy when compared to the expert [13]. A study evaluating the value of problem-based learning as compared with more conventional teaching methods concludes that problem-based learning produces better educational results [14]. Thus, in a clinical environment, an ongoing feedback process between the evaluating clinician and the detecting technician will help technicians learn to interpret scans with even greater levels of accuracy.

4.2. Educational versus Clinical Exposure. Differences in educational versus clinical exposure are made apparent in

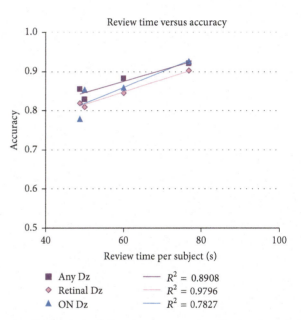

FIGURE 8: Amount of time novices spent reviewing images is compared with the accuracy of their assessments.

the present pilot study. From an educational standpoint, the novices may be ranked: A < B < C < D (refer to Methods). However, from a clinical exposure standpoint, the amount of contact time with patients and with review of typical clinical data may be ranked: A < C < D < B, as the pre-1st-year technician has had *4 years* of exposure to an ophthalmic environment and has collected clinical data from a typical cross section of the population. Assuming this technician is representative of the value of clinical learning, her performance edifies the findings of the value of problem-based learning in medical education [11, 14].

In some regards, the 1st-year student (C) may have had a relative challenge in identifying normal, as he spent a year in ophthalmic research, exposed to challenging cases of ophthalmic disease with subtle findings. This may have predisposed him to identify disease, even in subtle cases, but not to identify health (i.e., reduced specificity).

4.3. Interpreting Accuracy and the ROC Plots. The ROC plots enable a two-dimensional perspective on reviewer accuracy, at a glance. The Pre-1st-year optometry student who has experience as an ophthalmic technician (pink square, Figure 5) consistently outperformed the other novices. This performance supports the need for clinical exposure to general practice in order to help students contextualize their clinical observations. The 1st-year and nonoptometric reviewer have similar levels of clinical exposure. While they make different errors in reviewing the data in Figures 5(b) and 5(c) (one has more false positives with lower sensitivity; the other has fewer false positive with higher sensitivity), their performance is similar in terms of their accuracy (see Figure 7).

4.4. Time Invested on Image Review. The novices were asked to report on the amount of time spent reviewing the data and the number of sittings. Novices B and D took a longer amount of time reviewing each subject's data set (which consisted of 3 image files). There is an apparent correlation between the amount of time invested in image review and the accuracy of the overall categorization exercise. Interestingly, this correlation appears strongest for retinal disease ($R^2 = 0.98$), which requires a higher level of image scrutiny than the determination of optic nerve disease ($R^2 = 0.78$).

4.5. Challenges Predicting Optic Nerve Disease in the Presence of Retinal Disease. The reduced PPV *and* reduced sensitivity for patients with optic nerve disease, as compared to retinal disease, may be attributed to the challenges of assessing RNFL in the presence of an irregular outer retina, or even inner retinal disturbances, such as vitreoretinal adhesions. The interpretation of these challenging situations has been explored in detail, "interpreting the ganglion cell complex in the presence of retinal pathology" [1, 15].

5. Conclusions

The iWellnessExam™ offers the health care provider a very reliable technology for the clinical identification of eyes at risk. Novices can be trained in a short amount of time to effectively use the data from the iWellnessExam™ to screen for disease with a high rate of sensitivity, while maintaining high specificity. Accuracy of the novice reviewers covaries with both clinical exposure and time spent on image review per subject.

Future Directions

This study shows a small sample of novice reviewers with different levels of clinical and educational exposure. It would be insightful to undertake this review with a larger sample of students at various stages of optometric education. In the interest of public health, a similar study could be undertaken with training of nonophthalmic medical technicians, to explore the potential for the identification of eye disease in patients who do not seek routine eye care but do manage their health with primary medical providers. Indeed, it is often an eye exam which results in medical referrals following the identification of retinal pathology.

Conflict of Interests

Dr. Sherman has lectured for Optovue several times in 2015. None of the other authors have any conflict of interests regarding the publication of this paper.

References

[1] C. Awad, S. Slotnick, S. Nath, and J. Sherman, "Sensitivity and specificity of the iVue iWellnessExam™ in detecting retinal and optic nerve disorders," *Eye and Brain*, vol. 5, no. 1, pp. 9–21, 2013.

[2] A. Schulze, N. Pfeiffer, S. Gunther, and E. M. Hoffmann, "Measurement of retinal ganglion cell complex in glaucoma, ocular hypertension and healthy subjects with fourier domain optical coherence tomographic (rtvue 100, Optovue)," *ARVO Meeting Abstracts*, vol. 50, article 3323, 2009.

[3] M. Seong, K. Sung, S. Park, J. Choi, and M. Kook, "Glaucoma discrimination capability of macular inner retinal layer thickness assessed by spectral domain optical coherence tomography," *ARVO Meeting Abstracts*, vol. 50, article 3326, 2009.

[4] L. Alexander, "Maximizing the Use of Peripapillary Assessment of Retinal Nerve Fiber Layer (RNFL) and Ganglion Cell Complex (GCC) for Optic Neuropathy by Hemi-Field Comparison," Optovue, September 2015, http://www.optovue.com/wp-content/uploads/2015/11/Alexander-L-Maximizing-the-use-of-peripapillary-assessment-of-RNFL-and-GCC-for-optic-neuropathy-by-hemifield-comparison-optovue-white-paper.pdf.

[5] L. M. Sakata, J. DeLeon-Ortega, V. Sakata, and C. A. Girkin, "Optical coherence tomography of the retina and optic nerve—a review," *Clinical & Experimental Ophthalmology*, vol. 37, no. 1, pp. 90–99, 2009.

[6] J. Chen, X. Sun, and M. Wang, "Fourier-domain optical coherence tomography measurement of macular ganglion cell complex and peripapillary nerve fiber layer thickness in normal and glaucomatous human eyes," *Investigative Ophthalmology & Visual Science*, vol. 50, p. 3324, 2009, ARVO Meeting Abstracts.

[7] B. Konno Sr., T. S. Prata, V. C. Lima et al., "Macular ganglion cell complex versus peripapillary retinal nerve fiber layer analysis for assessment of early glaucoma," *ARVO Meeting Abstracts*, vol. 51, article 2742, 2010.

[8] September 2015, http://optovue.com/wp-content/uploads/2015/09/iVue-Brochure.pdf.

[9] A. Tomidokoro, M. Hangai, N. Yoshimura, and M. Araie, "Sensitivity and specificity of thickness measurements of macular ganglion cell layer and ganglion cell complex using spectral-domain OCT for diagnosis of preperimetric or early glaucoma," *Investigative Ophthalmology & Visual Science*, vol. 51, p. 216, 2010, ARVO Meeting Abstracts.

[10] N. R. Kim, E. S. Lee, G. J. Seong, J. H. Kim, H. G. An, and C. Y. Kim, "Structure-function relationship and diagnostic value of macular ganglion cell complex measurement using fourier-domain OCT in glaucoma," *Investigative Ophthalmology and Visual Science*, vol. 51, no. 9, pp. 4646–4651, 2010.

[11] S. T. Takagi, Y. Kita, F. Yagi, and G. Tomita, "Macular retinal ganglion cell complex damage in the apparently normal visual field of glaucomatous eyes with hemifield defects," *Journal of Glaucoma*, vol. 21, no. 5, pp. 318–325, 2012.

[12] C. P. Gracitelli, R. Y. Abe, and F. A. Medeiros, "Spectral-domain optical coherence tomography for glaucoma diagnosis," *The Open Ophthalmology Journal*, vol. 9, no. 1, pp. 68–77, 2015.

[13] K. Rose, M. Jong, F. Yusof et al., "Grader learning effect and reproducibility of Doppler Spectral-Domain Optical Coherence Tomography derived retinal blood flow measurements," *Acta Ophthalmologica*, vol. 92, no. 8, pp. e630–e636, 2014.

[14] A. Aziz, S. Iqbal, and A. U. Zaman, "Problem based learning and its implementation: faculty and student's perception," *Journal of Ayub Medical College Abbottabad*, vol. 26, no. 4, pp. 496–500, 2014.

[15] J. Sherman, S. Slotnick, and J. Boneta, "Discordance between structure and function in glaucoma: possible anatomical explanations," *Optometry*, vol. 80, no. 9, pp. 487–501, 2009.

Permissions

All chapters in this book were first published in JOPH, by Hindawi Publishing Corporation; hereby published with permission under the Creative Commons Attribution License or equivalent. Every chapter published in this book has been scrutinized by our experts. Their significance has been extensively debated. The topics covered herein carry significant findings which will fuel the growth of the discipline. They may even be implemented as practical applications or may be referred to as a beginning point for another development.

The contributors of this book come from diverse backgrounds, making this book a truly international effort. This book will bring forth new frontiers with its revolutionizing research information and detailed analysis of the nascent developments around the world.

We would like to thank all the contributing authors for lending their expertise to make the book truly unique. They have played a crucial role in the development of this book. Without their invaluable contributions this book wouldn't have been possible. They have made vital efforts to compile up to date information on the varied aspects of this subject to make this book a valuable addition to the collection of many professionals and students.

This book was conceptualized with the vision of imparting up-to-date information and advanced data in this field. To ensure the same, a matchless editorial board was set up. Every individual on the board went through rigorous rounds of assessment to prove their worth. After which they invested a large part of their time researching and compiling the most relevant data for our readers.

The editorial board has been involved in producing this book since its inception. They have spent rigorous hours researching and exploring the diverse topics which have resulted in the successful publishing of this book. They have passed on their knowledge of decades through this book. To expedite this challenging task, the publisher supported the team at every step. A small team of assistant editors was also appointed to further simplify the editing procedure and attain best results for the readers.

Apart from the editorial board, the designing team has also invested a significant amount of their time in understanding the subject and creating the most relevant covers. They scrutinized every image to scout for the most suitable representation of the subject and create an appropriate cover for the book.

The publishing team has been an ardent support to the editorial, designing and production team. Their endless efforts to recruit the best for this project, has resulted in the accomplishment of this book. They are a veteran in the field of academics and their pool of knowledge is as vast as their experience in printing. Their expertise and guidance has proved useful at every step. Their uncompromising quality standards have made this book an exceptional effort. Their encouragement from time to time has been an inspiration for everyone.

The publisher and the editorial board hope that this book will prove to be a valuable piece of knowledge for researchers, students, practitioners and scholars across the globe.

List of Contributors

Bingjie Wang, Renyuan Chu, Jinhui Dai, Xiaomei Qu and Hao Zhou
Key Myopia Laboratory of Chinese Health Ministry, Department of Ophthalmology, Eye & ENT Hospital, Fudan University, No. 83, Fenyang Road, Shanghai 200031, China

Rajeev K. Naidu
The University of Sydney, Camper down, NSW2006, Australia

Mengmeng Wang
Hebei Provincial Eye Hospital, Hebei Provincial Ophthalmology Key Lab, Hebei Provincial Institute of Ophthalmology, Xingtai, Hebei 054001, China

Lei Zuo
Department of Ophthalmology, Shanghai General Hospital, Nanjing Medical University, Shanghai 200080, China

Haidong Zou
Department of Ophthalmology, Shanghai General Hospital, Shanghai Jiao Tong University, Shanghai 200080, China

Jianhong Zhang and Xinfeng Fei
Department of Ophthalmology, Branch of Shanghai First People's Hospital, Shanghai 200081, China

Xun Xu
Department of Ophthalmology, Shanghai General Hospital, Nanjing Medical University, Shanghai 200080, China

Xiaoguang Cao, Xianru Hou and Yongzhen Bao
Peking University People's Hospital, Ophthalmology Department, Key Laboratory of Vision Loss and Restoration, Ministry of Education, Beijing Key Laboratory for the Diagnosis and Treatment of Retinal and Choroid Diseases, Beijing 100044, China

Maria Rosaria De Pascale, Linda Sommese and Claudio Napoli
U.O.C. Immunohematology, Transfusion Medicine and Transplant Immunology, Regional Reference Laboratory of Transplant Immunology, Azienda Ospedaliera Universitaria (AOU), Second University of Naples, 80100 Naples, Italy

Michele Lanza
Multidisciplinary Department of Medical, Surgical and Dental Sciences, Second University of Naples, 80100 Naples, Italy

A.M. Sherif, M. A. Ammar, Y. S.Mostafa, S. A. Gamal Eldin and A. A. Osman
Department of Ophthalmology, Faculty of Medicine, Cairo University, Cairo 12411, Egypt

Marketa Sobotova, Lenka Hecova, Renata Ricarova and Stepan Rusnak
Department of Ophthalmology, University Hospital Pilsen, Alej Svobody 80, 304 60 Plzen, Czech Republic

Jindra Vrzalova and Ondrej Topolcan
Department of Nuclear Medicine, Laboratory of Immunoanalysis, University Hospital Pilsen, Dr. E. Benese 13, 305 99 Plzen, Czech Republic
Central Radioisotopic Laboratory, Faculty of Medicine in Pilsen, Charles University in Prague, Dr. E. Benese 13, 305 99 Plzen, Czech Republic

Chan HeeMoon
Department of Ophthalmology, Seoul St. Mary's Hospital, The Catholic University of Korea College of Medicine, Seoul 06591, Republic of Korea

Jungwoo Han, Young-Hoon Ohn and Tae Kwann Park
Department of Ophthalmology, Soonchunhyang University College of Medicine, Bucheon Hospital, Bucheon 14584, Republic of Korea

Lara Pasovic
Department of Medical Biochemistry, Oslo University Hospital, Kirkeveien 166, P.O. Box 4956, Nydalen, 0424 Oslo, Norway
Faculty of Medicine, University of Oslo, Sognsvannsveien 9, 0372 Oslo, Norway

Jon Roger Eidet, Berit S. Brusletto and Torstein Lyberg
Department of Medical Biochemistry, Oslo University Hospital, Kirkeveien 166, P.O. Box 4956, Nydalen, 0424 Oslo, Norway

Tor P. Utheim
Department of Medical Biochemistry, Oslo University Hospital, Kirkeveien 166, P.O. Box 4956, Nydalen, 0424 Oslo, Norway
Department of Oral Biology, Faculty of Dentistry, University of Oslo, Sognsvannsveien 10, P.O. Box 1052, Blindern, 0316Oslo,Norway

Mehmet Bulut, Berna DoLan, Deniz Turgut Çoban, Muhammet Kazim Erol and Devrim Toslak
Antalya Training and Research Hospital, Ophthalmology Department, 07050 Antalya, Turkey

Aylin Yaman and Fatma KurtuluG
Antalya Training and Research Hospital, Neurology Department, 07050 Antalya, Turkey

Ebru Kaya BaGar
Department of Animal Science Biometry and Genetics Unit, Faculty of Agriculture, Akdeniz University, 07070 Antalya, Turkey

Hui Yang, Jing Lu, Xiujuan Zhao, Xiaohu Ding, ZhonghaoWang, Xiaoyu Cai, Yan Luo and Lin Lu
State Key Laboratory of Ophthalmology, Zhongshan Ophthalmic Center, Sun Yat-sen University, Guangzhou 510060, China

Hua Yan
Department of Ophthalmology, Tianjin Medical University General Hospital, No. 154, Anshan Road, Tianjin 300052, China

XiuWang, Xiaoxiao Lu, Jun Yang, Ruihua Wei, Liyuan Yang and Shaozhen Zhao
Tianjin Medical University Eye Hospital, Fukang Road No. 251, Nankai District, Tianjin 300384, China

XilianWang
Tianjin Beichen Hospital, Beiyi Road No. 7, Beichen District, Tianjin 300400, China

Medine AslJ YJldJrJm
Department of Ophthalmology, Bahcelievler State Hospital, 34180 Istanbul, Turkey

Burak Erden and Mustafa ElçioLlu
Department of Ophthalmology, Okmeydanı Education and Research Hospital, 34384 Istanbul, Turkey

Mehmet TetikoLlu
Department of Ophthalmology, Dumlupinar University School of Medicine, 43270 Kutahya, Turkey

Özlem Kuru
Department of Ophthalmology, Mus State Hospital, 49000 Mus, Turkey

Nobuko Enomoto, Ayako Anraku, Kyoko Ishida, Asuka Takeyama, Fumihiko Yagi and Goji Tomita
Department of Ophthalmology, Toho University, Ohashi Medical Center, 2-17-5 Ohashi, Meguro-ku 153-8515, Japan

Hyung Bin Hwang, Byul Lyu, Hye Bin Yim and Na Young Lee
Department of Ophthalmology, Incheon St. Mary's Hospital, College of Medicine, The Catholic University of Korea, 222 Banpo-daero, Seocho-gu, Seoul 137-701, Republic of Korea

Shida Chen
Laboratory of Immunology, National Eye Institute, National Institutes of Health, Bethesda, MD 20892, USA
Zhongshan Ophthalmic Center, Sun Yat-sen University, Guangzhou 510060, China

Defen Shen, Nicholas A. Popp, Jingsheng Tuo and Chi-Chao Chan
Laboratory of Immunology, National Eye Institute, National Institutes of Health, Bethesda, MD 20892, USA

Alexander J. Ogilvy and Mones Abu-Asab
Histology Core, National Eye Institute, National Institutes of Health, Bethesda, MD 20892, USA

Ting Xie
Stowers Institute for Medical Research, Kansas City, MO 64110, USA
Department of Anatomy and Cell Biology, University of Kansas School of Medicine, Kansas City, KS 66160, USA

Toshiyuki Oshitari, Yuta Kitamura, Sakiko Nonomura, Miyuki Arai, Yoko Takatsuna, Eiju Sato, Takayuki Baba and Shuichi Yamamoto
Department of Ophthalmology and Visual Science, Chiba University Graduate School of Medicine, Inohana 1-8-1, Chuo-ku, Chiba Prefecture, Chiba 260-8670, Japan

Ahmed M. Sherif, Nihal A. El-Gheriany, YehiaM. Salah El-Din, Lamiaa S. Aly and Amr A. Osman
Department of Ophthalmology, Faculty of Medicine, Cairo University, Cairo 11519, Egypt

Michael A. Grentzelos
Vardinoyiannion Eye Institute of Crete (VEIC), Faculty of Medicine, University of Crete, Heraklion, 71003 Crete, Greece

George D. Kymionis
Vardinoyiannion Eye Institute of Crete (VEIC), Faculty of Medicine, University of Crete, Heraklion, 71003 Crete, Greece
Bascom Palmer Eye Institute, University of Miami, Miller School of Medicine, Miami, FL 33136, USA

Dong Yoon Kim
Department of Ophthalmology, College of Medicine, Chungbuk National University, Cheongju, Republic of Korea

Soo Geun Joe
Department of Ophthalmology, Gangneung Asan Hospital, University of Ulsan, College of Medicine, Gangneung, Republic of Korea

Seunghee Baek
Department of Clinical Epidemiology and Biostatistics, Asan Medical Center, University of Ulsan, College of Medicine, Seoul, Republic of Korea

June-Gone Kim, Young Hee Yoon and Joo Yong Lee
Department of Ophthalmology, Asan Medical Center, University of Ulsan, College of Medicine, 88 Olympic-ro 43-gil, Songpa-gu, Seoul 138-736, Republic of Korea

List of Contributors

Xiaoliang L. Xu
Department of Pathology, Memorial Sloan-Kettering Cancer Center, 1275 York Avenue, New York, NY 10021, USA

Dan-Ning Hu
Department of Ophthalmology, The New York Eye and Ear Infirmary of Mount Sinai, Icahn School of Medicine at Mount Sinai, New York, NY 10003, USA

Codrin Iacob, Adrienne Jordan and Sandip kumar Gandhi
Department of Pathology, The New York Eye and Ear Infirmary of Mount Sinai, Icahn School of Medicine at Mount Sinai, New York, NY 10003, USA

Dennis L. Gierhart
ZeaVision LLC, Chesterfield, MO 63005, USA

Richard Rosen
Department of Ophthalmology, The New York Eye and Ear Infirmary of Mount Sinai, Icahn School of Medicine at Mount Sinai, New York, NY 10003, USA

Manqiong Yuan, Yaofeng Han and Ya Fang
State Key Laboratory of Molecular Vaccinology and Molecular Diagnostics, School of Public Health, Xiamen University, Xiamen 361102, China
Key Laboratory of Health Technology Assessment in Fujian Province University, School of Public Health, Xiamen University, Xiamen 361102, China

Cheng-I Chu
Department of Public Health, Tzu Chi University, Hualien 97004, Taiwan

Guanglin Shen and Xiaoping Ma
Department of Ophthalmology, Zhongshan Hospital, Fudan University, 180 Fenglin Road, Shanghai 200032, China

Anton Hommer
Private Office, Vienna, Austria

Douglas A. Hubatsch
Alcon Laboratories, Inc., Fort Worth, TX 76134, USA

Juan Cano-Parra
Hospital Municipal de Badalona, 08911 Barcelona, Spain

Dominika Wróbel-DudziNska, Ewa Kosior-Jarecka, Urszula Aukasik and Tomasz garnowski
Department of Diagnostics and Microsurgery of Glaucoma, Medical University, Chmielna 1, 20-079 Lublin, Poland

Janusz Kocki
Department of Clinical Genetics, Medical University, Radziwiłłowska 11, 20-080 Lublin, Poland

Agnieszka Witczak and JerzyMosiewicz
Department of Internal Diseases, Medical University, Staszica 16, 20-081 Lublin, Poland

Dorottya Pásztor, Bence Lajos Kolozsvári, Adrienne Csutak, András Berta, Beáta Andrea Kettesy and Mariann Fodor
Department of Ophthalmology, University of Debrecen, Debrecen 4012, Hungary

Ziad Hassan
Orbident Refractive Surgery and Medical Center, Debrecen 4012, Hungary

Péter Gogolák
Department of Immunology, University of Debrecen, Debrecen 4012, Hungary

Tomoichiro Ogawa, Takuya Shiba and Hiroshi Tsuneoka
Department of Ophthalmology, The Jikei University School of Medicine, 3-25-8 Nishishinbashi, Minato-ku, Tokyo 105-0003, Japan

Alice T. Epitropoulos
The Eye Center of Columbus, 262 Neil Avenue, Columbus, OH 43215, USA
The Ohio State University, Columbus, OH, USA

Yangshun Gu, Baisheng Xu, QinWu,1 Chixin Du, Nan Hong and Bo Jiang
Department of Ophthalmology, First Affiliated Hospital, College of Medicine, Zhejiang University, Hangzhou, Zhejiang 310003, China

Chunfei Feng
Department of Operation Room, First Affiliated Hospital, College of Medicine, Zhejiang University, Hangzhou, Zhejiang 310003, China

Yang Ni, Peng Li and Zhihua Ding
State Key Lab of Modern Optical Instrumentation, Department of Optical Engineering, Zhejiang University, Hangzhou, Zhejiang 310027, China

Li Chen, Yong Tao, Jing Feng and Yan Rong Jiang
Department of Ophthalmology, People's Hospital, Peking University, 11 Xizhimen South Street, Xicheng District, Beijing 100044, China
Key Laboratory of Vision Loss and Restoration, Beijing Key Laboratory of Diagnosis and Therapy of Retinal and Choroid Diseases, Ministry of Education, 11 Xizhimen South Street, Xicheng District, Beijing 100044, China

Samantha Slotnick
Private Practice, Scarsdale, NY 10583, USA
SUNY State College of Optometry, New York, NY 10036, USA
SUNY Eye Institute, Syracuse, NY 13202, USA

Catherine Awad
Nova Southeastern University College of Optometry, Fort Lauderdale, FL 33314, USA
University of Incarnate Word Rosenberg School of Optometry, San Antonio, TX 78229, USA

Sanjeev Nath
Eye Institute & Laser Center, New York, NY 10065, USA

Jerome Sherman
SUNY State College of Optometry, New York, NY 10036, USA
SUNY Eye Institute, Syracuse, NY 13202, USA
Eye Institute & Laser Center, New York, NY 10065, USA

CPSIA information can be obtained
at www.ICGtesting.com
Printed in the USA
BVOW10*1000110916
461715BV00003B/2/P